Immunology and Immune System Disorders

nova
Medicine & Health
New York

Immunology and Immune System Disorders

Mast Cells and their Role in Health and Disease
Ana I. Faustino, PhD (Editor), Paula A. Oliveira, PhD (Editor)
2022. ISBN: 978-1-68507-628-3 (Softcover)
2022. ISBN: 978-1-68507-690-0 (eBook)

The Innate Immune System in Health and Disease: From the Lab Bench Work to Its Clinical Implications. Volume 1
Jorge Morales-Montor, PhD (Editor)
2022. ISBN: 978-1-68507-507-1 (Hardcover)
2022. ISBN: 978-1-68507-644-3 (eBook)

The Innate Immune System in Health and Disease: From the Lab Bench Work to Its Clinical Implications. Volume 2
Jorge Morales-Montor, PhD (Editor)
2022. ISBN: 978-1-68507-510-1 (Hardcover)
2022. ISBN: 978-1-68507-649-8 (eBook)

Vaccines: Operation Warp Speed, Regulation and Safety
Oliver Huerta (Editor)
2021. ISBN: 978-1-53619-059-5 (Hardcover)
2020. ISBN: 978-1-53619-096-0 (eBook)

IgG4 Related Disease: Illustrated Pathology of Novel Systemic Disease
Syuichi Koarada, MD (Editor)
2020. ISBN: 978-1-53618-050-3 (Hardcover)
2020. ISBN: 978-1-53618-051-0 (eBook)

Basics and Fundamentals of Immunology
Manzoor Ahmad Mir, PhD (Editor)
2020. ISBN: 978-1-53616-639-2 (Hardcover)
2020. ISBN: 978-1-53616-640-8 (eBook)

More information about this series can be found at https://novapublishers.com/product-category/series/immunology-and-immune-system-disorders/

Kenan Demir, Selim Görgün and Bahar Uslu
Editors

Cytokines and Diseases

nova
Medicine & Health
New York

https://doi.org/10.52305/UKTK2910

NOTICE TO THE READER

Library of Congress Cataloging-in-Publication Data

ISBN: 979-8-88697-214-6

Published by Nova Science Publishers, Inc. † New York

Contents

Preface

Cytokines and Diseases will contribute to the pathogenesis, follow-up, and treatment processes of different clinical pictures and diseases in the light of current information obtained from the literature. This book aims to describe the type, effects, and kinetics of cytokine production, as well as to summarize the pathophysiology of the cytokine storm that occurs after bacterial sepsis or severe viral infection. It has been a summative review containing the most up-to-date data for academics participating in cytokine-based therapy studies, studies targeting cytokine production or effects, and clinical trials that arouse interest after the Covid-19 pandemic.

Chapter 1

Introduction to Cytokines

Burcu Bozkaya Yücel[1,*], MD and Soner Şahin[2], MD

[1]Department of Pediatric Rheumatology, Samsun Training and Research Hospital, Samsun, Turkey
[2]Department of Neurosurgery, Nişantaşı University, Faculty of Medicine, İstanbul, Turkey

Abstract

Cytokines are pleiotropic immunomodulatory polypeptides that function in both innate and adaptive immunity. They are glycosylated monomeric or polymeric peptide structures produced by various immune cells like macrophages, T-lymphocytes, B-lymphocytes, NK cells, dendritic cells, and stromal cells. They regulate biological events such as cellular communication, proliferation, differentiation, immune homeostasis, inflammation, and morphogenesis. Over the years, many different classifications of cytokines have been made. More recently, they have been classified based on structural similarities and cytokine receptor families. This chapter examines various aspects of cytokine biology in light of the current literature, cellular and molecular networks, and the relationship of cytokines with the diseases.

Keywords: cytokine, interleukin, inflammation, immunity

Introduction

The term "cytokine" comes from the Greek words (cyto: cell and kinos: movement) (Benveniste, 2014; Dembic, 2015; Klimov, 2019). In different studies conducted between 1960 and 1970, the undeniable role of T cells in antibody production was emphasized, and the hypothesis was that specific molecules would be released from T cells to stimulate B cells. The theory was true. When the T-cell culture supernatant was examined, many different molecular structures thought to have a stimulating role in the proliferation and differentiation of B cells were detected (Kishimoto, 2006). It was understood that these substances are mediators that regulate the immune response that allows the cells to communicate with each other.

---

* Corresponding Author's Email: bozkayaburcu@hotmail.com.

In: Cytokines and Diseases
Editors: Kenan Demir, Selim Görgün and Bahar Uslu
ISBN: 979-8-88697-214-6

With current knowledge, cytokines are low-molecular-weight (8-80 kDa), pleiotropic immunomodulatory substances that function in cellular responses (Chung, 2009; Dembic, 2015; Klimov, 2019). Cytokines are generally glycosylated monomeric or polymeric peptides and proteins (Dembic, 2015). They are produced and secreted by various cell types; in innate immunity, dendritic cells and macrophages stimulate natural killer (NK) cells with the cytokines they produce and cause the release of interferon-y (IFN-y), whereas, in adaptive immunity, the primary source of cytokines is secreted by T cells (Klimov, 2019; Chauhan, 2021) (Table 1).

Table 1. Cytokines secreted by immune system cells

Cell Type	**Cytokine**
Macrophages	IL-1α, IL-1β, IL-1Ra, IL-6, IL-10, IL-12, IL-23, TNF, TNF-α and TGF-β
Monocytes	TNF-α, IL-1α, IL-1β, IL-6, IL-10
Neutrophils	IL-1α, IL-1β, IL-4, IL-17, IL-27, IFN-γ, TGF-β
T Lymphocytes	IFN-γ, TNF-β, IL-2, IL-4, IL-5, IL-6, IL-9, IL-10, IL-13, IL-17A, IL-17F, IL-22
B Lymphocytes	IL-2, IL-4, IL-6, IL-10, IL-12, TGF-β1, TNF-α, IFN-γ
Natural killer cells (NK)	IL-5, IL-10, IL-13, IL-17A, IL-22, TNF-α and IFN-γ
Dendritic cells	TNF-α and different interleukins such as, IL-1, IL-4, IL-6, IL-10, IL-12, IL-15, IL-17, IL-23
Mast cells	IL-4, IL-13

Cytokines are signaling molecules that show their function depending on their biological activities. They may have an effect on an adjacent cell, characterized in cell-to-cell interaction (paracrine effect), or on the cells that secrete them (autocrine effect), and these soluble products can also show their efficacy (endocrine effect) by the blood circulation in which they participate. Cytokines are generally similar to hormones, although they differ in many ways (Levine, 2013; Abbas, 2019; Klimov, 2019):

Cytokines have a greater number of production sites, whereas a gland or tissue mainly produces hormones.

Cytokines act in a microenvironment.

In the absence of a cytokine, other cytokines can often substitute it (redundancy); however, a lack of a particular hormone is irreplaceable.

Cytokines have local and systemic effects. They have a wider range of action (pleiotropy) than hormones.

Cytokines regulate biological events such as cellular communication, proliferation, differentiation, immune homeostasis, inflammation, and morphogenesis and play an essential role in initiating, maintaining, or downregulating the immune response (Dembic, 2015). Cytokines are affected by many factors such as the oxygen level, hormones, nutrition, metabolites, and microbial agents, apart from the microenvironment in which they are secreted. In autoimmune, autoinflammatory and infectious diseases, especially recently in COVID-19 patients, multi-organ failure development and excessive secretion of proinflammatory cytokines occur. This clinical picture is seen as an increasing cause of mortality and is called a cytokine storm (Rodriguez, 2020).

Structure of Cytokines

Cytokines are usually glycosylated monomeric or polymeric polypeptides and proteins. They can be in the form of monomers, dimers, and trimers, but the most common forms are dimers and trimers. For example, interleukin-1 (IL-1) is a typical monomer, and IFN-γ, the representative of dimers, is a homodimer. When IFN-γ has two molecules located in antiparallel, it is called the active form (Dembic, 2015). Heterodimers that cross-share some of their molecules are mostly interleukins, the most exciting examples of which are reported as IL-12, IL-23, IL-27 and IL-35. Tumor necrosis factor (TNF) is an example of a trimer structure and consists of three monomers. There is a link between the N (amino)-terminal part of the former and the C (COOH)-terminal part of the other. The triangular structure is complete when the second monomer forms the link again extending to the C-part of the first monomer (Dembic, 2015; Klimov, 2019; Chauhan, 2021).

Classification of Cytokines

Previously, cytokines were classified according to the cell of origin (interleukins = leukocyte-derived, monokines = monocyte-derived, lymphokines = lymphocyte-derived) and are named by their functional role in inflammatory responses. In addition, cytokines do not show biological activity limited to a specific function. They are classified based on structural similarities and cytokine receptor families. Cytokines may also be classified by their functions (Chung, 2009; McInnes, 2013; Chauhan, 2021) (Table 2).

Table 2. Classification of cytokines by their functions

Function	Cytokine
Proinflammatory cytokines	IL-1 α/β, TNF- α/β, IL-6, IL-11, IL-18, IFN-γ
Anti-inflammatory cytokines	IL-10, TGF β, IL-1ra
Cytokines of neutrophil recruitment and activation	CXCL8/IL-8, IL-1 α/β, TNF- α/β, G-CSF, IL-17A, IL-17F
Cytokines of eosinophil recruitment and activation	IL-2, IL-3, IL-4, IL-5, GM-CSF, CCL5/RANTES, CCL11/eotaxin, CCL7/MCP-3, CCL13/MCP-4
Cytokines of T-cell recruitment	IL-16, CCL5/RANTES, CCL3/MIP-1 α, CCL4/MIP-1 β, TSLP, CCL17/TARC, CCL22/MDC
Growth factors	PDGF, VEGF, TGF-β, FGF, EGF, SCF

TGF transforming growth factor; GM-CSF granulocyte-macrophage colony-stimulating factor; MCP monocyte chemotactic protein; MIP macrophage inflammatory protein; RANTES regulated on activation, normal T-cell expressed, and secreted; TSLP thymic stromal lymphopoietin; MDC macrophage-derived chemokine; PDGF platelet-derived growth factor; VEGF vascular endothelial growth factor; FGF fibroblast growth factor; EGF epidermal growth factor; SCF stem cell factor.

TGF transforming growth factor; GM-CSF granulocyte-macrophage colony-stimulating factor; MCP monocyte chemotactic protein; MIP macrophage inflammatory protein; RANTES regulated on activation, normal T-cell expressed, and secreted; TSLP thymic stromal lymphopoietin; MDC macrophage-derived chemokine; PDGF platelet-derived growth factor; VEGF vascular endothelial growth factor; FGF fibroblast growth factor; EGF epidermal growth factor; SCF stem cell factor.

IL-1 Family

The IL-1 family is considered to play a role in the innate immune response. It is also associated with acute and chronic inflammatory states. The IL-1 family consists of seven proinflammatory molecules (IL-1α, IL-1β, IL-18, IL-33, IL-36α, β, γ) and four anti-inflammatory molecules (IL-1 receptor antagonist-1RA), IL-36R antagonist (IL-36RA), IL-37 and IL-38 (McInnes, 2013; Levine, 2013; Benveniste, 2014).

IL-1 is like a marker to show the severity of inflammatory diseases. In clinical studies, it is known that IL-1 participates in the pathogenesis of inflammatory processes such as rheumatoid arthritis (RA), osteoarthritis, gout and type 2 diabetes. When IL-1 signaling is high, it is involved in the occurrence of different inherited autoinflammatory diseases, including cryopyrin-associated periodic syndromes (CAPS), familial Mediterranean fever (FMF), and TNF-receptor-related periodic syndromes (TRAPS) (Chan, 2020).

IL-1α and IL-1β have high inflammatory activity in the reactions it participates in. IL-1α is found as a structural precursor molecule in individuals without the disease state. It is not biologically synthesized or processed (Garlanda, 2013; Marotto, 2019). IL-1α is localized on platelets, endothelial cells, and apoptotic bodies in the epithelial cells of the mucosa, skin, liver, kidney, and lungs. The precursor IL-1α activates its receptor on the adjacent cell and migrates to the cell surface (Dinarello, 2012). IL-1β, unlike IL-1α, is not constitutively expressed. L-1β produced by hematopoietic cells (monocytes, tissue macrophages, dendritic cells) activates toll-like receptors (TLR) or intracellular NOD-like receptors (NLRs). IL-1α or IL-1β itself, the IL-1β precursor (Pro-IL1β), is inactive and must be broken down by caspase-1, a cysteine protease that converts it to the active form (Dinarello, 2012; Marotto, 2019). Caspase-1 functions in the molecular platforms called inflammasomes that recognize signals such as pathogen-associated molecular patterns (PAMPs) and danger-associated molecular patterns (DAMPs). Activation of the NLRP3 inflammasome activates caspase-1. Activated caspase-1 cleaves the pro-IL-1β and pro-IL-18 to their active forms (Chung, 2009). IL-1β, which is converted to its active form, is released from cells, binds to the IL-1 receptor (IL-1R), and triggers the inflammatory cascade. They are termed "Alarmins" due to their ability to induce acute-phase reactant synthesis (Chauhan, 2021). This process causes the activation of inflammation-related genes such as COX2 and PLA2, PGE2 synthesis, the stimulation of acquired immunity, and the development of systemic events such as fever (Dinarello, 2012; Chan, 2020).

Various treatment approaches have been used for IL-1 inhibition, including receptor antagonism and IL-1 binding. Anti-IL-1 drugs include anakinra, canakinumab, rilonacept and gevokizumab. Anakinra and two other IL-1 inhibitors, canakinumab, and rilonacept are effective in the treatment of autoinflammatory diseases such as cryopyrin-associated periodic syndromes (CAPS), TNF receptor-associated periodic syndrome (TRAPS), mevalonate kinase deficiency (MKD), and colchicine resistant FMF due to their effects on inflammation (Urien, 2013; Goldbach-Mansky et al., 2008; De Benedetti et al., 2018). IL-1 inhibition plays a role in selected patients with acute gouty arthritis and the treatment of pseudogout. In COVID-19, anakinra has been shown to ameliorate the process of hyper-inflammation in lung involvement caused by SARS-COV-2 and the multisystem inflammatory syndrome (MIS-C) (CORIMUNO-19 Collaborative group, 2021; Kyriazopoulou et al., 2021; Fouriki et al., 2021).

IL-1Ra is an IL-1 receptor antagonist. It is also a natural inflammatory cytokine of this family. The cytokines IL-1α, IL-1β and IL-1Rα compete with each other for IL-1R binding. The binding function of the IL-1 receptor on cell surfaces also prevents the receptor from interacting with IL-1 (Dinarello, 2018). Interestingly, an imbalance between IL-1 and IL-1Ra may lead to the development of uncontrolled inflammation in the patient. DIRA (deficiency of the IL-1 receptor antagonist) is an autosomal recessive disease with loss-of-function mutations in the IL1Ra gene (ILR1N), leading to life-threatening systemic inflammation with symptoms of multifocal osteomyelitis, periostitis, and pustulosis. Treatment with the IL-1R antagonist anakinra results in dramatic improvement (Sözeri et al., 2018).

IL-18 is an immunoregulatory cytokine. Pro-IL-18 is inactive like Pro-IL-1β and needs to be cleaved by caspase-1. Active IL-18 is released from macrophages and dendritic cells and promotes the secretion of IFN-γ from NK cells (Dinarello, 2018). IL-18 is activated as a result of its binding to the IL-18 receptor complex and activation of nuclear factor-kB (NF-kB). This stimulation has been shown to result in the production and release of different cytokines and chemokines. Several autoinflammatory, autoimmune, and metabolic disorders are associated with the high production of IFN-γ and IL-18. SoJIA, MAS (Yasin, 2020), and adult-onset Still's disease (AOSD) (Girard, 2016) are characterized by high serum IL-18 concentrations (Dinarello, 2018; Kaplanski, 2018), and in the case of an imbalance between IL-18 and IL-18 binding protein (IL-18BP), other diseases such as avian flu, asthma resistant to corticosteroid drugs, and life-threatening sepsis have also been clinically described (Kaplanski, 2018). Different genetic polymorphisms in IL-18 or IL-18R may also cause allergic reactions, and metabolic and autoimmune disorders in the patient (Rex, 2020).

Type 1 Cytokine Family

Type 1 cytokines can be divided into two groups: cytokines with short and long chains. Short-chain type 1 cytokines can be subdivided based on their cytokine receptors. Among some long-chain cytokine 1 family members, the IL-6 family (signaling via gp130), IL-12, growth hormone, prolactin, erythropoietin, thrombopoietin, leptin, and granulocyte colony stimulating factor (GCSF) are identified. Some members of the type I cytokine family share the common cytokine receptor y chain (yc). It shares the y chain (yc) as a common cytokine receptor. These cytokines are shown as IL-2, IL-4, IL-7, IL-9, IL-13, IL-15, and IL-21. These cytokines activate JAK1, JAK2, JAK3 and TYK2 with their stimulation and can be observed in the downstream activation of the STAT3, STAT5A, STAT5B or STAT6 pathway (Kovanen, 2004). Some members of this family that share the β chain (βc) as the common cytokine receptor include IL-3, IL-5, and granulocyte-macrophage colony stimulating factor (GM-CSF). Cytokines share common βc receptor signaling throughout this process, via the JAK2 and STAT5A and STAT5B pathways (Levine, 2013; Chauhan, 2021).

X-linked severe combined immunodeficiency (SCID) is defined when type 1 cytokines that share γ receptor mutations in the γ chain as a common cytokine receptor are examined. A mutation in JAK3 can also result in hereditary SCID with autosomal recessive inheritance when combined with T cells and defective T-cell responses (Notarangelo et al., 2001).

IL-6 Family

IL-6 family cytokines, IL-6, IL-11, IL-27, IL-31, IL-35, ciliary neurotrophic factor (CNTF), leukemia inhibitory factor (LIF), oncostatin M (OSM), cardiotrophin 1 (CT-1), and cardiotrophin-like cytokine (CLC) are classified as a broad group. The IL-6 family of cytokines utilizes the IL-6 signal transducer glycoprotein 130 (gp130) and this structure is common to all but IL-31. IL-31, which binds a cytokine receptor complex that includes OSM-specific receptor subunit-β (OSMRβ) and IL-31 receptor subunit-α (IL-31Ra), is also reserved in this regard. IL-6 can bind to the gp130 subunit. Meanwhile, it is in a complex with the membrane-bound (mIL-6R) or soluble IL-6 receptor (sIL-6R) to induce intracellular signaling (Levine, 2013). IL-6-related cytokine receptor complexes transmit the intracellular signals they form through the Janus kinase-signal converter and JAK-STAT, which is called the activator of the transcription pathway, where receptor-associated JAKs (especially JAK1, JAK2 and TYK2) activate the transcription factors STAT1 and STAT3. Stimulation of the IL-6/JAK/STAT3 pathway mediates the transcription of many genes involved in proliferation, differentiation and transformation in this process (Jones, 2018).

When some other signaling pathways are investigated, it is reported that the SH2 protein tyrosine phosphatase 2 (SHP2), phosphoinositide 3-kinase (PI3K) and protein kinase B (PKB; also known as AKT) pathways function. SHP2 binds to phosphorylated gp130. It has also been shown to promote the activation of the RAS–RAF–MEK-ERK mitogen-activated protein kinase (MAPK) cascade (Rose-John, 2018). The MAPK cascade plays a role in cell growth and antibody synthesis.

Meanwhile, it activates various transcription factors while functioning (Rose-John, 2018; Uciechowski, 2020).

IL-6 family cytokines act on various immune reactions that regulate innate and adaptive immunity, such as inflammation, apoptosis, differentiation and the acute phase response. Meanwhile, it also has pleiotropic effects with multiple signaling pathways (Hunter, 2015; Uciechowski, 2020; Kang, 2020).

IL-6 regulates different oncogenic processes mediated by STAT3. It is also recognized as a pro-tumorigenic cytokine (Jones, 2018). IL-6 has been shown to play a role in the mechanisms of immune regulation and immune dysregulation in the pathogenesis of some diseases. Treatment strategies blocking IL-6 have been proven effective in chronic inflammatory diseases.

Tocilizumab, a humanized anti-IL-6R monoclonal antibody, inhibits both sIL-6R and mIL-6R and is licensed by the FDA for the treatment of RA, SoJIA and polyarticular juvenile idiopathic arthritis (pJIA), adult-onset Still's disease, idiopathic multicentric Castleman disease (iMCD), cytokine release syndrome, giant cell arteritis, and Takayasu arteritis. Siltuximab, an anti-IL-6 chimeric mAb, has been licensed to treat iMCD. IL-6 blockade was also among the treatment targets in uveitis, neuromyelitis optica (NMO), and recently COVID-19 pneumonia (Mullard, 2014; Choy, 2020).

Type II Cytokines

The type II cytokine family includes IFNs and IL-10 family members. Interferons are indispensable mediators in host defense against RNA and DNA viruses and tumor cells. In addition, IFNs modulate innate, in-vivo adaptive immune responses and autoimmunity. These are defined as low molecular weight proteins that protect uninfected cells from viral infections while also being prepared by infected host cells. They are produced very rapidly in the living organism in response to viral infection or other inducers. Structurally, members of this family are also represented as single trans-membrane (spreading) proteins with extracellular domains. Their ligands are six alpha-helical monomers or homodimers with 20-30% sequence identity (Chauhan, 2021).

When the structures of type I IFNs are examined in detail, it is seen that they are non-glycosylated proteins containing 165-200 amino acids with five alpha-helical bundles positioned by two disulfide bonds. IFN gene transcription is initiated via toll-like receptor (TLR) signaling. Type I IFNs show binding to receptors including IFN receptor 1 (IFNAR1) and IFN receptor 2 (IFNAR2). Meanwhile, it also induces phosphorylation of STAT1 and STAT2 (Renauld, 2003; Levine, 2013).

The only known type II IFN is IFN-γ. The IFN-γ protein is a glycosylated protein with 140 amino acids in its structure. IFN-γ acts by binding to a receptor complex consisting of the IFN-γ receptor (IFNGR1) and (IFNGR2). IFGRN1 specifically binds to JAK1, and IFGR2 binds to JAK2. Meanwhile, it leads to the activation of STAT1 to induce the transcriptional activation of genes activated by IFN-γ (Levine, 2013).

IL-10 family cytokines can be classified as IL-10, IL-19, IL-20, IL-22, IL-24, IL-26, IL-28, and IL-29. These cytokines are also referred to as type III IFN (IFN-λ) family members. In addition, IL-10 family cytokines activate the same signaling pathway as type I IFNs (Levine, 2013; Chauhan, 2021).

TNF Family

Two cytotoxic mediators were isolated in studies conducted in 1984. TNF (derived from macrophages – molecular mass 17 kDa) and another were named lymphotoxin (derived from lymphocytes – 20 kDa), TNF-α and TNF-β. Interestingly, these constructs were binding to the same receptor (Gray et al., 1984).

The TNF receptor family plays an important role in immune and inflammatory reactions. Some members of the TNF superfamily were found to have proliferative activity on hematopoiesis, apoptosis, differentiation and morphogenesis. In addition, these cytokines have been shown to be associated with various diseases, including cancer, and cardiovascular, neurological, pulmonary, autoimmune and metabolic disorders (Aggarwal, 2012). It is reported that TNF-α has two different effects on cancer, positive and negative (Balkwill, 2009).

TNF is considered as the prototypical cytokine of the superfamily. It acts on its functions through two receptors. TNFR1 and TNFR2 stimulate proinflammatory and anti-inflammatory pathways. TNF family ligands that bind to the death receptor (TNFR1) or a non-death receptor (TNFR2) also regulate mechanisms at the cellular level that can ultimately result in cell death (Aggarwal, 2003; Prashant, 2021).

The binding of TNFRs leads to the recruitment of cytoplasmic proteins termed the TNF receptor-associated factor (TRAF) family that link TRAF-interacting TNFRs to intracellular signaling pathways and activate the transcription factors of the NFκB family and various MAP kinase cascades (Xie, 2013; Park, 2018; Kucka, 2021) and TNF receptor-associated death domain (TRADD) leads to the activation of caspases that result in apoptosis (Hashem et al., 2016).

Various mutations occur in TNFRSF1A, which encodes TNFR1. These mutations cause TRAPS (tumor necrosis factor receptor associated periodic syndrome). Clinical manifestations of TRAPS may include periodic fever and serosal, synovial and cutaneous inflammatory manifestations. Meanwhile, IL-1 inhibition has been shown to be effective (Jarosz-Griffiths et al., 2019).

IL-17 Family

The IL-17A, IL-17B, IL-17C, IL-17D, IL-17E (IL-25) and IL-17F, amino acid sequence conformity and cytokine family members are classified according to their homology. When the IL-17 receptor family is classified, it is seen that it consists of 5 members (IL-17RA, RB, RC, RD and RE). It has been found to be important that they share a sequence homology, like ligands (Toy, 2006; Chunfang, 2013). This activates the downstream signaling pathways of IL-17R. In other words, it mediates the activation of NF-κB and mitogen-activated protein kinase (MAPK), leading to the stimulation of proinflammatory cytokines and chemokines in the system (Shalom-Barak, 1998). It is seen that IL-17A and IL-17F, which are the most striking members in this regard, can be secreted as homodimers and heterodimers (IL-17A/F) (Wright, 2007). Both IL-17A and IL-17F are produced by effector Th17 cells. It also contributes to stimulating the expression of cytokines and chemokines, including IL-1, TNF, IL-6, GM-CSF, macrophage chemotactic protein-1 and CXC chemokine ligand 10, which are considered to play a role in autoimmune and inflammatory diseases in terms of their clinical importance. IL-17E functions by binding to IL-17RA and 17RB (IL-25R) receptors, produced by immune cells, including Th2 cells, mast cells, macrophages, and eosinophils. Meanwhile, it also activates the NF-kB pathway (Weaver, 2007; Benveniste, 2014).

IL-17A cytokine secretion is detected in many clinics in many autoimmune and autoinflammatory diseases. Diseases in which it plays an important role include psoriasis, psoriatic arthritis and spondylarthritis. Anti-IL-17A blocking agents are used to treat many clinical problems, especially psoriasis, psoriatic arthritis, rheumatoid arthritis, ankylosing spondylitis, inflammatory bowel disease, multiple sclerosis, solid hematological cancer, and non-alcoholic fatty liver disease, and this subject is being improved by new research (Morales, 2020).

TGF-β Family

Transforming growth factor-β (TGF-β) is a vital cytokine that regulates various cellular processes such as family members, proliferation, differentiation, communication, apoptosis and tissue remodeling. When the isoforms (TGF-β1, -β2, -β3) of TGF-β, which is a polypeptide from the human TGF-β family, are examined, it is found that they contain activins, inhibins, sol proteins, nodal, myostatin, bone morphogenetic proteins (BMPs) and growth and differentiation factors (GDFs). (Levine, 2013; Aggarwal, 2012). TGF-β is the prototype member of the family. They were also defined by researchers as polypeptide hormones and hormone-like growth factors (Roberts, 1981). In addition, various functions of TGF-β, which are considered to be vital, such as wound healing, growth, development, cell differentiation and apoptosis have been reported (Shi, 2003).

TGF-β is actually expressed as a precursor protein and subsequently degraded by latent transforming growth factor β-binding proteins (LTBPs). TGF-β pro-peptide (latency-associated peptide-LAP) binds via disulfide bonds in the cell. LAP, TGF-β and LTBP form their complexes (LLC). LTBPs are involved in the maintenance of TGF-β latency. It also plays a role in targeting the latent growth factor to the extracellular matrix (ECM). LTBP-1 supports TGF-β activation by integrins and accompanies the LTBP-3 skeletal structure (Aggarwal, 2012; Robertson, 2015).

When the serine/threonine kinase activity is examined, the active TGF-β dimer structure signals through type I (TGF-βRI) and type II receptors (TGF-βRII). TGF-βRs are activated by non-Smad signaling pathways such as Smad (Sma and Mad Related Family) and MAP kinases, PI3K and Rho-ROCK1 (Levine, 2013; Souchelnytskyi, 1996; Kawabata, 1999).

When BMPs are examined in detail, it is determined that they play a role in bone development, bone remodeling and repair of various defects. This has led to more effective uses of BMPs for treatment processes. They have also been approved for the clinical use of bone tissue regeneration in orthopedics and dentistry clinics for recombinant human BMP-2 and BMP-7.

Conclusion

Cytokines are thought to be a key factor in unknown pathogenesis processes in different diseases caused by the immune response and immune dysregulation. The complexity of cytokines has been emphasized by various publications in the literature. This may be due to the fact that a particular cytokine is endowed with both proinflammatory and anti-inflammatory effects, depending on the cell and disease context in vivo. Cytokines are the cause or the consequence of the diseases. Conditions in which communication between tissues and the immune system is disrupted cause diseases. The biological functions and signal transduction pathways of some of the most recently discovered cytokines are still not fully elucidated. Research aiming to understand the pathophysiology of cytokines illuminates the disease etiologies and generates novel therapeutic strategies.

References

Abbas AK, Lichtman AH, Pillai S, Baker DL. (2020). *Basic immunology: Functions and Disorders of the Immune System,* Sixth edition. Elsevier, Philadelphia.

Aggarwal BB. (2003). Signalling pathways of the TNF superfamily: A double-edged sword. *Nature Rev Immunol,* 3:745-756.

Aggarwal BB, Gupta SC, Kim JH. (2012). Historical perspectives on tumor necrosis factor and its superfamily: 25 years later, a golden journey. *Blood,* 119(3):651-665. https://doi.org/10.1182/blood-2011-04-325225.

Balkwill F. (2009). Tumour necrosis factor and cancer. *Nat Rev Cancer,* 9:361-371. https://doi.org/10.1038/nrc2628.

Benveniste EN. (2014). Cytokines. In Aminoff MJ, Daroff RB. (eds) *Encyclopedia of the Neurological Sciences,* Second Edition. Academic Press, p 921-925 https://doi.org/10.1016/B978-0-12-385157-4.00175-5.

Bodmer JL, Schneider P, Tschopp J. (2002). The molecular architecture of the TNF superfamily. *Trends Biochem Sci,* 27(1):19-26. https://doi.org/10.1016/s0968-0004(01)01995-8.

Chan AH, Schroder K. (2020). Inflammasome signaling and regulation of interleukin-1 family cytokines. *The Journal of Experimental Medicine,* 217(1):e20190314. https://doi.org/10.1084/jem.20190314.

Chauhan P, Nair A, Patidar A, Dandapat J, Sarkar A, Saha B. (2021). A primer on cytokines. *Cytokine*, 145:155458.

Choy EH, De Benedetti F, Takeuchi T, Hashizume M, John MR, Kishimoto T. (2020). Translating IL-6 biology into effective treatments. *Nat Rev Rheumatol*, 16:335-345. https://doi.org/10.1038/s41584-020-0419-z.

Chunfang G, Ling W, Xiaoxia L. (2013). IL-17 family: Cytokines, receptors and signaling. *Cytokine,* 64(2):477-485. https://doi.org/10.1016/j.cyto.2013.07.022.

CORIMUNO-19 Collaborative group. (2021). Effect of anakinra versus usual care in adults in hospital with COVID-19 and mild-to-moderate pneumonia (CORIMUNO-ANA-1): A randomised controlled trial. *The Lancet Respiratory Medicine*, 9(3):295-304.

De Benedetti F, Gattorno M, Anton J, Ben-Chetrit E, Frenkel J, Hoffman HM, Koné-Paut I, Lachmann HJ, Ozen S, Simon A, Zeft A, Calvo Penades I, Moutschen M, Quartier P, Kasapcopur O, Shcherbina A, Hofer M, Hashkes PJ, Van der Hilst J, Hara R, Bujan-Rivas S, Constantin T, Gul A, Livneh A, Brogan P, Cattalini M, Obici L, Lheritier K, Speziale A, and Junge G. (2018) Canakinumab for the Treatment of Autoinflammatory Recurrent Fever Syndromes. *N Engl J Med*, 378(20):1908-1919. https://doi.org/10.1056/NEJMoa1706314.

Dembic Z. (2015). Introduction-Common Features about Cytokines. In: *The Cytokines of the Immune System the Role of Cytokines in Disease Related to Immune Response*. Elsevier, NewYork, p 1-16.

Dinarello CA. (2018). Overview of the IL-1 family in innate inflammation and acquired immunity. *Immunol Rev*, 281:8-27. https://doi.org/10.1111/imr.12621.

Dinarello CA, Simon A, van der Meer JWM. (2012). Treating inflammation by blocking interleukin-1 in a broad spectrum of diseases. *Nature Reviews Drug Discovery*, 11(8):633-652.

Fouriki A, Fougère Y, De Camaret C, Blanchard Rohner G, Grazioli S, Wagner N, Relly C, Pachlopnik Schmid J, Trück J, Kottanatu L, Perez E, Perez M-H, Schaffner D, Asner SA, Hofer M. (2021). Case Report: Case Series of Children with Multisystem Inflammatory Syndrome Following SARS-CoV-2 Infection in Switzerland. *Front Pediatr*, 8:594127. https://doi.org/10.3389/fped.2020.594127.

Garbers C, Heink S, Korn T, Rose-John S. (2018). Interleukin-6: designing specific therapeutics for a complex cytokine. *Nature reviews Drug discovery*, 17(6):395-412 https://doi.org/10.1038/nrd.2018.45.

Garlanda C, Dinarello CA, Mantovani A. (2013). The interleukin-1 family: Back to the future. *Immunity,* 39(6):1003-1018.

Girard C, Rech J, Brown M, Allali D, Roux-Lombard P, Spertini F, Schiffrin EJ, Schett G, Manger B, Bas S, Del Val G, Gabay C. (2016). Elevated serum levels of free interleukin-18 in adult-onset Still's disease. *Rheumatology*, 55(12):2237-2247.

Goldbach-Mansky R, Shroff SD, Wilson M, Snyder C, Plehn S, Barham B, Pham T-H, Pucino F, Wesley RA, Papadopoulos JH, Weinstein SP, Mellis SJ, Kastner DL. (2008). A pilot study to evaluate the safety and efficacy of the long-acting interleukin-1 inhibitor rilonacept (interleukin-1 Trap) in patients with familial cold autoinflammatory syndrome. *Arthritis Rheum,* 58(8):2432-42.

Gray PW, Aggarwal BB, Benton CV, Bringman TS, Henzel WJ, Jarrett JA, Leung DW, Moffat B, Ng P, Svedersky LP, Palladino MA, Nedwin GE. (1984). Cloning and expression of cDNA for human lymphotoxin, a lymphokine with tumour necrosis activity. *Nature*, 312(5996):721-724.

Hashem RM, Mohamed RH, Abo-El-matty DM. (2016). Effect of curcumin on TNFR2 and TRAF2 in unilateral ureteral obstruction in rats. *Nutrition,* 32(4):478-85.

Hunter C, Jones S. (2015). IL-6 as a keystone cytokine in health and disease. *Nat Immunol*, 16:448-457.

Jarosz-Griffiths HH, Holbrook J, Lara-Reyna S, McDermott MF. (2019). TNF receptor signalling in autoinflammatory diseases. *Int Immunol,* 31(10):639-648. https://doi.org/10.1093/intimm/dxz024.

Jones SA, Jenkins BJ. (2018). Recent insights into targeting the IL-6 cytokine family in inflammatory diseases and cancer. *Nat Rev Immunol,* 18:773-789. https://doi.org/10.1038/s41577-018-0066-7.

Kang S, Narazaki M, Metwally H, and Kishimoto T. (2020). Historical overview of the interleukin-6 family cytokine. *The Journal of Experimental Medicine,* 217(5):e20190347. https://doi.org/10.1084/jem.20190347.

Kaplanski G. (2018). Interleukin-18: Biological properties and role in disease pathogenesis. *Immunological Reviews*, 281(1):138-153. https://doi.org/10.1111/imr.12616.

Kawabata M, Miyazono K. (1999). Signal transduction of the TGF-beta superfamily by Smad proteins. *J Biochem*, 125(1):9-16.

Kian Fan Chung. (2009). Cytokines, In: Barnes PJ, Drazen JM, Rennard SI, Thomson NC. (eds). *Asthma and COPD*, Second edn. Academic Press, p 327-341 https://doi.org/10.1016/B978-0-12-374001-4.00027-4.

Kishimoto T. (2006). Interleukin-6: Discovery of a pleiotropic cytokine. *Arthritis Research and Therapy*, 8 (Suppl 2):S2. https://doi.org/10.1186/ar1916.

Klimow VV. (2019). Cytokines. In: Molecules of the Immune System from Basic to Clinical Immunology. *Springer Nature*, Switzerland, p 41- 49.

Kovanen PE, Leonard WJ. (2004). Cytokines and immunodeficiency diseases: Critical roles of the gamma(c)-dependent cytokines interleukins 2, 4, 7, 9, 15, and 21, and their signaling pathways. *Immunological Reviews*, 202:67-83. https://doi.org/10.1111/j.0105-2896.2004.00203.x.

Kucka K, Wajant H. (2021). Receptor Oligomerization and Its Relevance for Signaling by Receptors of the Tumor Necrosis Factor Receptor Superfamily. *Frontiers in Cell and Developmental Biology,* 8:615141. https://doi.org/10.3389/fcell.2020.615141.

Kyriazopoulou E, Panagopoulos P, Metallidis S, Dalekos GN, Poulakou G, Gatselis N, Karakike E, Saridaki M, Loli G, Stefos A, Prasianaki D, Georgiadou S, Tsachouridou O, Petrakis V, Tsiakos K, Kosmidou M, Lygoura V, Dareioti M, Milionis H, Papanikolaou IC, Akinosoglou K, Myrodia D-M, Areti Gravvani A, Stamou A, Theologia Gkavogianni T, Katrini K,Theodoros Marantos T, Trontzas IP,Syrigos K,Chatzis L, Chatzis S, Vechlidis N, Avgoustou C, Chalvatzis S, Kyprianou M, van der Meer JW, Eugen-Olsen J, Netea MG, Giamarellos-Bourboulis EJ. (2021). An open label trial of anakinra to prevent respiratory failure in COVID-19. *Elife,* 10:e66125. https://doi.org/10.7554/eLife.66125.

Levine SJ. (2013). Cytokines. In: Lennarz WJ, Lane MD. (eds) *Encyclopedia of Biological Chemistry,* Second edn. Academic Press, p 613-621.

McInnes IB. (2013). Cytokines. In: Firestein GS, Budd RC, Gabriel SE, McInnes IB, O'Dell JR (eds). *Kelley's Textbook of Rheumatology*, 9th edn. WB Saunders Pages, p 369-381 https://doi.org/10.1016/B978-1-4377-1738-9.00026-8.

Marotto D, Batticciotto A, Ceribelli A, Puttini Piercarlo S. (2019). The journey of canakinumab; on- and off-label indications. *Beyond Rheumatology*, 1(1):22-30.

Mullard A. (2014). Green light for Janssen's IL-6 Blocker. *Nat Biotechnol*, 32:607.

Notarangelo LD, Mella, P, Jones, A, de Saint Basile G, Savoldi G, Cranston T, Vihinen M, Schumacher RF. (2001). Mutations in severe combined immune deficiency (SCID) due to JAK3 deficiency. *Human Mutation,* 18(4):255-263 https://doi.org/10.1002/humu.1188.

Park HH. (2018). Structure of TRAF family: Current understanding of receptor recognition. *Front Immunol,* 9:1999. https://doi.org/10.3389/fimmu.2018.01999.

Renauld JC. (2003). Class II cytokine receptors and their ligands: key antiviral and inflammatory modulators. *Nat Rev Immunol*, 3(8):667-76. https://doi.org/10.1038/nri1153.

Rex D, Agarwal N, Keshava Prasad TS, Kandasamy RK, Subbannayya Y and Pinto SM. (2020). A comprehensive pathway map of IL-18-mediated signalling. *Journal of Cell Communication and Signalling*, 14(2):257-266. https://doi.org/10.1007/s12079-019-00544-4.

Richardson JS. (2008). The anatomy and taxonomy of protein structure. *Adv Protein Chem,* 34(1981):167-339. https://doi.org/10.1016/s0065-3233(08)60520-3.

Roberts AB, Anzano MA, Lamb LC, Smith JM and Sporn MB. (1981). New class of transforming growth factors potentiated by epidermal growth factor: Isolation from non-neoplastic tissues. *Proc Natl Acad Sci,* 78:5339-5343.

Robertson IB., Horiguchi M, Zilberberg L, Dabovic B, Hadjiolova K and Rifkin DB. (2015). Latent TGF-β-binding proteins. *Matrix Biology: Journal of the International Society for Matrix Biology*, 47:44-53.

Rodríguez Y, Novelli L, Rojas M, De Santis M, Acosta-Ampudia Y, Monsalve DM, Ramírez-Santana C, Costanzo A, Ridgway WM, Ansari AA, Gershwin ME, Selmi C, Anaya J-M. (2020). Autoinflammatory and autoimmune conditions at the crossroad of COVID-19. *Journal of Autoimmunity,* 114:102506.

Rose-John S. (2018). Interleukin-6 Family Cytokines. *Cold Spring Harbor Perspectives in Biology,* 10(2):a028415. https://doi.org/10.1101/cshperspect.a028415.

Ruiz de Morales J, Puig L, Daudén E, Cañete JD, Pablos JL, Olveira Martín A, González Juanatey C, Adán A, Montalbán X, Borruel N, Ortí G, Holgado-Martín E, García-Vidal C, Vizcaya-Morales C, Martín-Vázquez V, González-Gay MA. (2020). Critical role of interleukin (IL)-17 in inflammatory and immune disorders: An updated review of the evidence focusing in controversies. *Autoimmunity Reviews*, 19(1):102429.

Shalom-Barak T, Quach J, Lotz M. (1998). Interleukin-17-induced gene expression in articular chondrocytes is associated with activation of mitogen-activated protein kinases and NF-kappaB. *The Journal of biological chemistry*, 273(42):27467-27473.

Shi Y, Massagué J. (2003). Mechanisms of TGF-beta signaling from cell membrane to the nucleus. *Cell,* 113(6):685-700.

Souchelnytskyi S, ten Dijke P, Miyazono K, Heldin CH. (1996). Phosphorylation of Ser165 in TGF-beta type I receptor modulates TGF-beta1-induced cellular responses. *The EMBO Journal,* 15(22):6231-6240.

Sözeri B, Gerçeker-Türk B, Yıldız-Atıkan B, Mir S, Berdeli A. (2018). A novel mutation of interleukin-1 receptor antagonist (IL1RN) in a DIRA patient from Turkey: Diagnosis and treatment. *The Turkish Journal of Paediatrics*, 60(5):588-592.

Toy D, Kugler D, Wolfson M, Vanden Bos T, Gurgel J, Derry J, Tocker J, Peschon J. (2006). Cutting edge: Interleukin 17 signals through a heteromeric receptor complex. *Journal of Immunology,* (Baltimore, Md.: 1950) 177(1):36-39.

Uciechowski P, Dempke W. (2020). Interleukin-6: A Masterplayer in the Cytokine Network. *Oncology,* 98(3):131-137.

Urien S, Bardin C, Bader-Meunier B, Mouy R, Compeyrot-Lacassagne S, Foissac F, Florkin B, Wouters C, Neven B, Treluyer J-M, Quartier P. (2013). Anakinra pharmacokinetics in children and adolescents with systemic-onset juvenile idiopathic arthritis and autoinflammatory syndromes. *BMC Pharmacology and Toxicology*, 14:40.

Weaver CT, Hatton RD, Mangan PR, Harrington LE. (2007) IL-17family cytokines and the expanding diversity of effector T-cell lineages. *Annual Reviews of Immunology*, 25:821-852.

Wright JF, Guo Y, Quazi A, Luxenberg DP, Bennett F, Ross JF, Qiu Y, Whitters MJ, Tomkinson KN, Dunussi-Joannopoulos K, Carreno BM, Collins M, Wolfman NM. (2007). Identification of an interleukin 17F/17A heterodimer in activated human CD4+ T cells. *The Journal of Biological Chemistry,* 282(18):13447-13455.

Xie P. (2013). TRAF molecules in cell signaling and in human diseases. *Journal of Molecular Signaling*, 8(1):7.

Yasin S, Solomon K, Canna SW, Girard-Guyonvarc'h C, Gabay C, Schiffrin E, Sleight A, Grom AA, Schulert GS. (2020). IL-18 as therapeutic target in a patient with resistant systemic juvenile idiopathic arthritis and recurrent macrophage activation Syndrome. *Rheumatology*, (Oxford, England) 59(2):442-445.

Chapter 2

The Immune System

Duygu Keser[*]
Enka Technical School, Kocaeli, Turkey

Abstract

Immunity is described as resistance to diseases, particularly infectious diseases. It is possible to divide the immune system into two interrelated defense systems, the non-specific or innate immune system and the specific or adaptive immune system. These two systems work in close cooperation but take on different duties. Innate immunity is the first barrier for protecting against infections. Differently from the innate immune system, acquired immunity and the molecular basis of its adaptive mechanisms depend on recognizing the invading agent in a specific way and cause the formation of immune memory. The basic elements of the immune system are expressed in two groups. These are the central lymphoid organs comprising the bone marrow and thymus, and the peripheral lymphoid organs comprising the spleen, lymph nodes, and mucosal lymphoid tissue. The complement system is another aspect of the immune response. Cytokines are produced and secreted by various cells, regulating inflammatory and immunity events, such as inflammation, cell growth, healing, and injury. Because of this weakness of the individual's immune system, many disease symptoms appear, such as inflammatory disease, psychosomatic diseases, cancer, etc. Therefore, to strengthen the immune system, we have to care about our body.

Keywords: immune system, innate immune system, adaptive immune system, immune system organs, cytokine

Introduction

Immunity is defined as resistance to diseases, particularly infectious diseases. The immune system is an important and necessary system for the continuation of life because it represents a sum of all processes protecting a living organism against diseases, recognizing and destroying tumor cells and pathogens (Chinen et al., 2006).

---

[*] Corresponding Author's Email: dukeser@gmail.com.

In: Cytokines and Diseases
Editors: Kenan Demir, Selim Görgün and Bahar Uslu
ISBN: 979-8-88697-214-6

The immune system represents an organization of cells and molecules having specific roles in the defense against infections (Peter et al., 2000). The system performs the scanning of each foreign substance entering or contacting the body and distinguishes them from healthy body cells and tissues. Moreover, it detects cells and molecules with an abnormal appearance that occur in the body at certain intervals (Chinen et al., 2006; Paul 2003; Porth 2004). The immune system is carried out through interactions between cells and antigen receptors located on the surface of lymphocytes. These receptors are called cell surface receptors specializing as antigen recognition units. There are many cell surface molecules that have been determined (Stites and Terr 1991).

The human body protects against viruses, bacteria, and other foreign substances with physical barriers, including phagocytic cells in the blood and tissues and different blood-derived molecules. It consists of approximately a trillion cells named lymphocytes and approximately 100 million trillion molecules named antibodies that the lymphocytes generate and secrete. Pattern recognition represents the immune system's specific ability, and its duty is patrolling the body and guarding its identity. The immune system's cells and molecules reach the majority of tissues via the bloodstream, entering tissues by penetrating the capillary walls (Jernes 1973; IQQIG 2006).

It is possible to divide the immune mechanisms into two interrelated defense systems, the non-specific or innate immune system and the specific or adaptive immune system (Paul 2003). These two systems work in close cooperation but take on different duties (IQQIG 2006).

Non-Specific Defense: The Innate Immune System

In the evolutionary process, all multicellular organisms such as vertebrates, invertebrates, and even plants develop defense mechanisms to protect themselves against infections caused by microorganisms and to get rid of damaged or necrotic cells. The first defense system they developed consists of the structures that exist naturally in organisms and are ready to recognize and remove microbes and dead cells. Therefore, these host defense mechanisms are called natural resistance or natural immunity. All cells and molecules that make up innate immunity form the innate immune system (Abbas et al., 2014).

The innate immune system, the first stage of the defense system, distinguishes between things belonging to the organism and foreign things. However, it does not differentiate one type of pathogen from another (Litman et al., 2005). Non-specific resistance consists of two general lines of defense:

- The first line of defense; and
- The second line of defense (Fait et al., 1976) (Agerberth and Gudmundsson 2006).

When microorganisms come to the mucous membranes in the epithelial tissue of our skin, or respiratory, gastrointestinal, and urogenital tract, they encounter the first line of defense. The second line of defense includes chemical signals, antimicrobial peptides, antiphagocytic and natural killer cells, and fever associated with the response to inflammation (Fait et al., 1976) (Agerberth and Gudmundsson 2006).

The innate immune response most effectively directs the adaptive immune system with various microorganisms. Moreover, the innate immune system represents a key participant in the clearance of dead tissues and the onset of the repair process (Abbas et al., 2014).

The innate immune system performs its defense function with more limited responses in comparison with the more variable and specialized responses of adaptive immunity. In addition, the specificity of innate immunity differs in several ways from the specificity of lymphocytes, which is the foreign recognition vehicle of acquired immunity (Abbas et al., 2014).

Antiviral defense and inflammation constitute the two major responses of innate immunity. Inflammation is characterized by the condition when plasma proteins and leukocytes are accumulated and activated in the area of infection or tissue damage. The said proteins and cells together play a role in killing extracellular microorganisms and removing damaged tissue. The natural immune defense against intracellular viruses is ensured with natural killer cells and cytokines called type I interferon (Abbas et al., 2014).

Innate Immune System Cells

Various cell types defend and protect the body in the innate immune system (Beutler 2004).

Phagocytes: The duty of phagocytes is to digest the cell. Phagocytes circulate in the body for the purpose of digesting and eliminating possible threats such as viruses and bacteria (Iwasaki and Medzhitov 2015).

Macrophages: Macrophages represent phagocytic cells that are capable of moving along the capillary walls separate from the circulatory system. The ability of macrophages to circulate outside the circulatory system is essential since it ensures that macrophages capture pathogens in a short time. Furthermore, macrophages can release cytokines with the aim of signaling other cells toward a pathogen-containing area (Iwasaki and Medzhitov 2015).

Mast cells: Mast cells are present in connective tissue and mucous membranes. They are crucial for the inflammatory response and wound healing and defense against pathogens. In the case of the activation of mast cells, they secrete cytokines and granules that contain chemical molecules. Molecules, e.g., histamine, lead to the dilation of blood vessels, increasing the blood flow and their concentration at the infection site. The cytokines secreted in the said process act as messengers and cause other immune cells, e.g., macrophages and neutrophils, to move toward the infection site or be alert to circulating threats (Metz et al., 2013).

Neutrophils: Neutrophils represent phagocytic cells classified as granulocytes due to containing granules in their cytoplasm. The above-mentioned granules have high toxicity to fungi and bacteria, causing them to stop their growth or die on contact (Iwasaki et al., 2015). Approximately 50-60% of leukocytes in the blood are neutrophils. In general, the neutrophil count does not increase in viral infections, whereas a systemic infection or the presence of a systemic inflammatory response causes an increased neutrophil count in the blood. The damaged area response results in the accumulation of pus, which is a yellow, viscous liquid containing molecules including dead neutrophils, bacteria, and semi-digested neutrophils in the area (May and Marchesky 200; Langermans et al., 1994).

Eosinophils: Eosinophils are granulocytes that target multicellular parasites (Iwasaki and Medzhitov 2015). In multiple disease conditions, the migration of eosinophils from the bone marrow, localizing to affected sites, and activating as a response to tissue damage and infection are stimulated by inflammatory mediators, e.g., chemokines and cytokines (Davis and Rothenberg 2014).

Eosinophils secrete free radicals and toxic proteins, killing parasites and bacteria. The usage of free radicals and toxic proteins also leads to tissue damage in the course of allergic reactions. Therefore, the activation and release of toxins by eosinophils are very important for regulation to prevent tissue damage that is not necessary (Iwasaki and Medzhitov 2015).

Basophils: Basophils represent granulocytes responding to multicellular parasites. Basophils secrete histamine like mast cells. Basophils and mast cells are important factors in creating an allergic response because of histamine usage.

Natural Killer Cells: Rather than attacking pathogens in a direct manner, natural killer cells destroy the infected host cell for the purpose of stopping the infection's spread. Infected or compromised host cells are capable of signaling natural killer cells for destruction via the expression of specialized receptors and antigen presentation (Stone et al., 2010).

Dendritic cells: Dendritic cells represent antigen-presenting cells contacting external environments through the skin, the inner mucosal layer of the nose, the stomach and intestines, and lungs. Since dendritic cells are found in tissues, which constitute common points for initial infection, they are capable of identifying threats and acting as messengers for antigen presentation and the remaining part of the immune system. Moreover, dendritic cells may perform the function of a bridge between the innate and adaptive immune systems (Banchereau and Steinman 1998).

Specific Defense: The Adaptive Immune System

Specific immunity develops throughout the individual's lifetime. It distinguishes between those belonging to the organism and those that do not. White blood cells are called lymphocytes, an important building block in a specific defense. These cells contain T cells that contribute to cellular immunity and B cells that contribute to humoral immunity. Cellular immunity involves the generation of Tc cells. These cells have the ability to destroy antigen-carrying cells. Humoral immunity is characterized by a condition when B cells transform into plasma cells secreting immunoglobulins with antigen-specific activity (Porth 2004).

Unlike the innate immune system, acquired immunity and the molecular basis of its adaptive mechanisms depend on recognizing the invading agent in a specific way and cause the formation of immune memory. Because of this memory, the system acquires the capacity to react faster (Wolowczuk et al., 2008).

Lymphocytes

T and B lymphocytes constitute the cells of the adaptive immune system. There are about 2 trillion lymphocytes in the human body that make up 20-40% of white blood cells. Their total mass is approximately identical to the liver or brain. The peripheral bloodstream includes only 2% of all circulating lymphocytes. However, 98% of total lymphocytes move within tissues and the lymphatic system, involving the spleen and lymph nodes (Bloom and Fawcett 1994).

Lymphocytes develop from stem cells in the bone marrow. They mature in primary lymphoid organs (the thymus or bone marrow), then go to secondary lymphoid tissue through the blood and settle down there.

B Lymphocytes: B lymphocytes are responsible for humoral (antibody-based) immunity. Immunoglobulin-(Ig) molecules are found on the cell surfaces of B lymphocytes, and these molecules produce a specific receptor against the antigen. These surface immunoglobulins are IgM and IgD. A surface immunoglobulin receptor on a B lymphocyte binds only one kind of antigen. Therefore, in the immune system, there are ten thousand types of B lymphocytes ready for ten thousand possible specific receptors for various antigens. When the antigen enters the organism, it finds the B lymphocytes with a specific receptor for this type of antigen on their surface. This antigen stimulates the B lymphocytes. Then these stimulated B lymphocytes differentiate and transform into plasma cells. The plasma cells synthesize a large number of antibodies. Some of the stimulated B lymphocytes become memory cells. These memory B lymphocytes are long-lasting, and when they meet the same antigen again, they multiply rapidly and produce rapid and strong antibody responses (Stites 1991).

T Lymphocytes: T lymphocytes are responsible for the cellular type of immune response. T precursor cells made in the bone marrow become mature T lymphocytes in the thymus. During this maturation, many receptors are located on the surface of T lymphocytes (MacDonald et al., 2001). Different cell surface molecules characterize the differentiation of T lymphocytes. CD4, CD8, CD25, and CD44 are among the molecules. A lot of immature cells that enter the thymus are described as early T lineage progenitors (Benz et al., 2008; Bhandoola et al., 2003). T lymphocytes make up the most important part of the immune system. The cells do not directly depend on the antibody, and they form cell-directed and specific immunity (Bloom and Fawcett 1994).

Complement System

The complement system is described as a mechanism complementing other features of the immune response. Typically, the complement system works as a part of innate immunity. However, it is capable of working in cooperation with the adaptive immune system when needed.

The discovery of the complement system was made in the 1890s, when it was revealed to help or "complement" the killing of bacteria by heat-stable antibodies found in the normal serum (Walport 2001). The complement system involves more than 30 proteins. These proteins are found as soluble proteins in the blood or membrane-associated proteins. Activating the complement system causes a sequential cascade of enzymatic reactions (complement activation pathways), which leads to forming the potent anaphylatoxins C3a and C5a, eliciting many physiological responses in the range from chemoattraction to apoptosis. At first, it was considered that the complement system takes the primary part in innate immunity, in which a strong and quick response is mounted against invading pathogens. However, nowadays, it becomes more evident that the complement system also takes a significant part in adaptive immunity, which includes T and B cells that assist with eliminating pathogens (Dunkelberger and Song 2010) (Molina et al., 1996) and in maintaining immunologic memory that prevents pathogens from re-invasion. The complement system not only takes part in innate and adaptive immunity, but also plays a role in tumor growth, tissue regeneration (Qu et al., 2009), and human pathological conditions, e.g., age-related macular degeneration, atypical hemolytic uremic syndrome, etc. (Wagner and Frank 2010).

Complement activation in plasma consists of three different ways: classical, alternative, and lectin pathways. Proteins in the inactive zymogen form become active after some sequential reactions. C3 is the common endpoint in all three pathways. After C3, C3a, C3b, and C5a are formed, the membrane attack complex (MAK; C5b-9) and other activation products are formed (Dunkelberger and Song 2010).

The complement system is under tight control with many inhibitors limiting its activity in situ. This kind of mechanism does not allow the body to damage its own tissues (Rus et al., 2005).

Immune System Organs

The immune system's fundamental elements are expressed in two groups. These are the central lymphoid organs comprising the thymus and bone marrow, and the peripheral lymphoid organs comprising the lymph nodes, spleen, and mucosal lymphoid tissue. Lymphocytes mature in the thymus and bone marrow, and peripheral lymphoid organs fulfill their functions by working in a way that complements each other (Lake and Oski 1978).

Lymph nodes: There are approximately 600 lymph nodes in our body. The first meeting area of mononuclear phagocytes with foreign antigens is the lymph nodes. The gastrointestinal tract and respiratory system usually take antigens into the body. Afferent lymphatic channels bring antigens to the lymph from the area whose antigens resist them. The production of antibodies, the T-cell response, and cytokine generation occur in the lymph nodes. The lymph enlargement of the glands, the normal proliferation of cells or foreign or abnormal reactions occur as a result of cell infiltration (Cecen 2009).

Spleen: The spleen, a lymphoid organ, is significantly involved in the defense mechanism of the body. The spleen represents the destruction site of blood cells. Moreover, the spleen separates and eliminates blood cells covered with antibodies and damaged ones (Mebius and Kraal 2005). Lymphocyte production is an important duty of the spleen (Ramiro-Puig 2007). The lymphoid system is among the most essential organs in antifungal and antibacterial immune activities (Chadburn 2000).

Mucosal Lymphoid Tissue: Approximately half of the lymphocytes of the immune system are present in the mucosa-associated lymphoid tissue (MALT) (Croitoru 1994). MALT is found along all surfaces of mucosal tissues. Nasopharynx-associated lymphoid tissue (NALT), gut-associated lymphoid tissue (GALT), and bronchus-associated lymphoid tissue (BALT) are its most well-known examples. However, the descriptions of lacrimal duct-associated (LDALT), conjunctiva-associated (CALT), larynx-associated (LALT), and salivary duct-associated lymphoid tissue (DALT) have been made. The primary duty of MALT is generating and secreting IgA along the mucosal surfaces in antigen-specific, Th2-dependent reactions via Th1, and cytotoxic T-cell mediated reactions may also emerge, leading to immunotolerance afterward (Gormley 1998; Kiyono and Fukuyama 2004).

Bone Marrow: The bone marrow constitutes the tissue involving the center and the epiphysis of bones, the place of the production of novel blood cells. It has been considered for a long period of time that the bone marrow represents a hematopoietic organ. Nevertheless, it is a known fact that the generation and maturation of B cells occur in the bone marrow.

Furthermore, long-term lived plasma cells that produce antigen-specific antibodies are present in the bone marrow. In this way, the bone marrow makes a contribution to humoral immune responses. Bone marrow-derived cells, such as stromal cells and leukocytes, are capable of secreting numerous cytokines. IL-7 and IL-15 are generated by stromal cells and cells of hemopoietic lineage in the bone marrow. IL-7 represents a "stromal cytokine" generated by various stromal tissues, involving those in the bone marrow (Zhao et al., 2012).

Thymus: Despite the very high regenerative capacity of the thymus during fetal development, a decrease occurs in the regenerative capacity of the human postnatal thymus with time. The human thymus represents a lymphoepithelial organ where the development of T cells occurs in the course of fetal life. Following maturation and selection in the fetal thymic microenvironment, T cells migrate to peripheral lymphoid tissues, e.g., the spleen, lymph nodes, and gut, and form the peripheral T-cell repertoire (Haynes and Hale 1998).

Cytokines and the Immune Response

Cytokines are regulatory proteins with a 20-30 kD molecular weight, and they are produced during all phases of the immune response. They are active even at 10^{-5} to 10^{-6} molar concentrations. They exert their effects in a soluble form. Cytokines are generated and secreted by different cells, regulating inflammatory and immunity events, such as inflammation, cell growth, healing, and injury (Nororiha et al., 1995).

Cytokines are secreted in a very short time from stimulated cells, but they are not stored. Moreover, novo is produced by cytokines in response to a stimulus (Judith et al., 2007). They can be generated by various cells, e.g., B lymphocytes, macrophages, T lymphocytes and mast cells, fibroblasts, endothelial cells, various stromal cells, etc. (Seder and Ahmed 2003; Pleiotropic). They can show similar effects (redundant), agonist effects or antagonistic effects. Cytokines show their effect as a result of binding to particular receptors on target cells. They have autocrine, paracrine, and endocrine effects (Judith et al., 2007).

The impacts of cytokines on the immune system are as follows:

They differentiate and proliferate the lymphoid system and some other cells (Seder and Ahmed 2003).

They activate the cells playing a role in inflammation for going to the reaction zone.

At low concentrations, cytokines cause general infection signs such as fever, myalgia, general headache, acute-phase response, etc. However, with high concentrations of cytokines, shock and death occur.

They exhibit antiviral activity (Nachbaur et al., and Palladino et al., 2014).

Conclusion

The immune system represents a significant and essential system for the continuation of life because the immune system represents all processes protecting a living organism against diseases, recognizing and killing tumor cells and pathogens (Chinen 2006). The said protection involves physical barriers, phagocytic cells in the blood and tissues, and different blood-derived molecules (Paul 2003). It is possible to divide the above-mentioned mechanisms into two interrelated defense systems, the adaptive and innate immune systems (Schenten and Medzhitov 2011).

Natural immunity is innate and non-specific. The skin surface is the innate immune system's first defense line. Enzymes, the alternative complement system pathway, natural killer cells, acute-phase proteins, and cytokines ensure extra defense lines. More complex organisms have an adaptive immune system that is triggered by foreign antigens that have encountered natural immune system defenses. The adaptive immune system is specific to the foreign antigen itself. Moreover, it has an immunologic memory that allows for a more intense response when encountered again (Shames and Kishyama 2006). A warning to the adaptive immune system triggers complex events, including the activation of lymphocytes, antibodies and effective cell production, and eventually stimulates a sequence that results in the elimination of the organism (Dinarello 1999). The specific immunity provided by T and B lymphocytes has 5 important features. These are specificity, diversity, memory response, self-limitation, and recognizing what belongs or does not belong to the organism. Additionally, cytokines are very important in the immune system because of the formation of the immune response. Generally, the roles of cytokines are tissue homeostasis, cellular activation, differentiation, and relocation (Wolowczuk 2008).

The basic elements of the immune system are expressed in two groups. These are the central lymphoid organs comprising the thymus and bone marrow, and the peripheral lymphoid organs comprising the spleen, lymph nodes, and mucosal lymphoid tissue. The maturation of lymphocytes takes place in the thymus and bone marrow, and the peripheral lymphoid organs fulfill their functions by working in a way that complements each other (Lake and Oski 1978).

The immune system is the most important factor for our body. Immune system diseases emerge as one or more immune system abnormalities. Generally, these metabolisms are infection-prone (Bolander 2006; Combs 2008). Because of this weakness of the individual's immune system, many disease symptoms appear, such as inflammatory disease, psychosomatic diseases, cancer, etc. Therefore, in order to strengthen the immune system, we have to care about our body (Alonso-Aperte and Varela-Moreiras 2000).

References

Abbas A K, Litchman A, Pillai S (2014). *Basic of Immunology, Functions and disorders of the immune system*, 4th edn. Elsevier.

Agerberth B, Gudmundsson G (2006). Host antimicrobial defence peptides in human disease. *Curr. Top Microbiol. Immunol.* 306:67-90.

Alonso-Aperte E, Varela-Moreiras G (2000). Drugs–nutrient interactions: a potential problem during adolescence. *European Journal of Clinical Nutrition* 54(1): 69-74.

Banchereau J. and Steinman R M (1998). Dendritic cells and the control of immunity. *Nature* 392(6673):245-252.

Benz C, Martins V C, Radtke F, Bleul C C (2008). The stream of precursors that colonizes the thymus proceeds selectively through the early T lineage precursor stage of T cell development. *J. Exp. Med.* 205:1187–1199.

Beutler B, Innate immunity: an overview (2004) *Molecular immunology* 40(12):845-859.

Bhandoola A, Sambandam A, Allman D, Meraz A, Schwarz B (2003). Early T lineage progenitors: New insights, but old questions remain. *J. Immunol.* 171:5653–5658.

Bloom W, Fawcett D W (1994). *A Textbook of Histology*. 12th Ed., Chapmann and Hall, Newyork-London, p 124-144.

Bolander, F F (2006). Vitamins: not just for enzymes Current opinion in investigational drugs. *Europe PMC Plus* 7(10):912-915.

Cecen E (2009). Peripheral Lymphadenopathy in Childhood. *ADU Medicine Faculty Journal* 10(1):45–52.

Chadburn A (2000). The spleen: Anatomy and anatomical function. *Seminars in Hematology* 37(1): 13-21.

Chinen J, Finkelman F, Shearer W T (2006). Advances in basic and clinical immunology. *J. Allergy Clin. Immunol.* 118:489-95.

Croitoru K, Bienenstock J (1994). Characteristics and Functions of mucosa-associated lymphoid tissue. In: Ogra P L, Mestecky J, Lamm M E, Strober W, McGhee J R, and Bienenstock J (eds) Handbook of Mucosal Immunology, *Academic Press*, San Diego, p 141–51.

Davis B P and Rothenberg M E (2014). Eosinophils and Cancer. *Cancer Immunology Research* 2:1.

Dembic Z (2015). *The Cytokines of the Immune System: The Role of Cytokines in Disease Related to Immune Response*. Elseiver Press.

Dinarello C A (1999). Cytokines as endogenous pyrogens. *J. Infect. Dis.* 179(S2):294- 304.

Dunkelberger J R, Song W C (2010). Complement and its role in innate and adaptive immune responses. *Cell Res.* 20(1):34–50.

Fair W, Couch J, Wehner N (1976). Prostatic antibacterial factor. Identity and significance. *Urology* 7:169-77.

Gormley P D, Powell-Richards A O, Azuara-Blanco A, Donoso L A, Dua H S (1998). Lymphocyte subsets in conjunctival mucosa-associated lymphoid-tissue after exposure to retinal-S-antigen. *Int. Ophthalmol.* 2:77–80.

Haynes H, Hale L (1998) The Human Thymus a Chimeric Organ Comprised of Central and Peripheral Lymphoid Components. *Immunologic Research* 18/3:175-192.

IQWiG (Institute for Quality and Efficiency in Health Care) (2006) *The innate and adaptive immune systems*. Avaible via https://www.ncbi.nlm.nih.gov/books/NBK279396. Accessed 24 Dec 2021.

Iwasaki A, Medzhitov R (2015). Control of adaptive immunity by the innate immune system. *Nature immunology* 16(4):343-353.

Jernes K N (1973). The Immune System. *Scientific American* 229(1):52-63.

Judith A O, Punt J, Stranford S A (2007). *Kuby Immunology*, 7th edn. Macmillan, USA.

Kiyono H, Fukuyama S (2004). NALT- versus Peyer's-patch-mediated mucosal immunity. *Nat. Rev. Immunol.* 4: 699–710.

Lake A M, Oski F A (1978). Peripheral lymphadenopathy in childhood. Ten-year experience with excisional biopsy. *Am. J. Dis. Child.* 132:357-9.

Litman G, Cannon J, Dishaw L (2005). Reconstructing immune phylogeny: new perspectives. *Nat. Rev. Immunol.* 5:866-79.

MacDonald H R, Wilson A, Radtke F (2001). Notch1 and T-cell development: insights from conditional knockout mice. *Trends in Immunology* 22:155–160.

May R, Machesky L (2001). Phagocytosis and the actin cytoskeleton. *J. Cell Sci.* 114: 1061-1077.

Mebius R E, Kraal G (2005). Structure and function of spleen. *Nature Reviews Immunology* 5(8):606-616.

Metz M, Brockow K, Metcalfe D D, Galli S J (2013). *Mast cells, basophils, and mastocytosis, in Clinical Immunology* 284-297.

Molina H, Holers V M, Li B, Fung Y, Mariathasan S, Goellner J, Strauss-Schoenberger J, Karr R W, Chaplin D D (1996). Markedly impaired humoral immune response in mice deficient in complement receptors 1 and 2. *Proc. Natl. Acad. Sci. USA* 93(8):3357–3361.

Nachbaur D M, Herold M, Maneschg A, Huber H (1991). Serum levels of interleukin-6 in multiple myeloma and other hematological disorders: correlation with disease activity and other prognostic parameters. *Annals of Hematology* 62(2-3): 54-8.

Nororiha I L, Niemir Z, Stein H, Waldher R (1995). Cytokines and growth factors in renal disease. *Nephrol. Dial Transplant.* 10:775-786

Palladino C, Bruno B, and Boccadoro M (2014). Discovering the Meaning of Monoclonal Gammopathy of Undetermined Significance: Current Knowledge, Future Challenges. *Translational Medicine UniSa* 8:12–18.

Paul W E (2003). *Fundamental Immunology*, 5th edn. Lippincott Williams & Wilkins, USA.

Peter J D, Roitt I M (2000). The Immune System. *N. Engl. J. Med.* 343:37-49.

Porth C.M (2004). *Essentials of Pathophysiology: Concepts of Altered Health States*. Lippincott Williams&Wilkins, USA.

Ramiro-Puig E, Pérez-Cano F J, Ramírez-Santana C, Castellote C, Izquierdo-Pulido M, Permanyer J, Franch A, Castell M (2007). Spleen lymphocyte function modulated by a cocoa-enriched diet *Clin. Exp. Immunol.* 149(3): 535-542.

Rus H, Cudrici C, Niculescu F (2005). The role of the complement system in innate immunity. *Immunol. Res.* 33:103-12.

Schenten D, Medzhitov R (2011). The Control of Adaptive Immune Responses by the Innate Immune System. *Advances in Immunology* 109: 87-124.

Seder R A, Ahmed R (2003). Similarities and differences in CD4+ and CD8+ effector and memory T cell generation. *Nature immunology* 4(9):835-42.

Shames R S, Kishiyama J L (2006). Immune system diseases. In: McPee S (ed) Shepherd E, Suleymanlar G (translation eds) *Pathophysiology of diseases*, 4th edn. p 31-57.

Stites D P, Terr A (1991). *Basic and Clinical Immunology*, 7th edn, Appleton&Lange, Connecticut, p 16-44.

Stone K D, Prussin C, Metcalfe D D (2010). IgE, mast cells, basophils, and eosinophils. *Journal of Allergy and Clinical Immunology* 125(2):S73-S80.

Walport M J (2001). Complement. First of two parts. *N. Engl. J. Med.* 344(14):1058–1066.

Wolowczuk I, Verwaerde C, Viltart O, Delanoye A, Delacre M, Pot B (2008). Feeding Our Immune System: Impact on Metabolism. *Clin. Dev. Immunol*. 1:20.

Zhao E, Xu H, Wang L, Kryczek I, Wu K, Hu Y, Wang G, Zou W (2012). Bone marrow and the control of immunity. *Cellular & Molecular Immunology* 9: 11–19.

Chapter 3

Synthesis of Cytokines

Enes Çelik*, MD and Ayşen Bingöl, MD
Akdeniz University School of Medicine, Department of Pediatric Allergy and Immunology, Antalya, Turkey

Abstract

Cytokines are important small protein molecules for intercellular communication and have several functions. They are involved in various aspects of cell growth, activation and differentiation. More than 100 genes encoding cytokine-like activities have been identified. Cytokines include interferons, interleukins, chemokines, tumor necrosis factors, growth factors, and adipokines. They can also be classified according to their functions like proinflammatory and anti-inflammatory cytokines. They are mainly synthesized by blood cells, epithelial cells, and lymphoid tissues. The immune system responds according to the type and function of the cytokine produced.

Keywords: adipokines, chemokines, cytokines, growth factors, interferons, interleukins, tumor necrosis factors

Introduction

Cytokines are proteins that play a role in cell signaling and are usually smaller than 40 kDa in molecular weight (Chousterman et al., 2017). More than 100 genes encoding cytokine-like activities have been identified (Dinarello 2007). Cytokines exert endocrine, autocrine, and paracrine activities and affect many biological processes such as embryonic development, stem cell differentiation, immunological response to infection and antigens, pathogenesis of diseases, tissue homeostasis, and cognitive functions (Dinarello 2007; Chousterman et al., 2017).

Cytokines include interferons (IFNs), interleukins (ILs), chemokines, tumor necrosis factors (TNFs), growth factors, and adipokines. Cytokines can also be classified according to their functions. Table 1 shows the functional classes of cytokines (Dinarello 2007).

---

* Corresponding Author's Email: drenescelik@outlook.com.

In: Cytokines and Diseases
Editors: Kenan Demir, Selim Görgün and Bahar Uslu
ISBN: 979-8-88697-214-6

Table 1. Functional classes of cytokines

Class	Function	Examples
Proinflammatory cytokines	increase inflammatory mediators	TNF-α, IL-1α, IL-1β, IL-12, IL-18, IL-23
Anti-inflammatory cytokines	decrease inflammatory genes	TGF-β, IFN-α/β, IL-10, IL-13, IL-1Rα
Lymphocyte growth factors	clonal expansion, Th1/Th2/Th17 polarization	IL-2, IL-4, IL-7, IL-17, IL-15
Colony-stimulating factors	hematopoiesis, pro- and anti-inflammatory	G-CSF, GM-CSF, IL-3, IL-7
Th1 cytokines	increase Th1 response	IL-2, IL-12, IL-18, IFN-γ
Th2 cytokines	increase Th2 response and antibody production	IL-4, IL-5, IL-18, IL-25, IL-33
Th17 cytokines	increase Th17 and autoimmune responses	IFN-γ, IL-17, IL-23
Type I IFN	anti-viral, anti-inflammatory	IFN-α, IFN-β
Type II IFN	macrophage activation	IFN-γ
Adipokines	proinflammatory, pro-atherogenic	adiponectin, leptin, IL-1α, TNF-α, IL-6
Mesenchymal growth factors	fibrosis, pro-metastatic	FGF, TGF-β
Chemokines	increase cellular emigration and activation	CCL1, CCL2, CXCL1

*Adapted from (Dinarello 2007).

In this chapter, the synthesis of cytokines will be explained.

Interferons

IFNs are a family of cytokines with antiviral, antiproliferative, and antitumor activity and immunomodulatory effects (López de Padilla and Niewold 2016). They are classified into three main types based on their receptor specificity (Chousterman et al., 2017). Type 1 interferons include IFN-α (alpha), IFN-β (beta), IFN-ω (omega), IFN-τ (tau), IFN-δ (delta), and IFN-ε (epsilon), while IFN-γ (gamma) is type 2 and IFN-λ (lambda) is type 3 (Negishi et al., 2018).

IFNs produced from virus-infected cells act on neighboring uninfected cells to initiate antiviral immunity that inhibits virus replication (Sen and Williams 2019). All somatic nucleated cells induced by the presence of viral RNA or via other cell membrane receptors can produce type 1 IFNs, which in turn activate the Th1 response of the adaptive immune system (Dembic 2015a). In addition to being a critical part of the antiviral response, the type I IFN pathway has been shown to be overactive in many autoimmune diseases (López de Padilla and Niewold 2016).

Viral infection triggers a variety of pattern recognition receptors (PRRs) such as toll-like receptors (TLRs) (Sen and Williams 2019). TLRs were the first discovered PRRs that recognize pathogen-associated molecular patterns (PAMPs). TLRs located on the surface of the cell membrane or in endosomes activate the immune system by providing the gene induction of type 1 IFNs and proinflammatory cytokines (Negishi et al., 2018). Cells with activated TLR3 and TLR4 receptors can especially produce IFN-β (Negishi et al., 2012). Transcriptional regulation of the IFN-α and IFN-β genes is mainly controlled by interferon regulatory factors (IRFs), and signaling that activates nuclear factors IRF3 and IRF7 enables the synthesis of type I IFNs. It has also been determined that plasmacytoid dendritic cells are a subset of myeloid cells that express high amounts of TLR7 and TLR9 and secrete very high levels of type I IFNs (Colonna et al., 2004).

Type 2 interferon (IFN-γ) has less antiviral activity compared to IFN-α and IFN-β, and its immunomodulatory effects are more pronounced. Although mainly synthesized by $CD4^+$ T helper and $CD8^+$ cytotoxic T cells, they are also produced by natural killer (NK) cells, B cells, dendritic cells (DCs) and macrophages (Dembic 2015a; Chousterman et al., 2017; Negishi et al., 2018).

Type 3 interferon (IFN-λ), other names IL-28 and IL-29) has antiviral and immunomodulatory effects (Dembic 2015a). Similar to type 1 IFNs, they are synthesized by the recognition of various PAMPs (Negishi et al., 2018).

Interleukins

Proteins that bind to their specific receptors and function as communication between leukocytes are called ILs. Nearly 40 ILs have been identified (Akdis et al., 2011). While proinflammatory ILs are responsible for cell activation, tissue damage and necrosis, anti-inflammatory ILs aim to reduce and reverse the inflammatory process (Chousterman et al., 2017).

The main source of IL-1 is mononuclear phagocytic cells, and it is also produced by various cells such as keratinocytes, endothelial cells, osteoblasts, glial cells, synovial cells, and neutrophils (Commins et al., 2010). It is secreted as pro-IL-1 as a result of many proinflammatory stimuli such as cell damage, activated complement components, antigen-antibody complexes, leukotrienes, TNFs, granulocyte-macrophage colony stimulating factor (GM-CSF) and IL-1 itself (autocrine) (Dembic 2015b). IL-1α and IL-1β induce proinflammatory proteins and hematopoiesis and play a role in many autoimmune and inflammatory diseases (Dinarello 1996). IL-1Ra (receptor antagonist), on the other hand, suppresses inflammation by antagonizing IL-1 by being synthesized and released from similar cells in response to the same stimuli that cause IL-1 production (Eisenberg et al., 1990).

IL-2 is mainly produced by the activation of $CD4^+$ and $CD8^+$ T cells after antigen/TCR interaction and costimulation. It is also secreted by activated DCs, NK and NKT cells. IL-2 plays a role in the proliferation of T and B cells, the development of Treg cells, and the proliferation and differentiation of NK cells (Malek 2008). It has been reported to play a role in T-cell-mediated autoimmune and inflammatory diseases and some immune deficiencies (Commins et al., 2010).

IL-3 is synthesized by T cells, NK cells, macrophages, eosinophils, and mast cells (Hawwari et al., 2002). IL-3 is a hematopoietic growth factor and plays a role in the activation of basophils and eosinophils (Ihle 1992). The IL-3, IL-5, and GM-CSF receptors consist of a cytokine-specific α chain and a common β chain, resulting in a partial overlap of the functions of these cytokines (Martinez-Moczygemba and Huston 2003). The association of IL-3 with allergic diseases and malignancies has been reported (Celestin et al., 2001; Testa et al., 2002).

IL-4 is mainly produced by Th2 cells, but also by basophils, mast cells, NKT cells, eosinophils, type 2 innate lymphoid cells (ILC2s) and γ/δ T cells (Nelms et al., 1999; Zhu 2015). It plays a role in Th2 cell differentiation from antigen-stimulated naive T cells, the regulation of immunoglobulin class switching, increasing class II MHC molecule expression in B lymphocytes, increasing IL-4R and CD23 expression, tissue adhesion and inflammation, and B- and T-cell growth (Nelms et al., 1999; Junttila 2018). It has been found to be associated with allergic, inflammatory, and autoimmune diseases and malignancies (Dembic 2015b).

IL-5 is synthesized by Th2 cells, ILC2s, activated mast cells, eosinophils, Tc2 cells, NK cells, NKT cells and γ/δ T cells (Martinez-Moczygemba and Huston 2003; Akdis et al., 2011; Zhu 2015). IL-5 is an important factor in the development, growth, maturation and activation of eosinophils (Mould et al., 2000). It plays a role in increasing the chemotactic activity and adhesion capacity on eosinophils, the differentiation of myeloid cells, wound healing and remodeling (Akdis et al., 2011). It is one of the most important cytokines in the pathophysiology of allergic inflammation and asthma (Martinez-Moczygemba and Huston 2003).

IL-6 (formerly IFN-β2) is produced by monocytes, macrophages, endothelial cells, T and B cells, keratinocytes, fibroblasts and hepatocytes by various stimuli during systemic inflammation. It plays a role in the activation of leukocytes, the synthesis of acute-phase proteins from the liver, T-cell differentiation and activation, B-cell differentiation, immunoglobulin production and hematopoiesis (Akira et al., 1993). Its association with autoimmune diseases, chronic inflammatory diseases and some malignancies has been reported (Linker-Israeli et al., 1999).

IL-7 is produced by many stromal tissues, epithelial cells in the thymus and bone marrow, the intestinal epithelium, keratinocytes, hepatocytes, DCs, follicular DCs, B cells, monocytes and macrophages. It plays a role in the proliferation of Pre-B and Pro-B lymphocytes, megakaryocyte maturation, the synthesis of inflammatory mediators in monocytes, the survival of naive T lymphocytes and VDJ recombination (Fry and Mackall 2002). It has been shown to be associated with allergic and autoimmune diseases (Lundmark et al., 2007; Kelly et al., 2009).

IL-8 (also known CXCL8) is synthesized by a wide variety of cells such as neutrophils, lymphocytes, macrophages, monocytes, fibroblasts, endothelial and epithelial cells, keratinocytes, hepatocytes, synovial cells, chondrocytes, smooth muscle and skeletal muscle cells, and some tumor cells. Its production is stimulated by TNF-α, IL-1α, IL-1β and bacterial lipopolysaccharides (LPS) (Akdis et al., 2011). IL-8 acts as a chemoattractant for neutrophils, eosinophils, basophils, T lymphocytes, NK cells and GM-CSF (Burke et al., 2008). It induces the release of hematopoietic progenitor cells from the bone marrow to the peripheral blood (Laterveer et al., 1995). It also has angiogenic effects (Heidemann et al., 2003). Its level has been shown to increase in infections and chronic inflammatory conditions such as autoimmune diseases (Skov et al., 2008).

IL-9 is mainly secreted by Th2 and Th9 cells, and to a lesser extent by eosinophils and mast cells (Veldhoen et al., 2008). IL-9 production is induced by the cascade of IL-2, IL-4 and IL-10 cytokines, as well as by TGF-β in a different way (Houssiau et al., 1995; Veldhoen et al., 2008). IL-9 functions as a growth factor for T cells and mast cells, and plays a role in the inhibition of cytokine production from Th1 lymphocytes, IgE production, proliferation of $CD8^+$ T cells and mast cells, and chemokine and mucus secretion from bronchial epithelial cells (Akdis et al., 2011). It has been found to be associated with asthma, food allergy, helminth infections and Hodgkin lymphoma (Merz et al., 1991; Temann et al., 1998; Forbes et al., 2008; Licona-Limón et al., 2017).

IL-10 is produced by T cells, B cells, monocytes, macrophages and DCs (Nagalakshmi et al., 2004). IL-10 gene expression is controlled by the transcription factors Sp1 and Sp3 (Tone et al., 2000). IL-10 regulates the inflammatory response by showing an immunosuppressive effect (de Waal Malefyt et al., 1991). It has been reported to have a protective effect in autoimmune and allergic diseases (Akdis et al., 1998; Llorente et al., 2000).

IL-11 is synthesized by many stromal cells such as fibroblasts, epithelial cells, osteoblasts, synoviocytes, and chondrocytes (Leng and Elias 1997). Its production is induced by IL-1, TGF-β, IL-13 and TNF-α cytokines. IL-11 induces hematopoiesis and thrombocytopoiesis, induces acute-phase proteins, regulates macrophage activity, regulates neuronal differentiation, and functions in inflammation, bone and tissue remodeling (Leng and Elias 1997; Chen et al., 2005).

IL-12 is a proinflammatory cytokine produced by activated inflammatory cells such as monocytes, macrophages, DCs, B cells, neutrophils and microglia (Trinchieri 2003; Wang et al., 2012). Bacteria, fungi, parasites, viruses and their products induce IL-12 production (Trinchieri 2003). IL-12 induces IFN-γ production, NK cell activation, and Th1 differentiation and cytotoxicity (Wang et al., 2012). Thus, it shows immunomodulatory, antimicrobial and antitumor activity (Trinchieri 2003; Wang et al., 2012).

IL-13 is secreted by Th2 lymphocytes, mast cells, eosinophils, basophils, ILC2s and NKT cells, especially when triggered by an allergen or parasite (Zhu 2015; Junttila 2018). IL-13 antagonizes Th1 cytokines such as IFN-γ, TNF-α and IL-12, increases the expression of MHC II and CD23 in B lymphocytes, induces adhesion molecules such as CD11b, CD11c, and CD18, increases the production of IgE and IgG_4, plays a role in alternative macrophage activation, activates mast cells and eosinophils and prolongs their life span (Wynn 2003; Poulsen and Hummelshoj 2007; Junttila 2018). It is one of the important cytokines that play a role in asthma and other allergic inflammatory diseases (Zhu 2015).

IL-14 has been detected in T cells, T-cell clones and lymphoma cells. It has been reported that it plays a role in activated B-cell proliferation, lymphomas and autoimmunity (Delfraissy et al., 1986; Ambrus et al., 1993; Ford et al., 1995).

IL-15 is synthesized by immune cells such as activated T cells, monocytes, macrophages, DCs and nonimmune cells such as skeletal muscle cells and keratinocytes as a result of signals that trigger natural immunity (Giri et al., 1994; Saeed and Revell 2001).

IL-16 is produced by both immune and nonimmune cells such as T cells, DCs, eosinophils, mast cells, epithelial cells, and fibroblasts. It plays a role in chemotaxis, cell adhesion, migration and fusion (Cruikshank et al., 2000).

The IL-17 family consists of proinflammatory cytokines. While many innate and adaptive immune cells can produce IL-17 cytokines, the main source is Th17 cells (Cua and Tato 2010; Dong and Ma 2016).

IL-18 is synthesized by macrophages, dendritic cells, Kupfer cells, osteoblasts, keratinocytes, intestinal epithelial cells and synovial fibroblasts and plays a role in many autoimmune and inflammatory diseases (Gracie et al., 2003).

IL-19 is synthesized by monocytes, B cells, keratinocytes and airway epithelial cells as a result of stimuli such as LPS (Gallagher et al., 2004; Leigh et al., 2020).

IL-20 is produced by keratinocytes, monocytes, and endothelial and epithelial cells as a result of stimuli such as LPS and serves in the epidermal function (Blumberg et al., 2001; Hsing et al., 2006). IL-21 and IL-22 are synthesized by T cells and NKT cells, IL-23 by macrophages and DCs, and other ILs are synthesized by various tissues and cells according to their functions (Akdis et al., 2011).

Chemokines

Chemokines are a family of cytokines consisting of approximately 50 small proteins weighing 8-10 kDa that are critically important to the immune system (Mantovani 1999; Zhang et al., 2021). They are divided into four groups as CXC, CC, XC and CX_3C according to the disulfide bonds that hold the peptide together (Vinader and Afarinkia 2012).

Chemokines play a particular role in leukocyte trafficking and maturation, but also in collagen production, angiogenesis and hematopoiesis. Although chemokines act as intercellular signals, their sources and targets are various. It is possible that all cell types can produce chemokines under favorable conditions. Some chemokines are synthesized constitutively, some by induction, and some are synthesized both constitutively and inducibly. In addition, a cell can produce many chemokines in response to the same stimulus (Mantovani 1999; Vinader and Afarinkia 2012).

Tumor Necrosis Factors

TNF is a proinflammatory cytokine and plays an important role in cell survival, differentiation, proliferation, and death (Wang and Lin 2008). TNF is mainly synthesized by macrophages, but also by various cells such as mast cells, lymphocytes, fibroblasts, endothelial cells and neuronal cells (Wajant et al., 2003). TNF-α has a critical role in the production and regulation of inflammatory cytokines (Parameswaran and Patial 2010). In addition to its immunomodulatory activity, it also has different functions such as antitumor and metabolic effects (Mencoboni et al., 1992).

Growth Factors

This group includes TGF-β, thymic stromal lymphopoietin (TSLP), colony stimulating factor (CSF), stem cell factor (SCF), keratinocyte growth factor, ciliary neurotrophic factor, epidermal growth factor, fibroblast growth factor, hepatocyte growth factor, insulin-like growth factor (IGF), platelet derived growth factor, nerve growth factor, vascular endothelial growth factor and endothelins (Dembic 2015c).

TGF-β is synthesized by various cells such as eosinophils, T cells and monocytes (Commins et al., 2010). It has many effects that regulate cell function, differentiation, proliferation and migration. It plays a role in inflammation, immune homeostasis and wound repair (Taylor 2009).

TSLP is synthesized from the skin, lungs, intestines, and thymus. It regulates Th2 cell differentiation. It plays an important role in the pathogenesis of asthma and atopic dermatitis (He and Geha 2010).

SCF, CSF, M-CSF (macrophage-CSF), G-CSF (granulocyte-CSF) and GM-CSF are hematopoietic growth factors. They are produced from bone marrow stromal cells, fibroblasts, endothelial and epithelial cells (Wakefield et al., 1990; Broudy 1997).

IGF-I and IGF-II are mainly synthesized from the liver. Their synthesis by extrahepatic tissues also shows that they have autocrine and paracrine effects in addition to their endocrine effects (LeRoith et al., 1992).

Adipokines

The term adipokine is used for substances secreted by adipose tissue. Adiponectin, leptin, resistin, apelin, vaspin, omentin, visfatin, retinol binding protein-4, serum amyloid A, plasminogen activator inhibitor-1, and angiotensinogen are adipokines, and TNF-α and IL-6 secreted from macrophages in adipose tissue are also accepted as adipokines (Leal and Mafra 2013).

Conclusion

Cytokines are important molecules that provide intercellular communication. They are mainly synthesized by blood cells, epithelial cells, and lymphoid tissues. New researches on the synthesis of cytokines and the immune system will be a guide for a better understanding of homeostatic balance and the pathogenesis of diseases.

References

Akdis C A, Blesken T, Akdis M, et al. (1998) Role of interleukin 10 in specific immunotherapy. *J. Clin. Invest.* 102:98–106. https://doi.org/10.1172/JCI2250.

Akdis M, Burgler S, Crameri R, et al. (2011) Interleukins, from 1 to 37, and interferon-γ: receptors, functions, and roles in diseases. *J. Allergy Clin. Immunol.* 127:701–770. https://doi.org/10.1016/j.jaci.2010.11.050.

Akira S, Taga T, Kishimoto T (1993) Interleukin-6 in biology and medicine. *Adv. Immunol.* 54:1–78. https://doi.org/10.1016/s0065-2776(08)60532-5.

Ambrus J L J, Pippin J, Joseph A, et al. (1993) Identification of a cDNA for a human high-molecular-weight B-cell growth factor. *Proc. Natl. Acad. Sci. USA* 90:6330–6334. https://doi.org/10.1073/pnas.90.13.6330.

Blumberg H, Conklin D, Xu WF, et al. (2001) Interleukin 20: discovery, receptor identification, and role in epidermal function. *Cell* 104:9–19. https://doi.org/10.1016/s0092-8674(01)00187-8.

Broudy V C (1997) Stem Cell Factor and Hematopoiesis. *Blood* 90:1345–1364. https://doi.org/10.1182/blood.V90.4.1345.

Burke S M, Issekutz T B, Mohan K, et al. (2008) Human mast cell activation with virus-associated stimuli leads to the selective chemotaxis of natural killer cells by a CXCL8-dependent mechanism. *Blood* 111:5467–5476. https://doi.org/10.1182/blood-2007-10-118547.

Celestin J, Rotschke O, Falk K, et al. (2001) IL-3 induces B7.2 (CD86) expression and costimulatory activity in human eosinophils. *J. Immunol.* 167:6097–6104. https://doi.org/10.4049/jimmunol.167.11.6097.

Chen Q, Rabach L, Noble P, et al. (2005) IL-11 receptor alpha in the pathogenesis of IL-13-induced inflammation and remodeling. *J. Immunol.* 174:2305–2313. https://doi.org/10.4049/jimmunol.174.4.2305.

Chousterman BG, Swirski FK, Weber GF (2017) Cytokine storm and sepsis disease pathogenesis. *Semin. Immunopathol.* 39:517–528. https://doi.org/10.1007/s00281-017-0639-8.

Colonna M, Trinchieri G, Liu Y-J (2004) Plasmacytoid dendritic cells in immunity. Nat Immunol 5:1219–1226. https://doi.org/10.1038/ni1141.

Commins S P, Borish L, Steinke J W (2010) Immunologic messenger molecules: cytokines, interferons, and chemokines. *J. Allergy Clin. Immunol.* 125:53-72. https://doi.org/10.1016/j.jaci.2009.07.008.

Cruikshank WW, Kornfeld H, Center DM (2000) Interleukin-16. *J. Leukoc. Biol.* 67:757–766. https://doi.org/https://doi.org/10.1002/jlb.67.6.757.

Cua D J, Tato C M (2010) Innate IL-17-producing cells: the sentinels of the immune system. *Nat. Rev. Immunol.* 10:479–489. https://doi.org/10.1038/nri2800.

de Waal Malefyt R, Haanen J, Spits H, et al. (1991) Interleukin 10 (IL-10) and viral IL-10 strongly reduce antigen-specific human T cell proliferation by diminishing the antigen-presenting capacity of monocytes via downregulation of class II major histocompatibility complex expression. *J. Exp. Med.* 174:915–924. https://doi.org/10.1084/jem.174.4.915.

Delfraissy J F, Wallon C, Vazquez A, et al. (1986) B cell hyperactivity in systemic lupus erythematosus: selectively enhanced responsiveness to a high molecular weight B cell growth factor. *Eur. J. Immunol.* 16:1251–1256. https://doi.org/10.1002/eji.1830161011.

Dembic Z (2015a) Chapter 5 - Cytokines of the Immune System: Interferons. In: *Dembic Z (ed) The Cytokines of the Immune System.* Academic Press, Amsterdam, p 123–142.

Dembic Z (2015b) Chapter 6 - Cytokines of the Immune System: Interleukins. In: *Dembic Z (ed) The Cytokines of the Immune System.* Academic Press, Amsterdam, p 143–239.

Dembic Z (2015c) Chapter 8 - Cytokines Important for Growth and/or Development of Cells of the Immune System. In: *Dembic Z (ed) The Cytokines of the Immune System.* Academic Press, Amsterdam, p 263–281

Dinarello C A (1996) Biologic basis for interleukin-1 in disease. *Blood* 87:2095–2147.

Dinarello C A (2007) Historical insights into cytokines. *Eur. J. Immunol.* 37 Suppl 1:S34-45. https://doi.org/10.1002/eji.200737772.

Dong W, Ma X (2016) Regulation of Interleukin-17 Production. *Adv. Exp. Med. Biol.* 941:139–166. https://doi.org/10.1007/978-94-024-0921-5_7.

Eisenberg S P, Evans R J, Arend W P, et al. (1990) Primary structure and functional expression from complementary DNA of a human interleukin-1 receptor antagonist. *Nature* 343:341–346. https://doi.org/10.1038/343341a0.

Forbes EE, Groschwitz K, Abonia JP, et al. (2008) IL-9- and mast cell-mediated intestinal permeability predisposes to oral antigen hypersensitivity. *J. Exp. Med.* 205:897–913. https://doi.org/10.1084/jem.20071046.

Ford R, Tamayo A, Martin B, et al. (1995) Identification of B-cell growth factors (interleukin-14; high molecular weight-B-cell growth factors) in effusion fluids from patients with aggressive B-cell lymphomas. *Blood* 86:283–293.

Fry T J, Mackall C L (2002) Interleukin-7: from bench to clinic. *Blood* 99:3892–3904. https://doi.org/10.1182/blood.v99.11.3892.

Gallagher G, Eskdale J, Jordan W, et al. (2004) Human interleukin-19 and its receptor: a potential role in the induction of Th2 responses. *Int. Immunopharmacol.* 4:615–626. https://doi.org/10.1016/j.intimp.2004.01.005.

Giri JG, Ahdieh M, Eisenman J, et al. (1994) Utilization of the beta and gamma chains of the IL-2 receptor by the novel cytokine IL-15. *EMBO J.* 13:2822–2830.

Gracie J A, Robertson S E, McInnes I B (2003) Interleukin-18. *J. Leukoc. Biol.* 73:213–224. https://doi.org/10.1189/jlb.0602313.

Hawwari A, Burrows J, Vadas M A, Cockerill PN (2002) The human IL-3 locus is regulated cooperatively by two NFAT-dependent enhancers that have distinct tissue-specific activities. *J. Immunol.* 169:1876–1886. https://doi.org/10.4049/jimmunol.169.4.1876.

He R, Geha R S (2010) Thymic stromal lymphopoietin. *Ann. N Y Acad. Sci.* 1183:13–24. https://doi.org/10.1111/j.1749-6632.2009.05128.x.

Heidemann J, Ogawa H, Dwinell M B, et al. (2003) Angiogenic effects of interleukin 8 (CXCL8) in human intestinal microvascular endothelial cells are mediated by CXCR2. *J. Biol. Chem.* 278:8508–8515. https://doi.org/10.1074/jbc.M208231200.

Houssiau F A, Schandené L, Stevens M, et al. (1995) A cascade of cytokines is responsible for IL-9 expression in human T cells. Involvement of IL-2, IL-4, and IL-10. *J. Immunol.* 154:2624–2630.

Hsing C-H, Ho C-L, Chang L-Y, et al. (2006) Tissue microarray analysis of interleukin-20 expression. *Cytokine* 35:44–52. https://doi.org/10.1016/j.cyto.2006.07.006.

Ihle JN (1992) Interleukin-3 and hematopoiesis. *Chem. Immunol.* 51:65–106. https://doi.org/10.1159/000420755.

Junttila IS (2018) Tuning the Cytokine Responses: An Update on Interleukin (IL)-4 and IL-13 Receptor Complexes. *Front Immunol.* 9:888. https://doi.org/10.3389/fimmu.2018.00888.

Kelly E A B, Koziol-White C J, Clay K J, et al. (2009) Potential contribution of IL-7 to allergen-induced eosinophilic airway inflammation in asthma. *J. Immunol.* 182:1404–1410. https://doi.org/10.4049/jimmunol.182.3.1404.

Laterveer L, Lindley I J, Hamilton M S, et al. (1995) Interleukin-8 induces rapid mobilization of hematopoietic stem cells with radioprotective capacity and long-term myelolymphoid repopulating ability. *Blood* 85:2269–2275.

Leal V de O, Mafra D (2013) Adipokines in obesity. *Clin. Chim. Acta* 419:87–94. https://doi.org/10.1016/j.cca.2013.02.003.

Leigh T, Scalia R G, Autieri M V (2020) Resolution of inflammation in immune and nonimmune cells by interleukin-19. *Am. J. Physiol. Cell Physiol.* 319:C457–C464. https://doi.org/10.1152/ajpcell.00247.2020.

Leng S X, Elias J A (1997) Interleukin-11. *Int. J. Biochem. Cell Biol.* 29:1059–1062. https://doi.org/10.1016/s1357-2725(97)00017-4.

LeRoith D, McGuinness M, Shemer J, et al. (1992) Insulin-like growth factors. *Biol. Signals* 1:173–181. https://doi.org/10.1159/000109323.

Licona-Limón P, Arias-Rojas A, Olguín-Martínez E (2017) IL-9 and Th9 in parasite immunity. *Semin. Immunopathol.* 39:29–38. https://doi.org/10.1007/s00281-016-0606-9.

Linker-Israeli M, Wallace DJ, Prehn J, et al. (1999) Association of IL-6 gene alleles with systemic lupus erythematosus (SLE) and with elevated IL-6 expression. *Genes Immun.* 1:45–52. https://doi.org/10.1038/sj.gene.6363631.

Llorente L, Richaud-Patin Y, García-Padilla C, et al. (2000) Clinical and biologic effects of anti-interleukin-10 monoclonal antibody administration in systemic lupus erythematosus. *Arthritis Rheum.* 43:1790–1800. https://doi.org/10.1002/1529-0131(200008)43:8<1790::AID-ANR15>3.0.CO;2-2.

López de Padilla C M, Niewold T B (2016) The type I interferons: Basic concepts and clinical relevance in immune-mediated inflammatory diseases. *Gene* 576:14–21. https://doi.org/https://doi.org/10.1016/j.gene.2015.09.058.

Lundmark F, Duvefelt K, Iacobaeus E, et al. (2007) Variation in interleukin 7 receptor alpha chain (IL7R) influences risk of multiple sclerosis. *Nat. Genet.* 39:1108–1113. https://doi.org/10.1038/ng2106.

Malek TR (2008) The biology of interleukin-2. *Annu. Rev. Immunol.* 26:453–479. https://doi.org/10.1146/annurev.immunol.26.021607.090357.

Mantovani A (1999) The chemokine system: redundancy for robust outputs. *Immunol. Today*. 20:254–257. https://doi.org/10.1016/s0167-5699(99)01469-3.

Martinez-Moczygemba M, Huston D P (2003) Biology of common beta receptor-signaling cytokines: IL-3, IL-5, and GM-CSF. *J. Allergy Clin. Immunol.* 112:653–65; quiz 666. https://doi.org/10.1016/S0091.

Mencoboni M, Lerza R, Bogliolo G (1992) [Tumor necrosis factor: a cytokine with multiple actions]. *Recenti. Prog. Med.* 83:15–17.

Merz H, Houssiau F A, Orscheschek K, et al. (1991) Interleukin-9 expression in human malignant lymphomas: unique association with Hodgkin's disease and large cell anaplastic lymphoma. *Blood* 78:1311–1317.

Mould A W, Ramsay A J, Matthaei K I, et al. (2000) The effect of IL-5 and eotaxin expression in the lung on eosinophil trafficking and degranulation and the induction of bronchial hyperreactivity. *J. Immunol.* 164:2142–2150. https://doi.org/10.4049/jimmunol.164.4.2142.

Nagalakshmi M L, Murphy E, McClanahan T, de Waal Malefyt R (2004) Expression patterns of IL-10 ligand and receptor gene families provide leads for biological characterization. *Int. Immunopharmacol.* 4:577–592. https://doi.org/10.1016/j.intimp.2004.01.007.

Negishi H, Taniguchi T, Yanai H (2018) The Interferon (IFN) Class of Cytokines and the IFN Regulatory Factor (IRF) Transcription Factor Family. Cold Spring Harb Perspect Biol 10:. https://doi.org/10.1101/cshperspect.a028423.

Negishi H, Yanai H, Nakajima A, et al. (2012) Cross-interference of RLR and TLR signaling pathways modulates antibacterial T cell responses. *Nat. Immunol.* 13:659–666. https://doi.org/10.1038/ni.2307.

Nelms K, Keegan A D, Zamorano J, et al. (1999) The IL-4 receptor: signaling mechanisms and biologic functions. *Annu. Rev. Immunol.* 17:701–738. https://doi.org/10.1146/annurev.immunol.17.1.701.

Parameswaran N, Patial S (2010) Tumor necrosis factor-α signaling in macrophages. *Crit. Rev. Eukaryot. Gene. Expr.* 20:87–103. https://doi.org/10.1615/critreveukargeneexpr.v20.i2.10.

Poulsen L K, Hummelshoj L (2007) Triggers of IgE class switching and allergy development. *Ann. Med.* 39:440–456. https://doi.org/10.1080/07853890701449354.

Saeed S, Revell P A (2001) Production and distribution of interleukin 15 and its receptors (IL-15Ralpha and IL-R2beta) in the implant interface tissues obtained during revision of failed total joint replacement. *Int. J. Exp. Pathol.* 82:201–209. https://doi.org/10.1046/j.1365-2613.2001.iep0082-0201-x.

Sen G C, Williams B R G (2019) Lnc(ing) interferon production and action. *Cell Res.* 29:690–691. https://doi.org/10.1038/s41422-019-0207-y.

Skov L, Beurskens F J, Zachariae C O C, et al. (2008) IL-8 as Antibody Therapeutic Target in Inflammatory Diseases: Reduction of Clinical Activity in Palmoplantar Pustulosis. *J. Immunol.* 181:669 LP – 679. https://doi.org/10.4049/jimmunol.181.1.669.

Taylor A W (2009) Review of the activation of TGF-beta in immunity. *J. Leukoc. Biol.* 85:29–33. https://doi.org/10.1189/jlb.0708415.

Temann U A, Geba G P, Rankin J A, Flavell R A (1998) Expression of interleukin 9 in the lungs of transgenic mice causes airway inflammation, mast cell hyperplasia, and bronchial hyperresponsiveness. *J. Exp. Med.* 188:1307–1320. https://doi.org/10.1084/jem.188.7.1307.

Testa U, Riccioni R, Militi S, et al. (2002) Elevated expression of IL-3Ralpha in acute myelogenous leukemia is associated with enhanced blast proliferation, increased cellularity, and poor prognosis. *Blood* 100:2980–2988. https://doi.org/10.1182/blood-2002-03-0852.

Tone M, Powell M J, Tone Y, et al. (2000) IL-10 gene expression is controlled by the transcription factors Sp1 and Sp3. *J. Immunol.* 165:286–291. https://doi.org/10.4049/jimmunol.165.1.286.

Trinchieri G (2003) Interleukin-12 and the regulation of innate resistance and adaptive immunity. *Nat. Rev. Immunol.* 3:133–146. https://doi.org/10.1038/nri1001.

Veldhoen M, Uyttenhove C, van Snick J, et al. (2008) Transforming growth factor-beta "reprograms" the differentiation of T helper 2 cells and promotes an interleukin 9-producing subset. *Nat. Immunol.* 9:1341–1346. https://doi.org/10.1038/ni.1659.

Vinader V, Afarinkia K (2012) A beginner's guide to chemokines. *Future Med. Chem.* 4:845–852. https://doi.org/10.4155/fmc.12.49.

Wajant H, Pfizenmaier K, Scheurich P (2003) Tumor necrosis factor signaling. *Cell Death Differ.* 10:45–65. https://doi.org/10.1038/sj.cdd.4401189.

Wakefield P E, James W D, Samlaska C P, Meltzer M S (1990) Colony-stimulating factors. *J. Am. Acad. Dermatol.* 23:903–912. https://doi.org/10.1016/0190-9622(90)70313-7.

Wang X, Lin Y (2008) Tumor necrosis factor and cancer, buddies or foes? *Acta Pharmacol. Sin.* 29:1275–1288. https://doi.org/10.1111/j.1745-7254.2008.00889.x.

Wang Y, Fan KT, Li J-M, Waller E K (2012) The regulation and activity of interleukin-12. *Front Biosci.* (Schol Ed) 4:888–899. https://doi.org/10.2741/s306.

Wynn T A (2003) IL-13 effector functions. *Annu. Rev. Immunol.* 21:425–456. https://doi.org/10.1146/annurev.immunol.21.120601.141142.

Zhang H, Chen K, Tan Q, et al. (2021) Structural basis for chemokine recognition and receptor activation of chemokine receptor CCR5. *Nat. Commun.* 12:4151. https://doi.org/10.1038/s41467-021-24438-5.

Zhu J (2015) T helper 2 (Th2) cell differentiation, type 2 innate lymphoid cell (ILC2) development and regulation of interleukin-4 (IL-4) and IL-13 production. *Cytokine* 75:14–24. https://doi.org/10.1016/j.cyto.2015.05.010.

Chapter 4

Cytokines and Immune Regulation

Mehmet Akif Kaya*, **MD and Dilara Fatma Kocacik Uygun, MD**
Akdeniz University School of Medicine, Department of Pediatric Allergy and Immunology, Antalya, Turkey

Abstract

Cytokines are mediators consisting of different proteins that allow communication between cells. Cytokines act as positive or negative regulators in many phases of the immune response. Their activity depends on the density of other cytokines in the same micro-environment together with receptor expression on the surface of target cells. Cytokines play a critical role in regulating the type and size of immune response developed in response to internal and external stimuli.

Keywords: cytokines, immune regulation, cellular immunity, humoral immunity, antigen presentation

Introduction

Cytokines are mediators consisting of different proteins that allow communication between cells. Although they were first described as products of immune system cells and tasked with regulating the immune response, it is now known that many cytokines are produced by cells other than the immune system and used in cellular communication.

Cytokines, which act as regulators in every phase of the immune response, specify both the severity and the cytotoxic, humoral, cell-mediated, or allergic nature of this response.

In this section, cytokines that participate in immune regulation are grouped as the system-induced mononuclear phagocytic origin or T-lymphocyte origin, predominantly cytotoxic, humoral, cell-mediated, or allergic immunity, and immunosuppressive cytokines.

* Corresponding Author's Email: akifkaya@gmail.com.

In: Cytokines and Diseases
Editors: Kenan Demir, Selim Görgün and Bahar Uslu
ISBN: 979-8-88697-214-6

Antigen Presentation by Cytokines

Cytokines, which are mainly released by mononuclear phagocytic cells and other antigen-presenting cells (APCs), cause exacerbation of inflammation by stimulating cellular infiltration. The recognition, processing, and presentation of antigens by APCs to T-helper lymphocytes are carried out entirely through cytokines.

In addition, stereotypical components of pathogens stimulate natural immunity by increasing cytokine production with pattern recognition receptors on monocytes. These receptors help the immune system's ability to distinguish pathogenic proteins from non-pathogenic proteins. Cytokines produced by monocytes consist of tumor necrosis factor (TNF) and interleukin (IL) molecules known as IL-1, IL-6, IL-8, IL-12, IL-15, IL-18, and IL-23 (Kotsias et al., 2019).

Tumor Necrosis Factor (TNF)

TNF symbolizes two homologous proteins derived essentially from mononuclear phagocytes (TNF-a) and lymphocytes (TNF-β) (Beutler and Cerami 1989).

The active form of both cytokines is a homotrimer. Besides mononuclear phagocytes, TNF-a can also be produced by neutrophils, activated lymphocytes, natural killer (NK) cells, endothelial cells, and mast cells. The strongest stimulant of TNF production is the stimulation of monocytes by lipopolysaccharides through Toll-like receptor 2 (TLR2) and Toll-like receptor 4 (TLR4). The Toll-like receptor family stands for a large group of pattern recognition receptors that recognize the parts of pathogenic cells that are not present in mammalian cells, activating a natural immune response by releasing cytokines from mononuclear phagocytic cells (Vanamee and Faustman 2018).

TNF-a is a membrane-bound protein produced from resolvable active factors with TNF-a converting enzymes. TNF-β (at the same time known as lymphotoxin-a) is synthesized as a secretory protein that combines with LT-β, the third member of the same family, to form heterotrimers and bind to the cell surface. TNF-a and TNF-β are connected to two different receptors – TNFR I (p55) and TNFR II (p75) – with similar affinities, showing similar effects, if not identical ones (Tartaglia and Goeddel 1992).

TNFs induce anti-tumor immunity by stimulating the anti-tumoral functions of the immune system and by a direct cytotoxic effect on malignant cells. TNF interacts with endothelial cells to stimulate molecules known as intracellular adhesion molecule (ICAM)-1, vascular cell adhesion molecule (VCAM)-1, and E-selectin. Thereby, granulocytes are directed to the inflammation zone. TNF is a powerful neutrophil activator that mediates adhesion, chemotaxis, degranulation, and respirator explosion. The clinical use of TNF in the treatment of malignancy has lost its popularity in the past due to serious side effects. TNF is responsible for severe cachexia that develops after chronic infections and malignation. Furthermore, TNF increases vascular permeability, leading to a decrease in intravascular volume; it is the major endogenous mediator of toxic shock and sepsis (Jung et al., 2019).

IL-1

The IL-1 family consists of four different peptides. These are IL-1a, IL-1β, IL-1 receptor antagonist [IL-1ra] and IL-18 (Dinarello and Wolff 1993). IL-1a and IL-1β have similar biological activities. IL-1a, IL-1β, and IL-1ra are connected with affinities similar to two different IL-1 receptors. Type I receptors are responsible for the proinflammatory response that identifies with IL-1 (Mantovani et al., 2019).

The functions of type II receptors expressed in B cells, neutrophils, and bone marrow cells are in the opposite direction of type I receptors. The "capture" and sequestration of IL-1 by these inactive type II receptors lead to an anti-inflammatory response (Arend 1993).

Although IL-1 is mainly produced by mononuclear phagocytic cells, it can also be produced by many different cells such as endothelium, osteoblasts, synovial cells, neutrophils, glial cells, and keratinocytes. IL-1 production can be stimulated by microorganisms, bacterial endotoxins, antigens, and other cytokines.

IL-1a, IL-1β, and IL-18, members of the same family, are synthesized as a precursor form with weak activity. The conversion of these procytokines to the active form depends on their division by a specific enzyme called IL-1 converting enzyme (ICE) or caspase 1 (Cerretti et al., 1992).

The inflammatory activity of IL-1 depends on the activation of T lymphocytes by increasing IL-2 production and expression of IL-2 receptors. In the lack or absence of IL-1, a decrease in the inflammatory response or a condition of tolerance is observed. IL-1 also increases B-lymphocyte proliferation, leading to immunoglobulin synthesis. Fever, somnolence, lethargy, and anorexia that occur during the inflammatory response are linked to the interaction of IL1 in the central nervous system. When the cerebrospinal fluids of patients undergoing febrile convulsion were examined, a significant increase was shown in IL-1 levels and HMGB-1 levels secreted in response to IL-1 (Kaya et al., 2021). It also stimulates the synthesis of acute phase reactants such as amyloid, complement, and C-reactive peptide as a result of IL-1-hepatocyte interaction. IL-1 also stimulates the adherence of leukocytes to the endothelium by increasing the production of IL-1, ICAM-1, VCAM-1, and E-selectin. Although TNF and IL-1 activities have similar results, the fact that TNF has no direct effect on lymphocyte proliferation is their main difference.

IL1ra production is stimulated by many cytokines, including IL-4, IL-6, IL-13, and transforming growth factor-β (TGF-β). It is thought that the damage caused by the proinflammatory effects of IL-1 is curbed by IL1ra activity (Mantovani et al., 2019).

IL-6

The most important source of IL-6 is mononuclear phagocytic cells. Besides mononuclear phagocytic cells, it can also be produced by T and B lymphocytes, fibroblasts, endothelial cells, keratinocytes, hepatocytes, and bone marrow. B lymphocytes stimulated by IL-6 differentiate into mature plasma cells by producing immunoglobulin. IL-6 also mediates the activation and differentiation of T lymphocytes (Rose-John 2018).

In addition to lymphocyte activation, IL-6 is involved in the co-regulation of activities such as a secondary fever response to inflammation and the production of acute-phase proteins together with IL-1. IL-6 is considered to be the most important stimulant for the production of acute-phase proteins in hepatocytes. In addition to all these proinflammatory effects, IL-6 also has various anti-inflammatory effects. While IL-1 and TNF induce the synthesis of each other and also IL-6, IL-6 finishes this inflammatory cascade by inhibiting IL-1 and TNF synthesis. Moreover, IL-6 reinforces its anti-inflammatory effect by stimulating IL-1ra synthesis (Akira et al., 1993).

IL-12, 18, and 23

IL-12 is mainly released from monocytes and macrophages, as well as from B cells, dendritic cells, Langerhans cells, neutrophils, and mast cells (Tait Wojno et al., 2019). Its biologically active molecular form consists of two heterodimer units in the form of p40 and p35. The p40 subunit is homologous to the IL-6 soluble receptor, while the p35 subunit is homologous to IL-6. IL-12 induces proliferation, cytotoxic function, and cytokine production of natural killer cells. IL-12 also stimulates the proliferation of T-helper and cytotoxic T lymphocytes (Brunda 1994).

The main production place of IL-18 is the liver. In addition to the liver, it can be produced by the lung, pancreas, kidney, and skeletal system, but it is not secreted by lymphocytes, neutrophils, or NK cells (Dinarello 2000).

IL-18 activation requires a specific converting enzyme (ICE or caspase-1) similar to IL-1. Unlike other inflammatory cytokines, IL-18 is constitutively expressed regardless of need. However, its activity is regulated by the function of the transformative enzyme. Although IL-18 is structurally similar to IL-1, its biological activity is similar to IL-12 rather than IL-1. IL-12 and IL-18 stimulate the release of interferon-γ (IFN-γ) synergistically. IL-18 has an important role in cellular adhesion with ICAM-1 expression. IL-18 has been connected to its distinctive heterodimer IL-18R receptor. The expression of this receptor is also stimulated by IL-12 (Novick et al., 2001).

IL-23 is a recently discovered cytokine homologous to the p35 subunit of IL-12 that is secreted by active dendritic cells. Similar to IL-12 and IL-18, it strongly stimulates IFN-γ emissions. It is also estimated that it stimulates lymphocyte differentiation towards TH1 (Moschen et al., 2019).

IL-15

IL-15 has similar immune-regulatory activities to IL-2. Both cytokine receptors are β and the γ chain is commonly used, whereas IL-15 is distinguished from IL-2 by the use of the α chain in the receptor signal complex. Although these two cytokines have similar functions in terms of activity, they differ in their production locations. Active T lymphocytes, the most important source of IL-2, do not express IL-15; mononuclear phagocytic cells, epithelial cells, fibroblasts, and placenta are the main sources of IL-15. IL-15 is also a chemotactic and growth factor for T cells. IL-15 is involved in the growth and differentiation of B cells, as well as in the differentiation of NK cells (Zhang et al., 2021).

Cytotoxic Immunity

The immune response to virus-infected cells and neoplastic cells is firstly mediated by CD8+ cytotoxic T lymphocytes and NK cells. The main cytokines that activate this cytotoxic immunity are IL-2, IL-4, IL-5, IL-6, IL-7, IL-10, IL-11, IL-12, IL-15, TNF-α, TNF-β and interferons (Taniuchi 2018).

Interferons (IFN)

The IFN family consists of three members: IFN-α, IFN-β, and IFN-γ.

IFN-α is released from monocytes, macrophages, B lymphocytes, and NK cells. It has important roles in antiviral immunity with its ability to protect virus-infected cells from infection, suppress viral replication in infected cells, and stimulate antiviral immunity by cytotoxic T lymphocytes and NK cells. IFN-α also has effects such as upward regulation of class I MHC molecules and stimulation of antitumor activity. The effects of IFN-β and IFN-α are similar (Lazear et al., 2019).

IFN-γ is mainly produced by T lymphocytes and NK cells, and partly by macrophages. IFN- γ also has a moderate antiviral immunological effect. Their role in cellular and allergic immunity will be discussed in the next section.

IL-11

IL-11 acts as a stimulant in the bone marrow along with lymphocytes, erythrocytes, platelets, and other growth factors in the production of mast cells through hematopoietic stem cells. IL-11 also increases the production of acute-phase proteins and stimulates lymphoid cell differentiation. IL-11 is also an important stimulating factor for connective tissue cells such as fibroblasts. Studies are reporting that this function may have a role in bronchial remodeling seen in asthma (Zheng et al., 2001).

Humoral Immunity

IL-7 and IL-11, which act as lymphoid stem cell growth factors in the bone marrow, contribute to the maturation of B lymphocytes. IL-7, which is produced in the thymus stromal tissue together with the bone marrow, interacts with lymphoid precursors and plays a critical role in the development of B and T lymphocytes. Furthermore, IL-7 stimulates the proliferation of CD8+ T lymphocytes with NK cells and the disruptive effect of macrophages on tumor cells.

The isotype change of B lymphocytes after they are produced in the bone marrow, the transformation of mature B cells by activation into immunoglobulin secreting B cells, and their differentiation into plasma cells are under the control of T lymphocytes (Finkelman et al., 1990).

The cytokines that regulate the isotype change of B lymphocytes can be summarized as IL-4 and IL-13 for IgE isotype, TGF-β for IgA, and IL-10 for IgG4 production. Other cytokines involved in the regulation of humoral immunity by acting on the B cell are IL-1, IL-2, IL-5, IL-6, IL-12, IL-15, IL-21, and IFN-γ (Cyster and Allen 2019).

Cellular Immunity

IL-2

IL-2 secretion from T cells is induced as a result of the interaction of B7 molecules (B7-1: CD80 or B7-2: CD86), an integral membrane protein found in antigen-presenting cells, with CD28 on T cells. Simultaneously with IL-2 release, an increase in IL-2R expression is also observed. IL-1 and IL-6 cytokines are also involved in the formation of these responses. The binding of secreted IL-2 to T lymphocytes containing IL-2R induces clonal T-lymphocyte proliferation. Simultaneous expression of IL-2R along with IL-2 production is required for T-cell proliferation. This requirement enables T cells to participate in the specific immune response by activating them in an antigen-specific way. In addition to the T-cell growth factor role of IL-2, it is known to play a role in the activation of NK cells, B cells, cytotoxic T cells, and macrophages (Ross and Cantrell 2018).

IL-21

IL-21 is a newly identified cytokine with a similar structure to IL-2 and IL-15, usually produced by activated T cells. IL-21 receptors are expressed on activated B and T lymphocytes, and NK cells. Many functions such as activating NK cells and proliferation of B and T cells have been defined (Parrish-Novak et al., 2000).

Interferon Gamma

The basic cytokine of cellular immunity is IFN-γ. It is mainly produced by CD4+ T lymphocytes but it can also secrete CD8+ T cells and NK cells. IFN-γ increases MHC class I and II molecule expression. IFN-γ stimulates monocytes' antigen presentation and cytokine production. It also stimulates endothelial adhesion and phagocytosis. As a result of these activities, macrophages are collected in the inflammatory region, and their ability to kill intracellular pathogens increases (Farrar and Schreiber 1993). In addition to their effects on mononuclear phagocytes, IFN-γ also stimulates the cytotoxic activity of NK cells and neutrophils. Together with IL-1 and TNF, it stimulates the adhesion of granulocytes to endothelial cells as a result of the induction of ICAM-1. IFN-γ inhibits viral replication in a similar way to other interferons. In addition, the allergic immune response created through IL-4 is blocked by IFN-y (Lazear et al., 2019).

IL-16 and IL-17

Additional cytokines secreted by CD4+ T lymphocytes and contributing to cellular immunity are TNF-β, IL-16, and IL-17. IL-16 is a cytokine that is chemotactic for helper T lymphocytes, eosinophils, and monocytes, and uses the CD4 molecule as a receptor. Its production is regulated by TNF-α, TGF-β, IL-4, IL-9, IL-13, and histamine (Cruikshank et al., 1994).

IL-17 is a cytokine usually secreted by CD4+CD45RO+ memory T lymphocytes and eosinophils activated by T lymphocytes. IL-17, IL-6, IL-8, IL-11, and granulocyte-colony stimulating factor [G-CSF] activate macrophages, fibroblasts, and stromal cells by stimulating the secretion of prostaglandin E2 and nitric oxide along with many cytokines. It is known that this activation also plays a role in asthma remodeling (Amatya et al., 2017).

Anti-Inflammatory Cytokines

In addition to cytokines that stimulate a humoral, cellular and cytotoxic immune response, many cytokines such as TGF-β and the IL-10 family, as well as the previously mentioned IL-1ra, have predominantly anti-inflammatory effects.

TGF-β

TGF-β represents a large family of peptides that regulate cell growth, having both stimulating and suppressing effects on different cell types. Essentially, it is known to be produced by osteocytes, chondrocytes, platelets, fibroblasts, monocytes, and some T cells. It has been suggested that TGF-β, which produced helper T lymphocytes, represents a different phenotype called T repressor (Tr1) or T helper type 3 (TH3) cells (Sporn and Roberts 1992).

TGF-β is synthesized as an inactive precursor protein. It requires proteolytic division for its activation. TGF-β is an important fibrosis stimulator, involved in wound healing and scar formation. It also inhibits B lymphocytes, and CD4 and CD8 T lymphocytes in the immune system. B lymphocytes inhibit the secretion of immunoglobulin, which is the main function, and cytotoxic functions of phagocytes and NK cells. TGF-β produced by apoptotic T cells creates an immunosuppressive environment during apoptosis, preventing the development of inflammation and autoimmunity after apoptosis. TGF-β can also reduce allergic inflammation by inhibiting IgE synthesis and mast cell proliferation (Chen et al., 2001). In contrast to these anti-inflammatory effects, TGF-β is an important chemotactic for macrophages (Sonoda et al., 1989).

Family of IL-10

IL-10 can be produced by many cells, including TH1 and TH2 lymphocytes, CD8+ T lymphocytes, B lymphocytes, mast cells, and mononuclear phagocytic cells. IL-10 shows immunosuppressive effects by suppressing IFN-γ and TNF-α production by NK cells, IL-2 and IFN-γ by T helper 1 lymphocytes, IL-4 and IL-5 by T helper 2 lymphocytes, and TNF-α, IL-1β, IL-6, IL-8 and IL-12 by mononuclear phagocytes (Saraiva et al., 2020).

In addition to these, IL-10 inhibits the expression of MHC class II molecules, CD23, ICAM-1, and B7. Inhibition of B7 expression results in the deterioration of the relationship between antigen-presenting cells and CD4+ T lymphocytes. This inhibition of antigen presentation to helper T cells results in the inhibition of cytokine production of TH1 and TH2 cells. In allergic airway diseases such as asthma and allergic rhinitis, reduced IL-10 expression in airways has been shown to contribute to the development of the inflammatory environment by causing a decrease in tolerance to allergens and bioaerosols (Borish et al., 1996).

Besides, it takes part in the prevention of allergic diseases by inhibiting IL-10 eosinophil survival and IgE synthesis stimulated by IL-4. Unlike the inhibition of allergic inflammation of IL-10, it is known to act as an activating factor that stimulates cell proliferation and Ig secretion on B lymphocytes. IL-10 also acts as a growth co-factor for CD8+ T lymphocytes. In summary, IL-10 has a stimulating effect on the humoral and cytotoxic immune response and an inhibitory effect on the cellular and allergic immune response.

IL-19, a member of the IL-10 family, in the expression of monocytes is induced by lipopolysaccharide (LPS) and GM-CSF. IL-20, another member of the IL-10 family, identified in recent years, is expressed by keratinocytes (Gallagher et al., 2000).

IL-22, another new member of the IL-10 family, is released from T lymphocytes and mast cells. IL-22 expression is induced by IL-9 and LPS and stimulates the acute phase response. IL-24, the last member of the IL-10 family, is released as a result of inducing type 2 T helper cells with murine and IL-4 (Keir et al., 2020).

T-Helper Lymphocytes (TH)

T-helper lymphocytes (TH) are divided into 4 different subgroups according to their cytokine repertoire (Mosmann and Coffman 1989). Naive T lymphocytes (TH0) mainly produce IL-2 but have the potential to synthesize the characteristic cytokines of TH1 and TH2 lymphocytes. The cytokines identified with type 1 helper lymphocytes are interferon-γ and TNF-β, and these cells cannot produce IL-4 and IL-5. Unlike TH1, TH2 lymphocytes can also produce IL-4, IL-5, IL-9, and IL-25, but they cannot produce IFN-γ and TNF-β. Both groups of T-helper lymphocytes (TH1 and TH2) can produce GM-CSF, TNF-α, IL-2, IL-3, IL-10, and IL-13. TH1 lymphocytes activate other T lymphocytes and monocytes, taking part in both cellular and humoral immune responses. The production of IL-4, IL-5, and IL-13 by TH2 lymphocytes and the relative absence of IFN-γ, dominate the allergic immune response. TH3 lymphocytes produce TGF-β and IL-10, which are known for their immunosuppressive functions. This function of TH3 lymphocytes may be important in limiting and terminating the immune response (Zhu 2018).

One of the critical factors in determining the differentiation of T-helper lymphocytes in the direction of TH1/TH2 is the cytokine environment in which the T lymphocyte is activated. Cytokine IL-4 is the main determinant of differentiation in the direction of TH2 lymphocytes. This differentiation forms the main point in the pathogenesis of allergic diseases. The differentiation of T-helper lymphocytes towards TH1 lymphocytes is mediated by IL-12, IL-18, and IL-23 in the medium (Seder et al., 1992; Zhu 2018).

Allergen Immune Response and Cytokines

The cytokine profile differentiated in the direction of TH2 is evident in skin biopsies taken from the bronchial walls of asthma patients, nasal mucosa in allergic rhinitis, and positive epidermal prick test areas. Although TH1 cytokines are reduced proportionally in allergic inflammatory tissue, IFN-y can be detected. Cytokine secretion is stimulated as a result of the IFN-y stimulating helper T-cell function, and the expression of adhesion molecules increases and activates eosinophils, exacerbating allergic inflammation (Randolph et al., 1999).

The cytokine response of the immune system after contact with the allergen in individuals without atopic sensitization is even more complex. Healthy individuals living in the same environment with allergic individuals are exposed to allergens at similar concentrations. The absence of an inflammatory response to allergens is also ensured by the active participation of cytokines. It is known that this tolerance to allergens in non-allergic individuals depends on the differentiation of the immune system towards TH1 lymphocytes. However, the traditional TH1 lymphocyte response requires the onset of the inflammatory process by stimulating the production of proinflammatory cytokines and mononuclear phagocytes. Non-atopic individuals have control mechanisms that also curb this system. When non-allergic individuals and allergic patients were compared, a decrease in allergen-induced T-cell proliferation and a significant decrease in allergen-specific IgG antibody responses were shown in the first group (Platts-Mills et al., 2001). A contribution to this tolerance is decreased accessory cell function. When comparing the healthy lung and asthmatic lung, in the healthy lung, its expression on alveolar macrophages and dendritic cells is decreased. This reduction in the antigen-presenting system limits allergen presentation to T-helper lymphocytes, thereby limiting cellular activation and proliferation. When the airway cytokine levels of healthy individuals without known allergies are examined, it is known that concentrations of IL-10 and TGF-β, which are known to relieve the inflammatory response, have increased (von Bubnoff et al., 2001).

Conclusion

Cytokines are involved in the positive or negative regulation of cellular activities in almost every phase of the immune response and inflammation. Cytokines produced in response to immune damage determine both the severity and nature of the response to this damage. The deficiency, excess, or dysfunction of cytokines involved in immune regulation leads to clinical insufficiencies such as immunodeficiency, hypersensitivity and atopy.

References

Akira S, Taga T, Kishimoto T (1993) Interleukin-6 in biology and medicine. *Advances in immunology* 54:1–78. https://doi.org/10.1016/s0065-2776(08)60532-5.

Amatya N, Garg A v., Gaffen SL (2017) IL-17 Signaling: The Yin and the Yang. *Trends in Immunology* 38:310–322. https://doi.org/10.1016/j.it.2017.01.006.

Arend W P (1993) Interleukin-1 receptor antagonist. *Advances in immunology* 54:167–227. https://doi.org/10.1016/s0065-2776(08)60535-0.

Beutler B, Cerami A (1989) The biology of cachectin/TNF--a primary mediator of the host response. *Annual review of immunology* 7:625–55. https://doi.org/10.1146/annurev.iy.07.040189.003205.

Borish L, Aarons A, Rumbyrt J, et al., (1996) Interleukin-10 regulation in normal subjects and patients with asthma. *The Journal of allergy and clinical immunology* 97:1288–96. https://doi.org/10.1016/s0091-6749(96)70197-5.

Brunda M J (1994) Interleukin-12. *Journal of leukocyte biology* 55:280–8. https://doi.org/10.1002/jlb.55.2.280.

Cerretti D P, Kozlosky C J, Mosley B, et al., (1992) Molecular cloning of the interleukin-1 beta converting enzyme. *Science (New York, NY)* 256:97–100. https://doi.org/10.1126/science.1373520.

Chen W, Frank M E, Jin W, Wahl S M (2001) TGF-beta released by apoptotic T cells contributes to an immunosuppressive milieu. *Immunity* 14:715–25. https://doi.org/10.1016/s1074-7613(01)00147-9.

Cruikshank W W, Center D M, Nisar N, et al., (1994) Molecular and functional analysis of a lymphocyte chemoattractant factor: association of biologic function with CD4 expression. *Proceedings of the National Academy of Sciences of the United States of Americ*a 91:5109–13. https://doi.org/10.1073/pnas.91.11.5109.

Cyster J G, Allen C D C (2019) B Cell Responses: Cell Interaction Dynamics and Decisions. *Cell* 177:524–540. https://doi.org/10.1016/j.cell.2019.03.016.

Dinarello C A (2000) Interleukin-18, a proinflammatory cytokine. *European cytokine network* 11:483–6.

Dinarello C A, Wolff SM (1993) The role of interleukin-1 in disease. *The New England journal of medicine* 328:106–13. https://doi.org/10.1056/NEJM199301143280207.

Farrar M A, Schreiber R D (1993) The molecular cell biology of interferon-gamma and its receptor. *Annual review of immunology* 11:571–611. https://doi.org/10.1146/annurev.iy.11.040193.003035.

Finkelman F D, Holmes J, Katona I M, et al. (1990) Lymphokine control of in vivo immunoglobulin isotype selection. *Annual review of immunology* 8:303–33. https://doi.org/10.1146/annurev.iy.08.040190.001511.

Gallagher G, Dickensheets H, Eskdale J, et al., (2000) Cloning, expression and initial characterization of interleukin-19 (IL-19), a novel homologue of human interleukin-10 (IL-10). *Genes and immunity* 1:442–50. https://doi.org/10.1038/sj.gene.6363714.

Jung M K, Lee J S, Kwak J E, Shin E-C (2019) Tumor Necrosis Factor and Regulatory T Cells. *Yonsei Medical Journal* 60:126. https://doi.org/10.3349/ymj.2019.60.2.126.

Kaya M A, Erin N, Bozkurt O, et al. (2021) Changes of HMGB-1 and sTLR4 levels in cerebrospinal fluid of patients with febrile seizures. *Epilepsy Research* 169:106516. https://doi.org/10.1016/ j.eplepsyres.2020.106516.

Keir M E, Yi T, Lu T T, Ghilardi N (2020) The role of IL-22 in intestinal health and disease. *Journal of Experimental Medicine* 217(3): e20192195. https://doi.org/10.1084/jem.20192195.

Kotsias F, Cebrian I, Alloatti A (2019) Antigen processing and presentation. *International Review of Cell and Molecular Biology* 348:69–121.

Lazear H M, Schoggins J W, Diamond M S (2019) Shared and Distinct Functions of Type I and Type III Interferons. *Immunity* 50:907–923. https://doi.org/10.1016/j.immuni.2019.03.025.

Mantovani A, Dinarello C A, Molgora M, Garlanda C (2019) Interleukin-1 and Related Cytokines in the Regulation of Inflammation and Immunity. *Immunity* 50:778–795. https://doi.org/10.1016/ .immuni.2019.03.012.

Moschen A R, Tilg H, Raine T (2019) IL-12, IL-23 and IL-17 in IBD: immunobiology and therapeutic targeting. *Nature Reviews Gastroenterology & Hepatology* 16:185–196. https://doi.org/10.1038/s41575-018-0084-8.

Mosmann T R, Coffman R L (1989) TH1 and TH2 cells: different patterns of lymphokine secretion lead to different functional properties. *Annual review of immunology* 7:145–73. https://doi.org/10.1146/annurev.iy.07.040189.001045.

Novick D, Schwartsburd B, Pinkus R, et al., (2001) A novel IL-18BP ELISA shows elevated serum IL-18BP in sepsis and extensive decrease of free IL-18. *Cytokine* 14:334–42. https://doi.org/10.1006/cyto.2001.0914.

Parrish-Novak J, Dillon S R, Nelson A, et al. (2000) Interleukin 21 and its receptor are involved in NK cell expansion and regulation of lymphocyte function. *Nature* 408:57–63. https://doi.org/10.1038/35040504.

Platts-Mills T, Vaughan J, Squillace S, et al., (2001) Sensitisation, asthma, and a modified Th2 response in children exposed to cat allergen: a population-based cross-sectional study. *Lancet* (London, England) 357:752–756. https://doi.org/10.1016/S0140-6736(00)04168-4.

Randolph D A, Carruthers C J, Szabo S J, et al., (1999) Modulation of airway inflammation by passive transfer of allergen-specific Th1 and Th2 cells in a mouse model of asthma. *Journal of immunology* (Baltimore, Md : 1950) 162:2375–2383.

Rose-John S (2018) Interleukin-6 Family Cytokines. *Cold Spring Harbor Perspectives in Biology* 10:a028415. https://doi.org/10.1101/cshperspect.a028415.

Ross S H, Cantrell D A (2018) Signaling and Function of Interleukin-2 in T Lymphocytes. *Annual Review of Immunology* 36:411–433. https://doi.org/10.1146/annurev-immunol-042617-053352.

Saraiva M, Vieira P, O'Garra A (2020) Biology and therapeutic potential of interleukin-10. *Journal of Experimental Medicine* 217(1):e20190418. https://doi.org/10.1084/jem.20190418.

Seder RA, Paul WE, Davis MM, Fazekas de St Groth B (1992) The presence of interleukin 4 during in vitro priming determines the lymphokine-producing potential of CD4+ T cells from T cell receptor transgenic mice. *The Journal of experimental medicine* 176:1091–1098. https://doi.org/10.1084/jem.176.4.1091.

Sonoda E, Matsumoto R, Hitoshi Y, et al. (1989) Transforming growth factor beta induces IgA production and acts additively with interleukin 5 for IgA production. *The Journal of experimental medicine* 170:1415–20. https://doi.org/10.1084/jem.170.4.1415.

Sporn MB, Roberts AB (1992) Transforming growth factor-beta: recent progress and new challenges. *The Journal of cell biology* 119:1017–21. https://doi.org/10.1083/jcb.119.5.1017.

Tait Wojno E D, Hunter C A, Stumhofer JS (2019) The Immunobiology of the Interleukin-12 Family: *Room for Discovery. Immunity* 50:851–870. https://doi.org/10.1016/j.immuni.2019.03.011.

Taniuchi I (2018) CD4 Helper and CD8 Cytotoxic T Cell Differentiation. *Annual Review of Immunology* 36:579–601. https://doi.org/10.1146/annurev-immunol-042617-053411.

Tartaglia L A, Goeddel D V (1992) Two TNF receptors. *Immunology today* 13:151–3. https://doi.org/10.1016/0167-5699(92)90116-O.

Vanamee É S, Faustman D L (2018) Structural principles of tumor necrosis factor superfamily signaling. *Science Signaling* 11(511):eaao4910. https://doi.org/10.1126/scisignal.aao4910.

von Bubnoff D, Geiger E, Bieber T (2001) Antigen-presenting cells in allergy. *The Journal of allergy and clinical immunology* 108:329–39. https://doi.org/10.1067/mai.2001.117457.

Zhang S, Zhao J, Bai X, et al., (2021) Biological effects of IL-15 on immune cells and its potential for the treatment of cancer. *International Immunopharmacology* 91:107318. https://doi.org/10.1016/ j.intimp. 2020.107318.

Zheng T, Zhu Z, Wang J, et al., (2001) IL-11: Insights in asthma from overexpression transgenic modeling. *Journal of Allergy and Clinical Immunology* 108:489–496. https://doi.org/10.1067/mai.2001.118510.

Zhu J (2018) T Helper Cell Differentiation, Heterogeneity, and Plasticity. *Cold Spring Harbor Perspectives in Biology* 10:a030338. https://doi.org/10.1101/cshperspect.a030338.

Chapter 5

Cytokines and Genetics

Sevgi Durna Daştan[1], PhD and İnanç Baral[2,*], PhD
[1]Department of Biology, Faculty of Science, Sivas Cumhuriyet University, Sivas, Turkey
[2]Department of Biometrics and Genetics, Faculty of Veterinary Medicine, Sivas Cumhuriyet University, Sivas, Turkey

Abstract

Cytokines are called by different names, and can be indicated as interleukin, lymphokine, chemokine, interferon, and colony-stimulating factor. With a diverse array of functions, cytokines can act as either proinflammatory or anti-inflammatory elements, as well as function as growth factors and transcription factors on cells and tissues. There is limited knowledge of cytokine to cell interactions, and how cytokine signaling takes part in pathways for transcription and post-transcriptional processing. Molecular events that are next to cytokines may contain information to develop novel approaches to disease treatments. This chapter will review the genetics of noteworthy cytokines with regard to their expression, and regulation in both transcription and post-transcription levels. Also, epigenetics will be emphasized in contexts of chromosome accessing, DNA methylation, and histone acetylation. As the precise knowledge about cytokines increases, further research can be conducted in regard to effectively including such mechanisms in novel treatment approaches.

Keywords: cytokines, genetics, gene expression, cytokine mediators

Introduction

Cytokines as secreted proteins are known to be critical in both the regulation and control of wide ranges of immune responses such as the regulation of T-cell differentiation. Such regulations are actually depending on the intricate molecular interactions between cytokines and others (Huang and August 2015; Schmitt and Ueno 2015). Cytokine functioning requires coupling with cytokine receptors that are classified by their 3D structures, which initiates intracellular signal transduction to affect genes through their

* Corresponding Author's Email: inancbaral@gmail.com.

In: Cytokines and Diseases
Editors: Kenan Demir, Selim Görgün and Bahar Uslu
ISBN: 979-8-88697-214-6

functions as transcription factors to control cellular events (Parker and Papenfuss 2018). TNF, IL-6, and IL-1b, which are proinflammatory cytokines, are responsible for creating an effective inflammation response in cases of infections and tissue-level injuries. So far, strategies to block or inhibit these cytokines have proved to be effective in treatment approaches in autoimmune disorders (Kovalenko and Wallach 2016). IL-6 is a member of a 4-helix cytokine group that binds to IL-6 receptors located on membranes, which leads to the attachment of another membrane protein, i.e., glycoprotein-130 (gp130), to trigger intracellular JAK/STAT and Ras-Raf-MAPK signal pathways. The stated gp130 is a signal protein element of the gp130 cytokine family (Chalaris et al. 2016). Type I IFNs are known to be critical cytokines in cases of both antiviral and immunomodulatory responses, which include 13 subtypes of IFNa, a subtype of IFNb along with IFNε, IFNκ, and IFNɣ in humans. The activity of type I IFNs is dependent on the binding into a heterodimeric cell surface receptor composed of IFNaR1 and IFNaR2 units (Landolfo and De Andrea 2016). The IL-12/IL-23 cytokine family includes structurally homologous heterodimeric cytokines of IL-23, IL-12, IL-35, and IL-27 and when these cytokines bind into heterodimeric receptors, they enable different signaling and transcriptional activation pathways. Having different shared subunits both in cytokines and receptors is indicating significant plasticity in the IL-12/IL-23 cytokine group. Stimulation of TLRs enables antigen-presenting cells, namely, monocytes, dendritic cells, and macrophages to produce IL-12, IL-23, and IL-27. Different regulatory T- and B-cell (Treg and Breg, respectively) subsets produce IL-35. IL-12/IL-23 cytokine family members have their roles in the differentiation of different T-helper cell lines, which include Th-1, Th-17, Th-2, and Treg lines. The pathogenesis of a diverse set of autoimmune disorders contains IL-12 and IL-23, and targeting them with monoclonal antibodies revealed promising results. Members of this cytokine family can either act in a tumor milieu or directly on cancerous cells to regulate tumor growth profiles. Overall, the research on this family of cytokines advances the current understanding of immune functions regarding the immunoregulation, autoimmunity, and immunity against tumors (Pistoia 2016). The IL-17 family of cytokines is critically important in contexts of inflammation response, autoimmunity, and host defensive responses through their powerful proinflammatory traits. Over the years, significant results have been obtained in regard to IL-17 production patterns and their roles in diseases (Lai and Dong 2016). IL-10 is primarily noteworthy as a non-redundant critical cytokine to alleviate both acute and chronic inflammatory responses, which is striking in that IL-10 is necessary to maintain tolerance against host microbiota and in tight regulation of the infection. The IL-20 cytokine subfamily comes into play with their shared traits in structure, associated receptors, targets, and bioactivities (Rutz et al. 2014; Rutz and Ouyang 2016). Aside from the namesake IL-10 itself, distant relatives of IL-28A-B, and IL-29 make up the IL-10 family, and coupled with their IFNs, they constitute the type II cytokines. When evaluated, it is striking that mutations generally fall on the coding genes of cytokines and their shared receptors, along with other molecules that have parts in the same signaling pathway such as co-stimulant proteins. The great many autoimmune disorders are implied to be the end results of either excessive or suppressive expression profiles of certain cytokine genes, namely, TNFs, IL-2-2R-3-7-10-23R, IFNs, and TGFs among others (Murphy and Weaver 2017).

The Genetics of IL-1 and IL-1R Family Cytokines

To date it has been identified that there are seven agonists, three receptor antagonists, and one anti-inflammatory element in the IL-1 family of cytokines. The agonists are IL-36a-b-g, IL-1a/1b, IL-33, and IL-18; the receptor antagonists are IL-1Ra, IL-36Ra, and IL-38; and IL-37 is the anti-inflammatory cytokine. IL-1a and IL-33 are considered as alarmins, which alarm the system in cases of tissue injury. There are 11 members in the IL-1R family, which are IL-1R1, IL-1R2, IL-1R3, IL-1R4, IL-1R5, IL-1R6, IL-1R7, IL-1R8, IL-1R9, and IL-1R10 (Garlanda et al. 2013). Receptors share a motif that includes an extracellular chain of three Ig-like domains and an intracellular TIR domain, which is critical for MyD88 adaptor signaling and is shared among TLRs. When the stated TIR domain is excited with bacterial invasion or tissue damage, a conserved signaling pathway is activated to relocate NF-κB into the nucleus to activate MAPKs, which include p38, JNKs, and ERKs (Barton and Medzhitov 2003), that would lead to an enhancing of the innate immune response to intensify inflammation. Recent indications point to four signal receptor complexes, which are IL-1R, IL-18R, IL-33R, and the most recent IL-37R.

Genes of IL-1A and IL-1B are adjacent to each other located on the q arm of Chr2, and both are expressed as precursors without signal sequences that are 271 and 269 residues long, respectively, requiring post-processing. The IL-1A precursor directs itself to the nucleus to make complicated interactions with regulators, TFs, and the chromatin, making IL-1A one of the duality-of-function cytokines that can bind into both surface and DNA receptors, just like IL-33 and IL-37. However, in the case of physiological apoptotic signaling, IL-1A becomes unable to initiate an inflammatory response as it becomes bound to chromatin, but if a necrotic signal occurs, then chromatin-bound IL-1A relocates to the cytosol to initiate a neutrophil-mediated inflammatory response (Cohen et al. 2010; Rider et al. 2011; Garlanda and Jaillon 2016).

As a vital cytokine for type II immune and inflammatory responses, IL-33 is a sizable protein reaching 30 kDA, which includes a chromatin-binding N-terminal domain and a big, 18 kDA C-terminal region. Different cell lines, namely, stromal, parenchymal, and hematopoietic cells, express IL-33 either as essential or in response to induction. Also, IL-33 is critically stored in the nuclei of different cell lines, which include endothelia, epithelia, and keratinocytes that possibly release the cytokine in response to necrosis-inducing injury, making them similar to alarmins to develop a sterile inflammation response like the IL-1A. Aside from its 30 kDa full form, IL-33 can be processed by cleavers like calpain, serine proteases of neutrophils, cathepsin G, and elastase to provide more powerful and alternative forms (Lefrancais et al. 2012). Even though the pathway of action is not yet known, IL-33 can also bind into chromatin to become transcriptional suppressor.

On the other hand, the IL-18 precursor, which is a 24 kDa protein, is fundamentally expressed in monocytes/macrophages, endothelia, and epithelia, and evaluations revealed close structural associations both in protein and gene morphology between IL-18 and IL-37. Again, IL-37 requires IL-18A as its receptor, further suggesting association. IL-18 constitutes a signal complex with both IL-18RA and IL-18RB (co-receptor) to recruit myD88, IRAKs, and TRAF-6 to initiate NF-κB relocation to the nucleus.

There are four known members of the IL-36 family, which are IL-36a-b-g, and a receptor antagonist (IL-36Ra) with their genes clustered tightly in Chr2 where the genes for IL-1 and IL-1Ra are also present. These members are requiring the N-terminal sequence curtailing in the

A-X-Asp motif that is the present IL-1 family for activation, which leads to elevated bio-functioning on their part (Towne et al. 2011).

There are five known spliced variant forms of IL-37, with the variant called IL-37b being the best known among them, that is stimulated by the actions of IL-1b or TLRs, and possibly by the anti-inflammatory cytokine TGF-b (Nold et al. 2010). While IL-37 was not identified in the mouse genome, it was discovered that human IL-37 is functional in mice. Aside from its natural release in the case of cellular death, IL-37 is also presently chromatin-bound, possibly as a transcriptional suppressor, which is like IL-1a and IL-33. IL-37 serves to inhibit inflammatory responses caused by LPS or IL-1, and binds to IL-18RA; however, it uses IL-1R8 for inhibitory signaling (Nold et al. 2010, Nold-Petry et al. 2015).

The gene encoding IL-38 is found to be close to the genes of IL-1Ra and IL-36Ra, and has the same significant sequence as them with a most striking structural similarity to IL-1Ra. As of yet, it is known that dermal basal epithelia and tonsillar proliferative B cells are producing IL-38 with a 152-residue-long precursor, and with no cleavage site for caspase-1 action, as well as no signal sequence.

The Genetics of Tumor Necrosis Family (TNF) Cytokines

Ligands are associated with the TNFs identified by investigating mechanisms of activated leukocytes in the cases of tissue response against bacterial toxins and necrosis. TNF-associated bio-signaling is the end result of the enhancement of acting members in the pathways, generally conveying ligands. The TNF family is prominent in the development of immunity, and therefore, depends on the stimulation of other intricate connections between the immune elements that lead to either innate or adaptive immune responses. The primary mode of action provided by the TNF family is their triggering function on MAPK pathways, which leads to NF-κB activation and gene expression activation both in transcription and post-transcription levels. Their activation requires TRAF ubiquitin-ligase activation and IAP (inhibitor of apoptosis) ubiquitin-ligases, which in turn can be repressed by the deubiquitination mechanisms of various enzyme or proteins (Wertz and Dixit 2010; Walczak 2011). The functioning of TNFs by activating TFs of NF-κB is dual in nature as it has both immune regulation and developmental initiation effects, the latter of which was indicated by EDA (Lefebvre and Mikkola 2014). Currently, two differing signaling pathways are known for NF-κB activation, which are called the canonical and alternative pathways, respectively. In the former, RelA:p50 NF-κB dimers are activated, and require IKK-2 (IkB kinase-2) and the NEMO adaptor, which in the end leads to an innate inflammatory response. In the latter, RelB:p52 NF-κB dimers are activated, and require IKK-1 and NIK (NF-κB-inducing kinase), which in the end leads to the regulation of adaptive immunity by initiating both T- and B-cell development (Hayden and Ghosh 2004; Wallach and Kovalenko 2016).

The Genetics of IL-6 Family Cytokines

Cytokines are unique in their grouping in that, unlike other protein families that are grouped according to their primary structure homologies, they are grouped according to their characteristic 4-helix structural motif homology, which includes the pattern of the up-up-down-down sequence (Bazan 1989; 1990; Chalaris et al. 2016). This family contains IL-6, IL-11, CLC, CT-1, CNTF (ciliary neurotrophic factor), OSM, and LIF (leukemia-inhibiting factor) (Garbers et al. 2012; Heinrich et al. 2003). IL-6 is a typical cytokine that exhibits pleiotropy, and is essential in host immunity. Immune, hematologic, and acute-phase responses are all activated by IL-6 in the cases of infections or tissue injury, which trigger on-the-spot production of IL-6 by monocyte/macrophages (Tanaka et al. 2016). In response to a wide array of different stimulants, other cell lines can also produce IL-6, namely, mesenchymal cells, endothelia, fibroblasts, and even cancerous cells (Tanaka et al. 2016). IL-6 gene expression has multi-layered tight regulation involving various levels such as chromatin remodeling, transcription, transcript-exporting, prost-transcriptional modification, and translation. IL-6 transcription is also reported to be altered by a G/C SNP in -174 of flanking regions of the gene. IL-6 is also prone to epigenetic control by histone modifications and DNA methylations, which shows itself in the cellular differentiation process by the evident chromatin-remodeling (Tanaka et al. 2016).

IL-27 is a complex heterodimeric composition that involves EBI3, p28/IL-30, and a regular 4-helix pattern, and functions through the gp130/WSX-1 heterodimer (Pflanz et al. 2004), which includes it in the IL-6 family (Garbers et al. 2012). Nevertheless, IL-27 can be considered as a member of the IL-12 family, which includes heterodimeric IL-12, IL-23, and IL-35 (Garbers et al. 2012; Jones et al. 2012). IL-35, which is also known as EBI3/p35 complex, functions through using four different b-receptor complexes, which are IL-12Rb2/IL-12Rb2, IL-12Rb2/gp130, gp130/gp130, and IL-12Rb2/WSX-1 (Collison et al. 2012; Wang et al. 2014), and this implies a bridging effect as seen in the IL-6-12-27 families (Garbers et al. 2012). There are studies indicating allotypical variants of the IL-6R gene, and one of them is a coding SNP (rs2228145) observed in exon 9 (Asp358Ala), which when homozygous leads to the double expression of sIL-6R and suppressed CRP levels, resulting in decreased susceptibility to coronary disorders and myocardiac infarctions (Hingorani and Casas 2012). The stated coding SNP is in the cleavage site of ADAM17 that was mapped in the IL-6R stalk region of Gln357-Asp358 (Garbers et al. 2014). Additionally, sgp130 as an alternative splicing product can bind into the IL-6/sIL-6R complex, and function as a transitive signal transducer for IL-6 inhibition (Tanaka et al. 2000; Chalaris et al. 2016).

The Genetics of Interferons (IFNs)

IFNs are cytokines first described as natural antiviral substances, and grouped into 3 principal classes of type I, II, and III interferons (IFNI, IFNII, IFNIII, respectively), which are then divided into type I as IFNI1 (IL-29), IFNI2 (IL-28A), INFI3 (IL-28B), and INFI4 as the last (Donnelly and Kotenko 2010; Prokunina-Olsson et al. 2013). The distinction of IFNs is based on various parameters that include gene locations, amino acid sequences, associated receptors, stimulants, producers, and bio-activities. Encoding genes of IFNIs are observed as clusters in the p21 region of Chr9 of humans (and, of syntenic Chr4 of mice), and observed as intronless genes (Ivashkiv and Donlin 2014). The family of human IFNI contains 13 IFNa, a IFNb, a IFNε, a IFNκ, and IFNɣ. There is a 75 to 100% amino acid sequence similarity between IFNa subtypes; this reduces to 30% in IFNb, and further reduces to 15 to 30% in others with IFNa being the reference. Numerous (>100) different IRGs (IFN-regulated genes) are being regulated in two ways (enhancement or suppressing) by IFN binding and signal induction. IRGs are mainly responsible for the antiviral phenotype of cells, which is initiated by IFNs and may include cellular protection, proliferative inhibition, or modulation of immune responses (Schneider et al. 2014). The microarray method enabled the observing of the modified gene expression profiles of >2000 genes following IFN induction, which revealed the tightly regulated manner of IFN responses that implies specificity in involved genes and their mutually exclusive activation patterns. This outcome further supports the notion of predicting the precise response through finely tracking the nature, duration, context, and activation/deactivation profiles of pathways (Landolfo and De Andrea 2016). The gene responsible for IFN is designated in q12 of Chr15 in humans (Chr10 in mice) with 4 exons and 3 introns that are evolutionarily conserved across the species (Naylor et al. 1983; 1984; Bae et al. 2016). Notably among IFNs, IFN-ɣ is solely capable of modulating more than 2300 gene expressions in humans (Fenimore and Young 2016). The aforementioned IFN gene provides a ~1.2 kbp long transcript that would translate into a 166 residue long polypeptide, which is then truncated by 23 residues in the terminal to provide a 143 residue long mature and monomeric IFNg protein that is 17 kDa in weight (Derynck et al. 1982; 1983). Between the human and mouse products, the measured sequence similarities are 60-65% for mRNA, and 40% for the polypeptide, which supports the lesser co-sensitivity to the associated receptor between species (Gray and Goeddel 1983).

There is an identified unique SNP (T to A) in the IFNg locus at the þ874 (þ874 A/T) position in the initial intron of the human gene that correlates with the translation start site, which changes the translation product and is associated with certain clinical conditions (Bae et al. 2016). A tightly complicated regulatory system controls the IFN-ɣ gene expression, which is normally expressed by elements of the innate immunity, particularly from NK and NKT cells. The expression of IFN-ɣ is also evident in adaptive elements that include CD4+ Th-1 cells and CD8+ cytotoxic T-effector cells (CD4+ and CD8+ cells, respectively). Multiple levels of tight control are present for IFN-ɣ production, which include epigenetic regulation, chromosomal re-organization, membrane signaling, various TFs, mRNA integrity checks, and long non-coding RNA (LncRNA) interferences (Fenimore and Young 2016). In certain cell types, particular genomic regions become important regulatory domains for INF-ɣ expression, e.g., human genome 92-18 bp prior to TSS (transcription start site) is critical for only T cells and NKT cells, but not for the NK cells (Fenimore and Young 2016).

The Genetics of IL-12 and IL-23 Cytokines

Back in the year 1989, IL-12 was first discovered as an NK-stimulatory factor (Pistoia 2016), but it is now known that it is the p70 heterodimer formed by p40 and p35 with covalent disulfide bonding. Similarly, the formation of IL-12R is achieved by the heterodimerization of IL12Rb1 and IL-12Rb2, which is simultaneously required for potent binding sites to IL-12 (Pistoia 2016). Encoding genes for p35 (IL-12a) and p40 (IL-12b) are disparate from each other by being in different genomic regions. In humans, the locations for these genes are in 3p12-q13.2 for p35, and 5q31-33 for p40. These locations changes to Chr6 and Chr11, respectively in the mouse genome, and there is no sequence homology between the species (Noben-Trauth et al. 1996; Schweitzer et al. 1996; Zheng et al. 2016). The end product of p35 is 209 residues long and a 27.5 kDa heavy polypeptide that has a 7-cysteine residue sequence and 3 possible N-glycosylation cores, whereas the p40 end product is 328 residues long and 34.7 kDa in weight that has a 22 residue long signal sequence. The end products of p35 and p40 bind by forming disulfide bonds and are released through secretion by the producers. To have an activated IL-12, the same cell must simultaneously express p35 and p40 genes, and in this regard p40 is defining as it is limited to cells that should produce activated IL-12 (Zheng et al. 2016).

Research is pointing to the associations between autoimmune disorders and variations in the IL-12/IL-23 genes, and recent GWA (Genome-wide Association) studies accumulated large sets of data that require fine filtering to associate with particular diseases. A proposal for this regard was recently presented (van Wanrooij et al. 2012), in which the researchers revealed two SNP clusters of IL-12 linked to autoimmune disorders, which are the Th-1/Th-17 cluster and the Th-1/IL-35 cluster. They also revealed a third cluster of SNPs that is not part of either of the previous clusters. The former cluster typically indicates the ability of IL-23 to stabilize and promote pathogenic Th-17 cells (van Wanrooij et al. 2012). Both IL-12 and IL-23 share p40 as a common subunit, but IL-23 has its own specific subunit designated as p19, which has the common 4-helix motif and a ~15% sequence similarity to p35. The functioning of IL-23 requires a complex formed between IL-12Rβ1 and IL-23R, but IL-23R is mostly limited to specialized T cells and ILCs (Welsby and Goriely 2016). Here in the signaling, it is required that both TyK2 and JAK2 have activated and phosphorylated the STAT3. Specific p19 is the natural target of miRNA-107 from intestinal DCs and macrophages, but the presence of the microbiota effectively hinders its expression in favor of IL-23. In humans, the NOD2 signal pathway of DCs induces miRNA-29 expression that targets p40 directly, but also targets p19 in relative terms (Welsby and Goriely 2016).

The second identified cluster, Th-1/IL-35 is reported to have SNPs associated with certain diseases, which all include the IL-12A gene, but, the dominance of IL-12A without an IL-12B presence is indicating a dysregulation in IL-35 (van Wanrooij et al. 2012; Pistoia 2016). While the observed disease-associated SNPs are mostly located in non-coding regions, they may have indirect transcriptional regulation effects through enhancing, miRNA targeting, etc., to achieve reduced or increased expression profiles, which would lead to either resistance or susceptibility to assorted disorders.

IL-27 as a member of the IL-12 family has a unique subunit designated as p28, and a shared subunit of EBI3 with the IL-12 p35 subunit. IL-27 is mainly produced by monocytes/macrophages, and DCs, but, other cell lines can produce lesser amounts, which include the plasma cells, microglias, NK cells, endothelia, and placental trophoblasts. The production is triggered by different TLR agonists, which include LPS, poly(I:C), CpG, and both Gram-negative and Gram-positive bacteria (Liu et al. 2007). LPS specifically induces p28 expression through the MyD88/NF-κB pathway. In this regard, another note is that IFN-ɣ from both T cells and NK cells can activate IRGs (IFN-ɣ regulatory factors), which include IRF1-3-7-8, that can increase IL-27 expression both alone and coupled with LPS. Again, IRF8 directly binds to the p28 promoter region to stimulate p28 expression.

The Genetics of IL-17 Cytokines

The research on the IL-17 family revealed substantial advances in the field of immunology by furthering the current understanding of immune pathways and their clinical associations, notably through the discovery of the Th-17 cell line, which abolished the established Th-1 and Th-2 system. As of yet, 6 cytokines and 5 receptors are known. The known cytokines are IL-17A to F, and the known receptors are IL-17RA to E (Li et al. 2000; Starnes et al. 2002; Lee et al. 2001; Kawaguchi et al. 2001; Moseley et al. 2003). Accumulated knowledge implies that the IL-17 family has significant roles in diverse processes, which include stress responses, host immunity, and the pathogenesis of autoimmune, inflammatory, and cancerous diseases (Happel et al. 2003; Ferretti et al. 2003; Yang et al. 2014; Zhang et al. 2006). Back in 1993, IL-17A, the first of the IL-17 family, was cloned from rodent T cells, and designated as CTLA8 (Rouvier et al. 1993). Subsequent analyses in humans revealed a 63% amino acid sequence homology with rodent CTLA8, and a 72% homology with viral IL-17. CTLA8 was mapped to Chr1A and is 147 residues long (Rouvier et al. 1993), and human IL-17A was mapped to p12 of Chr6 and is 155 residues long (Moseley et al. 2003). The encoding gene of IL-17B is located in q32-24 of Chr5 in humans, and its expression is observable in various cells, namely, the pancreas and small intestines (Li et al. 2000). The encoding gene of IL-17C is located in q24 of Chr16 in humans, and its expression is observable mainly in the testes, prostate, thymus, colon, spleen, and skin (Liet al. 2000; Song et al. 2011; 2013; Ramirez-Carrozzi et al. 2011; Dong and Ma 2016). IL-17F is a disulfide-bonded homodimer obtained from a leukocyte-anchored pool, and its gene location is mapped to p12 of Chr6 (Lai and Dong 2016). The IL-17E gene was mapped to q11 of Chr1 (Lai and Dong 2016). The encoding gene of IL-17D was obtained by RACE-PCR and mapped to p11 of Chr13 (Starnes et al. 2002), all in humans.

The Genetics of IL-10 Cytokines

IL-10 was designated first as a suppressor of Th-1 cells and then as a Th-2 cell-associated cytokine (Moore et al. 2012; Murray 2016); however, further research revealed its ability to suppress active myeloid cells, and therefore, to produce cytokines/chemokines, and to regulate antigen presentation (Murray 2016). Studies revealed both direct and indirect relationships between certain disease phenotypes and more than a hundred different variants in both IL-10 and its pathway (Huttenhower et al. 2014; Jostins et al. 2012; Parkes et al. 2013). With the advent of IL-10 blocking the inflammatory cytokine/chemokine production, two differing postulations were proposed, which are the total blockade and the gene-specific blockade of the inflammatory response, respectively. Again, it was not clear whether IL-10 functions at transcription, or at post-transcription levels as in the case of certain chemokines (Murray 2016). This paradigm was solved in 2002 by microarray analyses, which revealed the IL-10 function through the gene-specific blockade mechanism, leaving TLR-induced and MyD88-dependent genes intact (Ramirez-Carrozzi et al. 2009). Further research revealed certain associations between IL-10 and mRNA stability, e.g., IL-10 enhancement of TTP (tristetraprolin, encoded by zfp36) expression in the STAT3 pathway (Murray 2016). Since TTP is one of the significant destabilizers for mRNA, and produced by active macrophages, it functions at distinct stages. When a high amount of transcript containing 30'UTR region is required, TTP is repressed by the p38 MAPK as long as the requirement stays (Kratochvill et al. 2011; Schaljo et al. 2009). DUSP1 from TLRs is synergistically involved in this response together with IL-10, where DUSP1 inactivates the already activated p38 MAPK, which implies the negative regulatory function of IL-10 on inflammation-associated MAPKs (Murray 2016). Aside from the namesake IL-10, the family also includes close relatives of IL-19-20-22-24-26, and distant relatives of IL-28A-B, and IL-29 (Rutz and Ouyang 2016). IL-10 forms non-covalent homodimer structures by binding two receptors, IL-10R1 and IL-10R2. Here the IL-10R1 is a defining unique receptor that has high affinity for IL-10, but IL-10R2 is more or less shared by IL-22-26-28A-28B-29 (Rutz et al. 2014; Ouyang et al. 2011), and, therefore, IL-10R1 is more specific, limited mainly to leukocytes, which again implies that IL-10 is uniquely targeting leukocytes. Both human and mouse genomes exhibit high homology for the IL-10 gene, which in both is located on Chr1 as it clusters directly next to genes of IL-19-20-24 (Rutz and Ouyang 2016). All members of this cytokine family have 5 exons, and 4 introns in their genes, and they have significant sequence similarities in conserved non-coding sequences (CNS) between humans and mice, which stresses out the biological prominence of IL-10 regulation (Jones and Flavel 2005; Rutz and Ouyang 2016). These CNS sites of IL-10 also contain hypersensitive regions for DNaseI digestion (HSS), which indicates that the chromatin remodeling and modifications, particularly at lysine residues on histone tails, are important regulatory mechanisms for IL-10 expression.

The Genetics of IL-20 Cytokines

The IL-20 subfamily includes IL-22, IL-24, IL-20, IL-19, and IL-26 as cytokines, which are actually parts of the IL-10 family, yet share both structural homology and associated receptors. Despite the severely limited sequence homology between members of class II receptors, e.g., a 22% sequence similarity between IL-10 and IL-22, they share a striking homology in genomic organization and structure (Rutz and Ouyang 2016; Renauld 2003). In evolutionary terms, gene duplication results in these receptors coming from a common ancestor, and this evolution probably occurred before vertebrate speciation, coinciding with the adaptive immunity. The genes of IL-19-20-24 share a genetic structure with IL-10 that has 5 exons, and 4 introns, which are mapped to q32 of Chr1 in humans. The genes of IL-22 and IL-26 are mapped to q15 of Chr12 in humans, adjacent to the IFN-g gene, but there are gene duplications for IL-22 in some strains of mice that are called IL-22b, but this is possibly transcriptionally inactive. On the other hand, mice lack the IL-26 gene, which is universally conserved across vertebrates. However, there are still gene remnants in the form of exons that are similar to those of humans in mice, which are, however, not composing a true gene. Structurally, IL-10 family members share the α-helix motif containing a 6-helix pattern (A to F) and connecting loop motifs. Further research revealed two structural subgrouping (Zdanov 2010), where the anti-parallel 6-helix motif in IL-19-20-22-24 defines the IL-20 subfamily with the resulting monomeric bundles (Rutz and Ouyang 2016).

The Genetics of IL-4 Cytokines

Type II cytokines and IL-4 have the capacity to function on non-immune elements of the body either via direct or indirect mechanisms, e.g., both IL-4 and IL-13 can directly affect lymphatic endothelia to suppress their proliferation and tube formation as seen in vitro, and to repress lymphangiogenesis as seen in vivo (Ho an Miaw 2016). Mechanisms of expression control of genes specific to Th-2 cells are investigated by using IL-4, and prior research revealed 5 different binding sites (P0, P1, P2, PRE-I/P4, and P5) in the IL-4 promoter for NFAT/AP-1, which together constitute the IL-4 promoter framework. The IL-4 promoter, which is ~400 bp long, has binding sites for both positive and negative TFs, which include C/EBP, NF-κB, and IRF4 as positive, and IRF1, and CIITA as negative factors. IL-4 expression from Th-2 cells is further stabilized by epigenetic regulations, but distinctions of these mechanisms are almost impossible because of the dependence on Th-2 differentiation. The encoding gene of IL-4 was located on Chr5 in humans, and on Chr11 in mice which is called the Th-2 locus, and the gene has 4 exons (Ho and Miaw 2016).

Cytokines and MicroRNAs

Cytokine expression can be regulated by miRNAs in a direct or indirect manner. Direct regulations contain the targeting of binding sequences by miRNAs, whereas indirect regulations contain ARE-BPs (adenine(uridine)-rich element binding proteins). Cytokines can also regulate miRNA expression as seen in proinflammatory cytokines (IL-1β, and TNF-α), where miRNA-146a, and -155 can be regulated. Notably, miRNA-146a expression exhibits a significant increase in various cells in response to the accumulation of proinflammatory cytokines. Supplying the cells with molecular mimics of miRNA-146a proved to be able to save cells from death, along with promotions in cellular proliferation, implying a curious relationship in chronic inflammation coupled with an extended survival of cells (Liu 2011). If cells start to undergo EMT (epithelial-mesenchymal transition) as a response to cytokine stimulation, TGF-β uses snail proteins to inhibit pri-miRNA-200c, which restores the inhibition of TF8 on the E-cadherin gene. This process is amplified by the actions of IL-1β and TNF-α, which enhance the expression of TGF-β receptor Type I (TBR-1) (Liu 2008). Again, EMT increases MMP production in cells that would lead to E-cadherin cleavage, which is stimulated by TGF-β1, IL-1β, and TNF-α (Liu 2011). Three principal ways are proposed for miRNA association with the pathogenesis: (1) blockade and/or inhibition of miRNA transcription; (2) excessive expression of miRNAs; and (3) either mutations or epigenetic modification in the 3'UTR (seed) of miRNAs. Since certain miRNAs are actually oncogenes, excessive expression of such miRNAs like miRNA-17-92 would result in unintended oncogenesis by shutting down the physiological apoptosis. Alterations of the seed region, however, would result in target overexpression, e.g., an SNP in the miRNA-146a seed region changes a pro-apoptotic function into an anti-apoptotic function (Jazdzewski et al. 2009). Similarly for HLA-G, an identified gene for asthma susceptibility, an SNP in the seed region would block the miRNA-148 binding, leading to increased susceptibility (Tan et al. 2007). The great majority of miRNAs are expressed in a wide array of different tissues, e.g., the lungs are the specific tissue for miRNA-195, and miRNA-200c, the skin is most prominent tissue for miRNA-203, and the heart is predominant for miRNA-1 (Liu 2011). Alterations in the expression profiles are implicated in the pathogenesis of a diverse array of diseases, but here we will focus on inflammatory associations and relations. Even though the miRBase miRNA database is growing day by day, there are a few registered miRNAs directly responsible in cytokine regulations, probably due to the general lack of 3'UTR binding sites in cytokines. The known cytokines that actually have a 3'UTR binding site for miRNAs are listed as IL-1A, IL-4, IL-7, IL-8, IL-10, IL-11, IL-12A, IL-12B, IL-13, IL-15, IL-16, IL-17A/D/F, IL-18, IL-22, IL-23A, IL-24, IL-25, IL-29, IL-33 and IL-34. Aside from direct binding, miRNAs control cytokine production through AREs, having an AUUUA pentamer, and a UUAUUAUU oktamer, that recruit ARE-Bps to either positively or negatively affect cytokine production (Anderson 2008), which are regulated by miRNAs such as TTP, AUF-1, and members of HUR. The majority of cytokines have ARE sites located in 3'UTR, which include IL-1A, IL-1B, IL-2, IL-3, IL-4, IL-5, IL-6, IL-7, IL-8, IL-10, IL-11, IL-12A, IL-12B, IL-17, IL-20 and IL-27, and there are more than 4000 genes in the ARE database that can be targeted for post-transcriptional modifications. There are also cytokines that can regulate miRNA expression as stimulators and promoters, as in the case of both IL-1β and TNF-α, which stimulate the expressions of miRNA-146a and miRNA-155 in many cell lines. Particularly, miRNA-146a is responsive to the development of an inflammatory response, and in turn takes part in the regulation of immune responses, chronicity of the inflammation, and cellular proliferation and/or differentiation.

Conclusion

Multiple layers exist for the regulation of cytokine expression profiles. Extracellular signals, TFs, posttranscriptional modifications, and epigenetics are all responsible for the intricate regulations. The arduous interactions network formed between cytokines (particularly by IL-1β and TNF-α) and miRNAs (particularly by miRNA-146a and miRNA-155) may reveal the precise mechanism involving the chronic inflammatory states seen in various diseases. The future perspectives should involve novel approaches in therapeutic strategies that include the specific miRNA targeting of specific cytokines especially for chronic inflammatory diseases and conditions.

References

Anderson P (2008) Post-transcriptional control of cytokine production. *Nat Immunol* 9(4):353-359.

Bae H, Barlow AT, Young H, Valencia JC (2016) Interferon g: An Overview of Its Functions in Health and Disease. In: Ratcliffe MJH, Hein W, Gordon JR, Guidos CJ, Rolink A (eds) *Encylopedia of Immunobiology*. Elsevier Ltd, p 494-500.

Barton GM, Medzhitov R (2003) Toll-like receptor signaling pathways. *Science* 300:1524-1525.

Bazan JF (1989) A novel family of growth factor receptors: a common binding domain in the growth hormone, prolactin, erythropoietin and IL-6 receptors, and the p75 IL-2 receptor beta-chain. *Biochem Biophys Res Commun* 164:788-795.

Bazan JF (1990) Haemopoietic receptors and helical cytokines. Immunol Today 11:350-354.

Chalaris A, Rose-John S, Garbers C (2016) The Biology of Interleukin-6, a Major Target in Anti-Inflammatory Therapies. In: Ratcliffe MJH, Hein W, Gordon JR, Guidos CJ, Rolink A (eds) *Encylopedia of Immunobiology*. Elsevier Ltd, p 476-484. ISBN: 978-0-12-374279-7.

Cohen I, Rider P, Carmi Y et al. (2010) Differential release of chromatin-bound IL-1alpha discriminates between necrotic and apoptotic cell death by the ability to induce sterile inflammation. *Proc Natl Acad Sci* USA 107:2574-2579.

Collison L, Delgoffe G, Guy C, Vignali K, Chaturvedi V, Fairweather D, Satoskar A, Garcia K, Hunter C, Drake C, Murray P, Vignali DA (2012) The composition and signaling of the IL-35 receptor are unconventional. *Nat Immunol* 13:290-299.

Derynck R, Leung DW, Gray PW, Goeddel DV (1982) Human interferon gamma is encoded by a single class of mRNA. *Nucleic Acids Res* 10(12):3605-3615.

Derynck R, Singh A, Goeddel DV (1983) Expression of the human interferon-gamma cDNA in yeast. *Nucleic Acids Res* 11(6):1819-1837.

Dong W, Ma X (2016) Regulation of Interleukin-17 Production. Pg: 139-166. In: Ma X, Cohen IR, Lajtha NSA, Lambris JD, Paoletti R (Eds) *Regulation of cytokine gene expression in immunity and diseases.* Volume: Advances in Experimental Medicine and Biology. Springer Press, p 139-166. ISBN 978-94-024-0921-5.

Donnelly RP, Kotenko SV (2010) Interferon-lambda: a new addition to an old family. *J Interferon Cytokine Res* 30:555-564.

Fenimore J, Young HA (2016) Regulation of IFN-γ Expression. Pg: 1-20. In: Ma X, Cohen IR, Lajtha NSA, Lambris JD, Paoletti R (eds) *Regulation of cytokine gene expression in immunity and diseases.* Volume: Advances in Experimental Medicine and Biology. Springer Press, p 1-20. ISBN 978-94-024-0921-5.

Ferretti S, Bonneau O, Dubois GR, Jones CE, Trifilieff A (2003) IL-17, produced by lymphocytes and neutrophils, is necessary for lipopolysaccharide-induced airway neutrophilia: IL-15 as a possible trigger. *J Immunol* 170:2106-2112.

Garbers C, Hermanns H, Schaper F, Müller-Newen G, Grötzinger J, Rose-John S, Scheller J (2012) Plasticity and cross-talk of Interleukin 6-type cytokines. *Cytokine Growth Factor Rev* 23:85-182.

Garbers C, Monhasery N, Aparicio-Siegmund S, Lokau J, Baran P, Nowell MA, Jones SA, Rose-John S, Scheller J (2014) The interleukin-6 receptor Asp358Ala single nucleotide polymorphism rs2228145 confers increased proteolytic conversion rates by ADAM proteases. *Biochim Biophys Acta* 1842:1485-1494.

Garlanda C, Jaillon S (2016) Cytokine and their receptors. In: Ratcliffe MJH, Hein W, Gordon JR, Guidos CJ, Rolink A (eds) *Encylopedia of Immunobiology,* Elsevier Ltd, p 438-446. ISBN: 978-0-12-374279-7.

Garlanda C, Dinarello CA, Mantovani A (2013) The interleukin-1 family: back to the future. *Immunity* 39: 1003-1018.

Gray PW, Goeddel DV (1983) Cloning and expression of murine immune interferon cDNA. *Proc Natl Acad Sci* USA 80(19):5842-5846.

Happel KI, Zheng M, Young E, Quinton LJ, Lockhart E, Ramsay AJ, Shellito JE, Schurr JR, Bagby GJ, Nelson S, Kolls JK (2003) Cutting edge: roles of Toll-like receptor 4 and IL-23 in IL-17 expression in response to Klebsiella pneumoniae infection. *J Immunol* 170:4432-4436.

Hayden MS, Ghosh S (2004) Signaling to NF-kappaB. *Genes Dev* 18: 2195-2224.

Heinrich P, Behrmann I, Haan S, Hermanns H, Müller-Newen G, Schaper F (2003) Principles of interleukin (IL)-6-type cytokine signalling and its regulation. *Biochem J* 374:1-20.

Hingorani AD, Casas JP (2012) The interleukin-6 receptor as a target for prevention of coronary heart disease: a mendelian randomisation analysis. *Lancet* 379:1214-1224.

Ho IC, Miaw SC (2016) Regulation of IL-4 Expression in Immunity and Diseases. In: Ma X, Cohen IR, Lajtha NSA, Lambris JD, Paoletti R (eds) *Regulation of cytokine gene expression in immunity and diseases,* Volume: Advances in Experimental Medicine and Biology. Springer Press. p 31-77. ISBN 978-94-024-0921-5.

Huang W, August A (2015) The signaling symphony: T cell receptor tunes cytokine-mediated T cell differentiation. *J Leukoc Biol* 97(3):477-485.

Huttenhower C, Kostic AD, Xavier RJ (2014) Inflammatory bowel disease as a model for translating the microbiome. *Immunity* 40:843-854.

Ivashkiv LB, Donlin LT (2014) Regulation of type I interferon responses. *Nat Rev Immunol* 14: 36-49.

Jazdzewski K, Murray EL et al. (2008) Common SNP in pre-miR-146a decreases mature miR expression and predisposes to papillary thyroid carcinoma. *Proc Natl Acad Sci* USA 105(20):7269-7274.

Jones EA, Flavell RA (2005) Distal enhancer elements transcribe intergenic RNA in the IL-10 family gene cluster. J Immunol 175 (11):7437-7446.

Jones L, Chaturvedi V, Uyttenhove C, Van Snick J, Vignali DA (2012) Distinct subunit pairing criteria within the heterodimeric IL-12 cytokine family. *Mol Immunol* 51:234-244..

Jostins L, Ripke S, Weersma RK, Duerr RH, McGovern DP, Hui KY, Lee JC, Schumm LP, Sharma Y, Anderson CA et al. (2012) Host-microbe interactions have shaped the genetic architecture of inflammatory bowel disease. *Nature* 491:119-124.

Kawaguchi M, Onuchic LF, Li XD, Essayan DM, Schroeder J, Xiao HQ, Liu MC, Krishnaswamy G, Germino G, Huang SK (2001) Identification of a novel cytokine, ML-1, and its expression in subjects with asthma. *J Immunol* 167:4430-4435.

Kratochvill F, Machacek C, Vogl C, Ebner F, Sedlyarov V, Gruber AR, Hartweger H, Vielnascher R, Karaghiosoff M, Rulicke T et al. (2011) Tristetraprolin-driven regulatory circuit controls quality and timing of mRNA decay in inflammation. *Mol Syst Biol* 7:560.

Lai Y, Dong C (2016) Interleukin-17 Family. In: Ratcliffe MJH, Hein W, Gordon JR, Guidos CJ, Rolink A (eds) *Encylopedia of Immunobiology*. Elsevier Ltd, p 534-543. ISBN: 978-0-12-374279-7.

Landolfo S, De Andrea M (2016) Interferon a/b. In: Ratcliffe MJH, Hein W, Gordon JR, Guidos CJ, Rolink A (eds) *Encylopedia of Immunobiology*. Elsevier Ltd, p 485-493. ISBN: 978-0-12-374279-7.

Lee J, Ho WH, Maruoka M, Corpuz RT, Baldwin DT, Foster JS, Goddard AD, Yansura DG, Vandlen RL, Wood WI, Gurney AL (2001) IL-17E, a novel proinflammatory ligand for the IL-17 receptor homolog IL-17Rh1. *J Biol Chem* 276:1660-1664.

Lefebvre S, Mikkola ML (2014) Ectodysplasin research–where to next? *Semin Immunol* 26:220-228.

Lefrancais E, Roga S, Gautier V et al. (2012) IL-33 is processed into mature bioactive forms by neutrophil elastase and cathepsin G. *Proc Natl Acad Sci* USA 109:1673-1678.

Li H, Chen J, Huang A, Stinson J, Heldens S, Foster J, Dowd P, Gurney AL, Wood WI (2000) Cloning and characterization of IL-17B and IL-17C, two new members of the IL-17 cytokine family. *Proc Natl Acad Sci* USA 97:773-778.

Liu J, Cao S, Herman LM, Ma X (2003) Differential regulation of interleukin (IL)-12 p35 and p40 gene expression and interferon (IFN)-gamma-primed IL-12 production by IFN regulatory factor 1. *J Exp Med* 198:1265-1276.

Liu J, Guan X, Ma X (2007) Regulation of IL-27 p28 gene expression in macrophages through MyD88- and interferon-gamma-mediated pathways. *J Exp Med* 204 (1):141-152.

Liu X (2011) MicroRNAs and Cytokines. In: Preedy VR and Hunter RJ (eds) *Cytokines, Modern Insights into Disease from Molecules to Man Series Science Publishers.* CRC Press, p 3-17. ISBN 13: 978-1-4398-7620-6.

Liu X (2008) Infl ammatory cytokines augments TGF-beta1-induced epithelial-mesenchymal transition in A549 cells by up-regulating TbetaR-I. Cell. Motil. *Cytoskeleton* 65(12):935-944.

Moore KW, Vieira P, Fiorentino DF, Trounstine ML, Khan TA, Mosmann TR (2012) Pillars article: homology of cytokine synthesis inhibitory factor (IL-10) to the Epstein-Barr virus gene BCRFI. *Science* 1990(248):1230-1234.

Moseley TA, Haudenschild DR, Rose L, Reddi AH (2003) Interleukin-17 family and IL-17 receptors. Cytokine Growth Factor Rev 14:155-174.

Murphy K, Weaver C (2017) Genomics-based approaches are providing new insight into the immunogenetic basis of autoimmunity. *Janeway's Immunobiology*. 9th edition. P 669-671. Garland Science. Taylor and Francis Group, New York. ISBN 978-0-8153-4505-3.

Murray P (2016) IL-10. In: Ratcliffe MJH, Hein W, Gordon JR, Guidos CJ, Rolink A (eds) *Encylopedia of Immunobiology*. Elsevier Ltd, p 544-553ISBN: 978-0-12-374279-7.

Naylor SL, Gray PW, Lalley PA (1984) Mouse immune interferon (IFN-gamma) gene is on chromosome 10. *Somat Cell Mol Genet* 10(5):531-534.

Naylor SL, Sakaguchi AY, Shows TB, Law ML, Goeddel DV, Gray PW (1983) Human immune interferon gene is located on chromosome 12. *J Exp Med* 157(3):1020-1027.

Noben-Trauth N, Schweitzer PA, Johnson KR, Wolf SF, Knowles BB, Shultz LD (1996) The interleukin- 12 beta subunit (p40) maps to mouse chromosome 11. *Mamm Genome* 7:392.

Nold MF, Nold-Petry CA, Zepp JA et al. (2010) IL-37 is a fundamental inhibitor of innate immunity. *Nat Immunol* 11:1014-1022.

Nold-Petry CA, Lo CY, Rudloff I et al. (2015) IL-37 requires the receptors IL-18Ralpha and IL-1R8 (SIGIRR) to carry out its multifaceted anti-inflammatory program upon innate signal transduction. *Nat Immunol* 16:354-365.

Ouyang W, Rutz S, Crellin NK, Valdez PA, Hymowitz SG (2011) Regulation and functions of the IL-10 family of cytokines in infl ammation and disease. *Annu Rev Immunol* 29(1):71-109.

Parker GA, Papenfuss TL (2017) Basic Immunobiology. In: Parker GA (ed) *Immunopathology in toxicology and drug development.* Humana Press, p 1-100. ISBN 978-3-319-47385-7.

Parkes M, Cortes A, van Heel DA, Brown MA (2013) Genetic insights into common pathways and complex relationships among immune-mediated diseases. *Nat Rev Genet* 14:661-673.

Pflanz S, Hibbert L, Mattson J, Rosales R, Vaisberg E, Bazan JF, Phillips JH, McClanahan TK, de Waal Malefyt R, Kastelein RA (2004) WSX-1 and glycoprotein 130 constitute a signal-transducing receptor for IL-27. *J Immunol* 172:2225-2231.

Pistoia V (2016) The IL-12/IL-23 Cytokine Family. Pg: 525-533. In: Ratcliffe MJH, Hein W, Gordon JR, Guidos CJ, Rolink A (eds) *Encylopedia of Immunobiology.* Elsevier Ltd, p 525-533. ISBN: 978-0-12-374279-7.

Prokunina-Olsson L, Muchmore B, Tang W et al. (2013) A variant upstream of IFNL3 (IL28B) creating a new interferon gene IFNL4 is associated with impaired clearance of hepatitis C virus. *Nat Genet* 45:164-171.

Ramirez-Carrozzi V, Sambandam A, Luis E, Lin Z, Jeet S, Lesch J, Hackney J, Kim J, Zhou M, Lai J, Modrusan Z, Sai T, Lee,W, Xu M, Caplazi P, Diehl L, de Voss J, Balazs M, Gonzalez JrL, Singh H, Ouyang W, Pappu R (2011) IL-17C regulates the innate immune function of epithelial cells in an autocrine manner. *Nat Immunol* 12:1159-1166.

Ramirez-Carrozzi VR, Braas D, Bhatt DM, Cheng CS, Hong C, Doty KR, Black JC, Hoffmann A, Carey M, Smale ST (2009) A unifying model for the selective regulation of inducible transcription by CpG islands and nucleosome remodeling. *Cell* 138:114-128.

Renauld JC (2003) Class II cytokine receptors and their ligands: key antiviral and inflammatory modulators. *Nat Rev Immunol* 3(8):667-676.

Rider P, Carmi Y, Guttman O et al. (2011) IL-1a and IL-1b recruit different myeloid cells and promote different stages of sterile inflammation. *J Immunol* 187:4835-4843.

Rouvier E, Luciani MF, Mattei MG, Denizot F, Golstein P (1993) CTLA-8, cloned from an activated T cell, bearing AU-rich messenger RNA instability sequences, and homologous to a herpesvirus saimiri gene. *J Immunol* 150:5445-5456.

Rutz S, Ouyang W (2016) Regulation of Interleukin-10 Expression. In: Ma X, Cohen IR, Lajtha NSA, Lambris JD, Paoletti R (Eds) *Regulation of cytokine gene expression in immunity and diseases.* Volume: Advances in Experimental Medicine and Biology. Springer Press, p 89-116. ISBN 978-94-024-0921-5.

Rutz S, Wang X, Ouyang W (2014) The IL-20 subfamily of cytokines- from host defence to tissue homeostasis. *Nat Rev Immunol* 14(12): 783-795.

Rutz S, Ouyang W (2016) The IL-20 Subfamily of Cytokines and Their Receptors. In: Ratcliffe MJH, Hein W, Gordon JR, Guidos CJ, Rolink A (eds) *Encylopedia of Immunobiology,* Elsevier Ltd, p 554-562. ISBN: 978-0-12-374279-7.

Schaljo B, Kratochvill F, Gratz N, Sadzak I, Sauer I, Hammer M, Vogl C, Strobl B, Muller M, Blackshear PJ et al. (2009) Tristetraprolin is required for full anti-inflammatory response of murine macrophages to IL-10. *J Immunol* 183:1197-1206.

Schmitt N, Ueno H (2015) Regulation of human helper T cell subset differentiation by cytokines. *Curr Opin Immunol* 34:130-136.

Schneider WM, Chevillotte MD, Rice CM (2014) Interferon-stimulated genes: a complex Web of host defenses. *Annu Rev Immunol* 32:513-545.

Schweitzer PA, Noben-Trauth N, Pelsue SC, Johnson KR, Wolf SF, Shultz LD (1996) Genetic mapping of the IL-12 alpha chain gene on mouse chromosome 3. *Mamm Genome* 7:394-395.

Song X, Qian Y (2013) IL-17 family cytokines mediated signaling in the pathogenesis of inflammatory diseases. *Cell Signal* 25:2335-2347.

Song X, Zhu S, Shi P, Liu Y, Shi Y, Levin SD, Qian Y (2011) IL-17RE is the functional receptor for IL-17C and mediates mucosal immunity to infection with intestinal pathogens. *Nat Immunol* 12:1151-1158.

Starnes T, Broxmeyer HE, Robertson MJ, Hromas R (2002) Cutting edge: IL-17D, a novel member of the IL-17 family, stimulates cytokine production and inhibits hemopoiesis. *J Immunol* 169:642-646.

Tanaka M, Kishimura M, Ozaki S, Osakada F, Hashimoto H, Okubo M, Murakami M, Nakao K (2000) Cloning of novel soluble gp130 and detection of its neutralizing autoantibodies in rheumatoid arthritis. *J Clin Invest* 106:137-144.

Tanaka T, Narazaki M, Masuda K (2016) Regulation of IL-6 in Immunity and Diseases. Pg: 78-100. In: Ma X, Cohen IR, Lajtha NSA, Lambris JD, Paoletti R (Eds) *Regulation of cytokine gene expression in immunity and diseases.* Volume: Advances in Experimental Medicine and Biology. Springer Press, p 78-100. ISBN 978-94-024-0921-5.

Tan Z, Randall G et al. (2007) Allele-specifi c targeting of microRNAs to HLA-G and risk of asthma. *Am J Hum Genet* 81(4):829-834.

Towne JE, Renshaw BR, Douangpanya J et al. (2011) Interleukin-36 (IL-36) ligands require processing for full agonist (IL-36alpha, IL-36beta, and IL-36gamma) or antagonist (IL-36Ra) activity. *J Biol Chem* 286:42594-42602.

Van Wanrooij RLJ, Zwiers A, Kraal G, Bourna GG (2012) Genetic variations in interleukin-12 related genes in immune-mediated diseases. *J Autoimm* 39:359-368.

Wallach D, Kovalenko A (2016) Roles of TNF and Other Members of the TNF Family in the Regulation of Innate Immunity. In: Ratcliffe MJH, Hein W, Gordon JR, Guidos CJ, Rolink A (eds) *Encylopedia of Immunobiology,* Elsevier Ltd, p 453-465. ISBN: 978-0-12-374279-7.

Walczak H (2011) TNF and ubiquitin at the crossroads of gene activation, cell death, inflammation, and cancer. *Immunol Rev* 244:9-28.

Wang RXX, Yu CRR, Dambuza IM, Mahdi RM, Dolinska M, Sergeey YV, Wingfield PT, Kim SHH, Egwuagu CE (2014) Interleukin-35 induces regulatory B cells that suppress autoimmune disease. *Nat Med* 20:633-641.

Wang Q, Liu J (2016) *Regulation and Immune Function of IL-27.* In: Ma X, Cohen IR, Lajtha NSA, Lambris JD, Paoletti R (eds) *Regulation of cytokine gene expression in immunity and diseases.* Volume: Advances in Experimental Medicine and Biology. Springer Press, p 190-211. ISBN 978-94-024-0921-5.

Welsby I, Goriely S (2016) Regulation of Interleukin-23 Expression in Health and Disease. In: Ma X, Cohen IR, Lajtha NSA, Lambris JD, Paoletti R (Eds) *Regulation of cytokine gene expression in immunity and diseases.* Volume: Advances in Experimental Medicine and Biology. Springer Press, p 167-189. ISBN 978-94-024-0921-5.

Wertz IE, Dixit VM (2010) *Signaling to NF-kappaB: regulation by ubiquitination.* Cold Spring Harb Perspect Biol 2:a003350.

Yang J, Sundrud MS, Skepner J, Yamagata T (2014) Targeting Th17 cells in autoimmune diseases. *Trends Pharmacol Sci* 35:493-500.

Zdanov A (2010) Structural analysis of cytokines comprising the IL-10 family. *Cytokine Growth Factor Rev* 21(5): 325-330.

Zhang Z, Zheng M, Bindas J, Schwarzenberger P, Kolls JK (2006) Critical role of IL-17 receptor signaling in acute TNBS-induced colitis. *Inflamm Bowel Dis* 12:382-388.

Zheng H, Ban Y, Wei F, Ma X (2016) Regulation of Interleukin-12 Production in Antigen-Presenting Cells. Pg: 117-138. In: Ma X, Cohen IR, Lajtha NSA, Lambris JD, Paoletti R (Eds) *Regulation of cytokine gene expression in immunity and diseases.* Volume: Advances in Experimental Medicine and Biology. Springer Press, p 117-138. ISBN 978-94-024-0921-5.

Chapter 6

Extreme Immune Response and Cytokine Storm

Metin Yadigaroğlu[1,*], MD and Nurçin Öğreten Yadigaroğlu[2], MD
[1]Samsun University Faculty of Medicine, Department of Emergency Medicine, Samsun, Turkey
[2]Karadeniz Technical University Faculty of Medicine, Department of Internal Medicine, Trabzon, Turkey

Abstract

The cytokine storm is a severe clinical pathology that occurs due to an extreme immune response and can cause mortality by multi-system involvement. As the name of the disease suggests, abnormally released cytokines play a role in the pathophysiology of the cytokine storm. Various criteria have been established to diagnose this disease, which can be included in the differential diagnosis with many clinical pathologies. Still, the biggest hurdle in managing the cytokine storm is delayed diagnosis. After diagnosis, appropriate treatment modalities were also established based on knowing the functions of the cytokines underlying the pathogenesis of the disease. Mortality rates, which were high in untreated cases, decreased significantly with appropriate treatments. In this section, the pathogenesis and clinic of the cytokine storm that occurs due to an abnormal immune response will be detailed.

Keywords: cytokine storm, pathogenesis, diagnosis, extreme immune response

Introduction

The extreme immune response is an immune pathology that results from the uncontrolled release of many and high levels of inflammatory mediators. In this immune pathology, cytokines play the leading role, and as a result, severe systemic inflammation, high ferritin in the blood, and hemodynamic instability occur. In untreated cases, progression to multi-organ failure and, as a result, death may be inevitable. This important clinic caused by cytokines is called the "cytokine storm." The term cytokine storm (CS) (also called hypercytokinemia or cytokine release syndrome) was first used for graft-versus-host (GVHD) disease in the early 1990s (Ferrara et al., 1993).

---

* Corresponding Author's Email: metin.yadigaroglu@samsun.edu.tr.

In: Cytokines and Diseases
Editors: Kenan Demir, Selim Görgün and Bahar Uslu
ISBN: 979-8-88697-214-6

Infectious and non-infectious conditions can cause an abnormally enhanced immune response, resulting in an unexpected cytokine release. Viral hemorrhagic fevers such as Ebola virus, hantavirus, pandemic pathogens such as smallpox, influenza, COVID-19, African trypanosomiasis, malignancies, rheumatic diseases, and congenital diseases or acquired immunodeficiencies, GVHD, and the use of some immunosuppressive drugs can be cited as examples that may cause hypercytokinemia (Zimmer et al., 1990; Clark 2007; Hu et al., 2021). The main factors causing the cytokine storm are the increase of proinflammatory cytokines such as interferon-gamma (IFN-y), tumor necrosis factor (TNF), and interleukins (IL-1, IL-6, IL-18), and the cells responsible for the release of these cytokines are macrophages, CD8+ T lymphocytes (cytotoxic T lymphocytes) and natural killer (NK) cells (Henter et al., 1991, Lachmann et al., 2011; Dinarello et al., 2013; Sieni et al., 2014; Avau et al., 2015; Brisse et al., 2015).

A prototype of the cytokine storm characterized by hyper inflammation is hemophagocytic lymphohistiocytosis (HLH). This disease is genetically based and autosomal recessive inherited, contains a monogenic mutation that prevents the function of NK cells and cytotoxic T lymphocytes, is either primary HLH or has no genetic basis, and causes immunological problems (such as malignancy, autoimmune disease, infection, drugs, etc.); this is classified as secondary HLH, which is due to two types. The autoimmunity-associated form of secondary HLH is also called macrophage activation syndrome (MAS). MAS is the picture of HLH that occurs in people with juvenile idiopathic arthritis (JIA) or other rheumatological diseases.

Regardless of all these nomenclatures, whether primary or secondary, HLH or MAS, these diseases are often triggered by an infection or other immune-activating condition, causing a cytokine storm. The most common clinical manifestations of cytokine storm are sepsis, septic shock, and multiple organ failure syndrome (MODs).

The cytokine storm, which occurs due to an excessive immune response, is a clinical condition that should be considered as it may cause increased morbidity and mortality. It is vital to take early precautions and establish appropriate treatment modalities in this context.

Pathophysiology

Cells involved in the formation of a cytokine storm are macrophages, cytotoxic T lymphocytes, and NK cells. Macrophages, which act as professional antigen presenters, present their antigens to lymphocytes. Cytotoxic T lymphocytes use class I histocompatibility proteins (MHC-1) to lyse foreign antigen-carrying cells such as macrophages. On the other hand, NK cells do this without the mediation of MHC-1. In the case of HLH, macrophages become overactive and secrete enough cytokines to cause tissue and organ damage. Cytotoxic T lymphocytes and NK cells are unable to eliminate activated macrophages. As a result, with excessive cytokine production, cell damage and multi-organ failure occur in the patient (Filipovicg et al., 2010).

Clinical Manifestations

The cytokine storm clinic is seen in the pediatric age group in primary HLH, which is genetically inherited, while secondary HLH is more common in older ages. However, this is not a rule. The disease usually begins with an acute or subacute fever of unknown origin. Then, uncontrollable systemic inflammation causes hepatitis by affecting the liver, encephalitis affecting the central nervous system, and life-threatening hemodynamic instability and MODs affecting the circulatory system. It may be accompanied by hepatomegaly, splenomegaly, lymphadenopathy, skin rashes, and impaired blood parameters. Coagulopathy, hyperferritinemia (> 500 mcg/L), bicytopenia, hemophagocytosis, high triglyceride, low fibrinogen, high soluble CD25, and an absence of, or low NK cell activity can be seen among the laboratory findings of the disease.

The clinical course of the disease begins acutely or sub-acutely over four weeks. In almost all cases, fever appears as a general symptom and is often refractory to treatment above 38.5°C. All organ systems may be affected in the following process. There may be skin involvement in the form of erythroderma, rash, and edema. Hematological involvement in the form of pterygia, purpura, ecchymosis, epistaxis, hematuria, and lymphadenopathy may be observed. Pulmonary involvement in pulmonary edema or acute respiratory distress may occur. This may be accompanied by cardiac involvement. Gastrointestinal system involvement in the form of hepatomegaly, splenomegaly, hematemesis, and melena may be seen. Acute renal failure may occur with renal involvement. Central nervous system involvement can be seen in the form of altered consciousness, seizures, encephalitis, and in progressive cases, coma. All these clinical signs and symptoms; Even if it is not specific if it suggests a cytokine storm in the differential diagnosis at this stage, will provide convenience to the clinician in terms of patient management.

Although the disease progresses with nonspecific symptoms and signs in its natural clinical course, age-related clinical presentation differences may occur. Especially in the cytokine storm clinic in the neonatal period, fever does not appear as in adults. Therefore, hepatomegaly and disturbances in blood parameters (such as cytopenia, coagulopathy) in the neonatal period should bring to mind the cytokine storm. However, one should be aware that the cytokine storm is a clinical emergency in any age group. In this context, the clinician should not forget that the cytokine storm is also essential to diagnose exclusion.

Relationship of Clinical Findings with Cytokines

Many of the clinical conditions mentioned above are explained by the effects of proinflammatory cytokines such as IFN-γ, TNF, IL-1β, IL-6, IL-10, and IL-18 (Henter et al., 1991, Lachmann et al., 2011; Dinarello et al., 2013; Sieni et al., 2014; Avau et al., 2015). Table 1 summarizes these cytokines and their clinical effects (Cron and Bahrens 2019).

In the cytokine storm, IFN-γ, IL-1β, IL-6, and TNF-α are cytokines that are responsible for fever and systemic disease. IL-1β, IFN-γ and TNF-α cytokines inhibit hematopoiesis and induce cytopenia (Arico et al., 2001). In addition, hemophagocytosis in the bone marrow also contributes to cytopenia. IFN-γ and TNF-α are the cytokines that contribute most to hemophagocytosis. Excessive release of these two cytokines may also impair liver functions and indirectly cause coagulation disorder that may even cause disseminated intravascular coagulopathy (DIC) (Eife et al., 1989; Marsh et al., 2010). While the elevation of IFN-γ causes cholestasis and low albumin, the elevation of IL-1β and TNF-α causes elevated serum levels of ferritin, an acute phase reactant (Clementi et al., 2002; Li et al., 2014; Alkhairy et al., 2015). Lipoprotein lipase activity suppressed by TNF-α also causes hypertriglyceridemia (Barilli et al., 2012). IL-6 elevation was also found to be associated with acute kidney injury (Jessen et al., 2013). Excessive elevation in IL-18 levels has been shown to be the cause of NK cell activity in the cytokine storm (Pagel et al., 2012). However, this information typically contradicts IL-18's activator for NK cells. High IL-6 levels also prevent NK cell activation by decreasing the expression of perforin and granzyme (Ueda et al., 2007). When NK cells cannot function effectively, deterioration of the current clinic is caused due to decreased cytotoxicity.

Table 1. Relationship between key cytokines and clinical features of cytokine storm syndrome

Key cytokines	**Clinical manifestations**
IFN-γ	Fever
	Depression of hematopoiesis
	Hemophagocytosis
	Macrophage activation
	Disseminated intravascular coagulation
	Hypoalbuminemia
TNF	Fever
	Cachexia
	Depression of hematopoiesis
	Hypertriglyceridemia
	Liver injury
	Disseminated intravascular coagulation
	Hypoalbuminemia
	Hyperferritinemia
	Neurological symptoms
IL-1β	Fever
	Acute-phase proteins
	Depression of hematopoiesis
	Hyperferritinemia
IL-6	Fever
	Acute-phase proteins
	Anemia
	Acute kidney Injury
IL-18	Liver injury
	NK cell dysfunction

As can be seen, many types of cytokines can contribute to the cytokine storm with different mechanisms and affect the clinic. Determining which disease causes this condition at the diagnosis stage is a problem that may challenge the clinician. Examples such as IL-18 levels being higher in Kawasaki Disease and a cytokine storm due to Epstein Barr Virus infection than a cytokine storm developing due to other diseases, and TNF levels being higher in a cytokine storm developing in lupus patients compared to other conditions causing a cytokine storm suggest that it may help the clinician in the diagnosis stage for the disease (Muralitharan et al., 2005). Since the underlying disease in a cytokine storm is mainly seen as an infection, malignancy, immunodeficiency, rheumatic or immunological pathology, its detection will be beneficial for the clinician in establishing appropriate treatment modalities.

Diagnostic Approach

In a cytokine storm, clinical and laboratory findings similar to sepsis with multi-organ failure or systemic inflammatory response syndrome (SIRS) dominate most patients. These patients may present to the hospital with an acute clinic, or they may worsen while they are hospitalized for different reasons. The patient's anamnesis and physical examination findings, and the results obtained from the tests to be requested are very important in the diagnostic approach.

Underlying diseases, the drugs used, and family history should be questioned in the anamnesis. The patient's vital signs such as fever, blood pressure, saturation, and respiratory rate should be recorded. In the physical examination, attention should be paid to rashes on the skin, signs of bleeding, the presence of lymphadenopathy and hepatosplenomegaly, and neurological findings. The first tests to be requested at the diagnostic stage; should be complete blood count, coagulation parameters (PT, aPTT, fibrinogen, D-dimer), and liver and kidney function tests (blood urea nitrogen, creatinine, ALT, AST, GGT, total bilirubin, albumin, and lactate dehydrogenase). Electrocardiography, echocardiography, and chest X-ray should be requested from patients for possible cardiopulmonary pathologies. Fasting serum triglyceride level and serum ferritin level should be ordered, and abdominal ultrasonography should be requested for hepatomegaly and/or splenomegaly, and brain computed tomography (BBT), and/or magnetic resonance imaging (MRI) should be requested for possible central pathologies. Blood and cerebrospinal fluid (CSF) cultures should be studied, and bone marrow biopsy should be performed if necessary.

If cytokine storm is considered as a preliminary diagnosis in the patient with the results obtained, immune phenotype tests can be examined in addition to these tests. These tests are: soluble IL-2 receptor alpha (sCD25 or sIL-2R), IL-18 and CXCL9 levels; lysosomal-associated membrane protein 1 (LAMP-1) level and NK cell functions determined by flow cytometry; cell surface expressions are determined by perforin and granzyme B proteins. In addition, serum immunoglobulin levels and lymphocyte subgroups can be determined.

According to immunophenotype tests, genetic tests may be requested in patients who do not have a genetic mutation in their family history. For example, PRF gene mutation analysis can be performed if the perforin level is low, and if the CD107-alpha level is low, UNC13D, STX11, STXBP2, and RAB27A mutation analyses can be performed. The heterozygous presence of any of these gene mutations in an adult with symptoms of cytokine storm is diagnostic (Bader et al., 2007, Murphy 2013). However, all these tests are available in specialized laboratories, which creates a handicap for the diagnostic process. For this reason, criteria have been determined to be used in the diagnostic process for the disease. These criteria can be listed as follows (Janka 2012; Locatelli et al., 2020):

- Fever above ≥ 38.5°C
- Splenomegaly

- Presence of cytopenia in the peripheral blood in at least two series (hemoglobin < 9 g/dl in adults or < 10 g/dl in newborns, platelet < 100.000/microL, absolute neutrophil count < 1000/microL)
- High fasting triglyceride (>265 mg/dL) or low fibrinogen (< 150 mg/dL)
- High ferritin (> 500 ng/mL)
- Low or absence of NK cell activity
- Soluble CD25 (soluble IL-2 receptor alpha [sIL-2R]) is over 2 standard deviations
- Hemophagocytosis in the bone marrow, lymph node, spleen, or liver.

The presence of five of these criteria, consisting of eight items, is significant in the diagnostic process, but since a cytokine storm has a high mortality rate, meeting all these diagnostic criteria should not delay the treatment process. For example, high triglyceride levels may not be seen in a patient without accompanying hepatic failure, or a high initial neutrophil count or reactive thrombocytosis may delay reaching the above diagnostic criteria in patients with cytokine storm secondary to infection (Okamoto et al., 2009). For all these reasons, these criteria have been modified so that the clinician can make more precise and faster decisions about cytokine storm. According to this; If three of the symptoms and signs of fever, splenomegaly, cytopenia, and hepatitis are present and they are accompanied by any one of hemophagocytosis, hyperferritinemia, hypofibrinogenemia, and NK cell dysfunction, it is sufficient for the diagnosis (Filipovich 2009; Jordan et al., 2011). These criteria are the most common clinics among the criteria listed above. However, it should not be forgotten that central nervous system involvement, kidney involvement, and respiratory problems may also be present in the clinic.

Calculation of the "Hscore" is another method that can help the clinician evaluate the diagnosis probability for HLH disease, which is seen as the basic prototype of the cytokine storm (Fardet et al., 2014). According to the "Hscore" system, which evaluates the presence of an underlying immunosuppression status, maximum fever level, hepatomegaly, splenomegaly, complete blood count parameters (hemoglobin, leukocytes, platelets), ferritin, triglyceride, fibrinogen, ALT, and AST levels, and hemophagocytosis in the bone marrow; a score of ≥ 250 supports cytokine storm with a probability of 99%, while a score of ≤ 90 reduces this rate to 1%.

Since the cytokine storm affects many systems at the same time, a differential diagnosis with many diseases should be made. These differential diagnoses include sepsis, malignancy, Kawasaki disease, encephalitis, thrombotic thrombocytopenic purpura, hemolytic uremic syndrome, and transfusion-related graft versus host disease. However, it should not be forgotten that even these diseases in the differential diagnosis may eventually cause cytokine storm.

The way to successfully treat cytokine storm syndrome is to suspect the disease in the early period and start treatment without delay. Suspected patients for diagnosis should be consulted with hematology and oncology specialists in the early period. The underlying pathology can be investigated in patients with a stable clinical status while making a treatment plan. Cytotoxic therapy should be avoided in these patients. Etoposide and reduced doses of dexamethasone over two months are recommended in patients whose general condition deteriorates, and many organ systems are affected. Intrathecal methotrexate and hydrocortisone treatment are given in addition to this treatment in patients with central nervous system involvement (Henter et al., 2002; Trottestam et al., 2011). As a supportive treatment, it aims to correct the blood and bleeding parameters of the patient, provide infection control, and stabilize vital signs, if any. At this stage, HLA typing and genetic testing should be requested from all patients and eligible family members for possible hematopoietic cell transplantation because hematopoietic cell transplantation is recommended in patients with HLH gene mutation and treatment-resistant clinic, who are unresponsive to initial treatment, and have untreatable hematological malignancy. In patients with recurrent or resistant disease, the IFN-γ blocking antibody "emapalumab" and dexamethasone treatment are recommended. An anti-CD52 monoclonal antibody, alemtuzumab, is recommended as an alternative to emapalumab (Jiang et al., 2009, Strout et al., 2010).

The prognosis of the disease is relatively poor in untreated cases. Patients with the HLH gene mutation have a 2-month survival without treatment (Henter et al., 1991; Janka et al., 2012). More than half of adequately treated patients survive more than six years (Henter et al. 2002; Trottestam et al., 2011). In addition, young age, central nervous system involvement, and lack of remission before hematopoietic cell transplantation are poor prognostic factors (Trottestam et al., 2011). Relapse occurs mainly in patients with gene mutations and often in the first year after the acute attack (Jordan et al., 2011).

Conclusion

The extreme immune response may occur in many clinical conditions, both genetic and acquired, and may cause the life-threatening cytokine storm. Knowing the mechanisms of action of cytokines in the pathogenesis of the disease and its reflection on the clinic is a cornerstone for managing the disease. In this way, possible mortality will be prevented with the appropriate treatment modality.

References

Alkhairy O K, Perez-Becker R, Driessen G J Abolhassani H, van Montfrans J, Borte S, Choo S, Wang N, Tesselaar K, Fang M, Bienemann K, Boztug K, Daneva A, Mechinaud F, Wiesel T, Becker C, Dückers G, Siepermann K, van Zelm C M, Rezaei N, van der Burg M, Aghamohammadi A, Seidel G M, Niehues T, Hammarström L (2015). Novel mutations in TNFRSF7/CD27: Clinical, immunologic, and genetic characterization of human CD27 deficiency. *The Journal of allergy and clinical immunology* 136(3):703–712.e10.

Arico M, Imashuku S, Clementi R Hibi S, Teramura T, Danesino C, Haber D A, Nichols K E (2001). Hemophagocytic lymphohistiocytosis due to germline mutations in SH2D1A, the X-linked lymphoproliferative disease gene. *Blood* 97(4):1131–1133.

Avau A, Put K, Wouters C H, Matthys P. (2015). Cytokine balance and cytokine-driven natural killer cell dysfunction in systemic juvenile idiopathic arthritis. *Cytokine & growth factor reviews* 26(1):35–45.

Bader P, Niethammer D, Willasch A, Kreyenberg H, Klingebiel T (2005). How and when should we monitor chimerism after allogeneic stem cell transplantation? *Bone marrow transplantation* 35(2):107–119.

Barilli A, Rotoli B M, Visigalli R, Bussolati O, Gazzola C G, Gatti R, Dionisi-Vici C, Martinelli D, Goffredo M B, Font M, Mariani F, Luisetti M, Dall'Asta V (2012). Impaired phagocytosis in macrophages from patients affected by lysinuric protein intolerance. *Molecular genetics and metabolism* 105(4):585–589.

Brisse E, Wouters C H, Matthys P (2015). Hemophagocytic lymphohistiocytosis (HLH): A heterogeneous spectrum of cytokine-driven immune disorders. *Cytokine & growth factor reviews* 26(3):263–280.

Clark I A (2007). The advent of the cytokine storm. *Immunology and cell biology* 85(4):271–273.

Clementi R, Emmi L, Maccario R, Liotta F, Moretta L, Danesino C, Aricó M (2002). Adult onset and atypical presentation of hemophagocytic lymphohistiocytosis in siblings carrying PRF1 mutations. *Blood* 100(6): 2266–2267.

Dinarello C A, Novick D, Kim S, Kaplanski G (2013). Interleukin-18 and IL-18 binding protein. *Frontiers in immunology* 4:289.

Eife R, Janka G E, Belohradsky B H, Holtmann H (1989). Natural killer cell function and interferon production in familial hemophagocytic lymphohistiocytosis. *Pediatric hematology and oncology* 6(3):265–272.

Fardet L, Galicier L, Lambotte O, Marzac C, Aumont C, Chahwan D, Coppo P, Hejblum G (2014). Development and validation of the HScore, a score for the diagnosis of reactive hemophagocytic syndrome. *Arthritis & rheumatology* (Hoboken, N.J.) m66(9):2613–2620.

Ferrara J L, Abhyankar S, Gilliland D G (1993). Cytokine storm of graft-versus-host disease: a critical effector role for interleukin-1. *Transplantation proceedings* 25(1 Pt 2):1216–1217.

Filipovich A H (2009). Hemophagocytic lymphohistiocytosis (HLH) and related disorders. *Hematology*. American Society of Hematology. *Education Program* 127–131.

Filipovich A, McClain K, Grom A (2010). Histiocytic disorders: recent insights into pathophysiology and practical guidelines. *Biology of blood and marrow transplantation: journal of the American Society for Blood and Marrow Transplantation* 16(1 Suppl): S82–S89.

Henter J I, Elinder G, Söder O, Hansson M, Andersson B, Andersson U (1991). Hypercytokinemia in familial hemophagocytic lymphohistiocytosis. *Blood* 78(11):2918–2922.

Henter J I, Samuelsson-Horne A, Aricò M, Egeler M R, Elinder G, Filipovich H A, Gadner H, Imashuku S, Komp D, Ladisch S, Webb D, Janka G, Histocyte Society (2002). Treatment of hemophagocytic lymphohistiocytosis with HLH-94 immunochemotherapy and bone marrow transplantation. *Blood* 100(7):2367–2373.

Hu B, Huang S, Yin L (2021). The cytokine storm and COVID-19. *Journal of medical virology* 93(1):250–256.

Janka G E (2012). Familial and acquired hemophagocytic lymphohistiocytosis. *Annual review of medicine* 63:233–246.

Jessen B, Bode S F, Ammann S, Chakravorty S, Davies G, Diestelhorst J, Frei-Jones M, Gahl W A, Gochuico B R, Griese M, Griffiths G, Janka G, Klein C, Kögl T, Kurnik K, Lehmberg K, Maul-Pavicic A, Mumford A D, Pace D, Parvaneh N, Rezaei N, de Saint Basile G, Schmitt-Graeff A, Schwarz K, Karasu G T, ZiegerB, Zur Stadt U, Aichele P, Ehl S (2013). The risk of hemophagocytic lymphohistiocytosis in Hermansky-Pudlak syndrome type 2. *Blood* 121(15):2943–2951.

Jiang L, Yuan C M, Hubacheck J, Janik J E, Wilson W, Morris J C, Jasper G A and Stetler-Stevenson M (2009). Variable CD52 expression in mature T cell and NK cell malignancies: implications for alemtuzumab therapy. *British journal of haematology* 145(2):173–179.

Jordan M B., Allen C E, Weitzman S, Filipovich A H, McClain K L (2011). How I treat hemophagocytic lymphohistiocytosis. *Blood* 118(15):4041–4052.

Lachmann H J, Quartier P, So A, Hawkins P N (2011). The emerging role of interleukin-1β in autoinflammatory diseases. *Arthritis and rheumatism* 63(2):314–324.

Li F Y, Chaigne-Delalande B, Su H, Uzel G, Matthews H and Lenardo M J (2014). XMEN disease: a new primary immunodeficiency affecting Mg2+ regulation of immunity against Epstein-Barr virus. *Blood* 123(14):2148–2152.

Locatelli F, Jordan M B, Allen C, Cesaro S, Rizzari C, Rao A, Degar B, Garrington T P, Sevilla J, Putti M-C, Fagioli F, Ahlmann M, Dapena Diaz J-L, Henry M, De Benedetti F, Grom A, Lapeyre G, Jacqmin P, Ballabio M, de Min C (2020). Emapalumab in Children with Primary Hemophagocytic Lymphohistiocytosis. *N. Engl. J. Med.* 382:1811.

Marsh R A, Madden L, Kitchen B J, Mody R, McClimon B, Jordan M B, Bleesing J J, Zhang K, Filipovich A H (2010). XIAP deficiency: a unique primary immunodeficiency best classified as X-linked familial hemophagocytic lymphohistiocytosis and not as X-linked lymphoproliferative disease. *Blood* 116(7): 1079–1082.

Masaki Shimizu (2019). *Clinical Features of Cytokine Storm Syndrome*. In: Randy Q. Cron, Edward M. Behrens (eds) Cytokine Storm Syndrome. Springer, Birmingham, AL, USA and Philadelphia, PA, USA, p 36.

Muralitharan S, Al Lamki Z, Dennison D, Christie B S, Wali Y A, Zachariah M, Romana M, Bayoumi R, Krishnamoorthy R (2005). An inframe perforin gene deletion in familial hemophagocytic lymphohistiocytosis is associated with perforin expression. *American journal of hematology* 78(1):59–63.

Murphy K M (2013) Chimerism analysis following hematopoietic stem cell transplantation. *Methods in molecular biology* (Clifton, N.J.) 999:137–149.

Okamoto M, Yamaguchi H, Isobe Y, Yokose N, Mizuki T, Tajika K, Gomi S, Hamaguchi H, Inokuchi K, Oshimi K, Dan K (2009). Analysis of triglyceride value in the diagnosis and treatment response of secondary hemophagocytic syndrome. *Internal medicine* (Tokyo, Japan) 48(10):775–781.

Pagel J, Beutel K, Lehmberg K, Koch F, Maul-Pavicic A, Rohlfs A–K, Al-Jefri A, Beier R, Ousager L B, Ehlert K, Gross-Wieltsch U, Jorch N, Kremens B, Pekrun A, Sparber-Sauer M, Mejstrikova E, Wawer A, Ehl S, zur Stadt U, Janka G (2012). Distinct mutations in STXBP2 are associated with variable clinical presentations in patients with familial hemophagocytic lymphohistiocytosis type 5 (FHL5). *Blood* 119(25):6016–6024.

Sieni E, Cetica V, Hackmann Y, Coniglio M L, Da Ros M, Ciambotti B, Pende D, Griffiths G, Aricò M (2014). Familial hemophagocytic lymphohistiocytosis: when rare diseases shed light on immune system functioning. *Frontiers in immunology* 5:167.

Strout M P, Seropian S, Berliner N (2010). Alemtuzumab as a bridge to allogeneic SCT in atypical hemophagocytic lymphohistiocytosis. Nature reviews. *Clinical oncology* 7(7):415–420.

Trottestam H, Horne A, Aricò M, Egeler R M, Filipovich A H, Gadner H, Imashuku S, Ladisch S, Webb D, Janka G, Henter J-I, Histiocyte Society (2011). Chemoimmunotherapy for hemophagocytic lymphohistiocytosis: long-term results of the HLH-94 treatment protocol. *Blood* 118(17):4577–4584.

Ueda I, Kurokawa Y, Koike K, Ito S, Sakata A, Matsumora T, Fukushima T, Morimoto A, Ishii E, Imashuku S (2007). Late-onset cases of familial hemophagocytic lymphohistiocytosis with missense perforin gene mutations. *American journal of hematology* 82(6):427–432.

Zimmer L, Apuri S, Eroglu Z Kottschade L A, Forschner A, Gutzmer R, Schlaak M, Heinzerling L, Krackhardt A M, Loquai C, Markovic S N, Joseph R W, Markey K, Utikal J S, Weishaupt C, Goldinger S M, Sondak V K, Zager J S, Schadendorf D, Khushalani N I (2017). Ipilimumab alone or in combination with nivolumab after progression on anti-PD-1 therapy in advanced melanoma. *European journal of cancer* (Oxford, England: 1990) 75:47–55.

Chapter 7

Cytokines in Sepsis and Septic Shock

Çağatay Erman Öztürk[1,*], MD and Selin Eyüpoğlu[2], MD
[1]Samsun Training and Research Hospital, Samsun, Turkey
[2]Giresun Training and Research Hospital, Giresun, Turkey

Abstract

Inflammation, cytokine release, endothelial damage, coagulation system activation, and microvascular blood flow decrease in sepsis cause organ failure. Prolonged inflammation, apoptosis, and T-cell exhaustion cause sepsis-associated immune paralysis. This immunosuppressive state predisposes to secondary infections. Immunomodulatory treatment options can increase life expectancy.

Keywords: cytokine, sepsis, septic shock

Introduction

Sepsis is a life-threatening organ dysfunction resulting from an excessive and abnormally irregular host response to infection according to the Sepsis-3 diagnostic criteria. If a patient with sepsis requires a vasopressor to keep the mean arterial pressure above 65 mmHg despite adequate fluid resuscitation, and if the serum lactate level is above 2 mmol/L, the patient is in septic shock. Mortality is high in patients with sepsis and septic shock (Singer 2016).

Bacterial, viral and fungal agents can cause infections. The immune system creates pro-inflammatory and anti-inflammatory responses against infection with innate and adaptive immunity. Prolonged inflammation in sepsis causes immune paralysis, endothelial damage, coagulation system activation, organ failure and secondary infections.

---

* Corresponding Author's Email: cageroz@gmail.com.

In: Cytokines and Diseases
Editors: Kenan Demir, Selim Görgün and Bahar Uslu
ISBN: 979-8-88697-214-6

Pathophysiology

Leukocytes are activated by pattern recognition receptors (PRRs) and these receptors can be activated by exogenous pathogen-associated molecular patterns (PAMPs) and endogenous injury-associated molecular patterns (DAMPs).

Four types of PRRs are known: Toll-like receptors (TLRs), nod-like receptors (NLRs), RIG-like receptors (RLRs), and C-type lectin receptors (CLR). The most known TLR is TLR4, a ligand of lipopolysaccharide (LPS). TLRs activate nuclear factor-kB (NF-kB). NLRs are intracellular PRRs. After the interaction of TLRs, NLRs and its ligand, inflammatory cytokines are released. CLR produces ROS, and binds to viruses, fungi and leishmania, and RLRs bind to viral RNA.

Cytokines are small proteins <40 kDa. They act by binding to their specific receptors. Interleukins, chemokines, tumor necrosis factor, interferons and growth factors are cytokines. Chemokines (CKs) bind with G proteins. They help leukocyte migration, and cell release from the bone marrow and spleen. Growth factors contribute to the cytokine storm. In sepsis, granulocyte-macrophage colony-stimulating factor (GM-CSF), macrophage colony-stimulating factor (M-CSF) and granulocyte colony-stimulating factor (G-CSF) are released (Chousterman 2017).

Tumor necrosis factor (TNF)-α, interleukin (IL)-1, IL-6, IL-12, IL-17, and interferon (INF)-β are proinflammatory cytokines. IL-10, transforming growth factor (TGF)-β, and IL-4 are anti-inflammatory cytokines.

TNF-α

TNF works with receptor (TNFR) 1 and TNFR2, and is released from macrophage and dendritic cells. After its release, immune cells are activated and they release mediators. Increased vascular permeability leads to pulmonary edema. It also causes fire. It activates macrophages, causes their differentiation, and prolongs life span. They trigger the release of other proinflammatory cytokines from activated macrophages. They increase the extravasation of neutrophils into the tissue. They increase the release of intercellular adhesion molecule (ICEM)-1 and vascular cell adhesion molecule (VCAM)-1 and chemokine in the endothelium. TNF triggers the procoagulant effect (Schulte 2013).

Anti-TNF therapy can reduce sepsis mortality (Chousterman 2017).

IL-1

This is released from activated macrophages and works with IL-1 receptor type 1 (IL-1R1) and IL-1R2. Like TNF-α, it causes fever, pulmonary edema, and increased vascular permeability, and triggers the coagulation cascade. They increase the release of other proinflammatory mediators from macrophages (Schulte 2013).

Elevated IL-1β is associated with poor prognosis in sepsis (Chousterman 2017).

IL-6

This can be released from immune cells, mesenchymal cells, endothelium and fibroblasts with infection and tissue damage (Odabaşı 2020). It activates B and T cells. It is responsible for fever, leukocytosis and the acute-phase response. It triggers coagulation, depresses myocardium and suppresses TNF-α and IL-1 release. It decreases T-regulatory (Tregs) cell growth and increases IL-10 production (Schulte 2013). It is responsible for antibody production and leads to bone resorption. VEGF production increases angiogenesis and vascular permeability. It causes lipolysis, and affects the release of insulin from the pancreas (Kang 2019).

High IL-6 levels in sepsis cause poor prognosis (Chousterman 2017).

IL-12

This is released from dendritic cells, macrophages and lymphocytes (Chousterman 2017). It increases the production of INF-γ by T cells and NK cells. It enables the transformation of T cells into TH1 cells (Schulte 2013).

INF-γ

This is released from activated NK, TH1 and CD8+ T cells. It has an antiviral effect. It is effective against intracellular pathogens. It can be tried in the treatment of immunoparalysis (Schulte 2013).

IL-15

This has been shown to increase INF-γ production by affecting NK cells in sepsis (Guo 2017).

IL-10

This is an anti-inflammatory cytokine, released from monocytes, macrophages, and B, T and NK cells. It inhibits TNF-α, IL-1, IL-6, INF-γ, and GM-CSF release. It increases the production of the IL-1 receptor antagonist (IL-1Ra) and soluble TNF receptors (sTNFRs). It can prevent the conversion of sepsis to septic shock (Schulte 2013).

High IL-10 levels indicate sepsis-associated immunosuppression (Chousterman 2017).

TGF-β

This is related to fibrosis, tissue damage repair, and immunosuppression in sepsis. It suppresses the release of IL-1, TNF-α, and high mobility group box-1 (HMGB1). It increases the production of IL-1Ra and sTNFRs. It suppresses IL-2 production from T lymphocytes, and supports T-regulatory cell development. It prevents NO-related hypotension in endotoxemia. It prevents cardiac myositis damage (Schulte 2013).

IL-4

This is released from T cells (Chousterman 2017). It inhibits the development of TH1 from T lymphocytes, and induces the development of TH2. It increases IL-4 release from TH2 and inhibits proinflammatory cytokine release (Schulte 2013).

After the effects of DAMPs and PAMPs in sepsis, proinflammatory cytokines, adhesion molecules, and procoagulant factors are released from the endothelium with the activation of the NF-κβ pathway. Nitric oxide (NO) production increases with inducible nitric oxide synthase (iNOS) upregulation.

Vascular cell adhesion molecule-1 (VCAM-1), platelet endothelial cell adhesion molecule-1 (PECAM-1) and intercellular cell adhesion molecule-1/2 (ICAM-1/2) are responsible for leukocyte adhesion, rolling and crawling. Adhesion molecule levels were found to be high in patients with severe organ failure in sepsis.

After the endothelium is stimulated, it secretes tissue factor (TF). TF initiates the coagulation cascade, and microvascular thrombosis occurs. Microvascular blood flow is reduced after sepsis-associated coagulopathy. Glycocalyx damage causes endothelial apoptosis, hyperpermeability and interstitial leakage. Microcirculatory dysfunction also causes organ failure in sepsis (Joffre 2020).

In septic shock, inflammation, endothelial dysfunction, intravascular coagulation, and hemodilution also affect the development of thrombocytopenia (Bedet 2018).

In a cytokine storm, fever, dyspnea, tachypnea, an increased IL-6 level, CRP, and an increase in ferritin are observed. Inflammatory cytokines cause cytokine release syndrome (CRS). A cytokine storm can cause ARDS. CRS T cells can trigger exhaustion, apoptosis and lymphopenia. A decreased lymphocyte count and dysfunction may lead to immunosuppression. High NKG2A expression may be an indicator of T-cell exhaustion (Odabaşı 2020).

Immune cell apoptosis, mainly lymphocytes, regulatory T (Treg) cell expression, PD-1 expression in T cells, and cellular exhaustion lead to immune suppression. Decreased monocyte HLA-DR expression is an indicator of immunosuppression (Cao 2019).

Spec et al. reported that PD-1 expression, which indicates T-cell exhaustion, increased in candida bloodstream infection (Spec 2016).

Mortality was found to be higher in elderly surgical intensive care patients compared to younger patients. In these patients, elevated soluble programmed death ligand-1 (sPD-L1), persistent lymphopenia, was evidence of prolonged inflammation and immunosuppression (Brakenridge 2018).

Immunomodulatory Therapy

If proinflammatory cytokine levels are high, anti-cytokine treatments may be more effective (Chousterman 2017). It was thought that patients with high plasma cytokine levels in septic shock would benefit from corticosteroid therapy (Bentzer 2016). Monalizumab (anti-NKG2A monoclonal antibody) may be effective in viral infections by increasing IFN-γ production (Odabaşı 2020).

In patients with sepsis and a diagnosis of macrophage activation-like syndrome (MALS), ferritin, IL-6, IL-18, and IFN-γ levels are high, and the IL-10/TNF-α ratio is low. In these patients, the IL-1β blocker anakinra can be tried in the treatment (Karakike 2019). Anti-IL-6 antibodies (Ab) (tocilizumab), anti-IL-6 receptor antibody and soluble gp130Fc can inhibit IL-6 signaling (Kang 2019).

It has been shown that procalcitonin affects cytokine release by acting as a mediator in sepsis with calcitonin gene-related peptide (CGRP) receptor signaling. The CGRP receptor antagonist olcegepant has been shown to increase survival in sepsis by suppressing the proinflammatory effect of procalcitonin in mice (Baranowsky 2021).

IL-7 increases the lymphocyte count and decreases apoptosis. Recombinant human IL-7 (CYT107) has a positive effect on the lymphocyte count and functions. Anti-PD-1 also acts similarly to IL-7 (Francois 2018). Inhibition of the PD-1/PD-L1 pathway has been shown to increase HLA-DR expression in sepsis-associated immunosuppression (Hotchkiss 2019).

PD-1/PD-L1 blockade, which reduces apoptosis, and the use of IL-7 in the treatment of sepsis-induced immunosuppression may be considered (Cao 2019; Odabaşı 2020).

Conclusion

Sepsis progresses with organ failure and has high mortality. In sepsis and septic shock, a cytokine storm causes endothelial dysfunction, coagulopathy, microvascular blood flow disruption, and immunosuppression. In addition to antimicrobial agents, intravenous fluids, vasopressor therapy and supportive therapy, immunomodulatory agents can be investigated as additional treatment options.

References

Baranowsky, A., Appelt, J., Kleber, C., Lange, T., Ludewig, P., Jahn, D., Pandey, P., Keller, D., Rose, T., Schetler, D., Braumüller, S., Huber-Lang, M., Tsitsilonis, S., Yorgan, T., Frosch, K. H., Amling, M., Schinke, T., & Keller, J. (2021) Procalcitonin Exerts a Mediator Role in Septic Shock Trough the Calcitonin Gene-Related Peptide Receptor. *Crit. Care Med.* 49(1):e41-e52. https//doi.org/10.1097/CCM.0000000000004731.

Brakenridge, S. C., Efron, P. A., Storz, J. A., et al. (2018) The impact of age on the innate response and outcomes after severe sepsis/septic shock in trauma and surgical intensive care unit patients. *J. Trauma Acute Care Surg.* 85(2):247-255. https//doi.org/10.1097/TA.0000000000001921

Bedet, A., Razazi, K., Boissier, F., Surenaud, M., Hue, S., Giraudier, S., Brun-Buisson, C., & Mekontso Dessap, A. (2018) Mechanisms of thrombocytopenia during septic shock: a multiplex cluster analysis of endogenous sepsis mediators. *Shock* 49(6):641-648. https//doi.org/10.1097/SHK.0000000000001015.

Bentzer, P., Fjell, C., Walley, K. R., Boyd, J., & Russell, J. A. (2016) Plasma cytokine levels predict response to corticosteroids in septic shock. *Int. Care Med.* 42:1970-1979. https//doi.org/10.1007/s00134-016-4338-z.

Cao, C., Yu, M., Chai, Y. (2019) Pathological alteration and therapeutic implications of sepsis-induced immune cell apoptosis. *Cell Death Dis.* 10:782.

Chousterman, B. G., Swirsky, F. K., Webwr, G. F. (2017) Cytokine storm and sepsis disease pathogenesis. *Semin. Immunopath*ol. 39:517-528. https//doi.org/10.1007/s00281-017-0639-8.

Francois, B., Jeannet, R., Daix, T., Walton, A. H., Shotwell, M. S., Unsinger, J., Monneret, G., Rimmelé, T., Blood, T., Morre, M., Gregoire, A., Mayo, G. A., Blood, J., Durum, S. K., Sherwood, E. R., & Hotchkiss, R. S. (2018) Interleukin-7 restores lymphocytes in septic shock: the IRIS-7 randomised clinical trial. *JCI* insight.

Guo, Y., Luan, L., Patil, N. K., Wang, J., Bohannon, J. K., Rabacal, W., Fensterheim, B. A., Hernandez, A., & Sherwood, E. R. (2017) Interleukin-15 Enables Septic Shock by Maintaining Natural Killer Cell Integrity and Function. *J. Immunol.* 198(3):1320-1333. https://doi.org/10.4049/jimmunol.1601486.

Hotchkiss, R. S., Colston, E., Yende, S., Angus, D. C., Moldawer, L. L., Crouser, E. D., Martin, G. S., Coopersmith, C. M., Brakenridge, S., Mayr, F. B., Park, P. K., Ye, J., Catlett, I. M., Girgis, I. G., & Grasela, D. M. (2019) Immune checkpoint inhibition in sepsis: a Phase 1b randomized, placebo-controlled, single ascending dose study of anti-PD-L1(BMS-936559). *Crit. Care Med.* 47(5):632-642. https//doi.org/10.1097/CCM.0000000000003685.

Joffre, J., Hellman, J., Ince, C., & Ait-Oufella, H. (2020) Endothelial Responses in Sepsis. *Am. J. Respir. Crit. Care Med.* 202(3):361-370. https//doi.org/10.1164/rccm.201910-1911TR.

Karakike, E., Giamarellos-Bourboulis, E. J. (2019) Macrophage Activation-Like Syndrome: A Distinct Entity Leading to Early Death in Sepsis. *Front. Immunol.* 10:55. https//doi.org/ 10.3389/fimmu.2019.00055.

Odabaşı, Z., Cinel, I. (2020) Consideration of Severe Coronavirus Disease 2019 As Viral Sepsis and Potential Use of Immune Checkpoint Inhibitors. *Crit. Care Explor.* 2(6):e0141. https//doi.org/10.1097/CCE.0000000000000141.

Schulte, W., Bernhagen, J., Bucala, R. (2013) Cytokines in Sepsis: Potent Immunoregulators and Potential Therapeutic Ttargets-An Updated View. *Mediators of inflammation* 2013:165974. http://doi.org./10.1155/2013/165974.

Shankar-Hari, M., Phillips, G. S., Levy, M. L., Seymour, C. W., Liu, V. X., Deutschman, C. S., Angus, D. C., Rubenfeld, G. D., Singer, M., & for the Sepsis Definitions Task Force. (2016) The third international consensus definitions for sepsis and septic shock (Sepsis-3). *JAMA* 315:801-810.

Spec, A., Shindo, Y., Burnham, C. A. D., Wilson, S., Ablordeppey, E. A., Beiter, E. R., Chang, K., Drewry, A. M., & Hotchkiss, R. S. (2016) T cell from patients with Candida sepsis display a suppressive immunophenotype. *Crit. Care* 20:15. https//doi.org/10.1186/s13054-016-1182-z.

Chapter 8

Cytokines and Patient Prognosis Monitoring

Tuğçehan Sezer Akman*, **MD**
Alaca State Hospital, Department of Anesthesiology and Reanimation, Çorum, Turkey

Abstract

Systemic inflammatory response refers to an exaggerated inflammatory response of the body that may occur against any stress factor without infection and is usually present in the etiology of all severe diseases. Cytokines are responsible for the regulation of this immune inflammatory response. Checking the levels of proinflammatory and anti-inflammatory cytokines identified for various diseases may be helpful in monitoring the prognosis, predicting disease outcomes, and treatment planning.

Keywords: cytokines, inflammation, prognosis

Introduction

SIRS (systemic inflammatory response syndrome) refers to an exaggerated defensive response of the body against harmful stress factors in cases such as acute inflammation, infection, surgery, trauma, malignancy or ischemia-reperfusion in order to eliminate the endogenous or exogenous source by limiting it (Chakraborty and Burns, 2021). The etiology of almost all severe diseases is accompanied by SIRS (Liu et al., 2020). While tumor necrotic factor alfa [TNF-α], interferon g [IFN-g], interleukin 1a [IL-1a], IL-1b, IL-6, IL-8, IL-12, and IL-17, which are proinflammatory cytokines, produce an effective inflammatory response for the removal of pathogens, transforming growth factor b [TGF-b], IL-10, IL-4 and IL-13, which are anti-inflammatory cytokines, and cytokine inhibitors (soluble TNF-RI and II, soluble IL-1ra) play a significant role in balancing the inflammatory response (Angurana et al., 2021).

However, the dysregulated release of acute and chronic phase reactants and the irregularity in the balance of pro- and anti-inflammatory pathways constitute the basis of SIRS (Chakraborty and Burns, 2021). Although the primary goal is to defend the body, the dysregulated cytokine storm may initiate a major inflammatory cascade that can lead to

* Corresponding Author's Email: tgchnszr@gmail.com.

In: Cytokines and Diseases
Editors: Kenan Demir, Selim Görgün and Bahar Uslu
ISBN: 979-8-88697-214-6

reversible or irreversible end-organ damage and even death (Chakraborty and Burns, 2021). One of the most likely causes of the rapid progression of the disease is cytokine storm (Liu et al., 2020). Individualized clinical care can be achieved to predict the early prognosis and protect the organ functions by predicting the severity of diseases and mortality rates with inflammatory parameters (Angurana et al., 2021).

Cytokines and Prognosis Monitoring in Respiratory Tract Diseases

Relationship between Cytokines and Respiratory Syncytial Virus (RSV)

Human respiratory syncytial virus (hRSV) is the primary cause of bronchiolitis and also one of the most important causes of respiratory tract infections in children. It has been associated with recurrent wheezing and the development of asthma. While it can be mildly overcome, it may sometimes progress with high morbidity that may require hospitalization/admission to the intensive care unit. The early prediction of high-risk patients will be beneficial for the improvement of disease management and clinical outcomes (Vazguez et al., 2019).

The suboptimal immune response to the virus during disease is Th-2-like responses with the production of cytokines and results in the collection of numerous proinflammatory immune cells. These markers which can be used as prognostic markers are IFN-α, IL-6, TSLP, IL-8, IL-33 and periostin. IL-12, IL-13 and IL-3 may be potential biomarkers. However, more studies are needed. IL-33 is responsible for initiating the innate and adaptive Th2 type immune response. A study conducted with mice demonstrated that the severity of the disease course did not change when IL-33 was neutralized during hRSV infection, but the development of hRSV infection was accelerated and had a more serious course in patients treated with IL-33 (Vazguez et al., 2019). It was revealed that when IL-33 was rapidly secreted in the lungs of RSV-infected neonatal mice, there was an increase in lung ILC-2 (group 2 natural lymphoid cells), but the same response did not occur in adult mice. IL-33 was shown to be the cause of Th2-biased immunopathophysiology after reinfection with RSV (Saravia et al., 2015).

In their study on 52 RSV-infected children, Brand et al. indicated that the joint evaluation of the CD 4 T-cell count and IL-8 and CCL-5 plasma concentrations was associated with the severity of disease and could be used in the evaluation (Brand et al., 2013). Low TNF-α and IL-6 plasma levels are correlated with increased hospitalization in infants (Brown et al., 2015).

Bont et al. examined in-vivo cytokine levels in the nasopharyngeal aspirates of infants with lower respiratory tract infection caused by RSV and demonstrated that the IFN gamma levels decreased in severely ill patients (Bont et al., 2001).

In the tracheal aspirate samples of infants with severe RSV infection, it was observed that the IL-6 and IL-17 levels increased (Van Drunen Little-van den Hurk and Watkiss, 2012). Furthermore, in mice infected with RSV, the IL-6, IL-17, and IL-23 levels increased, and the inflammation and viral load decreased when anti-IL-17 antibody treatment was administered (Mukherjee et al., 2011).

Relationship between Cytokines and SARS-CoV-2

Viral damage and uncontrolled inflammation contribute to the severity of COVID-19. In severely ill patients, inflammatory markers such as CRP, ferritin, and D-dimer, the neutrophil/lymphocyte ratio, inflammatory cytokines, and chemokines were high (Del Valle et al., 2020).

It was demonstrated that the IL-6 level was closely associated with gender, age, blood oxygen saturation, body temperature, and underlying diseases in individuals infected with severe acute respiratory syndrome coronavirus 2 (SARS-Cov-2). More severe inflammation was observed in patients who were male and elderly and had a high fever and especially COPD. The IL-6 level reflects the inflammation status during viral infection. It has been demonstrated that individuals with IL-6 levels 30 times higher than normal have a worse prognosis compared to those with normal values (Wu et al., 2021). IL-6 can be used as a treatment target in COVID-19 patients. Furthermore, it was shown that the severity of acute renal failure (ARF), one of the serious complications of COVID-19, was proportional to the IL-6 level, which revealed that the IL-6 level could also be an indicator of the progression of ARF (Wu et al., 2021).

In addition to IL-6, many other cytokines may be associated with COVID-19. In the study examining 12 types of cytokines, IL-10 was identified as a cytokine that could be most closely correlated with IL-6 (Wu et al., 2021). The study performed by Del Valle et al. showed that the levels of many cytokines were also high and contributed to tissue damage, apart from IL-6 in cytokine release syndrome. TNF-α, which plays a significant role in acute inflammatory reactions, IL-1, which is a proinflammatory cytokine, and IL-8, which enables neutrophil activation, are among these cytokines. In a study in which 1484 patients with suspected or evidence of COVID-19 were examined, the patients' serum IL-6, IL-8, TNF-α, and IL-1β levels were measured during their admission, and these results were associated with the clinical and laboratory markers of the disease severity and the outcome. It was found that high IL-6 and TNF-α serum levels were the predictors of disease severity and survival independently of other biomarkers. IL-6 was argued to be one of the most reliable prognostic factors in determining survival (Del Valle et al., 2020).

The COVID-19-associated cytokine response differs slightly from the classical cytokine storm associated with sepsis and CAR (chimeric antigen receptor-modified) T cells and progresses with high cytokine levels, which may last for days or weeks, and a relative lack of coordination between cytokines, which increases the possibility of developing strategies for alleviating the disease with anti-cytokine treatments.

A rational therapeutic approach based on the guidance of cytokine levels can be provided (Del Valle et al., 2020).

Relationship between Cytokines and Asthma

In asthma characterized by chronic airway inflammation, proinflammatory cytokines regulated by Th2 cells play a critical role. It was considered that the measurements of cytokine levels in peripheral blood might have a prognostic value in children with asthma exacerbation. It was found that IL-4 and IL-5 levels were high during exacerbations and that there was no difference between the levels of patients in the stable phase of asthma without attacks and healthy participants.

IL-4 and IL-5 levels were argued to play a significant role in airway inflammation and activation (Le-Thi-Thu and Nguyen-Thi-Dieu, 2016).

In a study examining the role of inflammation in obesity-associated asthma, this relationship could not be explained by inflammation; however, specifically CRP, TNF-α, IL-6, adiponectin, and neuropeptide Y (NPY) were found to be independently associated with the prevalence of asthma.

IL-6 and NPY were associated with the IL-4 marker of allergic airway inflammation in asthma, and it was indicated that there was a need for further studies so that they could be used as prognostic markers of asthma (Lu et al., 2015).

Cytokines and Prognosis Monitoring in Oncology Patients

The progression of cancer does not only depend on genetic changes involved in the origin of the tumor and paracrine interactions in the tumor microenvironment. The systemic interactions between the tumor and the host may mimic physiological processes such as inflammation and wound healing. This similarity was also reflected in histopathological images in the tumor microenvironment (McAllister and Weinberg, 2014). The role of the systemic inflammatory response in the development of tumorigenesis, malignant spread and cachexia is associated with cytokines (Dolan et al., 2019). It has been argued that the increase in the circulating neutrophil/lymphocyte ratio, which is an indicator of systemic inflammation, has prognostic importance in various cancer types, especially in advanced colon and pancreatic cancers. The Glasgow Prognostic Score (GPS) is a measurement of systemic inflammation that measures the circulating CRP and albumin and is used as an independent prognostic indicator for cancer patients (McAllister and Weinberg, 2014).

Two recent meta-analysis studies have demonstrated that CRP, albumin, neutrophils and platelets, which are the clinical markers of a systemic inflammatory response, have a prognostic value for patients with operable and advanced cancer. The aggressiveness of the disease and the development of cachexia have also been found to be associated with the activation of the systemic inflammatory response (Dolan and McMillan, 2020).

Inflammation is considered to be a distinguishing characteristic of cancer (Gunawardene et al., 2019). IL-6 is an essential component in the paraneoplastic cytokine pattern and plays a significant role in both the genesis and regulation of inflammation. In a number of independent clinical series, IL-6 and IL-10 were associated with the prognosis in different types of cancer (Lippitz and Harris, 2016, Lippitz, 2013). While a high IL-6 level represents the activation of the immunostimulatory system, a high IL-10 level represents systemic immunoparalysis in patients with advanced cancer (Lippitz, 2013). Both cytokines have specific prognostic effects since their high concentrations are associated with a negative prognosis in different types of cancer (Lippitz, 2013).

Although it may seem like a contradiction, it is a useless attempt for stimulation simultaneous with the suppression of the immune system function and reflects its fatal state (Lippitz, 2013).

In 100 articles including a total of 11,583 cancer patients, the relationship between IL-6 and survival was examined, and most of these studies reported a correlation between IL-6 and the increasing tumor stage or metastases. In 86% of patients reported in 23 different cancer types, a correlation between the serum IL-6 level and survival was documented. The increase in serum IL-6 level can be considered as a systemic late-stage phenomenon independently of the initial tumor histology (Lippitz and Harris, 2016). The relationship between high serum IL-6 levels and poor prognosis was demonstrated in 16 independent cancer types, and it was also found to be correlated with the tumor size and stage in patients with lung, colorectal, gastric, breast, and renal cell cancers, bone sarcoma, melanoma, nasopharyngeal and hepatocellular cancer (Lippitz, 2013).

The IL-10 level was found to be high in 13 different cancer types and was identified as a marker of advanced disease stage or poor prognosis in diffuse large B-cell lymphoma, Hodgkin's lymphoma, bone sarcomas, gastric, pancreatic and colon cancers, hepatocellular cancer, melanoma, renal cell cancer, and non-small cell lung cancer (Lippitz, 2013).

In the study carried out by Torres et al. on patients with pancreatic ductal adenocarcinoma, the panel of 5 serum cytokines consisting of PD-ECGF, EGVEGF/PK1, NRG1-beta1/HRG1-beta1, IL-29 and B7-1/CD80 was detected for the first time, and this kit was argued to be effective both as an auxiliary tool in predicting the prognosis of the disease and in identifying new targets in treatment (Torres et al., 2015).

Colorectal cancers were especially associated with the GPS, a systemic inflammation-based prognostic scoring system. It was argued that systemic inflammation caused by circulating cytokines might increase the probability of metastatic residuals in the microenvironment (Gunawardene et al., 2019). In a systematic review study in which cytokines that could be used as prognostic factors in colorectal cancers were identified, 570 records were reviewed, and seven studies evaluating multiple cytokines were found. The seven studies included were usually based on the selections including IL-6, IL-8, IL-1β, and TNF-α cytokines, and systemic inflammation and colorectal cancer outcomes were associated with each other (Gunawardene et al., 2019).

It was suggested that the shift toward Th2 lymphocyte-derived immunosuppressive cytokines (IL-4, IL-5, IL-6, IL-9, IL-10, IL13) was effective in the development of colorectal cancer with an impaired cytotoxic response. Th1 lymphocytes synthesize anti-tumor lymphocytes such as IL-2, IL-15, and IFN-gamma (Czajka-Francus et al., 2020). The soluble IL-2 receptor functions as an IL-2 antagonist, and there is an inverse relationship between serum IFN-gamma levels (Lippitz, 2013). In patients with colorectal cancer, while Th1-derived cytokines decrease, Th2-derived cytokines are expected to be at normal and increased concentrations. Furthermore, in an advanced cancer stage or poor prognosis, while the concentration of IL-2 decreased, an increase was observed in the soluble IL-2 receptor concentration (Lippitz, 2013; Czajka-Francus et al., 2020). However, there are studies revealing that IL-1 beta, IL-2, IL-4, IL-5, IL-6, IL-8, IL-9, and IL-17 A levels increase in patients with colorectal cancer (Czajka-Francus et al., 2020, Yamaguchi et al. 2019), which proves that Th1 and Th2 cytokines may vary in patients with colorectal cancer and at different cancer stages (Czajka-Francus et al., 2020). In colorectal cancer patients with distant metastases CCL2, IL-4, IL-6, IL-7, IL-8, IL-1RA and PDGF-BB cytokine levels were also found to be high (Kantola et al., 2012).

IL-7 and IL-8 cytokines are important in the development of colon cancer, and IL-8 is known to have a role in angiogenesis, tumor growth, metastasis development, and resistance to chemotherapy. IL-8 is considered to be a negative prognostic factor for colorectal cancer (Czajka-Francus et al., 2020).

If the functional concentrations of IL-2, IL-12, IFN-gamma, and HLA-DR can be maintained, it can be a positive prognostic indicator (Lippitz, 2013). There is a need for new prognostic markers to provide optimized treatment in colorectal cancers and reduce chemotherapy toxicity and cost.

The CA-125 marker used in ovarian cancer also increases in benign tumors and is devoid of sufficient sensitivity and specificity in the differentiation of malignant and benign tumors. The IL-7 level has been suggested to be used together with CA-125 as a marker in ovarian cancer (Lambeck et al., 2007).

It was determined that serum TGF-β1 levels were high in lung, breast, colorectal, and bladder cancers, glioblastoma multiforme, and hepatocellular, renal cell and gastric carcinoma, and they were interpreted as a sign of poor prognosis in breast cancer, gastric carcinoma, and lung adenocarcinoma. Moreover, TGF-β1 was considered to be an indicator of metastasis in malignant melanoma, renal cell, colorectal, breast, gastric and non-small cell lung cancer (Lippitz, 2013).

Significantly decreased HLA-DR expression in monocytes was reported in head and neck cancers, glioblastoma, lung cancer, malignant melanoma, colon cancer, and pancreatic carcinoma. It was found that the decreased HLA-DR expression on monocytes or tumor tissue was an indicator of poor prognosis and advanced disease stage in 12 different independent types of cancer (Lippitz, 2013).

MIF (macrophage migration inhibitory factor) is a proinflammatory cytokine with a significant role in innate immunity. High MIF expression is an indicator of a negative prognostic effect in gastric, breast, nasopharyngeal, head and neck, and esophageal squamous cell cancers, glioma and hepatocellular cancer. The overexpression of a single type of MIF implies that there is continuous inflammation in the cancer microenvironment (Lippitz, 2013).

The determination of the disease state by a cytokine panel rather than a single marker will make it possible to evaluate the immunological state more reliably. Creating models with reliable prognostic specificity, including as few cytokines as possible while creating cytokine sets specific to different cancers and stages, paves the way for easier and cost-effective clinical practices (Czajka-Francus et al., 2020).

Cytokines and Prognosis Monitoring in Cardiovascular System Diseases

Atherosclerosis refers to a multifactorial process that occurs in the arterial wall due to an excessive inflammatory response to harmful stimuli. Acute coronary syndrome (ACS) occurs with the rupture or erosion of the stable plaque (Heeschen et al., 2003). Atherosclerosis is the main cause of ischemic heart diseases (Amin et al., 2020). Atherosclerotic plaque becomes unstable as a result of the formation of inflammation in the vessel wall, proteolytic erosion of the connective tissue matrix, increased proinflammatory cytokine production and apoptosis, triggered by active macrophages and T cells (Heeschen et al., 2003). Furthermore, it was demonstrated that TNF-α, IL-1, and IL-6 triggered the proatherogenic gene expression (Amin et al., 2020).

Coronary plaque rupture is one of the most important causes of acute coronary syndrome. The rupture of the plate depends on its content. Macrophages are the primary inflammatory cells in the atherosclerotic plaque, and plaques rich in macrophage content are more prone to rupture (Moreno et al., 1994). T lymphocytes and active macrophages in the atherosclerotic area initiate the acute phase response with cytokine production and secretion and ensure the continuation of inflammation (Nakashima et al., 1998). Highly sensitive C-reactive protein

(HS-CRP) is synthesized in atherosclerotic plaques and is an important indicator of inflammation in unstable angina pectoris.

In addition, HS-CRP is considered to be an indicator of poor prognosis in unstable angina pectoris and ACS (Adukauskine et al., 2016).

It has been suggested that the IL-6 level is also an indicator of the intensity and sensitivity of plaque inflammation (Plutzky, 2001). It has been shown in studies that high levels of fibrinogen, which is one of the acute phase proteins, is a marker of atherosclerotic plaque formation and progression, and can also predict cardiovascular events that may develop (Kunutsor et al., 2016; Poredos and Jezovnik, 2015).

In patients with ACS, IL-10, which is an anti-inflammatory cytokine, is expected to decrease, in addition to an increase in CRP, serum amyloid A, and IL-6 levels. A high IL-10 serum level in patients with ACS was found to be associated with good outcomes. A low IL-10 level is not only an indicator of ACS triggering plaque instability but also an indicator of poor prognosis after the occurrence of an ischemic event (Kaptoge et al., 2014). Furthermore, the increased level of IL-10 in patients who could be discharged after ACS was considered as an indicator of a positive clinical course in the 6-month follow-up period (Heeschen et al., 2003).

In the study carried out in patients with coronary heart disease, IL-6, IL-18, MMP-9 (matrix metalloproteinase 9), Scd40-L (soluble CD-40 ligand), and TNF-α levels were studied, and it was concluded that many different proinflammatory cytokines were independent risk factors for coronary diseases (Kaptoge et al., 2014).

It was shown that there was an increase in the plasma levels of cytokines such as TNF, IL-1, and IL-6 in patients with heart failure (Gullestad et al., 2012). Some cytokines may be useful biomarkers to predict the prognosis. It was demonstrated that high CRP levels were correlated with the severity of disease in 4202 patients with heart failure, and they were found to be independently associated with morbidity and mortality (Anand et al., 2005). The role of CRP in cardiovascular disease primarily aims to demonstrate increased inflammatory activity, not its pathologic state in the disease. Pentraxin 3 produced at the inflammation site was found to be correlated with an increased risk of cardiac events in patients with heart failure (Gullestad et al., 2012).

Cytokines also play a significant role in post-cardiac arrest syndrome (PCAS). The excessive release of cytokines after cardiac arrest leads to ischemia-reperfusion injury, and myocardium and brain dysfunction. Interleukins, TNF, and matrix metalloproteinases have a prognostic role in PCAS. High levels of inflammatory cytokines were associated with mortality and poor neurological outcomes (Jou et al., 2020). In reperfusion injury, while TNF-α and IL-1 beta are primarily secreted, IL-6, IL-8, and IL-10 are secondarily secreted. In PCAS, serum and cerebrospinal fluid IL-6 and IL-8 levels peaked in the early period, and they were found to be associated with mortality as well as neurological/cardiological clinical outcomes. MMP-9 increases brain edema and complement activation due to damage to the blood-brain barrier. It was also found to be associated with poor clinical outcomes and mortality (Jou et al., 2020).

In patients with idiopathic and familial pulmonary arterial hypertension, it was observed that the blood levels of IL-2, IL-6, IL-8, IL-10, and IL-12p70 cytokines had a significant impact on survival, and it was concluded that they could be used in risk classification (Soon et al., 2010).

Conclusion

The inflammatory response that accompanies the etiology of diseases is regulated by cytokines. Following up the disease with a specified cytokine panel will indicate the patient's immunological state more reliably. The clinician can utilize cytokine monitoring while evaluating and classifying the patient's current state, predicting the disease outcome, and preparing a treatment plan. To this end, it is necessary to create disease-specific cytokine kits through further studies and pave the way for easier and cost-effective clinical practices.

References

Adukauskienė D, Čiginskienė A, Adukauskaitė A, Pentiokinienė D, Šlapikas R, Čeponienė I. (2016). Clinical relevance of high sensitivity C-reactive protein in cardiology. *Medicina,* (Kaunas, Lithuania) 52(1):1-10.

Amin MN, Siddiqui SA, Ibrahim M, Lukman H, Ahammed S, Kabir A, and Sultana F. (2020). Inflammatory cytokines in the pathogenesis of cardiovascular disease and cancer. *SAGE Open Medicine*, 8:2050312120965752.

Angurana SK, Bansal A, Muralidharan J, Aggarwal R, Singhi S. (2021). Cytokine Levels in Critically Ill Children with Severe Sepsis and Their Relation with the Severity of Illness and Mortality. *Journal of Intensive Care Medicine*, 36(5):576-583.

Anand IS, Latini R, Florea VG, Kuskowski MA, Rector T, Masson S, Signorini S, Mocarelli P, Hester A, Glazer R, Cohn JN, Val-HeFT Investigators. (2005). C-reactive protein in heart failure: Prognostic value and the effect of valsartan. *Circulation,* 112(10):1428-1434.

Bont L, Heijnen CJ, Kavelaars A, van Aalderen WM, Brus F, Draaisma JM, Pekelharing-Berghuis M, van Diemen-Steenvoorde RA, Kimpen JL. (2001). Local interferon-gamma levels during respiratory syncytial virus lower respiratory tract infection are associated with disease severity. *The Journal of Infectious Diseases*, 184(3):355-358.

Brand HK, Ferwerda G, Preijers F, de Groot R, Neeleman C, Staal FJT, Warris A, Hermans PWM. (2013). CD4+ T-cell counts and interleukin-8 and CCL-5 plasma concentrations discriminate disease severity in children with RSV infection. *Pediatric Research,* 73(2):187-193.

Brown PM, Schneeberger DL, Piedimonte G. (2015). Biomarkers of respiratory syncytial virus (RSV) infection: Specific neutrophil and cytokine levels provide increased accuracy in predicting disease severity. *Paediatric Respiratory Reviews*, 16(4):232-240.

Chakraborty RK, Burns B. (2021). Systemic Inflammatory Response Syndrome. In: *StatPearls* [Internet]. StatPearls Publishing.

Czajka-Francuz P, Francuz T, Cisoń-Jurek S, Czajka A, Fajkis M, Szymczak B, Kozaczka M, Malinowski KP, Zasada W, Wojnar J, Chudek J. (2020). Serum cytokine profile as a potential prognostic tool in colorectal cancer patients - one center study. *Reports of practical oncology and radiotherapy: Journal of Greatpoland Cancer Center in Poznan and Polish Society of Radiation Oncology,* 25(6):867-875.

Del Valle DM, Kim-Schulze S, Huang HH, Beckmann ND, Nirenberg S, Wang B, Lavin Y, Swartz TH, Madduri D, Stock A, Marron TU, Xie H, Patel M, Tuballes K, Van Oekelen O, Rahman A, Kovatch P, Aberg JA, Schadt E, Jagannath S, Mazumdar M, Charney AW, Firpo-Betancourt A, Mendu DR, Jhang J, Reich D, Sigel K, Cordon-Cardo C, Feldmann M, Parekh S, Merad M and Gnjatic S. (2020). An inflammatory cytokine signature predicts COVID-19 severity and survival. *Nature Medicine*, 26(10):1636-1643.

Dolan RD, Laird B, Klepstad P, Kaasa S, Horgan PG, Paulsen Ø, McMillan DC. (2019). An exploratory study examining the relationship between performance status and systemic inflammation frameworks and cytokine profiles in patients with advanced cancer. *Medicine*, 98(37):e17019.

Dolan RD, McMillan DC. (2020). The prevalence of cancer associated systemic inflammation: Implications of prognostic studies using the Glasgow Prognostic Score. *Critical Reviews in Oncology/Hematology*, 150:102962.

Gullestad L, Ueland T, Vinge LE, Finsen A, Yndestad A, Aukrust P. (2012). Inflammatory cytokines in heart failure: Mediators and markers. *Cardiology*, 122(1):23-35.

Gunawardene A, Dennett E, Larsen P. (2019). Prognostic value of multiple cytokine analysis in colorectal cancer: A systematic review. *Journal of Gastrointestinal Oncology*, 10(1):134-143.

Heeschen C, Dimmeler S, Hamm CW, Fichtlscherer S, Boersma E, Simoons ML, Zeiher AM, CAPTURE Study Investigators. (2003). Serum level of the antiinflammatory cytokine interleukin-10 is an important prognostic determinant in patients with acute coronary syndromes. *Circulation,* 107(16):2109-2114.

Jou C, Shah R, Figueroa A, Patel JK. (2020). The Role of Inflammatory Cytokines in Cardiac Arrest. *Journal of Intensive Care Medicine*, 35(3):219-224.

Kantola T, Klintrup K, Väyrynen JP, Vornanen J, Bloigu R, Karhu T, Herzig K-H, Näpänkangas J, Mäkelä J, Karttunen TJ, Tuomisto A and Mäkinen MJ. (2012). Stage-dependent alterations of the serum cytokine pattern in colorectal carcinoma. *British Journal of Cancer,* 107(10):1729-1736.

Kaptoge S, Seshasai SR, Gao P, Freitag DF, Butterworth AS, Borglykke A, Di Angelantonio E, Gudnason V, Rumley A, Lowe GDO, Jørgensen T, Danesh J. (2014). Inflammatory cytokines and risk of coronary heart disease: New prospective study and updated meta-analysis. *European Heart Journal*, 35(9):578-589.

Kunutsor SK, Kurl S, Zaccardi F, Laukkanen JA. (2016). Baseline and long-term fibrinogen levels and risk of sudden cardiac death: A new prospective study and meta-analysis. *Atherosclerosis,* 245:171-180.

Lambeck AJ, Crijns AP, Leffers N, Sluiter WJ, ten Hoor KA, Braid M, van der Zee AGJ, Daemen T, Nijman HW, Kast WM. (2007). Serum cytokine profiling as a diagnostic and prognostic tool in ovarian cancer: A potential role for interleukin 7. *Clinical Cancer Research: An Official Journal of the American Association for Cancer Research,* 13(8):2385-2391.

Le-Thi-Thu H, Nguyen-Thi-Dieu T. (2016). Study of the cytokine concentrations in unselected peripheral blood in children with asthma. *J Fran Viet Pneu*, 22(7):1-66.

Lippitz BE. (2013). Cytokine patterns in patients with cancer: A systematic review. *The Lancet Oncology*, 14(6):e218-e228.

Lippitz BE, Harris RA. (2016). Cytokine patterns in cancer patients: A review of the correlation between interleukin 6 and prognosis. *Oncoimmunology,* 5(5):e1093722.

Liu QQ, Cheng A, Wang Y, Li H, Hu L, Zhao X, Wang T, He F. (2020). Cytokines and their relationship with the severity and prognosis of coronavirus disease 2019 (COVID-19): A retrospective cohort study. *BMJ Open*, 10(11):e041471.

Lu Y, Van Bever HP, Lim TK, Kuan WS, Thiam Goh DY, Mahadevan M, Sim TB, Ho R, Larbi A, Ng TP. (2015). Obesity, asthma prevalence and IL-4: Roles of inflammatory cytokines, adiponectin and neuropeptide Y. *Pediatric Allergy and Immunology: Official Publication of the European Society of Pediatric Allergy and Immunology*, 26(6):530-536.

McAllister SS, Weinberg RA. (2014). The tumour-induced systemic environment as a critical regulator of cancer progression and metastasis. *Nature Cell Biology*, 16(8):717-727.

Moreno PR, Falk E, Palacios IF, Newell JB, Fuster V, Fallon JT. (1994). Macrophage infiltration in acute coronary syndromes. Implications for plaque rupture. *Circulation,* 90(2):775-778.

Mukherjee S, Lindell DM, Berlin AA, Morris SB, Shanley TP, Hershenson MB, Lukacs NW. (2011). IL-17-induced pulmonary pathogenesis during respiratory viral infection and exacerbation of allergic disease. *The American Journal of Pathology*, 179(1):248-258.

Nakashima Y, Raines EW, Plump AS, Breslow JL, Ross R. (1998). Upregulation of VCAM-1 and ICAM-1 at atherosclerosis-prone sites on the endothelium in the ApoE-deficient mouse. *Arteriosclerosis, Thrombosis and Vascular Biology*, 18(5):842-851.

Plutzky J. (2001). Inflammatory pathways in atherosclerosis and acute coronary syndromes. *The American Journal of Cardiology*, 88(8A):10K-15K.

Poredoš P, Ježovnik MK. (2015). Markers of preclinical atherosclerosis and their clinical relevance. *VASA Zeitschrift fur Gefasskrankheiten [VASA Journal of Vascular Diseases],* 44(4):247-256.

Saravia J, You D, Shrestha B, Jaligama S, Siefker D, Lee GI, Harding JN, Jones TL, Rovnaghi C, Bagga B, DeVincenzo JP, Cormier SA. (2015). Respiratory Syncytial Virus Disease Is Mediated by Age-Variable IL-33. *PLoS Pathogens*, 11(10):e1005217.

Soon E, Holmes AM, Treacy CM, Doughty NJ, Southgate L, Machado RD, Trembath RC, Jennings S, Barker L, Nicklin P, Walker C, Budd DC, Pepke-Zaba J, Morrell NW. (2010). Elevated levels of inflammatory cytokines predict survival in idiopathic and familial pulmonary arterial hypertension. *Circulation*, 122(9):920-927.

Torres C, Linares A, Alejandre MJ, Palomino-Morales RJ, Caba O, Prados J, Aránega A, Delgado JR, Irigoyen A, Martínez-Galán J, Ortuño FM, Rojas I and Perales S. (2015). Prognosis Relevance of Serum Cytokines in Pancreatic Cancer. *BioMed Research International,* 2015:518284.

Van Drunen Littel-van den Hurk S, Watkiss ER. (2012). Pathogenesis of respiratory syncytial virus. *Current Opinion in Virology*, 2(3):300-305.

Vázquez Y, González L, Noguera L, González PA, Riedel CA, Bertrand P and Bueno SM. (2019). Cytokines in the Respiratory Airway as Biomarkers of Severity and Prognosis for Respiratory Syncytial Virus Infection: An Update. *Frontiers in Immunology*, 10:1154.

Wu J, Shen J, Han Y, Qiao Q, Dai W, He B, Pang R, Zhao J, Luo T, Guo Y, Yang Y, Wu Q, Jiang W, Zhang J, Zhang M, Li N, Li W and Xia X. (2021). Upregulated IL-6 Indicates a Poor COVID-19 Prognosis: A Call for Tocilizumab and Convalescent Plasma Treatment. *Frontiers in Immunology*, 12:598799.

Yamaguchi M, Okamura S, Yamaji T, Iwasaki M, Tsugane S, Shetty V, Koizumi T. (2019). Plasma cytokine levels and the presence of colorectal cancer. *Plos One*, 14(3):e0213602.

Chapter 9

Autoimmune Diseases and Cytokines

Dilek Gun Bilgic[1,*], MD and Abdulkadir Bilgic[2], MD
[1]Manisa Celal Bayar University, Faculty of Medicine, Department of Medical Genetics, Manisa, Turkey
[2]Manisa State Hospital, Department of Orthopedics and Traumatology, Manisa, Turkey

Abstract

Cytokines are small cell-signaling molecules. Their receptors are located on the immune cells. Cytokines play a critical role in immune cell differentiation, migration, and function. Cytokines are widely researched for their role in autoimmune diseases. In recent years, targeted therapeutic agents targeting cytokines have been used in the treatment of autoimmune disorders.

Keywords: autoimmune diseases, cytokines, interleukins, monoclonal antibodies

Introduction

Autoimmune diseases are important diseases that affect a large number of people. While some autoimmune diseases are common, such as Hashimoto's thyroiditis, some are less common, such as Guillain-Barre syndrome. Autoimmune diseases, as the name suggests, are the result of a reaction of the immune system against the organism itself. While autoimmune diseases can sometimes be controlled with a simple treatment such as thyroxine administration in Hashimoto's disease, at other times they can be difficult to treat and life-threatening such as vasculitis.

What are Autoimmune Diseases?

Autoimmune diseases result from loss of self-tolerance. The body's immune system attacks and damages healthy body tissue. These conditions can affect almost any part of the human body.

* Corresponding Author's Email: dr_dgun@yahoo.com.

In: Cytokines and Diseases
Editors: Kenan Demir, Selim Görgün and Bahar Uslu
ISBN: 979-8-88697-214-6

The etiopathogenesis of autoimmune diseases has not yet been fully elucidated. Microorganisms, and genetic and environmental factors may play a role (Smatti et al., 2019). There are more than 80 types of autoimmune disorders. Common autoimmune disorders include: Hashimoto thyroiditis, Sjögren syndrome, Addison disease, Multiple sclerosis, systemic lupus erythematosus, dermatomyositis, Graves' disease, myasthenia gravis, pernicious anemia, reactive arthritis, rheumatoid arthritis, celiac disease, and type I diabetes (Autoimmune Disorders n.d.).

Cellular communication in the tissue or between different tissues is achieved through small molecules such as hormones, chemokines, and cytokines. A series of signal transduction begins that results in the regulation of gene expression in the nucleus. Cytokines which include interleukins, tumor necrosis factors, interferons, and chemokines, or transforming growth factor-related family factors are responsible for communication between immune cells populations (Szewczak and Donskow-Łysoniewska, 2020).

What Are Cytokines?

The term "cytokine", was suggested by Stanley Cohen after it was discovered that cytokines are also produced by cells other than lymphocytes (lymphokines) or monocytes (monokines) (Cohen et al., 1974; Flanagan et al., 1973). Cytokines have many functions. They are involved in the generation of blood cells, inflammation, immune regulation, chemotaxis, cellular growth, and differentiation. Depending on the cells they regulate, they can show either pro- or anti-inflammatory effects. Endogenous antagonists regulate the action of some cytokines (Chetaille Nézondet et al., 2020). Cytokines are grouped into superfamilies based on the receptor types with which they interact.

The major cytokine families are:

the type I/II cytokines,
the TNF family,
the IL-1 family,
the IL-17 cytokines,
the stem cell factor/receptor tyrosine kinase (STF/RTK) cytokines,
the transforming growth factor (TGF)-β family cytokines, and
the chemokines.

Type I/II Cytokines

The interleukin family, interferons (IFNs), IFN-like cytokines, colony-stimulating factors, hormones, and growth factors belong to type I/II cytokines. These families send messages through the Janus kinase (JAK) and signal transducer and the activator of transcription (STAT) pathways.

The common γ-chain cytokines include IL-2, IL-4, IL-7, IL-9, IL-15, and IL-21. The common β-chain cytokines include IL-3, IL-5, and granulocyte-macrophage colony-stimulating factor (GM-CSF).

Type I, hormone-like cytokines include erythropoietin, thrombopoietin, G-CSF, growth hormone and leptin.

Other type I cytokines are IL-6, IL-11, IL-27, IL-12, IL-23, and IL-35 (Schwartz et al., 2016). IL-4 takes a role in allergy and asthma. Dupilumab is a monoclonal antibody that inhibits the function of both interleukin IL-4 and IL-13 and is for the therapy of atopic dermatitis, asthma, and chronic rhinosinusitis with nasal polyposis (Ricciardolo et al., 2021). The monoclonal antibodies, mepolizumab and reslizumab inhibit IL-5 and are used for asthma (Calzetta et al., 2021). Tocilizumab is a monoclonal antibody to the IL-6 receptor which is used in the therapy of rheumatoid arthritis and is broadly relevant for many autoimmune diseases. In addition, due to an accentuated inflammatory response in COVID-19, several studies in the current literature about COVID-19-related respiratory failure have reported the benefits of tocilizumab and sarilumab (Angriman et al., 2021).

The monoclonal antibodies, ustekinumab and secukinumab (inhibitor) inhibit cytokines IL-12 and IL-17 respectively and, are used for the severe form of psoriasis (Simionescu et al., 2021). Type II cytokines include IFN-α, IFN-β, IFN-γ, IL-28, IL-29, IL-10, IL-19, IL-20, and IL-22. Anifrolumab is a monoclonal antibody antagonist of the type 1 interferon receptor (IFNAR). It is used for the treatment of autoimmune disorders, including systemic lupus erythematosus (SLE) and lupus nephritis.

Cytokines not only have proinflammatory effects but also anti-inflammatory actions. For example, IL-2 assists immune tolerance via upregulating the FOXP3 protein. But, in contrast with this, targeting IL-2 in MS is beneficial (Huss et al., 2015). On the other hand, while daclizumab is effective in the treatment of MS, it can cause autoimmune findings such as hair loss and skin discoloration (Giovannoni et al., 2014). Similarly, some other cytokines may show proinflammatory effects as well as anti-inflammatory effects. IL-10, IL-22 and IL-35 are examples of cytokines with anti-inflammatory effects. IL-10 inhibits T-cell-dendritic cell/macrophage signaling (Ouyang et al., 2011) and negatively regulates NLRP3 inflammasome activation to improve synovial inflammation in animal models (Greenhill et al., 2014).

TNF Family

The TNF family acts in the inflammation and immune response. The family has nearly 15 cytokines (Chu, 2013). Important members of this family are: TNFR1 and TNF-α-related apoptosis-inducing ligand (TRAIL) CD27, CD30, CD40, CD134, CD137, and Fas. These cytokines play a role in the development/suppression of many autoimmune diseases (Croft et al., 2012; Vinay and Kwon, 2011).

Some autoimmune diseases are treated with compounds targeting TNF family members (Vinay and Kwon, 2009). The TNFR1 signaling pathway is activated by the ligation of TNF-α and in the cytoplasm, complex I activates NF-κB, which causes an immune response, inflammation, tissue degeneration, and cell proliferation. Rheumatoid arthritis (RA) (Choy and Panayi, 2001), psoriatic arthritis (PsA), inflammatory bowel disease (IBD) (Adegbola et al., 2018), psoriasis (PS) (Celis et al., 2019), autoimmune uveitis, and Crohn's disease (CD) (Lis et al., 2014) are some of the autoimmune diseases related to TNFα. Infliximab is a recombinant monoclonal antibody specific for all forms of TNF-α in humans and inhibits the binding of TNF-α to its soluble and transmembrane receptors. Infliximab was recently approved by the

FDA for RA. In 1998, it was approved for the treatment of CD. Other approved diseases include ankylosing spondylitis (AS), PsA, CD and PS. Etanercept, adalimumab, certolizumab, and golimumab are other drugs blocking TNFα and approved by the FDA for the treatment of a series of autoimmune diseases (Jang et al., 2021).

The Role of IL-17 and Related Cytokines in Inflammatory Autoimmune Diseases

The immune system prevents self-reactive T cells from harming the organism. Regulatory T cells suppress self-reactive T cells. If there is an imbalance between these two cells in favor of self-reactive T cells, the risk of autoimmune disease increases. The IL-17 family is against extracellular and intracellular pathogens. Members of the IL-17 family are produced by a group of T helper cells known as T helper 17 cells in response to their stimulation with IL-23 (Happel et al., 2005). They play a role in the pathogenesis of some autoimmune diseases. An abnormal immune response predisposes to autoimmune diseases. An increased level of IL-17 results in the excessive generation of Th17 cells causing autoimmune diseases. It has been shown that IL-17A and IL-17F can enhance the expression of proinflammatory genes. IL-17 acts synergistically with these cytokines via upregulating some proinflammatory genes such as TNFα, IL-1, CXCL1, CCL20, IL-6, and G-CSF, and matrix metalloproteases through the activation of the NF-κB, MAPK and C/EBP pathways (Zhu and Qian, 2012). The activation of IL-17R results in the signaling of the adaptor protein Act1 and the tumor necrosis factor receptor-associated factor (TRAF) (Kuwabara et al., 2017). Autoimmune diseases such as RA, ankylosing spondylitis, psoriasis, and MS, clinical studies on humanized anti-IL-23 antibodies, humanized anti-IL-17 antibodies, and humanized IL-17R antibodies have been performed and the results have shown the benefits of these agents (Kopp et al., 2015; Kuwabara et al., 2017; Leonardi et al., 2008).

Effect of SCF on Inflammatory Cells

Stem cell factor (SCF), also termed mast cell growth factor or Kit ligand, binds the c-kit protooncogene product (Huang et al., 1990). Mast cells and eosinophils produce SCF (Hartman et al., 2001) and its c-Kit receptor at the cell membrane (Yuan et al., 1997). SCF by itself stimulates mast cell development, chemotaxis, degranulation, and mast cell adhesion (Columbo et al., 1992). The direct effects of SCF on eosinophils include the development of eosinophils which is enhanced by granulocyte colony stimulating factor G-CSF (Metcalf et al., 2002).

As SCF is upregulated in inflammatory conditions, it may be a potential therapeutic target for the inflammatory diseases in which mast cells or eosinophils increase such as asthma and allergic rhinitis (Reber et al., 2006).

TGF-β

Transforming growth factor beta (TGF-β) belongs to a transforming growth factor superfamily. TGF-β plays a regulatory role in the formation, maturation, proliferation and apoptosis of various cell types; additionally, in limiting autoimmunity; tumor surveillance; physiological immune response and tolerance. It also has functions such as inflammation and fibrosis development (Morikawa et al., 2016). Smads are activated in response to stimulation of the TGF-β receptors (TβRs) and maintain signaling within the cell. TGF-β plays a crucial role in the proper function of the human immune system. Pathologies in its function are involved in the disease mechanism of thyroid autoimmunity (Yang et al., 2010). The major histocompatibility complex (MHC) is a group of molecules that are important in initiating immune responses via presenting extracellular foreign proteins. They are found on antigen-presenting cells such as dendritic cells, mononuclear phagocytes, some endothelial cells, and B cells. TGF-β prevents the maturation of dendritic cells and, inhibits the upregulation of MHC class II. TGF-β deficiency contributes to Graves' disease's pathogenesis via an increase of the expression of MHC (major histocompatibility complex) class II antigens; inhibition of the suppressive activity of Tregs (T regulatory cells); alteration of Th1 cell- and Th2 cell-regulated responses; increased T-cell and B-cell proliferation, maturation, and differentiation; and increased production of antibodies (Ganesh et al., 2011). A decrease in serum TGF-β concentrations was found in Hashimoto's thyroiditis, causing the above-mentioned effects (Chen et al., 2000).

Chemokines

Chemokines are small, chemotactic cytokines that interact with specific seven-transmembrane G-protein coupled receptors (GPCRs). Approximately 50 chemokines have been identified to date. They are considered to be responsible for the development of inflammatory diseases and cancer. Hence, their functional inhibition for treating these diseases has been sought in many studies (Shachar and Karin, 2013). The MCP chemokine family members, including CCL2, CCL7, and CCL8, have a high homology which is considered to be an influential chemotactic factor for leukocytes, particularly monocytes and macrophages (Taghavi et al., 2019). The ligation of CCL2 with its receptor, CCR2, can induce different signaling pathways, including the JAK2/signal transducer and activator of transcription 3 (STAT3), mitogen-activated protein kinase (MAPK), and phosphatidylinositol-3-kinase (PI3K). Several previous studies reported that CCL2 increased significantly in the synovium fluid of patients with RA (Koch et al., 1992). In one study, ABN912 (human anti-CCL2 monoclonal antibody) was administered to patients with RA and a dose-dependent increase in ABN912-complex total CCL2 levels in peripheral blood was reported. Also, there were no significant benefits in RA patients treated with ABN912 compared to the placebo-treated group (Haringman et al., 2006; Miyabe et al., 2019, 2020).

This observation may be relevant for a variety of antibody-based therapies. Various chemoattractant factors are overexpressed by resident cells in the RA synovium, and this may be related to ongoing signalization owing to other cytokines. Tofacitinib/baricitinib, inhibitors of the JAK/STAT signaling pathway were found to be beneficial in RA via a reduction of inflammation and RA complications (Bechman et al., 2019).

Conclusion

In conclusion, recent advances in cytokine research and the increased development of inhibitory monoclonal antibodies lead to new therapeutic approaches in the treatment of autoimmune diseases. The overlap of the pathogenesis of different autoimmune diseases gives the chance to try new molecules in the treatment of each disease.

References

Adegbola SO, Sahnan K, Warusavitarne J, Hart A, Tozer P. (2018). Anti-TNF Therapy in Crohn's Disease. *International Journal of Molecular Sciences Multidisciplinary Digital Publishing Institute,* 19:2244.

Angriman F, Ferreyro BL, Burry L, Fan E, Ferguson ND, Husain S, Keshavjee SH, Lupia E, Munshi L, Renzi S, Ubaldo OGV, Rochwerg B, Sorbo LD. (2021). Interleukin-6 receptor blockade in patients with COVID-19: placing clinical trials into context. *The Lancet Respiratory Medicine Elsevier,* 9:655-664.

Bechman K, Subesinghe S, Norton S, Atzeni F, Galli M, Cope AP, Winthrop KL, Galloway JB. (2019). A systematic review and meta-analysis of infection risk with small molecule JAK inhibitors in rheumatoid arthritis. *Rheumatology,* 58:1755-1766.

Calzetta L, Aiello M, Frizzelli A, Bertorelli G, Ritondo BL, Rogliani P, Chetta A. (2021). The Impact of Monoclonal Antibodies on Airway Smooth Muscle Contractility in Asthma: A Systematic Review. *Biomedicines Multidisciplinary Digital Publishing Institute*, 9:1281.

Celis R, Cuervo A, Ramírez J, Cañete JD. (2019). Psoriatic Synovitis: Singularity and Potential Clinical Implications. *Front Med,* (Lausanne) 6:14.

Chen K, Wei Y, Sharp GC, Braley-Mullen H. (2000). Characterization of thyroid fibrosis in a murine model of granulomatous experimental autoimmune thyroiditis. *Journal of Leukocyte Biology,* 68:828-835.

Chetaille Nézondet A-L, Poubelle PE, Pelletier M. (2020). The evaluation of cytokines to help establish diagnosis and guide treatment of autoinflammatory and autoimmune diseases. *Journal of Leukocyte Biology*, 108:647-657.

Choy EH, Panayi GS. (2001). Cytokine pathways and joint inflammation in rheumatoid arthritis. *N Engl J Med*, 344:907-916.

Chu W-M. (2013). Tumor necrosis factor. *Cancer Letters,* 328:222-225.

Cohen S, Bigazzi PE, Yoshida T. (1974). Commentary. Similarities of T cell function in cell-mediated immunity and antibody production. *Cell Immunol*, 12:150-159.

Columbo M, Horowitz EM, Botana LM, MacGlashan DW, Bochner BS, Gillis S, Zsebo KM, Galli SJ, Lichtenstein LM. (1992). The human recombinant c-kit receptor ligand, rhSCF, induces mediator release from human cutaneous mast cells and enhances IgE-dependent mediator release from both skin mast cells and peripheral blood basophils. *The Journal of Immunology American Association of Immunologists,* 149:599-608.

Croft M, Duan W, Choi H, Eun S-Y, Madireddi S, Mehta A. (2012).. TNF superfamily in inflammatory disease: Translating basic insights. *Trends in Immunology*, 33:144-152.

Deeks ED. (2021). Anifrolumab: First Approval. *Drugs,* 81:1795-1802.

Flanagan TD, Yoshida T, Cohen S. (1973). Production of macrophage migration inhibition factors by virus-infected cell cultures. *Infect Immun*, 8:145-150.

Ganesh BB, Bhattacharya P, Gopisetty A, Prabhakar BS. (2011). Role of Cytokines in the Pathogenesis and Suppression of Thyroid Autoimmunity. *Journal of Interferon and Cytokine Research,* Mary Ann Liebert Inc publishers 31:721-731.

Giovannoni G, Gold R, Selmaj K, Havrdova E, Montalban X, Radue E-W, Stefoski D, McNeill M, Amaravadi L, Sweetser M, Elkins J, O'Neill G. (2014). Daclizumab high-yield process in relapsing-remitting multiple sclerosis (SELECTION): A multicentre, randomised, double-blind extension trial. *The Lancet Neurology*, 13:472-481.

Greenhill CJ, Jones GW, Nowell MA, Newton Z, Harvey AK, Moideen AN, Collins FL, Bloom AC, Coll RC, Robertson AA, Cooper MA, Rosas M, Taylor PR, O'Neill LA, Humphreys IR, Williams AS, Jones SA. (2014). Interleukin-10 regulates the inflammasome-driven augmentation of inflammatory arthritis and joint destruction. *Arthritis Res Ther*, 16:419.

Happel KI, Dubin PJ, Zheng M, Ghilardi N, Lockhart C, Quinton LJ, Odden AR, Shellito JE, Bagby GJ, Nelson S, Kolls JK. (2005). Divergent roles of IL-23 and IL-12 in host defense against Klebsiella pneumoniae. *Journal of Experimental Medicine*, 202:761-769.

Haringman JJ, Gerlag DM, Smeets TJM, Baeten D, van den Bosch F, Bresnihan B, Breedveld FC, Dinant HJ, Legay F, Gram H, Loetscher P, Schmouder R, Woodworth T, Tak PP. (2006). A randomized controlled trial with an anti-CCL2 (anti–monocyte chemotactic protein 1) monoclonal antibody in patients with rheumatoid arthritis. *Arthritis and Rheumatism,* 54:2387-2392.

Hartman M-L, Piliponsky AM, Temkin V, Levi-Schaffer F. (2001). Human peripheral blood eosinophils express stem cell factor. *Blood,* 97:1086-1091.

Huang E, Nocka K, Beier DR, Chu T-Y, Buck J, Lahm H-W, Wellner D, Leder P, Besmer P. (1990). The hematopoietic growth factor KL is encoded by the SI locus and is the ligand of the c-kit receptor, the gene product of the W locus. *Cell,* 63:225-233.

Huss DJ, Mehta DS, Sharma A, You X, Riester KA, Sheridan JP, Amaravadi LS, Elkins JS, Fontenot JD. (2015). In Vivo Maintenance of Human Regulatory T Cells during CD25 Blockade. *The Journal of Immunology American Association of Immunologists*, 194:84-92.

Jang D, Lee A-H, Shin H-Y, Song H-R, Park J-H, Kang T-B, Lee S-R, Yang S-H. (2021). The Role of Tumor Necrosis Factor Alpha (TNF-α) in Autoimmune Disease and Current TNF-α Inhibitors in Therapeutics. *International Journal of Molecular Sciences Multidisciplinary Digital Publishing Institute,* 22:2719.

Koch AE, Kunkel SL, Harlow LA, Johnson B, Evanoff HL, Haines GK, Burdick MD, Pope RM, Strieter RM. (1992). Enhanced production of monocyte chemoattractant protein-1 in rheumatoid arthritis. *J Clin Invest American Society for Clinical Investigation*, 90:772-779.

Kopp T, Riedl E, Bangert C, Bowman EP, Greisenegger E, Horowitz A, Kittler H, Blumenschein WM, McClanahan TK, Marbury T, Zachariae C, Xu D, Hou XS, Mehta A, Zandvliet AS, Montgomery D, van Aarle F, Khalilieh S. (2015). Clinical improvement in psoriasis with specific targeting of interleukin-23. *Nature,* 521:222-226.

Kuwabara T, Ishikawa F, Kondo M, Kakiuchi T. (2017). The Role of IL-17 and Related Cytokines in Inflammatory Autoimmune Diseases. *Mediators of Inflammation Hindawi,* 2017:e3908061.

Leonardi CL, Kimball AB, Papp KA, Yeilding N, Guzzo C, Wang Y, Li S, Dooley LT, Gordon KB. (2008). Efficacy and safety of ustekinumab, a human interleukin-12/23 monoclonal antibody, in patients with psoriasis: 76-week results from a randomised, double-blind, placebo-controlled trial (PHOENIX 1). *The Lancet,* 371:1665-1674.

Lis K, Kuzawińska O, Bałkowiec-Iskra E. (2014). Tumor necrosis factor inhibitors - state of knowledge. *Arch Med Sci*, 10:1175-1185.

Metcalf D, Mifsud S, Di Rago L. (2002). Stem Cell Factor Can Stimulate the Formation of Eosinophils by Two Types of Murine Eosinophil Progenitor Cells. *Stem Cells,* 20:460-469.

Miyabe Y, Lian J, Miyabe C, Luster AD. (2019). Chemokines in rheumatic diseases: Pathogenic role and therapeutic implications. *Nat Rev Rheumatol*, 15:731-746.

Miyabe Y, Miyabe C, Iwai Y, Luster AD. (2020). Targeting the Chemokine System in Rheumatoid Arthritis and Vasculitis. *JMA Journal*, 3:182-192.

Morikawa M, Derynck R, Miyazono K. (2016). TGF-β and the TGF-β Family: Context-Dependent Roles in Cell and Tissue Physiology. *Cold Spring Harb Perspect Biol,* 8:a021873.

Ouyang W, Rutz S, Crellin NK, Valdez PA, Hymowitz SG. (2011). Regulation and Functions of the IL-10 Family of Cytokines in Inflammation and Disease. *Annual Review of Immunology*, 29:71-109.

Reber L, Da Silva CA, Frossard N. (2006). Stem cell factor and its receptor c-Kit as targets for inflammatory diseases. *European Journal of Pharmacology*, 533:327-340.

Ricciardolo FLM, Bertolini F, Carriero V. (2021). The Role of Dupilumab in Severe Asthma. *Biomedicines Multidisciplinary Digital Publishing Institute*, 9:1096.

Schwartz DM, Bonelli M, Gadina M, O'Shea JJ. (2016). Type I/II cytokines, JAKs, and new strategies for treating autoimmune diseases. *Nat Rev Rheumatol,* 12:25-36.

Shachar I, Karin N. (2013). The dual roles of inflammatory cytokines and chemokines in the regulation of autoimmune diseases and their clinical implications. *Journal of Leukocyte Biology,* 93:51-61.

Simionescu AA, Danciu BM, Stanescu AMA. (2021). State-of-the-Art Review of Pregnancy-Related Psoriasis. *Medicina,* (Kaunas) 57:804.

Szewczak L, Donskow-Łysoniewska K. (2020). Cytokines and Transgenic Matrix in Autoimmune Diseases: Similarities and Differences. *Biomedicines Multidisciplinary Digital Publishing Institute,* 8:559.

Taghavi Y, Hassanshahi G, Kounis NG, Koniari I, Khorramdelazad H. (2019). Monocyte chemoattractant protein-1 (MCP-1/CCL2) in diabetic retinopathy: Latest evidence and clinical considerations. *J Cell Commun Signal*, 13:451-462.

Vinay DS, Kwon BS. (2011). The tumour necrosis factor/TNF receptor superfamily: Therapeutic targets in autoimmune diseases. *Clinical and Experimental Immunology,* 164:145-157.

Vinay DS, Kwon BS. (2009). TNF superfamily: Costimulation and clinical applications. *Cell Biology International,* 33:453-465.

Yang L, Pang Y, Moses HL. (2010). TGF-β and immune cells: An important regulatory axis in the tumor microenvironment and progression. *Trends in Immunology*, 31:220-227.

Yuan Q, Austen KF, Friend DS, Heidtman M, Boyce JA. (1997). Human Peripheral Blood Eosinophils Express a Functional c-kit Receptor for Stem Cell Factor that Stimulates Very Late Antigen 4 (VLA-4)–mediated Cell Adhesion to Fibronectin and Vascular Cell Adhesion Molecule 1 (VCAM-1). *Journal of Experimental Medicine*, 186:313-323.

Zhu S, Qian Y. (2012). IL-17/IL-17 receptor system in autoimmune disease: Mechanisms and therapeutic potential. *Clinical Science*, 122:487-511.

Chapter 10

Cytokines and Infectious Diseases

Mustafa Usanmaz*, **MD and Meltem Karslıoğlu, MD**
Samsun Gazi State Hospital, Samsun, Turkey

Abstract

Immune defense mechanisms have an important role in the pathogenesis of infections caused by infectious agents. Inflammatory and proinflammatory cytokines mediate the emergence of many infectious diseases. Today, the treatment of infectious diseases includes those aimed at reducing and preventing tissue damage caused by immune system components, as well as specific treatment for the organism.

Keywords: cytokines, inflammatory, infectious diseases

Introduction

Cytokines are powerful signaling molecules that are important to life. Cytokines are low-molecular-weight proteins. They play a mediating role in intercellular communication. Today there are many different proteins known as cytokines (Dinarello 2007). There are proinflammatory and anti-inflammatory cytokines. Cytokines are also classified according to their domains; if the cytokine acts on the cell that secretes it, it is classified as autocrine, if it acts around the place where it is released, it is paracrine, and if the cytokine acts on distant parts of the body, it is classified as endocrine. Many cytokines act locally paracrine and autocrine. Only certain blood cytokines, such as erythropoietin (EPO), transforming growth factor beta (TGF-β), and monocyte colony stimulating factor (M-CSF), have the ability to act at a distance.

Macrophages and lymphocytes are the cells responsible for cytokine production, but they can also be produced by epithelial and endothelial cells, polymorphonuclear leukocytes (PMN), connective tissue, and adipocytes. The presence of cytokines is required for the functions of macrophages (Unanue and Beller 1976; Huynh and Kay 2007).

* Corresponding Author's Email: m_usanmaz@yahoo.com.

In: Cytokines and Diseases
Editors: Kenan Demir, Selim Görgün and Bahar Uslu
ISBN: 979-8-88697-214-6

Sepsis and Cytokines

Sepsis is defined as the systemic inflammatory response to infection. The pathophysiology of sepsis includes microbial pathogens and inflammatory response. Studies have shown that the humoral system is activated and various cytokines are released as a result of infection and traumatic damage to the tissues. The result is the systemic inflammatory response, hemostatic changes, and the occurrence of organ damage (Bone 1991; Cohen 2002; Hotchkiss and Karl 2003). Some antigens and toxins initiate inflammation. This antigenic structure and toxins stimulate circulating mononuclear phagocytic cells by binding to the CD14 receptor. Tumor necrosis factor (TNF), interleukin 1 (IL-1), IL-6, IL-8, and platelet-activating factor (PAF) are released from monocytes. By activating IL-1 and IL-6 T cells, they cause the secretion of γ-interferon, IL-2, IL-4, and granulocyte-monocyte colony stimulating factors (GM-CSF) (Bone 1991; Cohen 2002) Table 1.

Inflammatory mediators in sepsis. BPI, bacterial/permeability promoting protein; CRP, C-reactive protein; IFN-g, interferon gamma; ICAM, intracellular adhesion molecule; LBP, lipopolysaccharide binding protein; IL-1Ra, interleukin-1 receptor antagonist; NO, nitric oxide; PAF, platelet activating factor; sIL-2r, soluble IL-2 receptor; sTNFr, soluble TNF receptor; PDGF, platelet-released growth factor; TGF-b, transforming growth factor; VCAM, vascular cell adhesion molecule; TNF, tumor necrosis factor

These cytokines are important and useful in local infections, but their excessive synthesis and release result in damage to the endothelial cells. Damage to the endothelium results in hemodynamic changes and organ failure (Table 2).

Nitric oxide (NO) secreted by the endothelial cell, formerly known as the endothelial depressing factor, is responsible for the widespread vasodilation in sepsis. The inflammatory response in sepsis is attempted to be balanced by mediators, some molecules, and cytokines that have opposite effects. Examples of counter-inflammatory cytokines are soluble TNF receptors and IL-1 receptor antagonists. IL-10 is the prototype of anti-inflammatory cytokines (Bone 1991; Cohen 2002; Hotchkiss and Karl 2003).

Table 1. Cytokines and their secreted cells in sepsis

Host cell	Proinflammatory mediators	Regulatory mediators	Anti-inflammatory mediators
Monocyte/macrophage	TNF-α, IL-1, IL-8, IFN-g, tissue factor, prostanoids, leukotrienes, PAF, NO	IL-6, IL-12	IL-1Ra, sTNFr, TGF-b
Neutrophils	integrin expression, superoxide, TNF-α, IL-1		BPI, defensins, acyclooxyacylhydrola
Lymphocytes	IFN-g, TNF-α	IL-12	IL-4, IL-10, sIL-2r
Endothelial cells	selectin, VCAM, ICAM, NO, tissue factor		
Platelets	serotonin	PDGF	
Plasma components	coagulation cascade, complement activation, bradykinin	CRP, LBP	

Table 2. Immune mediators, cytokines and their domains

Cytokines TNF-α, IL-1, IL-6, IL-18, IL-12, IL-15, MIF, HMGB-1	Neutrophil, lymphocyte, endothelial activation, coagulation/complement system activation, adhesion molecules, prostaglandin, nitric oxide synthetase, acute phase proteins, fever
Chemokines IL-8, MIP-1_, MIP-1_, MCP-1, MCP-3	Mobilization and activation of inflammatory cells, macrophage activation
Lipid Mediators Thromboxane A2, PAF, Prostaglandins, Leukotrienes Tissue factor (TF)	Activation of vascular endothelium and extrinsic coagulation pathway, vasoconstriction/vasodilation
Oxygen Radicals Superoxide and hydroxyl radicals NO	Antimicrobial effect, vasoconstriction/vasodilation

Table 3. Proinflammatory and anti-inflammatory cytokines in sepsis

Proinflammatory Cytokines	**Anti-Inflammatory Cytokines**
TNF-α	IL-1 Ra
IL-1	IL-4
IL-6	IL-10
IL-8	IL-13
PAF	sTNFR

After the first encounter of the microorganism and the host, a widespread activation begins in the innate immune system, including humoral and cellular immunity. At this point, mononuclear cells play a key role by releasing classical proinflammatory cytokines [such as interleukin (IL)-1, IL-6, and TNF]. TNF and IL-1 form the prototype of inflammatory cytokines and are highly effective in the formation of septic shock due to LPS (Bone 1991)

In sepsis, the target organ is the vascular endothelium and almost all mediators act on the vessels. Endotoxin, TNF-α, IL-1, PAF, leukotrienes, thromboxane A2 and nitric oxide (NO) increase endothelial permeability. In addition, proinflammatory cytokines such as IL-1 and IL-6 strongly trigger coagulation. IL-10 regulates coagulation by inhibiting tissue factor release from monocytes (Cohen 2002; Cavaillon and Adib-Conquy 2003; Bernard 2003).

Cytokine Storm

A cytokine storm is a highly fatal systemic inflammatory syndrome that can be triggered by various pathogens and treatments, cancer and autoimmune diseases, and includes excessive circulating cytokine levels and the hyperactivation of immune cells.

Interconnected complex cell types, signaling pathways, and cytokines are involved in the cytokine storm. Interleukin-1, interleukin-6, Interferon-γ, interleukin-18, and TNF are key cytokines that often have high levels in the cytokine storm (Schulert and Zhang 2016). Interferon-γ is a potent macrophage activator that is primarily secreted by activated T cells and NK cells. Interferon-γ causes fever, headache, dizziness, chills, and fatigue in the clinic (Vadhan and Nathan 1986). Fever is an important clinical feature of the cytokine storm and can be elicited through different mechanisms by interleukin-1, interleukin-6, or TNF. The interleukin-1-receptor antagonist anakinra is an effective agent for the treatment of certain cytokine storms (Eloseily and Weiser 2020). Interleukin-6, which is one of the important mediators of the cytokine storm, can signal in two ways: the classical cis signal and the trans signal. Activation of cis signaling results in hyper inflammation, vascular hyperpermeability, leakage, pulmonary dysfunction and hypotension, that may contribute to the cytokine storm (Kang and Tanaka 2019).

TNF may increase systemic inflammation by inducing fever and cellular apoptosis; It activates the release of interleukin-6 and can help to regulate immunity (Faulkner and Cooper 2005).

Cytokines in Viral Infections

Virus infections induce the expression of cytokines with a proinflammatory response. A strong host response is initiated at the onset of a viral infection. A cellular reaction is thought to initiate, in which cytokine production is triggered when viral surface proteins interact with cellular surface proteins. Many viral proteins not present in the infectious particle can also affect cellular signaling, leading to cytokine production (Burysek and Yeow 1999; Burysek 1999).

Herpes Simplex Virus

HSV causes some diseases such as eye, herpes, encephalitis and, genital infections. In primary HSV infection, the host responds by producing a range of cytokines. These include tumor necrosis factor alpha (TNF-α), IFN-α/β, interleukin-1β (IL-1β), IL-2, IL-6, IL-10, IL-12, IL-13, IFN-γ and granulocyte macrophage colony stimulating factor (GM-CSF) (Ellermann-Eriksen 1993; Ghanekar and Zheng 1996; Halford and Gebhardt 1996).

Cytomegalovirus

The cytokine profile of the CMV infection is typically proinflammatory production of IL-1β, IL-6, IL-12, TNF-α, IFN-α/β and IFN-γ (Peterson et al., 1992; Tay and Welsh 1997).

Epstein-Barr Virus

Infectious mononucleosis infection occurs after EBV transmission. EBV also plays a role in the pathogenesis of diseases such as Hodgkin's disease, Burkitt's lymphoma, and nasopharyngeal carcinoma. EBV infection progresses with high fever, lymphadenopathy and splenomegaly. Cytokines and chemokines produced during EBV infection include IL-1β, IL-1 receptor antagonist (IL-1Ra), IL-6, IL-8, IL-18, TNF-α, IFN-α/β, IFN-γ, monokine induced by IFN-γ (Mig), IFN-γ-inducible protein 10 (IP-10), and GM-CSF (D'Addario and Ahmad 1999; Lay and Tsao 1997; Lotz and Tsoukas 1996).

Influenza Virus

Influenza virus can cause infection in the respiratory tract after oral or nasal entry. The virus has an RNA genome and a membrane containing hemagglutinin (HA) and neuraminidase (NA). NA promotes viral release by breaking down sialic acids (Scholtissek 1991). Influenza virus infection progresses with fever, muscle pain and cough. Some cytokines and chemokines are induced during an influenza virus infection. These include IL-1, IL-2, IL-6, IL-8, IL-10, IL-15, IL-18, transforming growth factor β (TGF-β), TNF-α, IFN-α/β, IFN-γ, and GM-CSF (Hayden and Fritz 1998; Hennet and Ziltener 1992; Hofmann and Sprenger 1997).

Hepatitis B Virus

As with most viral infections, the main mediators of hepatic pathology in HBV infection are cell-mediated immunity and inflammation rather than cytopathic effects of the virus (Chisari and Ferrari 1995). It has been shown that HBV infection is associated with the production of a broad spectrum of proinflammatory cytokines and chemokines such as IL-1β, IL-6, IL-8, IL-12, TNF-α and IFN-γ (al-Wabel and al-Janadi 1993; Geneva-Popova and Murdjeva 1999; Gonzalez-Amaro and Garcia-Monzon 1991), as well as IL-10 which has been shown to be involved as an anti-inflammatory cytokine in HBV infection. It has been shown that IFN-γ is predominantly produced by Th1 cells in cytokine production (Hsu and Chang 1999). The role of hepatocytes in the production of TNF-α and IL-6 has been demonstrated (Gonzalez-Amaro and Garcia-Monzon 1991; Lee and Park 1998).

Human Immunodeficiency Virus

HIV is a retrovirus which infects CD4 T lymphocytes and monocytes/macrophages. In HIV infection, proinflammatory cytokines include IL-1, IL-2, IL-6, TNF-α, IFN-a/β, and IFN-γ, while anti-inflammatory cytokines include IL-4, IL-10, and IL-13 (Graziosi and Gantt 1996; Oberlin E and Amara 1996). Following acute viremia, a clinical state of increased CD4 T lymphocyte turnover occurs. This results in the immune system, especially T lymphocytes, being unable to keep up with excessive cell death, resulting in an immune deficiency and AIDS condition. Although HIV does not kill macrophages, it causes their dysfunction (Toso and Ferbas 1990).

Sars COV-2

During SARS-CoV-2 infection, there is an increase in neutrophils and other immune cells, and a detectable decrease in T cells (CD4+ and CD8+). The reduction of T cells is accompanied by an increased production of IL-6 and IL-8 (Zhang and Bastard 2020). IFNs, ILs, TNFs, and colony stimulating factors (CSFs) are the major cytokines involved in the generation of cytokine storms during COVID-19. Proinflammatory cytokines are IL-6, IL-12, IL-1β, IFN, and TNF, and anti-inflammatory cytokines/factors are IL-4, IL-7, IL-10, and TGFβ (Ding and Wang 2003; Song and Li 2020). In the case of excessive secretion of cytokines such as IFN-γ, clinical symptoms such as headache, dizziness, fever and fatigue may occur. TNF-α also causes symptoms such as fatigue, fever, and malaise, but can additionally lead to heart failure, damage to the lungs, and leakage of vessels (Shimabukuro-Vornhagen and Gödel 2018). The secretion of IL-6 triggers coagulation by causing leakage in the vessels and the occlusion of small blood vessels (Hunter and Jones 2015; Tanaka and Narazaki 2016). Cytokine storm is a fatal immune system disorder characterized by the sudden increase and hyperactivity of NK cells and T cells, especially macrophages, and excessive secretion of inflammatory cytokines and many chemical mediators (Osterholm 2005). Excessive secretion of proinflammatory cytokines causes apoptosis of the epithelial and endothelial cells in the lungs, resulting in vascular leakage, alveolar edema, and hypoxia. Overproduction of proinflammatory factors (IL-1β, IL-6, IL-8, and GM-CSF) and chemokines (IP-10, CCL2, CCL3, and CCL-5) causes lung tissue scarring and eventual death (Reghunathan and Jayapal 2005). The progression of cytokines has an important place in the immunopathogenesis of COVID-19. The first immune reaction occurs as a result of the entry of viral antigens into lung epithelial cells (Channappanavar and Fehr 2016). When viral particles enter lung epithelial cells, the apoptotic mechanism is induced and lung injury occurs and different chemokines are secreted. After the secretion of chemokines, neutrophils, alveolar macrophages, and dendritic cells gather in the lungs. Toll-like receptors (TLRs) on alveolar macrophages recognize viral particles. As a result, the secretion of proinflammatory cytokines such as IL-6, IL-18, and IL-1β, and TNF-α is activated. Other immune cells such as T cells, B cells, NK cells, and macrophages are also activated by these proinflammatory cytokines (Brisse and Wouters 2016; Schulert and Grom 2015). A defect in type-1 IFN immunity causes a delayed immune response against SARS-CoV-2 (Zhang and Bastard 2020). As a result of this delayed response, viral particles multiply uncontrollably and interferons are activated (Blanco-Melo and Nilsson-Payant 2020). Excess protein in the immune system means more cytokines and cytokine storms. The result is a hyperinflammatory reaction. These hyper-activated immune cells infiltrate the alveolar epithelium and cause severe vascular pathology and edema leading to ARDS. Multiple organ damage occurs if the inflammatory reaction spreads to other areas (Zhong and Tang 2020).

An increase in cytokine production is clinically manifested as high fever, vascular leakage, pleural effusion, and the formation of blood clots. Acute respiratory distress syndrome (ARDS) occurs due to excessive cytokine production (Drosten and Seilmaier 2013). High amounts of IFNs (IFN- γ), interleukins, and IFN-induced proteins (IP-10) have been identified in COVID-19 patients (Rakib and Nain 2021).

The clinical manifestations in SARS-CoV-2 infection are usually caused by the activation of different cytokines. When there is an increase in interferon levels, fever, malaise and chills can be seen, whereas when TNF levels are high, acute symptoms such as vascular damage and lung contusions can be seen (Rabaan and Al-Ahmed 2020). High levels of interleukins can lead to diffuse intravascular coagulation (DIC), a characteristic manifestation of a cytokine storm (Pathan and Hemingway 2004).

Bacterial Infections and Cytokines

Type-1 Interferons (IFN)

These are formed by 20 polypeptides of approximately 18 kDl. They limit the spread of pathogens, especially viruses, by secreting from the infected cell. They provide a balance between proinflammatory and anti-inflammatory pathways by limiting cytokine production, contributing to antigen presentation and functions of natural killer cells. In addition, they provide the development and preservation of immunological memory.

Type I IFNs are protective especially in viral infections and play an active role in bacterial infections. They can be produced by many different cell types such as natural killer cells, monocytes, macrophages, neutrophils, fibroblasts, hepatocytes, astrocytes, and endothelial cells, especially due to intracellular pathogens and bacterial toxins. In a study, it was observed that long-term prophylaxis with IFN-γ in addition to anti-infective agents increased quality of life and long-term survival, especially in people with chronic granulomatous disease. However, more evidence is needed for long-term prophylactic treatment (Ivashkiv and Donlin 2014; Martire and Rondelli 2008).

Tumor Necrosis Factor (TNF)

Tumor necrosis factor alpha is a 17-kD polypeptide produced by monocytes, macrophages, and T lymphocytes. It is synthesized after exposure to the cell wall and the lipopolysaccharide endotoxin of Gram-positive bacteria. It plays a role in the formation of fever response and granuloma formation with IL-1. A study also showed that TNF-α increased rapidly after endotoxin and Gram-negative bacteria infusion was given to animals and humans (Michie and Manogue 1988; Cannon and Tompkins 1990; Martich and Danner 1991).

In bacterial meningitis, high TNF-α concentrations are found in the CSF, and this has not been found to be correlated with systemic concentrations. This situation also supports that TNF-α is synthesized from different regions.

In sepsis, it is responsible for the formation of many signs and symptoms, and sepsis-like symptoms occur in the endotoxin infusion given to create a similar picture, and these effects are significantly reduced in patients who are administered anti-TNF antibodies.

TNF-α plays an active role in facultative intracellular bacterial infections and granuloma formation. It has been shown that exogenous TNF-α administration in Legionella pneumophilia infections reduces mortality (Blanchard and Friedman 1989; Blanchard and Djeu 1988; Ohga and Ueda 1991).

An increase in bacterial proliferation was demonstrated in mice infected with Listeria monocytogenes and subsequently administered anti-TNF agents. Again, more TNF-α was found in serum samples obtained from people with tuberculoid leprosy, which is known to be caused by Mycobacterium leprae and has a better prognosis than lepromatous leprosy (Opal et al., 1991; Silva and Bayston 1990).

TNF-α given as an infusion before the infection develops has been shown to decrease the induction of cytokine receptors and reduce mortality and morbidity in bacterial infections that may develop afterwards (Wallach and Holtmann 1988).

Interleukin-1

In terms of IL-la and IL-lß, they are recognized by the same receptors. They are produced by monocytes, macrophages, microglial cells, astrocytes, endothelial cells, and fibroblasts. Their synthesis is induced by endotoxins with lipopolysaccharide structures, Gram-positive cell wall structures, and other bacterial products. TNF-α and IL-1 can also induce their own production (Dinarello 1991).

In high-dose IL-1 infusion, a hemodynamic pattern similar to sepsis, such as hypotension and leukopenia, may occur. If TNF-α is given simultaneously, this effect appears more strongly (Okusawa and Gelfand et al., 1988).

In the picture of bacterial meningitis, it increases the transmission of neutrophils in the systemic circulation to the CSF and the permeability of the blood-brain barrier. A correlation was found between the concentration of IL-lß in the CSF and the degree of meningeal inflammation, the development of neurological sequelae, and mortality (Mustafa and Lebel MH 1989; Waage and Halstensen 1989).

It is very effective in the formation of a host response in the invasion of intracellular bacteria such as Listeria monocytogenes. It has been shown to reduce endotoxin-induced effects in experimental mice which have been given prior IL-1 treatment, and it has also been shown to reduce mortality in Klebsiella pneumonia, Listeria monocytogenes, and Pseudomonas aeruginosa infections (Van Deuren and Marcel 1992).

Interleukin-6

This is a 21-26 kD glycoprotein. It induces acute-phase protein secretion and B-cell differentiation in hepatocytes during infection (Schindler and Mancilla 1990).

It is detected in the circulation shortly after the experimental endotoxin infusion and reaches a maximum level within 3 hours. Like 558-613 TNF-α and IL-1, there are no obvious signs of sepsis after experimental infusion, but sepsis can also be detected at high concentrations and is associated with disease severity and a correlated APACHE-2 score (Van Deuren and Marcel 1992).

In bacterial meningitis, it reaches detectable levels in the CSF and is correlated with the leukocyte count. A high concentration of IL-6 is detected in the CSF associated with the leukocyte count and a low blood/CSF glucose ratio (Waage and Halstensen 1989; Nadal and Leppert 1989; Arditi and Manogue 1990; Rusconi and Panzzi 1991).

Bacteria and bacterial fimbriae, which are the source of urinary tract infection, stimulate the release of cytokines (IL-1α, IL-1β, IL-8, especially IL-6) in kidney epithelial cells (Hedges and Svanborg 1994).

In E. coli-induced pyelonephritis, a rapid decrease in IL-6 was shown after antibiotic treatment. However, this net decrease was not observed in patients who received empirical antibiotic treatment before reproduction (Horcajada and Velasco 2004).

IL-6 was also found to be significantly higher in patients with pneumococcal pneumonia at admission. Considering that CRP is affected by many factors, it has also been shown that IL-6 is more beneficial in the follow-up of community-acquired pneumonia. However, it is known that systemic corticosteroid therapy applied in many pneumonia patients also reduces the cytokine response (Endeman et al., 2011).

Interleukin-8

This is a small peptide with a molecular weight of 6-8 kDa. Due to its ability to activate neutrophils, an experimental IL-8 injection causes immediate neutrophilia. Again, after an experimental lipopolysaccharide injection, it reaches high concentrations in the plasma, similar to IL-6, and its increased concentrations were associated with survival in sepsis caused by bacterial infection (Van Deurenand Marcel 1992).

Interleukin-1 Receptor Antagonist

This is an 18-21 kD glycoprotein produced by monocytes. It increases in the first 24 hours after the experimental endotoxin infusion (Granowitz and Santos 199l). It has been shown to increase the survival of Gram-negative and positive-induced septicemia (Ohlsson and Bjòrk 1990) in patients with invasive meningococcal disease. After treatment with third-generation cephalosporins, the most significant decrease in cytokines was observed in IL-1Ra levels (Endeman and Meijvis 2011; Beran and Lawrence 2009).

Fungi and Cytokines

Due to the widespread use of broad-spectrum antibiotics, the increase in the immunosuppressive population, and the development of invasive treatment technology, the incidence of fungal infections is increasing and systemic treatment is required. In addition to treatment, neutrophils, macrophages, and cytokines constitute the first line of body defense against pathogens (Wang and Yang 2020).

First, the cellular immune system is stimulated against fungi and mycoses. Th1 cells provide a protective host defense against fungi by producing cytokines (IL-12), which basically stimulate the cellular immune response and phagocyte activation, such as IFN-γ.

An increase in IL-4 and IL-5 levels is an indicator of a poor prognosis, especially in rapidly progressing common or recurrent endemic mycoses (Blanco 2008).

Again, IL-4 triggers a Th1 response, which is protective, and Th2 reactivity, which prevents fungal allergy. Likewise, newborns with IL-12/IL-23/IFN-γ disorders are more susceptible to endemic mycoses due to an insufficient immune response (Zerbe 2005).

In disseminated candidosis cases, IL-17 increases neutrophil mobilization and contributes to the formation of a granuloma structure against fungi. Together with IL-23, neutrophil apoptosis is also reduced (Huang 2004).

Increased susceptibility to Candida albicans has been observed in IL-17 receptor deficient mice. Again, the IL-17 level was found to be higher in patients with candidemia compared to healthy subjects (Wang and Yang 2020).

IL-10, TGF-beta and IL-4 are involved in the prevention of allergic reactions against fungi. The Th1-type cellular immune response functions to eliminate fungi, and the Th2 immune response is often responsible for allergic reactions, or for instance IL-3 and IL-4. It is responsible for the elimination of fungi through the release of cytokines (Blanco and Garcia 2008; Romani 2008).

Conclusion

Cytokines are peptide agents that play a major role in intercellular communication and activate the immune system. They are produced by immune element cells such as macrophages, BT lymphocytes, mast cells and endothelium, fibroblasts, and various stromal cells and participate in the system. They can be produced simultaneously by more than one cell type (Stedman 2006).

Interleukins (IL) play an important role in the activation and differentiation, proliferation, maturation, migration, and adhesion of immune system cells. They are both anti-inflammatory and proinflammatory. Due to these properties, they have been the subject of many clinical studies and are widely used on animals (Vaillant and Qurie 2020).

Cytokines play an important role in the formation and suppression of signs and symptoms in many infective diseases and even in determining treatment strategies. For this reason, more comprehensive, multidisciplinary studies are required in terms of both examination and treatment.

References

al-Wabel A., al-Janadi M., Raziuddin S. (1993) Cytokine profile of viral and autoimmune chronic active hepatitis. *J Allergy Clinic Immunol* 92:902-908.

Arditi M., Manogue K. R., Caplan M., Yogev R. (1990) Cerebrospinal fluid cachectin/tumor necrosis factor-a and platelet-activating factor concentrations and severity of bacterial meningitis in children. *J Infect Dis* 162:139-47.

Beran O., Lawrence D. A., Andersen N. O. Dzupova, J. Kalmusova, M. Musilek, M. Holub (2009) Sequential analysis of biomarkers in cerebrospinal fluid and serum during invasive meningococcal disease. *European Journal of Clinical Microbiology and Infectious Diseases* 28(7):793-799.

Bernard G. R. (2003) Drotrecogin alfa (activated) (recombinant human activated protein C) for the treatment of severe sepsis. *Crit care Med* 31:85-93.

Blanchard D. K., Djeu J. Y., Klein T. W., Friedman H., Stewart II W. E. (1988) Protective effects of tumor necrosis factor in experimental Legionella Pneumophilia infections of mice via activation of PMN function. *J Leukocyte Biol* 43:429-35.

Blanchard D. K., Friedman H., Klein T. W., Djeu J. Y. (1989) Induction of interferon-gamma and tumor necrosis factor by Legionella pneunioplnha: augmentation of human neutrophil bactericidal activity. *J Leukoc Biol* 45:538-45.

Blanco J. L., Garcia M. E. (2008) Immune response to fungal infections. *Vet Immunol Immunopathol* 125:47-70.

Blanco-Melo D., Nilsson-Payant B. E., Liu W. C., Uhl S., Hoagland D., Møller R., Jordan T. X., Oishi K., Panis M., Sachs D., Taia T. Wang, Robert E. Schwartz, J. K Lim, Randy A. Albrecht, Benjamin R. tenOever (2020) Imbalanced Host Response to SARS-CoV-2 Drives Development of COVID-19. *Cell* 181:1036-1045. https://doi.org/10.1016/j.cell.2020.04.026.

Bone R. C. (1991) The pathogenesis of sepsis. *Ann Intern Med* 115:457.

Brisse E., Wouters C. H., Matthys P. (2016) Advances in the pathogenesis of primary and secondary haemophagocyticlymphohistiocytosis: Differences and similarities. *br. J. Haematol* 174:203=217 https://doi.org/10.1111/bjh.14147.

Burysek L., Yeow W. S., Lubyova B., Kellum M., Schafer S. L., Huang Y. Q., Pitha P. M. (1999) Functional analysis of human herpesvirus 8-encoded viral interferon regulatory factor 1 and its association with cellular interferon regulatory factors and p300. *J Virol* 73:7334-7342.

Burysek L., Yeow W. S., Pitha P. M. (1999) Unique properties of a second human herpesvirus 8-encoded interferon regulatory factor (vIRF-2) *J Hum Virol* 2:19-32.

Cannon J. G., Tompkins R. G., Gelfand J. A., Michie H. R., Stanford G. G., Van Der Meer J. W., Dinarello C. A. (1990) Circulating interleukin-1 and tumor necrosis factor in septic shock and experimental endotoxin fever. *Journal of Infectious Diseases* 161(1):79-84.

Cavaillon J. M., Adib-Conquy M., Fitting C., Adrie C., Payen D. (2003) Cytokine cascade in sepsis *Scand J Infect Dis* 35(9):535-44.

Channappanavar R., Fehr A. R., Vijay R., Mack M., Zhao J., Meyerholz D. K., Perlman S. (2016) Deregulated Type I Interferon and Inflammatory Monocyte-Macrophage Responses Cause Fatal Pneumonia in SARS-CoV-Infected Mice. *Cell Host Microbe* 19: 181-193. https://doi.org/10.1016/j.chom.2016.01.007.

Chisari F. V., Ferrari C. (1995) Hepatitis B virus immunopathology. *Springer Semin Immunopathol* 17:261-281.

Cohen J. (2002) The immunopathogenesis of sepsis. *Nature* 420:885-91.

D'Addario M., Ahmad A, Xu J. W., Menezes J. (1999) Epstein-Barr virus envelope glycoprotein gp350 induces NF-κB activation and IL-1β synthesis in human monocytes-macrophages involving PKC and P13-K. *FASEB J* 13:2203-2213.

Dinarello C. A. (1991) Interleukin-1 and interleukin-1 antagonism. *Blood* 8:1627-52.

Dinarello C. A. (2007) Historical view of cytokines. *Eur J Immunol* 37:(Annex 1):S34-45. https://doi.org/10.1002/eji.200737772.

Ding Y., Wang H., Shen H., Li Z., Geng J., Han H., Cai J., Li X., Kang W., Weng D., Yaodan Lu, Dehua Wu, Li He, Kaitai Yao (2003) The clinical pathology of the severe acute respiratory syndrome (SARS): A report from China. *J Pathol* 200:282-289. https://doi.org/10.1002/path.1440.

Drosten C., Seilmaier M., Corman V. M., Hartmann W., Scheible G., Sack S., Guggemos W., Kallies R., Muth D., Junglen S., Marcel A. Müller, Walter Haas, Hana Guberina, Tim Röhnisch, Monika Schmid-Wendtner, Souhaib Aldabbagh, Ulf Dittmer, Hermann Gold, Petra Graf, Frank Bonin, Andrew Rambaut, Clemens-Martin Wendtner (2013) Clinical features and virological analysis of a case of Middle East respiratory syndrome coronavirus infection. *Lancet Infect Teeth* 13:745-751. https://doi.org/10.1016/S1473-3099(13)70154-3.

Ellermann-Eriksen S. (1993) Autocrine secretion of interferon-α/β and tumor necrosis factor-α synergistically activates mouse macrophages after infection with herpes simplex virus type 2. *J Gene Virol* 74:2191-2199.

Eloseily E. M., Weiser P., Crayne C. B., Hilary Haines, Melissa L. Mannion, Matthew L. Stoll, Timothy Beukelman, T. Prescott Atkinson, Randy Q. Cron (2020) Benefit of anakinra in treating pediatric secondary hemophagocytic lymphohistiocytosis. *Arthritis Rheumatol* 72:326-334.

Endeman H. S. C. A., Meijvis S. C. A., Rijkers G. T., van Velzen-Blad H., Van Moorsel C. H. M., Grutters J. C., Biesma D. H. (2011) Systemic cytokine response in patients with community-acquired pneumonia. *European Respiratory Journal* 37(6):1431-1438.

Faulkner L., Cooper A., Fantino C., Altmann D. M., Sriskandan S. (2005) The mechanism of superantigen-mediated toxic shock: not a simple Th1 cytokine storm. *J Immunol* 175:6870-6877.

Geneva-Popova M., Murdjeva M. (1999) Study on proinflammatory cytokines (IL-1β, IL-6, TNF-α) and IL-2 in patients with acute hepatitis B. *Folia Med* 41:78-81.

Ghanekar S., Zheng L., Logar A., Navratil J., Borowski L., Gupta P., Rinaldo C. (1996) Cytokine expression by human peripheral blood dendritic cells stimulated in vitro with HIV-1 and herpes simplex virus. *J Immunol* 157:4028-4036.

Gonzalez-Amaro R., Garcia-Monzon C., Garcia-Buey L., Moreno-Otero R., Alonso J. L., Yague E., Pivel J. P., Lopez-Cabrera M., Fernandez-Ruiz E., Sanchez-Madrid F. (1994) Induction tumor necrosis chronic Factor α production by human hepatocytes in viral hepatitis. *J Exp Med* 179:841-848.

Granowitz E. V., Poutsiaka D. D., Cannon J. G., Wolff S. M., Dinarello C. A., Santos A. A., Wilmore, D. W. (1991) Production of interleukin-1-receptor antagonist during experimental endotoxaemia. *The Lancet* 338(8780):1423-1424.

Graziosi C., Gantt K. R., Vaccarezza M., Demarest J. F., Daucher M., Saag M. S., Shaw G. M., Quinn T. C., Cohen O. J., Welbon C. C., Pantaleo G., Fauci A. S. (1996) Kinetics of cytokine expression during primary human immunodeficiency virus type 1 infection. *Proc Natl Acad Sci USA* 93:4386-4391.

Halford W. P., Gebhardt B. M., Carr D. J. (1996) Persistent cytokine expression in trigeminal ganglion latently infected with herpes simplex virus type 1. *J Immunol* 157:3542-3549.

Hayden F. G., Fritz R. S., Lobo M. C., Alvord W. G., Strober W., Straus S. E. (1998) Local and systemic cytokine responses during experimental human influenza A virus infection. Relation to symptom formation and host defense. *J Clin Investig* 101:643-649.

Hedges S., Svanborg C. (1994) The mucosal cytokine response to urinary tract infections. *International journal of antimicrobial agents* 4(2):89-93.

Hennet T., Ziltener H. J., Frei K., Peterhans E. (1992) A kinetic study of immune mediators in the lungs of mice infected with influenza A virus. *J Immunol* 149:932-939.

Hofmann P., Sprenger H., Kaufmann A., Bender A., Hasse C., Nain M., Gemsa D. (1997) Susceptibility of mononuclear phagocytes to influenza A virus infection and possible role in the antiviral response. *J Leukoc Biol* 61:408-414.

Horcajada J. P., Velasco M., Filella X., Luisa Alvarez, Elisa De Làzzari, Jose Luis Marín, Blanca Collvinent, Alex Smithson, Jose Antonio Martínez, Mariana Noguero, Jordi Vila, Josep Mensa (2004) Evaluation of inflammatory and renal-injury markers in women treated with antibiotics for acute pyelonephritis caused by Escherichia coli. *Clinical and Diagnostic Laboratory Immunology* 11(1):142-146.

Hotchkiss R. S., Karl I. E. (2003) The Pathophysiology and treatment of sepsis. *N Engl J Med* 348/2:138-150.

Hsu H. Y., Chang M. H., Ni Y. H., Lee P. I. (1999) Cytokine release of peripheral blood mononuclear cells in children with chronic hepatitis B virus infection. *J Pediatr Gastroenterol Nutr* 29:540-545.

Huang W., Na L., Fidel P. L., Schwarzenberger P. (2004) Requirement of interleukin-17A for systemic anti-Candida albicans host defense in mice. *The Journal of infectious diseases*190(3):624-631. https://doi.org/10.1086/422329.

Hunter C. A., Jones S. A. (2015) IL-6 as a keystone cytokine in health and disease. *Nature immunology* 16(5):448-457. https://doi.org/10.1038/ni.3153.

Huynh K. K., Kay J. G., Stow J. L., Grinstein S. (2007) Fusion, fission, and secretion during phagocytosis. *Physiology (Bethesda, Md)* 22:366-372. https://doi.org/10.1152/physiol.00028.2007.

Ivashkiv L. B., Donlin L. T. (2014) Regulation of type I interferon responses. *Nat Rev Immunol* 14(1):36-49. https://doi.org/10.1038/nri3581.

Kang S., Tanaka T., Narazaki M., Kishimoto T. (2019) Targeting Interleukin-6 Signaling in Clinic. *Immunity* 50(4):1007-1023. https://doi.org/10.1016/j.immuni.2019.03.026.

Lay J. D., Tsao C. J., Chen J. Y., Kadin M. E., Su I. J. (1997) Upregulation of tumor necrosis factor-alpha gene by Epstein-Barr virus and activation of macrophages in Epstein-Barr virus-infected T cells in the pathogenesis of hemophagocytic syndrome. *The Journal of clinical investigation* 100(8):1969-1979. https://doi.org/10.1172/JCI119728.

Lee Y., Park U. S., Choi I., Yoon S. K., Park Y. M., Lee Y. I. (1998) Human interleukin 6 gene is activated by hepatitis B virus-X protein in human hepatoma cells. *Clinical cancer research: an official journal of the American Association for Cancer Research* 4(7):1711-1717.

Lotz M., Tsoukas C. D., Fong S., Dinarello C. A., Carson D. A., Vaughan J. H. (1996) Release of lymphokines after Epstein Barr virus infection in vitro. I. Sources of and kinetics of production of interferons and interleukins in normal humans. *J Immunol* 136:3636-3642.

Martich G. D., Danner R. L., Ceska M., Suffredini A. F. (1991). Detection of interleukin 8 and tumor necrosis factor in normal humans after intravenous endotoxin: the effect of antiinflammatory agents. *The Journal of experimental medicine* 173(4):1021-1024. https://doi.org/10.1084/jem.173.4.1021.

Martire B., Rondelli R., Soresina A., Pignata C., Broccoletti T., Finocchi A., Paolo Rossi, Marco Gattorno, Marco Rabusin, Chiara Azzari, Rosa M Dellepiane, Maria C Pietrogrande, Antonino Trizzino, Paolo Di Bartolomeo, Silvana Martino, Luigi Carpino, Fausto Cossu, Franco Locatelli, Rita Maccario, Paolo Pierani, Maria C Putti, Achille Stabile, Luigi D Notarangelo, Alberto G Ugazio, Alessandro Plebani, Domenico De Mattia, IPINET (Italian Network for Primary Immunodeficiencies (2008) Clinical features, long-term follow-up and outcome of a large cohort of patients with chronic granulomatous disease: an Italian multicenter study. *Clinical immunology* 126(2):155-164.

Michie H. R., Manogue K. R., Spriggs D. R., Revhaug A., O'Dwyer S., Dinarello C. A., Anthony Cerami, Sheldon M. Wolff, Wilmore D. W. (1988) Detection of circulating tumor necrosis factor after endotoxin administration. *New England Journal of Medicine* 318(23):1481-1486.

Mustafa M. M., Lebel M. H., Ramilo O., Olsen K. D., Reisch J. S., Beutler B., McCracken G. H. Jr. (1989) Correlation of interleukin-1 beta and cachectin concentrations in cerebrospinal fluid and outcome from bacterial meningitis. *The Journal of pediatrics* 115(2):208-213. https://doi.org/10.1016/s0022-3476(89)80067-8.

Nadal D., Leppert D., Frei K., Gallo P., Lament H., Fontana A. (1989) Tumor necrosis factor-α in infectious meningitis. *Arch Dis Childh* 64:1274-1279.

Oberlin E., Amara A., Bachelerie F., Bessia C., Virelizier J. L., Arenzana-Seisdedos F., Schwartz, O., Heard J. M., Clark-Lewis I., Legler D. F., Loetscher M., Baggiolini M., Moser B. (1996) The CXC chemokine SDF-1 is the ligand for LESTR/fusin and prevents infection by T-cell-line-adapted HIV-1. *Nature* 382(6594):833-835. https://doi.org/10.1038/382833a0.

Ohga S., Ueda K., Yoshikai Y., Takeda Y., Hiromatsu K., Nomoto K. (1991) Kinetics of fever and its related cytokines in mice after intraperitoneal infection with Listen monocytogenes. *J Therm Biol* 16:103-107.

Ohlsson K., Bjòrk P., Bergenfeldt M., Hageman R., Thompson R. C. (1990) Interleukin-1 receptor antagonist reduces mortality from endotoxin shock. *Nature* (London) 348:550-552.

Okusawa S., Gelfand J. A., Ikejima T., Conolly R. J., Dinarello C. A. (1988) Interleukin 1 induces a shock-like state in rabbits. Synergism with tumor necrosis factor and the effects of cyclooxygenase inhibition. *J Clin Invest* 81:1162-1172.

Opal S. M., Cross A. S., Sadoff J. C., H. H. Collins, N. M. Kelly, G. H. Victor, J. E. Palardy, M. W. Bodmer (1991) Efficacy of antilipopolysaccharide and anti-tumor necrosis factor monoclonal antibodies in a neutropenic rat model of Pseudomonas sepsis. *J Clin Invest* 88:885-90.

Osterholm M. T. (2005) Preparing for the next pandemic. *The New England journal of medicine* 352(18):1839-1842. https://doi.org/10.1056/NEJMp058068.

Pathan N., Hemingway C. A., Alizadeh A. A., Stephens A. C., Boldrick J. C., Oragui E. E., McCabe C., Welch S. B., Whitney A., O'Gara P., Nadel S., Relman D. A., Harding S. E., Levin M. (2004) Role of interleukin 6 in myocardial dysfunction of meningococcal septic shock. *Lancet* (London, England) 363(9404):203-209. https://doi.org/10.1016/S0140-6736(03)15326-3.

Peterson P. K., Gekker G., Chao C. C., Schut R., Verhoef J., Edelman C. K., Erice A., Balfour H. H. Jr. (1992) Cocaine amplifies HIV-1 replication in cytomegalovirus-stimulated peripheral blood mononuclear cell cocultures. *Journal of immunology* (Baltimore, Md.: 1950) 149(2):676-680.

Rabaan A. A., Al-Ahmed S. H., Sah R., Tiwari R., Yatoo M. I., Patel S. K., Pathak M., Malik Y. S., Dhama K., Singh K. P., Bonilla-Aldana D. K., Haque S., Martinez-Pulgarin D. F., Rodriguez-Morales A. J., Leblebicioglu H. (2020) SARS-CoV-2/COVID-19 and advances in developing potential therapeutics and vaccines to counter this emerging pandemic. *Annals of clinical microbiology and antimicrobials* 19(1):40. https://doi.org/10.1186/s12941-020-00384-w.

Rakib A., Nain Z., Sami S. A., Mahmud S., Islam A., Ahmed S., Siddiqui A., Babu S., Hossain P., Shahriar A., Nainu F., Emran T. B., Simal-Gandara J. (2021) A molecular modelling approach for identifying antiviral selenium-containing heterocyclic compounds that inhibit the main protease of SARS-CoV-2: an in silico investigation. *Briefings in bioinformatic* 22(2):1476-1498. https://doi.org/10.1093/bib/bbab045.

Reghunathan R., Jayapal M., Hsu L. Y., Chng H. H., Tai D., Leung B. P., Melendez A. J. (2005) Expression profile of immune response genes in patients with Severe Acute Respiratory Syndrome. *BMC immunology* 6(2):1-11. https://doi.org/10.1186/1471-2172-6-2.

Rusconi F., Parizzi F., Garlaschi L., Assael B. M., Sironi M., Ghezzi P., Mantovani A. (1991) Interleukin 6 activity in infants and children with bacterial meningitis. The Collaborative Study on Meningitis. *The Pediatric infectious disease journal* 10(2):117-21. https://doi.org/10.1097/00006454-199102000-00008.

Schindler R., Mancilla J., Endres S., Ghorbani R., Clark S. C., Dinarello C. A. (1990) Correlations and interactions in the production of interleukin-6 (IL-6), IL-1, and tumor necrosis factor (TNF) in human blood mononuclear cells: IL-6 suppresses IL-1 and TNF. *Blood* 75(1): 40-47.

Scholtissek C. (1991) Synthesis and function of influenza A virus glycoproteins. *Behring Institute Mitteilungen* (89):46-53.

Schulert G. S., Grom, A. A. (2015) Pathogenesis of macrophage activation syndrome and potential for cytokine- directed therapies. *Annual review of medicine* 66:145-159. https://doi.org/10.1146/annurev-med-061813-012806.

Schulert G. S., Zhang M., Fall N., Husami A., Kissell D., Hanosh, A., Zhang K., Davis K., Jentzen J. M., Napolitano L., Siddiqui J., Smith L. B., Harms P. W., Grom A. A., Cron, R. Q. (2016) Whole-Exome Sequencing Reveals Mutations in Genes Linked to Hemophagocytic Lymphohistiocytosis and Macrophage Activation Syndrome in Fatal Cases of H1N1 Influenza. *The Journal of infectious diseases* 213(7):1180-1188. https://doi.org/10.1093/infdis/jiv550.

Shimabukuro-Vornhagen A., Gödel, P., Subklewe, M., Stemmler, H. J., Schlößer H. A., Schlaak, M., Kochanek M., Böll B., von Bergwelt-Baildon M. S. (2018) Cytokine release syndrome. *Journal for immunotherapy of cancer* 6(1):56. https://doi.org/10.1186/s40425-018-0343-9.

Silva A. T., Bayston K. F., Cohen J. (1990) Prophylactic and therapeutic effects of a monoclonal antibody to tumor necrosis factor-alpha in experimental gram-negative shock. *The Journal of infectious diseases* 162(2):421-427.

Song P., Li W., Xie J., Hou Y., You C. (2020) Cytokine storm induced by SARS-CoV-2. Clinica chimica acta; *international journal of clinical chemistry* 509:280-287. https://doi.org/10.1016/j.cca.2020.06.017.

Stedman T. L. (2006) Cytokine. In: *Stedman's Medical Dictionary,* 28th edn. Wolters Kluwer Health, Lippincott Williams & Wilkins.

Tanaka T., Narazaki M., Kishimoto T. (2016) Immunotherapeutic implications of IL-6 blockade for cytokine storm. *Immunotherapy* 8(8):959-970. https://doi.org/10.2217/imt-2016-0020.

Tay C. H., Welsh R. M. (1997) Distinct organ-dependent mechanisms for the control of murine cytomegalovirus infection by natural killer cells. *Journal of virology* 71(1):267-275. https://doi.org/10.1128/JVI.71.1.267-275.1997.

Toso J. F., Ferbas J. J., Rappocciolo G., Armstrong J. A., Ho M., Rinaldo C. R. Jr. (1990) Stimulation of IFN-alpha production in HLA-DR+, light density peripheral blood mononuclear cells by human immunodeficiency virus. *Journal of experimental pathology* 5(3):123-125.

Unanue E. R., Beller D. I., Calderon J., Kiely J. M., Stadecker M. J. (1976) Regulation of immunity and inflammation by mediators from macrophages. *The American journal of pathology* 85(2):465-478.

Vadhan-Raj S., Nathan C. F., Sherwin S. A., Oettgen H. F., Krown S. E. (1986) Phase I trial of recombinant interferon gamma by 1-hour i.v. *infusion Cancer Treat Rep* 0:609-614.

Vaillant A. A. J., Qurie A. (2020) Interleukin. In: *StatPearls* [Internet]. Avaible via https://www.ncbi.nlm.nih.gov/books/NBK499840/.

Waage A., Brandtzaeg P., Halstensen A., Kierulf P., Espevik T. (1989) The complex pattern of cytokines in serum from patients with meningococcal septic shock. Association between interleukin 6, interleukin 1, and fatal outcome. *The Journal of experimental medicine* 169(1):333-338. https://doi.org/10.1084/jem.169.1.333.

Wallach D., Holtmann H., Engelmann H., Nophar Y. (1988) Sensitization and desensitization to lethal effects of tumor necrosis factor and IL-1. *J Immunol* 140:2994-9.

Wang Q., Yang M., Wang C., Cui J., Li X., Wang C. (2020) Diagnostic efficacy of serum cytokines and chemokines in fungal bloodstream infection in febrile patients. *Journal of clinical laboratory analysis* 34(4):e23149.

Zerbe C. S., Holland S. M. (2005) Disseminated histoplasmosis in persons with interferon-gamma receptor 1 deficiency. Clinical infectious diseases: an official publication of the Infectious *Diseases Society of America* 41(4):e38-e41. https://doi.org/10.1086/432120.

Zhang Q., Bastard P., Liu Z., Le Pen J., Moncada-Velez M., Chen J., Ogishi M., Sabli I., Hodeib, S., Korol C., Rosain J., Bilguvar K., Ye J., Bolze A., Bigio B., Yang R., Arias A. A., Zhou Q., Zhang Y., Onodi F., S. Korniotis, L. Karpf, Q. Philippot, M. Chbihi, L. Bonnet-Madin, K. Dorgham, N. Smith, W. M. Schneider, B. S. Razooky, H. H. Hoffmann, E. Michailidis, L. Moens, J. Eun Han, L. Lorenzo, L. Bizien, P. Meade Anna-Lena Neehus, A. C. Ugurbil, A. Corneau, G. Kerner, P. Zhang, F. Rapaport, Y. Seeleuthner, J. Manry, C. Masson, Y. Schmitt, A. Schlüter, T. Le Voyer, T. Khan, J. Li, J. Fellay, L. Roussel, M. Shahrooei, M. F. Alosaimi, D. Mansouri, H. Al-Saud, F. Al-Mulla, F. Almourfi, S. Zaid Al-Muhsen, F. Alsohime, S. Al Turki, R. Hasanato, D. van de Beek, A. Biondi, L. Rachele Bettini, M. D'Angio,' P. Bonfanti, L. Imberti, A. Sottini, S. Paghera, E. Quiros-Roldan, C. Rossi, A. J. Oler, M. F. Tompkins, C. Alba, I. Vandernoot, J. C. Goffard, G. Smits, I. Migeotte, F. Haerynck, P. Soler-Palacin, A. Martin-Nalda, R. Colobran, P. E. Morange, S. Keles, F. Çölkesen, T. Ozcelik, K. Kart Yasar, S. Senoglu, Ş. Nur Karabela, C. Rodríguez-Gallego, G. Novelli, S. Hraiech, Y. Tandjaoui-Lambiotte, X. Duval, C. Laouénan, COVID-STORM Clinicians; COVID Clinicians; Imagine COVID Group; French COVID Cohort Study Group; CoV-Contact Cohort; Amsterdam UMC COVID-19 Biobank; COVID Human Genetic Effort; NIAID-USUHS/TAGC COVID Immunity Group; A. L. Snow, C. L. Dalgard, J. D. Milner, D. C. Vinh, T. H. Mogensen, N. Marr, A. N. Spaan, B. Boisson, S. Boisson-Dupuis, J. Bustamante, A. Puel, M. J. Ciancanelli, I. Meyts, T. Maniatis, V. Soumelis, A. Amara, M. Nussenzweig, A. García-Sastre, F. Krammer, A. Pujol, D. Duffy, R. P. Lifton, S. Y. Zhang, G. Gorochov, V. Béziat, E. Jouanguy, V. Sancho-Shimizu, C. M. Rice, L. Abel, L. D. Notarangelo, A. Cobat, Helen C. Su, Casanova J. L. (2020) Inborn errors of type I IFN immunity in patients with life-threatening COVID-19. *Science* (New York) 370:(6515), eabd4570. https://doi.org/10.1126/science.abd4570.

Zhong J., Tang J., Ye C., Dong L. (2020) The immunology of COVID-19: is immune modulation an option for treatment? *The Lancet Rheumatology* 2(7):e428-e436. https://doi.org/10.1016/S2665-9913(20) 30120-X.

Chapter 11

Cytokines and Rheumatoid Arthritis

Ferhat Arık*, MD

Tomarza State Hospital, Department of Internal Medicine, Kayseri, Turkey

Abstract

Rheumatoid arthritis is a chronic rheumatic disease with synovial involvement, cartilage and bone destruction, and an increase in morbidity. There is inflammation in the joints caused by T and B cells, macrophages, and cytokines synthesized by fibroblasts. Normally, the balance of proinflammatory and inflammatory cytokines changes in favor of proinflammatory cytokines. Interleukin (IL)-1, IL-6, IL-7, IL-18, IL-33 and tumor necrosis factor-alpha (TNF-α), the importance of which has increased recently, are the cytokines that are mainly responsible for the development of the disease. An increase in bone resorption occurs because of proinflammatory cytokine increase and collagenase, prostaglandin and osteoclast activation. The approach of suppressing cytokines in treatment is important in suppressing disease activity.

Keywords: rheumatoid arthritis, interleukin-11, interleukin-6, tumor necrosis factor, interleukin-17

Introduction

Rheumatoid arthritis (RA) is a chronic rheumatic disease with synovial involvement, cartilage and bone destruction, and an increase in morbidity. The disease is characterized by cartilage erosion, synovial joint damage and fibrous ankylosis. The pathogenesis of RA is not clear, but it is thought to develop with the contribution of multiple immunological, genetic and environmental factors (Lee and Weinblatt 2001). More than 100 genes are responsible for the pathophysiology of the disease, the most important being those responsible for the human leukocyte antigen and major histocompatibility complex. Since the incidence of disease is 12-15% in identical twins, environmental factors are thought to be effective in the pathophysiology. The most important known environmental factor is smoking (Lundström et al. 2009). Genetic or environmental factors result in an increased cytokine response, for

---

* Corresponding Author's Email: ferhatarik@gmail.com.

In: Cytokines and Diseases
Editors: Kenan Demir, Selim Görgün and Bahar Uslu
ISBN: 979-8-88697-214-6

example increased smoking causes an increased cytokine response from macrophages (Makrygiannakis et al. 2008). After encountering an antigen, cytokine synthesis is carried out by T and B cells, macrophages, and fibroblasts. Cytokines are secreted by these cells that encounter the antigen. Cytokines are peptides that affect cell growth, maturation, differentiation and function. Cytokines have paracrine or autocrine effects on cells, thus playing an important role in the initiation and maintenance of rheumatoid arthritis (Goldring and Marcu 2009). TNF-α, interleukin-1 (IL-1) and IL-6, which are important in the pathogenesis, as well as IL-8, IL-13, IL-15, and IL-17, which have recently increased in importance, have also been shown in the synovium in the joint involved in RA (Tak and Bresnihan 2000). Among these cytokines detected in the RA synovium, the proinflammatory cytokines are IL-1, IL-6, IL-15, IL-17, IL-12, and IL-18, while the anti-inflammatory cytokines are TGFB, IL-4, IL-10, IL11 and IL-13 (Vervoordeldonk and Tak 2002). In a synovial fluid analysis in RA, it was found that IL-6 and TNF-α increased in parallel with disease activation (Tak et al. 1997). TNF-α is the main cytokine of inflammation, while IL-1 is the key cytokine in cartilage and bone resorption (Tak and Bresnihan 2000). Cytokines have proinflammatory and anti-inflammatory functions. In normal physiology, proinflammatory and anti-inflammatory cytokines are in balance, while proinflammatory cytokines are dominant in RA (Dinarello 1996).

IL-1 Family (IL-1F)

IL-1F functions from the first line of the natural inflammatory response (Ballak et al. 2015). Family members have both proinflammatory and anti-inflammatory properties. The IF-1 family includes IL-1α, IL-1β, IL-1Ra, IL-33 and IL-18.

IL-1 is a cytokine with a molecular weight of 10000 Daltons. Although it was initially identified in 1940 with its endogenous pyrogen feature, it is involved in many stages of immunity. It has many effects such as T-cell differentiation, neutrophilia, an increase in acute phase proteins, anorexia, and an increase in prostaglandin (Cohn 1968; Dinarello 2011).

IL-1 plays an important role in the initiation and progression of RA disease by causing vascular endothelial cell activation, osteoclast activation, an increase in polymorphonuclear cells and an increase in prostaglandin synthesis (Duff 1993). Bone and cartilage destruction in RA begins at the junction of the synovium, cartilage and bone. Although it is not clear which cytokine initiates the deterioration and loss of cartilage tissue, it is thought that the destruction is due to the activation of metalloproteinases by cytokines, especially IL-1 and TNF-α (Allard et al. 1987; Chu et al. 1992).

IL-1α is a proinflammatory cytokine found in hepatocytes, platelets, endothelial cells, keratinocytes, monocytes, and B lymphocytes (van de Veerdonk and Netea 2013). IL-1α found in platelets is effective in the development of atherosclerosis and has been associated with stroke pathology (Thornton et al. 2010). IL-1β is secreted from many cells, especially monocytes, macrophages and lymphocytes (Dinarello 2011). IL-1ra shows its effect by binding to the IL-1 receptor and blocking the effects of IL-1. Although it is found in the synovium of RA patients, its level is not high enough to inhibit IL-1.

In studies conducted after its discovery in the 1980s, IL-1Ra shows its effect by irreversibly blocking the receptor through the IL-1 receptor (Arend 1990). It has been shown that IL-1Ra is found together with IL-1 in the synovium in RA (Deleuran et al. 1992). In RA patients treated with IL-1Ra, the effects of IL-1 are inhibited by a decrease in osteoclast activity and a decrease in the amount of metalloproteinase. By reducing bone resorption, IL-1Ra helps to prevent destruction in the joints of RA patients (Schiff 2000). IL-1ra therapy is used successfully in RA. It is used in combination with methotrexate in the next-stage treatment of patients who have failed treatment with methotrexate (Cohen et al. 2004).

One of the members of the IL-1 family is IL-18. Its main source is macrophages and it shows its effect by increasing TNF-α from macrophages (Dai et al. 2004). However, although it is known as a proinflammatory cytokine, it inhibits osteoclasts. IL-8 exerts its effect by increasing the activation of two anti-inflammatory cytokines, IL-10 and TGF-B. The increased IL-10 and TGF-B reduce the effect of synovial IF-γ. In this case, although there is inflammation in the Th1 phenotype, the IF-γ levels are not high (Dayer 1999).

One of the members of the IL-1 family is IL-33 which is produced in many cells such as smooth muscle cells, epithelial cells, and primarily macrophages and dendric cells (Verri et al. 2010). When the patient and control groups were compared, it was shown that the amount of IL-33 was significantly higher in the serum analysis of RA patients. Anti-CCP and IL-33 levels were found to increase in parallel in the serum of RA patients (Hong et al. 2011). IL-33 is involved in the progression of RA by causing cartilage and bone destruction (Xu et al. 2013).

Tumor Necrosis Factor (TNF)

TNF-α is mainly produced by macrophages, and TNF-α and IL-1 together are the most important cytokines in the pathogenesis of RA. IL-1 and TNF-α show their effects by increasing the GM-CSF and also cause an increase in TNF-α IL-1, IL-2, IL-8, matrix metalloproteinases and prostaglandin production (Brennan, Maini, & Feldmann 1992). High levels of TNF-α were detected in synovial samples taken from patients with RA (Brennan et al. 1992). An increase of TNF-α causes synovial hyperplasia, leukocytosis, cartilage destruction, metalloproteinase activation and matrix destruction with effects similar to IL-1 (Maini, Elliott, Brennan, Williams and Feldmann 1997).

Treatment with anti-TNF-α drugs appears to be effective when treatment with methotrexate alone is not sufficient (which TNF inhibitor for rheumatoid arthritis? 2010).

IL-17

IL-17 is a cytokine produced by T cells (TH-17). Its receptor is found in many cells (Aarvak et al. 1999). It has been shown to be in synovium samples in RA patients. It causes IL-17, IL-6 and IL-8 to be released from stromal cells and also increases prostaglandin secretion (Laan et al. 1999). This cytokine also increases bone resorption by increasing synovial inflammation and osteoclast activation. Although it is thought to act together with IL-1 in cartilage destruction, IL-1 inhibition does not prevent IL-17 from causing cartilage destruction (Chabaud et al. 2001). Although the IL-17 blockade shows potential in treatment, moderate success has been achieved with existing treatments (Genovese et al. 2010).

IL-6

IL-6 is produced by synovial fibroblasts and macrophages and has both proinflammatory and anti-inflammatory properties. It is one of the most important cytokines in the initiation and development of RA. It is abundant in synovial fluid during active disease and correlates with disease activation (Duff 1993). IL-6 is mainly released by T cells, activates T and B cells, and contributes to pannus formation by increasing vascular endothelial growth factor (VEGF). It causes an increase in bone resorption by osteoclast activation (Choy et al. 2020). It shows its anti-inflammatory effects by increasing IL-1RA and suppressing inflammatory cytokines. However, as a result of the inhibition of IL-6, there is a decrease in disease progression and a slowdown in bone destruction (Choy et al. 2020).

Conclusion

In the development of RA, intense inflammation and cytokine release occur as a result of genetic and environmental factors. The immune mechanism that occurs is extremely complex and new information about the initial development of the disease continues to emerge. Cytokines are an important part of the immune system and the target of the latest treatments. As effective cytokines and their effects emerge in RA, developments towards the treatment of the disease will also emerge.

References

Aarvak T, Chabaud M, Miossec P, Natvig JB (1999) IL-17 is produced by some proinflammatory Th1/Th0 cells but not by Th2 cells. *J. Immunol*. 162(3):1246-1251.

Allard SA, Muirden KD, Camplejohn KL, Maini RN (1987) Chondrocyte-derived cells and matrix at the rheumatoid cartilage-pannus junction identified with monoclonal antibodies. *Rheumatol. Int*. 7(4):153-159.

Arend WP (1990) Interleukin-1 receptor antagonist: discovery, structure and properties. *Prog. Growth Factor Res*. 2(4):193-205.

Ballak DB, Stienstra R, Tack CJ, Dinarello CA, van Diepen JA (2015) IL-1 family members in the pathogenesis and treatment of metabolic disease: Focus on adipose tissue inflammation and insulin resistance. *Cytokine* 75(2):280-290.

Brennan FM, Maini RN, Feldmann M (1992) TNF alpha--a pivotal role in rheumatoid arthritis? *Br. J. Rheumatol*. 31(5):293-298.

Chabaud M, Lubberts E, Joosten L, van Den Berg W, Miossec P (2001) IL-17 derived from juxta-articular bone and synovium contributes to joint degradation in rheumatoid arthritis. *Arthritis Res*. 3(3):168-177.

Choy EH, De Benedetti F, Takeuchi T, Hashizume M, John M R, Kishimoto T (2020) Translating IL-6 biology into effective treatments. *Nat. Rev. Rheumatol*. 16(6):335-345.

Chu CQ, Field M, Allard S, Abney E, Feldmann M, Maini RN (1992) Detection of cytokines at the cartilage/pannus junction in patients with rheumatoid arthritis: implications for the role of cytokines in cartilage destruction and repair. *Br. J. Rheumatol*. 31(10):653-661.

Cohen SB, Moreland LW, Cush JJ, Greenwald MW, Block S, Shergy WJ, Study G (2004) A multicentre, double blind, randomised, placebo controlled trial of anakinra (Kineret), a recombinant interleukin 1 receptor antagonist, in patients with rheumatoid arthritis treated with background methotrexate. *Ann. Rheum. Dis*. 63(9):1062-1068.

Cohn ZA (1968) The structure and function of monocytes and macrophages. *Adv. Immunol*. 9:163-214.

Dai SM, Matsuno H, Nakamura H, Nishioka K, Yudoh K (2004) Interleukin-18 enhances monocyte tumor necrosis factor alpha and interleukin-1beta production induced by direct contact with T lymphocytes: implications in rheumatoid arthritis. *Arthritis Rheum.* 50(2):432-443.

Dayer JM (1999) Interleukin-18, rheumatoid arthritis, and tissue destruction. *J. Clin. Invest.,* 104(10):1337-1339.

Deleuran BW, Chu CQ, Field M, Brennan FM, Katsikis P, Feldmann M, Maini RN (1992). Localization of interleukin-1 alpha, type 1 interleukin-1 receptor and interleukin-1 receptor antagonist in the synovial membrane and cartilage/pannus junction in rheumatoid arthritis. *Br. J. Rheumatol.* 31(12):801-809.

Dinarello CA (1996) Biologic basis for interleukin-1 in disease. *Blood* 87(6):2095-2147.

Dinarello CA (2011) A clinical perspective of IL-1β as the gatekeeper of inflammation. *Eur. J. Immunol.* 41(5):1203-1217.

Dinarello CA (2011) Interleukin-1 in the pathogenesis and treatment of inflammatory diseases. *Blood* 117(14):3720-3732.

Duff GW (1993) Cytokines and anti-cytokines. *Br. J. Rheumatol.* 32(Suppl 1):15-20.

Genovese C, Van den Bosch F, Roberson S A, Bojin S, Biagini IM, Ryan P, Sloan-Lancaster, J (2010) LY2439821, a humanized anti-interleukin-17 monoclonal antibody, in the treatment of patients with rheumatoid arthritis: A phase I randomized, double-blind, placebo-controlled, proof-of-concept study. *Arthritis Rheum.* 62(4):929-939.

Goldring MB, Marcu KB (2009) Cartilage homeostasis in health and rheumatic diseases. *Arthritis Res. Ther.* 11(3):224.

Hong YS, Moon SJ, Joo YB, Jeon CH, Cho ML, Ju JH, Min JK (2011) Measurement of interleukin-33 (IL-33) and IL-33 receptors (sST2 and ST2L) in patients with rheumatoid arthritis. *J. Korean Med. Sci.* 26(9):1132-1139.

Laan M, Cui ZH, Hoshino H, Lotvall J, Sjostrand M, Gruenert DC, Linden A (1999) Neutrophil recruitment by human IL-17 via C-X-C chemokine release in the airways. *J. Immunol.* 162(4):2347-2352.

Lee DM, Weinblatt ME (2001) Rheumatoid arthritis. *Lancet* 358(9285):903-911. https://doi.org/10.1016/s0140-6736(01)06075-5.

Lundström E, Källberg H, Alfredsson L, Klareskog L, Padyukov L (2009) Gene-environment interaction between the DRB1 shared epitope and smoking in the risk of anti-citrullinated protein antibody-positive rheumatoid arthritis: all alleles are important. *Arthritis Rheum.* 60(6):1597-1603.

Maini R N, Elliott M, Brennan F M, Williams R O, Feldmann M (1997) TNF blockade in rheumatoid arthritis: implications for therapy and pathogenesis. *APMIS* 105(4):257-263.

Makrygiannakis D, Hermansson M, Ulfgren AK, Nicholas AP, Zendman AJ, Eklund A, Catrina AI (2008) Smoking increases peptidylarginine deiminase 2 enzyme expression in human lungs and increases citrullination in BAL cells. *Ann. Rheum. Dis.* 67(10):1488-1492.

Schiff MH (2000) Role of interleukin 1 and interleukin 1 receptor antagonist in the mediation of rheumatoid arthritis. *Ann. Rheum. Dis.* 59(Suppl 1):103-108.

Tak PP, Bresnihan B (2000) The pathogenesis and prevention of joint damage in rheumatoid arthritis: advances from synovial biopsy and tissue analysis. *Arthritis Rheum.* 43(12):2619-2633.

Tak PP, Smeets TJ, Daha MR, Kluin PM, Meijers KA, Brand R, Breedveld, FC (1997) Analysis of the synovial cell infiltrate in early rheumatoid synovial tissue in relation to local disease activity. *Arthritis Rheum.* 40(2):217-225.

Thornton P, McColl BW, Greenhalgh A, Denes A, Allan SM, Rothwell NJ (2010) Platelet interleukin-1alpha drives cerebrovascular inflammation. *Blood* 115(17):3632-3639.

van de Veerdonk FL, Netea MG (2013) New Insights in the Immunobiology of IL-1 Family Members. *Front. Immunol.* 4:167.

Verri WA, Jr Souto, FO, Vieira SM, Almeida SC, Fukada SY, Xu D, Cunha FQ (2010) IL-33 induces neutrophil migration in rheumatoid arthritis and is a target of anti-TNF therapy. *Ann. Rheum. Dis.* 69(9):1697-1703.

Vervoordeldonk MJ, Tak PP (2002) Cytokines in rheumatoid arthritis. *Curr. Rheumatol. Rep*. 4(3):208-217. https://doi.org/10.1007/s11926-002-0067-0.

Which TNF inhibitor for rheumatoid arthritis? (2010) *Med. Lett. Drugs Ther*. 52(1338):38-39.

Xu WD, Zhang M, Zhang YJ, Ye DQ (2013) IL-33 in rheumatoid arthritis: potential role in pathogenesis and therapy. *Hum. Immunol*. 74(9):1057-1060.

Chapter 12

Obesity and Cytokines

Düriye Sıla Karagöz Özen*, **MD**
Samsun Research and Training Hospital, Department of Internal Medicine, Samsun, Turkey

Abstract

Obesity is a growing global public health problem. The positive balance between energy intake and energy expenditure results in obesity. The body mass index (weight/height2) is a widely used criterion to define obesity, but lean people with an increased body mass index due to increased muscle mass are not qualified as being obese. An increase in body mass index above the normal levels is related to high cardiovascular risk. Adipose tissue is a large endocrine organ. It also affects inflammatory processes by secreting many peptide hormones, mainly leptin, resistin, and adiponectin. Healthy lean adipocytes contain anti-inflammatory cells that secrete anti-inflammatory cytokines such as IL-4 and IL-10. But expanding white adipose tissue starts to secrete proinflammatory cytokines such as interleukin (IL) 1β, IL-6, and tumor necrosis factor α (TNFα).

Keywords: obesity, IL-1β, IL-6, TNFα, cancer

Introduction

Obesity is a major public health problem with an exponentially increasing prevalence. Bodyweight is controlled by neural and hormonal factors. The positive balance between energy intake and energy expenditure results in obesity. Actually, obesity is an increase in adipose tissue mass. Although the body mass index (weight/height2) is a widely used criterion to define obesity, lean people with an increased body mass index due to increased muscle mass are not qualified as being obese.

According to data of the National Health and Nutrition Examination Survey (NHANES), the prevalence of obesity among adults in the USA is around 42.4% (NHANES 2020). The World Health Organization (WHO) stated that the prevalence of obesity increases in developing countries and complications begin to appear when the intra-abdominal adipose

* Corresponding Author's Email: silakaragoz@yahoo.com.

In: Cytokines and Diseases
Editors: Kenan Demir, Selim Görgün and Bahar Uslu
ISBN: 979-8-88697-214-6

tissue mass increases even at lower body mass index (BMI) levels. Furthermore, both obesity and malnutrition cause unexpected complications in low-income countries (WHO 2021).

A BMI of 30 and above is defined as obesity, and many studies have shown that cardiovascular risk increases as BMI increases (Table 1). Especially hypertension and glucose intolerance are determinants of cardiovascular risk. Another parameter associated with increased cardiovascular risk is the waist/hip ratio. A ratio higher than 0.9 in women and more than 1 in men is associated with increased cardiovascular risk (Liu et al., 2019). However, it should be kept in mind that the upper limits of the waist circumference vary according to gender and ethnicity. Visceral intra-abdominal adipose tissue hyperplasia is associated with systemic complications. Here, the role of cytokines released from adipose tissue is important. In a recent study about hospitalization and death in patients with heart failure, the hospitalization rates were higher in the obese high inflammation group than in the patients with low inflammation (Saleh et al., 2020).

Table 1. Weight status according to BMI in adults

Status	**Body mass index (kg/m^2)**	**Obesity level**
Underweight	< 18.5	None
Healthy weight	18.5-24.9	None
Overweight	25-29.9	None
Obesity	30.0-34.9	I
Obesity	35.0-39.9	II
Extreme obesity	≥ 40	III

Adipose tissue is a large endocrine organ. It affects the inflammatory processes by secreting many peptide hormones, mainly leptin, resistin, and adiponectin. Healthy lean adipocytes contain anti-inflammatory cells that secrete anti-inflammatory cytokines such as IL-4 and IL-10. But expanding white adipose tissue starts to secrete proinflammatory cytokines such as interleukin (IL) 1β, IL-6, and tumor necrosis factor α(TNFα) (Deng et al., 2016). When the relationship between cytokines and obesity is investigated, it is seen that cytokines play a role in the development of obesity and obesity-related complications. IL 1β, IL-6, IL-8, 1IL-10, monocyte chemoattractant protein 1, interferon-γ, and TNFα are particularly important cytokines that are secreted from adipose tissue (Deng et al., 2016).

The Role of Cytokines in the Development of Obesity

Hormones, neural signals, and environmental and cultural factors influence appetite regulation. The main hormone which regulates appetite on the hypothalamus is leptin which is secreted from adipocytes. It is known that genetic obesity syndromes are seen in individuals with decreased leptin hormone or leptin resistance at the receptor level. Besides leptin, insulin, cortisol, and gut peptides (cholecystokinin, ghrelin, peptide YY) also affect appetite on the hypothalamus.

Neural pathways include vagal stimulation that develops with gastrointestinal system distension. As mentioned earlier, obesity results from an imbalance between energy intake and expenditure. Although the basal metabolic rate varies from person to person, it is the major determinant of energy expenditure. In other words, most of our daily energy expenditure is fixed. Decreased adiponectin, a hormone released from adipocytes, is also associated with obesity.

A low-level systemic inflammation develops in obesity. It has been shown that a high fat diet causes hypothalamic leptin resistance in mice, and cytokines play a role here (Thaler et al., 2012). Following a high caloric intake, the hypothalamic inflammation process begins, and IL-1, TNF α, and the suppressor of cytokine signaling 3 (SOCS3) gene expression increase. These cytokines cause hypothalamic leptin resistance and stimulate fat storage (Thaler et al., 2012).

Brown and white adipocytes have different effects on energy metabolism. Previously, it was shown that a reduced brown adipose tissue mass may be related to an increased visceral white adipose tissue mass (Wang et al., 2015). Pescador et al., showed that metformin reduces the levels of proinflammatory cytokines like TNF α and IL-6 in brown adipose tissue (Pescador et al., 2021).

There are many studies related to IL-6 and obesity. Different results were obtained in these studies. In a study conducted with obese and fit adult men, leptin levels were found to be significantly higher in obese men, but no significant difference was found between the TNF-alpha and IL-6 levels in both groups. Also, that study showed that the use of tocilizumab, which blocks IL-6, had no effect on lipolysis in the fit group and slightly suppressed lipolysis in the obese group. It was shown that fatty acid mobilization decreased in both groups (Trinh et al., 2021). Maculewicz et al., showed that IL-6 gene polymorphism does not have an important role in low-grade obesity (Maculewicz et al., 2021).

In a study examining the metabolic aspects of 3 groups fed with a standard diet, a high-fat diet, and pomegranate juice, IL-1 beta, and TNF alpha were found to be significantly higher in the high-fat diet group, while IL-10 was found to be low (Michicotl-Meneses et al., 2021). These findings suggest that obesity is associated with a low level of inflammation and cytokines are involved in this process.

The Role of Cytokines in the Relationship Between Obesity and Insulin Resistance

The IL-6 level is associated with insulin resistance in obese individuals, and it was shown that IL-6 secretion from adipose tissue in obese individuals increases through TNFα and IL-1β. It was shown that high levels of IL-6, TNFα, and IL-1β released from adipose tissue in obese individuals were associated with insulin resistance (Al-Roub et al., 2021).

TNFα is another important cytokine that is related to insulin resistance in obese individuals. It came into prominence with low-grade inflammation emerging in both obesity and metabolic syndrome. Gonzalez-Gay et al., scrutinized this issue in 27 non-diabetic patients who were followed up with the diagnosis of rheumatoid arthritis and received anti-TNF infliximab treatment. They found that insulin sensitivity increased when measurements were made before infliximab infusion (0 minutes) and immediately after infusion (120 minutes) (Gonzalez-Gay et al., 2006).

Obesity also causes an increase in resistin levels which activates the suppressor of cytokine signaling 3 (SOCS3) and results in insulin resistance (Gallagher and LeRoith 2015).

The other proinflammatory cytokine IL-1β was investigated relating to the effects on insulin resistance in obese people. Accumulating data introducing the IL-1 association with insulin resistance in obese individuals has led to the investigation of the effects of anti-IL-1 therapies on insulin resistance. It has been shown that canakinumab and gevokizumab treatments, which are IL-1 receptor antagonists, have positive effects on glycemic control in diabetic individuals (Cavelti-Weder et al., 2012; Ridker et al., 2012; Hensen et al., 2013). However, further studies are needed to investigate the effectiveness and safety of anti-interleukin therapies in obesity and insulin resistance.

In mice, IL-18 has been shown to increase insulin sensitivity and even reverse TNFα-induced insulin resistance (Zorrilla et al., 2007). In humans, there is insufficient evidence to say that insulin resistance in the obese is improved with IL-18 treatment. Ballak et al., demonstrated the effects of the IL-1 family on obesity and insulin resistance in various ways. In that paper, not only IL-1 beta, alfa, and IL-18 but also IL-33 and IL-37 were evaluated (Ballak et al., 2015). The general fact about this subject is that we need more studies about the reliability of anti-IL-1 treatment regimens for insulin resistance in obese individuals.

It was shown that inositol-requiring enzyme 1α (IRE1α) might have an important role in obesity-induced inflammation. IRE1α deficiency was found to be related to diminished levels of proinflammatory cytokines such as TNFα or IL-1β (Shan et al., 2017).

As mentioned above, proinflammatory cytokines which are secreted from the visceral adipose tissue are major determinants of low-grade inflammation in obese people. The number of proinflammatory macrophages increased in subcutaneous adipose tissue in obese people with non-alcoholic fatty liver disease when compared to lean people (Fuchs et al., 2021). A high fat diet causes high levels of TNFα and IL-1β and metformin treatment is found to be related to diminished gene expression for these proinflammatory cytokines (Li et al., 2021).

The Role of Cytokines in the Obesity-Cancer Relationship

Obesity is a risk factor for cancer of the breast, ovary, endometrium, kidney, esophagus, colon, rectum, and pancreas. It is an independent risk factor for mortality in prostate cancer. Many studies are showing that an increase in visceral fat tissue and waist circumference is associated with cancer etiology and mortality in cancer patients (Kyrgiou et al., 2017; Fang et al., 2018). In these studies, the importance of cytokines and adipokines secreted from adipose tissue in the relationship between obesity and cancer was examined.

Adipose tissue is a large endocrine organ that is capable of secreting numerous cytokines and hormones (MacDougald and Burant 2007). Leptin and adiponectin are the major adipocyte-driven hormones, and they have opposite effects on cancer. Increased leptin levels are related to an increased risk of cancer while adiponectin is protective against cancer. Leptin stimulates macrophages to secrete IL-1, IL-6, IL-12, and TNFα and this results in an increased production of reactive oxygen species (ROS) (Carbone et al., 2012). ROS induce gene mutations and the proliferation of mutated cells, along with the activation of transcription factors in pre-malignant cells, various steps in cancer, and enhanced development. IL-6, IL-1β, and TNF α are major adipocyte-derived cytokines that have an impact on tumorigenesis (Hanahan and Weinberg 2011).

Leptin is a hormone secreted from adipose tissue which reduces appetite by acting on the hypothalamus. Although the leptin level increases in obese patients, there is a problem of binding to the hypothalamic leptin receptor. There are long and short isoforms of leptin receptors. Increased leptin in obese individuals binds to its long isoform receptor, activating intracellular signaling pathways associated with tumor growth and metastases, especially in breast cancer (Surmacz 2013).

Resistin is a proinflammatory cytokine released from macrophages. The increase in resistin causes insulin resistance by activating the suppressor of cytokine signaling 3 (SOCS3). Studies are showing that the level of resistin is high in cancer patients, but there is not enough evidence to say that it causes an increased risk independent of insulin resistance (Gallagher and LeRoith 2015).

In another recent study in premenopausal women with breast cancer, IL-6 and TNF-α levels in breast tissue were found to be high in patients with a larger waist circumference (≥86 cm), regardless of body mass index (Chang et al., 2021).

IL-6 has important roles in tumor cell development, growth, and spread (Naugler and Karin 2008). It was shown that IL-6 changes the Janus kinase/STAT pathway to start cancer cell development and angiogenesis. Increased levels of IL-6 in plasma were found to be related to disease aggressiveness and poor prognosis (Ghosh and Ashcraft 2013).

As mentioned above, TNFα levels are increased in obesity and like IL-6, TNFα is involved in cellular transformation, proliferation, invasion, angiogenesis, and metastasis in cancer (Balkwill 2009; Grivennikov and Karin 2011).

Conclusion

Cytokines and hormones released from adipose tissue are determinants of both insulin resistance and metabolic syndrome as well as cardiovascular risk. IL-1β, IL-6, and TNFα have been shown to be associated with insulin resistance and complications in obese individuals. Again, due to the increased incidence of cancer in obese people, studies focus on the roles of these common cytokines. There are insufficient data about the use of anti-cytokine therapies in the treatment of obesity and obesity-related complications such as cancer and metabolic syndrome. However, this issue seems to be important for future studies.

References

Al-Roub A, Al Madhoun A, Akhter N, Thomas R, Miranda L, Jacob T, Al-Ozairi E, Al-Mulla F, Sindhu S, Ahmad R (2021). IL-1β and TNFα Cooperativity in Regulating IL-6 Expression in Adipocytes Depends on CREB Binding and H3K14 Acetylation. *Cells* 10(11):3228.

Balkwill F (2009). Tumour necrosis factor and cancer. Nature reviews. *Cancer* 9(5):361–371.

Ballak D B, Stienstra R, Tack C J, Dinarello C A, van Diepen J A (2015). IL-1 family members in the pathogenesis and treatment of metabolic disease: Focus on adipose tissue inflammation and insulin resistance. *Cytokine* 75(2): 280–290.

Carbon F, La Rocca C, Matarese G (2012). Immunological functions of leptin and adiponectin. *Biochimie* 94(10):2082–2088.

Cavelti-Weder C, Babians-Brunner A, Keller C, Stahel M A, Kurz-Levin M, Zayed H, Solinger A M, Mandrup-Poulsen T, Dinarello C A, Donath M Y (2012). Effects of gevokizumab on glycemia and inflammatory markers in type 2 diabetes. *Diabetes care* 35(8):1654–1662.

Chang S L, Tchernof A, Durocher F, Diorio C (2021). Associations of Biomarkers of Inflammation and Breast Cancer in the Breast Adipose Tissue of Women with Combined Measures of Adiposity *Journal of obesity* 2021:3620147. https://doi.org/10.1155/2021/3620147.

Deng T, Lyon C J, Bergin S, Caligiuri M A and Hsueh W A (2016). Obesity, Inflammation, and Cancer. *Annual review of pathology* 11:421–449.

Fang X, Wei J, He X, Lian J, Han D, An P, Zhou T, Liu S, Wang F, Min J (2018). Quantitative association between body mass index and the risk of cancer: A global Meta-analysis of prospective cohort studies. *International journal of cancer*, 143(7):1595–1603.

Fuchs A, Samovski D, Smith G I, Cifarelli V, Farabi S S, Yoshino J, Pietka T, Chang S-W, Ghosh S, Myckatyn T M, Klein S (2021). Associations Among Adipose Tissue Immunology, Inflammation, Exosomes and Insulin Sensitivity in People with Obesity and Nonalcoholic Fatty Liver Disease. *Gastroenterology* 161(3):968–981.

Gallagher E J, LeRoith D (2015). Obesity and Diabetes: The Increased Risk of Cancer and Cancer-Related Mortality. *Physiological reviews* 95(3):727–748.

Ghosh S, Ashcraft K (2013). An IL-6 link between obesity and cancer. *Frontiers in bioscience* (Elite edition) 5:461–478.

Gonzalez-Gay M A, De Matias J M, Gonzalez-Juanatey C, Garcia-Porrua C, Sanchez-Andrade A, Martin J, Llorca J (2006). Anti-tumor necrosis factor-alpha blockade improves insulin resistance in patients with rheumatoid arthritis. *Clinical and experimental rheumatology* 24(1):83–86.

Grivennikov S I, Karin M (2011). Inflammatory cytokines in cancer: tumour necrosis factor and interleukin 6 take the stage. *Annals of the rheumatic diseases* 70(Suppl 1):i104–i108.

Hanahan D, Weinberg D A (2011). Hallmarks of cancer: the next generation. *Cell* 144(5):646–674.

Hensen J, Howard C P, Walter V, Thuren T (2013). Impact of interleukin-1β antibody (canakinumab) on glycaemic indicators in patients with type 2 diabetes mellitus: results of secondary endpoints from a randomized, placebo-controlled trial. *Diabetes & metabolism* 39(6):524–531.

Kyrgiou M, Kalliala I, Markozannes G, Gunter M J, Paraskevaidis E, Gabra H, Martin-Hirsch P, Tsilidis K K (2017). Adiposity and cancer at major anatomical sites: umbrella review of the literature. *BMJ* (Clinical research ed.) 356:j477.

Li X, Cai Y, Luo J, Ding J, Yao G, Xiao X, Tang Y, Liang Z (2021). Metformin attenuates hypothalamic inflammation via downregulation of RIPK1-independent microglial necroptosis in diet-induced obese mice. *Cell death discovery* 7(1):338.

Liu L, Gao B, Wang J, Yang C, Wu S, Wu Y, Chen S, Li Q, Zhang H, Wang G, Chen M, Pop-Busui R, Zhao M-H, Zhang L (2019). Joint association of body mass index and central obesity with cardiovascular events and all-cause mortality in prediabetic population: A prospective cohort study. *Obesity research & clinical practice* 13(5):453–461.

MacDougald O A, Burant C F (2007). The rapidly expanding family of adipokines. Cell metabolism 6(3):159–161 https://doi.org/10.1016/j.cmet.2007.08.010.

Maculewicz E, Antkowiak B, Antkowiak O, Mastalerz A, Białek A, Cywińska A, Borecka A, Humińska-Lisowska K, Garbacz A, Lorenz K, Szarska E, Michałowska-Sawczyn M, Dziuda Ł, Cięszczyk P (2021) IL-6 Polymorphisms Are Not Related to Obesity Parameters in Physically Active Young Men, *Genes* 12(10):1498.

Michicotl-Meneses M M, Del Rocío Thompson-Bonilla M, Reyes-López C A, García-Pérez B E, López-Tenorio I I, Ordaz-Pichardo C, Jaramillo-Flores M E (2021). Inflammation Markers in Adipose Tissue and Cardiovascular Risk Reduction by Pomegranate Juice in Obesity Induced by a Hypercaloric Diet in Wistar Rats. *Nutrients* 13(8):2577.

Naugler W E, Karin M (2008). The wolf in sheep's clothing: the role of interleukin-6 in immunity, inflammation and cancer. *Trends in molecular medicine* 14(3):109–119.

NHANES database. https://www.cdc.gov/nchs/about/factsheets/factsheet_nhanes.htm Accessed 19 Dec 2021.

Pescador Francisco V, Vázquez P, Esquinas E M, González-Páramos C, Valdecantos M P, García-Martínez I, Urrutia A A, Ruiz L, Escalona-Garrido C, Foretz M, Viollet B, Fernández-Moreno M Á, Calle-Pascual A L, Obregón M J, Aragonés J, Valverde Á M (2021). Metformin reduces macrophage HIF1α-dependent proinflammatory signaling to restore brown adipocyte function in vitro. *Redox biology* 48:102171. https://doi.org/10.1016/j.redox.2021.102171.

Ridker P M, Howard C P, Walter V, Everett B, Libby P, Hensen J and Thuren T (2012). Effects of interleukin-1β inhibition with canakinumab on hemoglobin A1c, lipids, C-reactive protein, interleukin-6, and fibrinogen: a phase IIb randomized, placebo-controlled trial. *Circulation* 126(23):2739–2748.

Saleh Z, Lennie T A, Darawad M W, Alduraidi H, Elshatarat R, Almansour I, Moser D (2020). The health outcomes of inflammation and obesity in patients with heart failure. *Heart & lung: the journal of critical care* 49(6):896–901.

Shan B, Wang X, Wu Y, Xu C, Xia Z, Dai J, Shao M, Zhao F, He S, Yang L, Zhang M, Nan F, Li J, Liu J, Liu J, Jia W, Qiu Y, Song B, Han J-D J, Rui L, Duan S-Z, Liu Y (2017). The metabolic ER stress sensor IRE1α suppresses alternative activation of macrophages and impairs energy expenditure in obesity. *Nature immunology* 18(5):519–529.

Surmacz E (2013). Leptin and adiponectin: emerging therapeutic targets in breast cancer. *Journal of mammary gland biology and neoplasia* 18(3-4):321–332.

Thaler J P, Yi C-X, Schur E A, Guyenet S J, Hwang B H, Dietrich M O, Zhao X, D A Sarruf D A, Izgur V, Maravilla K R, Nguyen H T, Fischer J D, Matsen M E, Wisse B E, Morton G J, Horvath T L, Baskin D G, Tschöp M H, Schwartz M W (2012). Obesity is associated with hypothalamic injury in rodents and humans. *The Journal of clinical investigation* 122(1):153–162.

Trinh B, Peletier M, Simonsen C, Plomgaard P, Karstoft K, Pedersen B K, Hall G, Ellingsgaard H (2021). Blocking endogenous IL-6 impairs mobilization of free fatty acids during rest and exercise in lean and obese men. *Cell reports Medicine* 2(9):100396.

Wang Q, Zhang M, Xu M, Gu W, Xi Y, Qi L, Li B, Wang W (2015). Brown adipose tissue activation is inversely related to central obesity and metabolic parameters in adult human. *PloS one* 10(4):e0123795.

WHO Databese (2021) https://www.who.int/health-topics/obesity Accessed 18 Dec 2021.

Zorrilla E P, Sanchez-Alavez M, Sugama S, Brennan M, Fernandez R, Bartfai T, Conti B (2007) Interleukin-18 controls energy homeostasis by suppressing appetite and feed efficiency. *Proceedings of the National Academy of Sciences of the United States of America* 104(26): 11097–1110.

Chapter 13

Cytokines and COVID-19

Aydin Aydinli*, MD
Istanbul Okan University, Medical Faculty, Department of Medical Microbiology, Istanbul, Turkey

Abstract

The COVID-19 pandemic has affected humanity all over the world since December 2019. Among many viral diseases, perhaps there has not been any other viral disease on which there has been so much research in such a short time. In addition to the characteristics of the virus, detailed studies on the etiopathogenesis of the disease it causes expand our horizons every day. We know that the disease is not only a viral pneumonia but develops as a multisystem disease. As in all infectious diseases, the role of cytokines in the clinical manifestation of the disease is very important in COVID-19 viral pneumonia. Even the "cytokine storm" situation that occurs with uncontrollable cytokine release is almost mentioned together with COVID-19. The effective suppression of cytokine release may be beneficial in the treatment of the disease.

Keywords: COVID-19, coronavirus, cytokines, cytokine storm

Introduction

In the period from December 2019 to the present, humanity has encountered a new mutation of the coronavirus that causes respiratory tract infections, and this epidemic, which has turned into a pandemic, has not only turned into a viral pneumonia, but also into a viral disease that threatens life and causes the most deaths. After the declaration of the pandemic, life in all countries has been taken up with the diagnosis of this new disease, deaths, hospital occupancy rates, treatment difficulties, and vaccination problems and the secondary problems it brings. It was reported that patients with viral pneumonia were detected on 8 December 2019 in the city of Wuhan, Hubei province of China. In the clinical evaluations of the cases, fever, respiratory distress and a bilateral infiltrative appearance in the chest x-rays were present. Within a few days, it was revealed that these patients originated from the Huanan seafood market, which sold

* Corresponding Author's Email: aydin.aydinli@okan.edu.tr.

In: Cytokines and Diseases
Editors: Kenan Demir, Selim Görgün and Bahar Uslu
ISBN: 979-8-88697-214-6

wild animals such as bats, snakes, and poultry. Chinese authorities reported that they had identified a new coronavirus on January 7, 2020. Five days later, the genome sequence of the new coronavirus was reported to the World Health Organization (WHO). After a rapid spread of the epidemic to other countries, the WHO declared the new coronavirus epidemic as a pandemic on 12 March 2020, and the new virus was named SARS-CoV-2 or COVID-19 (Tang et al., 2020). From the start date to today more than 200 countries and regions have reported their positive tests and number of deaths to the WHO. As of 30 November 2021, the total number of COVID-19 cases worldwide has been nearly 260 million and deaths have exceeded 5,2 million (WHO 2021).

Actually, we know that COVID-19 is not only a respiratory disease, but can be defined as a disease with multi-organ involvement. Although the immune pathogenesis of the disease has not been fully resolved, many possible mechanisms such as the systemic inflammatory response, excessive T-cell activation and angiotensin converting enzyme 2 (ACE2) receptor mechanisms and the antibody reaction against lung cells are known to play a role in the immune pathogenesis of the disease. The virus is cytotoxic in the first days of infection. Alveolar damage and diffuse thickening of the alveols are observed in biopsy specimens of patients infected with COVID-19. The lungs also show impaired cell membrane structures of virus-containing cells and severe endothelial damage. Virus particles can be seen in epithelial cells with electron microscopy, and direct toxicity of the virus can be observed with this method (Maciej et al., 2020).

Coronaviruses

Coronaviruses are single-stranded and positive-sense, 29.9 kb in length – the biggest RNA viruses, and the "corona" name comes from the spike-like structures on their envelope (Song et al., 2020; Kumar and Al Khodor 2020). SARS-CoV-2 (COVID-19) is a new member of the Sarbecovirus sub-genus within the beta coronavirus genus. Based on sequence homology, human coronaviruses (SARS-CoV, SARS-CoV-2, MERS-CoV, HCoV-229E and HCov-NL63) have animal origins. All of the coronaviruses are considered to have originated as beta coronaviruses from bats. The HCoV-OC43 and HKU1 probably originated from rodents. COVID-19 has a substantial structural resemblance to SARS-CoV and MERS-CoV and other coronaviruses. The virion of COVID-19 is just about 50-200 nm in diameter and it has 14 different ORFs (open reading frames) encoding 27 different proteins similar to other coronaviruses. ORF1a/b is coding two big proteins: *polyprotein/1a* and *polyprotein/1ab. Polyprotein 1a* and *1ab* are the non-structural proteins of the virus (NSP). These two polyproteins transform into 16 nonstructural proteins (NSP1-16) that make up the viral replication-transcriptional complex. NSP1-16 transforms membranes originating from the endoplasmic reticulum (ER) into vesicles that will later form the bilayer envelopes of the virus. Viral replication and transcription take place inside these vesicles, thanks to the replication-transcriptional complex formed by NSPs. Other ORFs encode four major structural proteins: the membrane (M), spike (S), envelope (E), and nucleocapsid (N) proteins. These four different structural proteins of the coronavirus have important functions. The S protein, which forms spikes on the viral surfaces, binds to the target cell membrane. The M protein gives the virion its shape and binds to the nucleocapsid and plays an important role in budding out of the cell. The E protein is involved in the pathogenesis of the virus and its budding, again. The N protein can bind to viral RNA and package the genome in the virion via the NSP3 protein (Kumar et al., 2020).

COVID-19 is primarily transmitted by respiratory droplets with breathing, coughing, sneezing, and sometimes loud talking, and also with direct or indirect contact. COVID-19 enters into host cells by the virus' spike glycoprotein (S protein). S glycoprotein binds to the angiotensin-converting enzyme 2 (ACE-2) receptors on the cell surface for entry into the cells. Angiotensin-converting-enzyme-2 (ACE-2), an important known metalloproteinase, acts as a receptor for the COVID-19 virus. COVID-19 utilizes the membrane bound form of ACE-2. After this binding, ACE-2 will be internalized and its membrane expression reduced. ACE-2 is also a significant regulator of bradykinin, and its decreased expression in the lung results in local vascular seepage leading to angioedema around the affected lung tissue. TMPRSS2 is a host serine protease that cleaves the S protein into S1 and S2 parts, allowing it to associate with the cell membrane, enter the cell, and initiate replication. Some proteins like TMPRSS2 such as furin and human endosomal cysteine proteases have a potential cleavage capacity of protein S. The transmembrane serine protease-2 (TMPRSS2) and ACE-2 are co-expressed by many cell types, both for entry of the viruses into nasal (goblet and ciliated cells) and lower airway bronchial epithelial cells and pneumocytes (type II pneumocytes-AT2 cells), immune cells in the lung, endothelial cells, neurons, enterocytes, cardiomyocytes, the small intestines, hepatocytes, and kidney cells. The ACE-2 enzyme also plays a role in acute lung injury, and may lead to the entry of the virus into the lung, which leads to COVID-19 pneumonia. Many studies have focused on this enzyme for the treatment and reduction of organ damage. When we look at the molecular details of the mechanism used by the virus to enter the host cell, it is seen that the host receptor/co-receptor relationship of the spike protein is important, and many studies focus on this subject (Mengyuan et al., 2020).

Similar to S protein activation, valosin-containing protein (VCP) and other factors also play a role in the COVID-19 infection process. Interferon-inducible transmembrane protein-like factors are involved in the host-pathogen interaction as antiviral factors in infections with RNA viruses such as coronaviruses (Wong et al., 2015).

Receptors for COVID-19

COVID-19 virus can also use the CD147 receptor to enter T cells. CD147 is a transmembrane immunoglobulin-like receptor that exists in secreted form and also acts as a receptor for HIV-1. Firstly, COVID-19 enters the host cell, releases its own RNA into the host cell's cytoplasm, and uses host cell systems to translate the poly proteins pp1a and pp1b. Post-translationally, they migrate from the endoplasmic reticulum to the Golgi apparatus, where mature virions are assembled in budding and leave the cell by exocytosis. Many systems of the innate immunity are found in infected cells, which are at different stages of replication and responsible for the production of virus-recognizing and type I (IFN-alpha and beta) and type III interferons and proinflammatory cytokines. Type I and type III interferons are produced by epithelial cells in viral infections. Many cells have type I interferon receptors. However, it is known that the effects of type III interferons are generally on epithelial cells and are less inflammatory, and they are also activated more rapidly than type I interferons. Interferons are one of the most potent antiviral components of innate immunity. Interferons also activate other innate and adaptive immune mechanisms. However, these responses appear to be reduced or dysregulated in COVID-19 infections. Coronaviruses block interferon signaling at various levels. Meanwhile, some non-structural proteins that inhibit the induction of interferons (via inhibition of IRF3 and IRF7) and interferon communication (such as inhibition of STAT1 signaling) are also produced by coronaviruses. A decreased antiviral response by inhibiting the interferon pathway causes an increased viral load, excessive inflammation due to the proinflammatory response, and eventually aggravation of the disease. A recent study showed that COVID-19 infection in humans induces weak interferon responses from infected pneumocytes that are even weaker than SARS-CoV infection (Sokolowska et al., 2020).

Classically, cytotoxic CD8+ T cells act on infected cells by direct neutralization, while CD4+ T cells assist B cells to initiate antibody production. T cells act in the enhancement of immunological memory in the form of virus-specific CD8+ and CD4+ T cells, as demonstrated in previous studies in SARS-CoV infection. The numbers of CD4+ and CD8+ T cells are below normal levels in most of the COVID-19 cases, and these numbers have been shown to be at the lowest levels in severe cases. In severe cases of COVID-19 infection, it has been reported that adaptive responses are delayed when the virus takes a long time to clear from the body. Moreover, a raised cytokine response from infected cells can also induce the apoptosis of T cells (Tay et al., 2020).

Cytokines and the COVID-19 Relationship

Cytokines are proteins secreted by cells of the innate and adaptive immune systems. They transmit signals by binding to specific receptors on cell surfaces and act on cytokine producing cells or other target cells. They have pivotal roles in the function of a variety of cells. As a generalization, cytokines and growth factors are quite similar, but cytokines are molecules that act on leukocytes and are involved in host defense, while growth factor acts on other somatic cell types. While hormones act by going to different distant organs through the blood, cytokines usually have a local effect. In summary, cytokines are produced in response to microorganisms and non-infectious antigens. Different cytokines stimulate various immune responses in different cells involved in immunity and inflammation (Warren 2008).

Cytokines have been shown to play a role in the development of inflammation, as they are very important inflammatory mediators (Mahmud-Al-Rafat et al., 2020). In severe cases of COVID-19, cytokine storms have been shown to lead to significant increases in cytokines such as IL-2, IL-7, IL-10, GSCF, and TNF-α (Mahmudpour et al., 2020). In the case of a cytokine storm, infections and the elimination of negative feedback on the immune system result in an overproduction of inflammatory cytokines with a biological activity that is quite different from that of many tissues and cells. These cytokines provide positive feedback on other cells of the immune system and recruit them to sites of inflammation, increasingly leading to the exacerbation of inflammation and organ damage. Interferons (IFN), tumor necrosis factor (TNF), interleukins (IL), the chemokine family, colony stimulating factors (CSF) and growth factors (GF) are the most well-known cytokines. On the basis of their functions, IL-1β, IL-6, IL-12, TNF and IFN-γ are proinflammatory factors; and IL-4, IL-10, IL-13 and TGF-β are classified as anti-inflammatory factors. A cytokine storm is a major cause of acute respiratory distress syndrome (ARDS) which is a systemic and severe inflammatory response associated with multiple organ failure (Song et al., 2020).

It would not be wrong to say that in addition to viral factors, some immunological factors are also clinically effective in the development of the disease. Locally or systemically, various proinflammatory cytokines like IL-1, IL-1β, IL-2, IL-6, IL-18, interferon-γ, TNF-α and macrophage colony stimulating factor (M-CSF) can cause the over-reaction of the immune systems with the release of high amounts of cytokines into the circulation and this is called cytokine release syndrome (CRS) or an uncontrolled "cytokine storm." We can say that this condition is an "increased inflammatory response," in which there is excessive production of proinflammatory cytokines by monocytes. In addition, adaptive immune system disorders occur due to CD4+ lymphocyte depletion. With the hyperactivation of monocytes, the excessive release of IL-6 occurs. An increase in the erythrocyte sedimentation rate (ESR), CRP, IL-1β, IL-6, IL-8, IL-2R and TNF-α levels in patients admitted to the intensive care unit due to severe COVID-19; acute respiratory distress syndrome (ARDS), disseminated intravascular coagulation (DIC), and coagulation disorders/hypercoagulation may also occur (Siddiqi et al., 2021; Singh et al., 2020). Previous studies have shown that the serum levels of proinflammatory cytokines such as IL1B, IL6, IL12, IFN-y, IP10 and MCP1 are associated with pulmonary inflammation and extensive lung injury in SARS patients. It has been reported that proinflammatory cytokines such as IFN-γ, TNF-a, IL-15 and IL-17 increase in MERS-CoV infection. High amounts of IL1B, IFN-γ, IP10 and MCP1 are also present in COVID-19 patients, possibly leading to activated T-helper-1 (T_{H1}) cell responses (Huang et al., 2020). Studies have shown that the storm caused by COVID-19 is associated with increased anti-inflammatory cytokines IL-4 and IL-10 released by T-helper-2 (T_{H2}) cells, in contrast to the cytokine storm in SARS disease (Tan et al., 2020). In severe COVID-19 infections, total T-cell counts, as well as CD4+ and CD8+ T cell counts, were also significantly lower than in milder cases. This indicates that there is progressive T-cell reduction in COVID-19 patients associated with disease severity (Sanz et al., 2011).

In cases of COVID-19, the overproduction of cytokines can damage the lung and lead to the death of the patient. Neutralizing anti-TNF-α, -IL1 and -IL6 antibodies, which have been used in the treatment of diseases such as cancer, type II diabetes and leukemia in previous studies, can be used to reduce lung damage (Dinarello et al., 2012; Shi et al., 2020).

According to some studies, increased levels of IL-6 may serve as a potential marker for predicting COVID-19 disease progression (Wang et al., 2020).

Conclusion

Unfortunately, the resurgence of COVID-19 cases due to new mutants in many countries is causing health professionals and epidemiologists to warn that we are still in the middle stages of the pandemic. A complete return to our normal lifestyle will only be possible, if the available vaccines are offered equally to everyone. At the same time, some effective therapeutic drugs and/or methods are urgently needed to contain the ongoing COVID-19 pandemic and perhaps save the lives of millions of people and give hope. The fight against the COVID-19 pandemic demonstrates the need for increased research and studies to better equip humanity for any future pandemics. Therefore, one of the most important molecular studies is based on cytokines and COVID-19 relationships.

References

Dinarello C. A., Simon A., van der Meer J. W. (2012) Treating inflammation by blocking interleukin-1 in a broad spectrum of diseases. *Nat Rev Drug Discov* 11(8):633-652.

Huang C., Wang Y., Li X. Lili Ren, Jianping Zhao, Yi Hu, Li Zhang, Guohui Fan, Jiuyang Xu, Xiaoying Gu, Zhenshun Cheng, Ting Yu, Jiaan Xia, Yuan Wei, Wenjuan Wu, Xuelei Xie, Wen Yin, Hui Li, Min Liu, Yan Xiao, Hong Gao, Li Guo, Jungang Xie, Guangfa Wang, Rongmeng Jiang, Zhancheng Gao, Qi Jin, Jianwei Wang, Bin Cao, (2020) Clinical features of patients infected with 2019 novel coronavirus in Wuhan, China. *Lancet* 395:497-506.

Kumar M. and Al Khodor S. (2020) Pathophysiology and treatment strategies for COVID-19. *J Transl Med* 18:353.

Maciej M. K., Piotr Trzonkowski, Magdalena Łasińska-Kowara, Andrzej Mital, Tomasz Smiatacz, Miłosz Jaguszewski (2020) COVID-19 Toward a comprehensive understanding of the disease. *Cardiology Journal* 27(2):99-114.

Mahmud-Al-Rafat M., Muzammal Haque Asim, Andrew W. Taylor-Robinson, Apurba Majumder, Abdul Muktadir, Hasneen Muktadir, Mahbubul Karim, Imran Khan, Mohammad Mainul Ahasan, Morsaline Billah (2020) A combinational approach to restore cytokine balance and to inhibit virus growth may promote patient recovery in severe COVID-19 cases, *Cytokine* 136:155228.

Mahmudpour M., Jamshid Roozbehb, Mohsen Keshavarza, Shokrollah Farrokhic, Iraj Nabipourad (2020) COVID-19 cytokine storm: The anger of inflammation. *Cytokine* 133:155151.

Mengyuan L., Ting Wang, Yun Zhou, Yutong Zhao, Yan Zhang, and Dr. Jianping Li (2020) Potential role of ACE-2 in coronavirus disease 2019 (COVID-19) prevention and management. *Journal of Translational Internal Medicine* 8:9-19.

Sanz F., Gimeno C., Lloret T., Nuria Tormo, Marisa Briones, Estrella Fernández, Angela Cervera, María Carmen Aguar, Eusebi Chiner, José Blanquer (2011) Relationship between the presence of hypoxemia and the inflammatory response measured by C-reactive protein in bacteremic pneumococcal pneumonia. *Eur Respir J* 38(suppl 55):2492.

Shi Y., Wang Y., Shao C., Jianan Huang, Jianhe Gan, Xiaoping Huang, Enrico Bucci, Mauro Piacentini, Giuseppe Ippolito & Gerry Melino (2020) COVID-19 infection: the perspectives on immune responses. *Cell Death Differ* 27(5):1451-1454.

Siddiqi H. K., Peter Libby and Paul M. Ridkera (2011) COVID-19- A vascular disease. *Trends in Cardiovascular Medicine* 31:1-5.

Singh S. P., Pritam M., Pandey B., Thakur Prasad Yadav (2020) Microstructure, pathophysiology and potential therapeutics of COVID-19: A comprehensive review. *J Med Virol* 93(1):275-299. https://doi.org/10.1002/jmv.26254.

Sokolowska M., Lukasik Z., Agache I. Cezmi A Akdis, Deniz Akdis, Mübeccel Akdis, Weronika Barcik, Helen A Brough, Thomas Eiwegger, Andrzej Eljaszewicz, Stefanie Eyerich, Wojciech Feleszko, Cristina Gomez-Casado, Karin Hoffmann-Sommergruber, Jozef Janda, Rodrigo Jiménez-Saiz, Marek Jutel, Edward F. Knol, Inge Kortekaas Krohn, Akash Kothari, Joanna Makowska, Marcin Moniuszko, Hideaki Morita, Liam O'Mahony, Kari Nadeau, Cevdet Ozdemir, Isabella Pali-Schöll, Oscar Palomares, Francesco Papaleo, Mary Prunicki, Carsten B. Schmidt-Weber, Anna Sediva, Jürgen Schwarze, Mohamed H. Shamji, Gerdien A. Tramper-Stranders, Willem van de Veen, Eva Untersmayr (2020) Immunology of COVID-19: mechanisms, clinical outcome, diagnostics and perspectives-a report of the European Academy of Allergy and Clinical Immunology (EAACI). *AllergyOct* 75(10):2445-2476.

Song P, Li W, Xie J, Yanlong Hou, and Chongge You (2020) Cytokine storm induced by SARS-CoV-2. *Clinica Chimica Acta* 509:280-287.

Tan W., Zhao X., Ma X., Wenling Wang, Peihua Niu, Wenbo Xu, George F. Gao, Guizhen Wu (2020) A novel coronavirus genome identified in a cluster of pneumonia cases-Wuhan, China 2019-2020. *China CDC Wkly* 24 2(4):61-62.

Tang D., Comish P., Kang R. (2020) The hallmarks of COVID-19 disease. *PLOS Pathogens* 16(5):e1008536.

Tay M. Z., Poh C. M., Rénia L. Paul A. MacAry, Lisa F. P. Ng, (2020) The trinity of COVID-19: immunity, inflammation and intervention. *Nat Rev Immunol* 20(6):363-374.

Wang C., Fei D., Li X., Mingyan Zhao, Kaijiang Yu (2020) IL-6 may be a good biomarker for earlier detection of COVID-19 progression. *Intensive Care Med* 8:1-2.

Warren L. (2008) Type I cytokines and Interferons and their receptors. In: Paul W. E. (ed) *Fundamental Immunology*, Sixth edn. Lippincott Williams and Wilkins, Wolters Kluwer, Philadelphia, p 706-749.

WHO (2021) *Coronavirus disease (COVID-2019) situation reports.* https://covid19.who.int/ Accessed 30 Nov 2021.

Wong H. H., Kumar P., Tay F. P. Dimitri Moreau, Ding Xiang Liu, Frédéric Bard (2015) Genome-Wide Screen Reveals Valosin Containing Protein Requirement for Coronavirus Exit from Endosomes. *J Virol* 89(21):11116-11128.

Chapter 14

Cytokines and Aids

Dilek Ozer[1,*] and Hakan Odabasi[2]

[1]Corlu State Hospital, Department of Medical Microbiology, Tekirdag, Turkey
[2]University of Health Sciences, Sancaktepe Training and Research Hospital, Department of Medical Microbiology, Istanbul, Turkey

Abstract

The relationship between HIV and the human immune system is very complex. HIV uses many ways to survive within infected people. HIV changes the immune system response in its favor. By disrupting cytokine regulation, it activates the immune system in a way that facilitates its own replication. This persistent immune activation plays an important role in HIV pathogenesis.

Keywords: Human Immunodeficiency Virus (HIV), HIV-1, HIV-2, AIDS, cytokines

Introduction

Cytokines are low-molecular-weight, soluble proteins, secreted by many cells. They have important tasks in nearly every biological process by their influence on other cells or themselves. One of these tasks is the regulation of the signaling network of immune system cells. If this signaling network regulation fails, the immune system works irregularly and ineffectively. Acquired immunodeficiency syndrome (AIDS) is the final stage of HIV infection characterized by a failed immune response with dysregulation of the cytokines (Parkin and Cohen 2001).

Extensive research finds that HIV changes cytokine production, especially in T cells, in order to increase virus replication and disturb the immune response. So, it is necessary to examine the T cells to understand why the characteristics of the cytokine network in HIV-infected individuals are different from other viral infections and why it progresses into AIDS (Reuter et al. 2012).

[*] Corresponding Author's Email: drdilekibis@gmail.com.

In: Cytokines and Diseases
Editors: Kenan Demir, Selim Görgün and Bahar Uslu
ISBN: 979-8-88697-214-6

Therefore, in this part of the book, we will mainly talk about the relationship between T cells and cytokines during HIV/AIDS. We will briefly touch on other cells involved in the pathogenesis of HIV/AIDS.

HIV Types and Progression into AIDS

Two major types of HIV have been recognized: HIV-1 and HIV-2. As HIV-1 is more prevalent worldwide, when we say HIV, we are generally referring to HIV-1. Table 1 gives some similarities and significant differences between HIV-1 and HIV-2.

Table 1. Similarities and differences between HIV-1 and HIV-2 (adopted from Nyamweya et al. 2013)

Characteristics	**Comparison**
Basic gene arrangement	Similar
Transmission ways	Similar
Intracellular replication pathways	Similar
Transmissibility	HIV-1 >HIV-2
Rate of progression	HIV-1 >HIV-2
Average levels of immune activation	HIV-1 >HIV-2
Plasma viral loads	HIV-1 >HIV-2
Probability progression into AIDS	HIV-1 >HIV-2
Distribution in the world	HIV-1 worldwide HIV-2 mostly limited to West Africa
Immune response protectability	Cellular responses to HIV-2 are more protective and produce more IL-2
CD4 counts during progression	HIV-2 >HIV-1

CD4+ T-Cell Cytokine Response to HIV/AIDS

CD4+ T cells play a key role in the activation of immune system cells. Therefore, they have a crucial place in the control and clearance of infections. As they are highly heterogeneous, separation of the groups is difficult. Thanks to the latest developments in structural biology, CD4+ T cells can be separated into six groups: T helper 1 (Th1), T helper 2 (Th2), T helper 17 (Th17), T helper 22 (Th22), regulatory T cells (Treg) and T follicular helper cells (Tfh) (Chatzileontiadou et al. 2020).

The immune system often uses the Th1 subset response against viral infections. Th1 cell differentiation requires interleukin 12 which is secreted by antigen presenting cells (APCs). IL-10 is known to inhibit APCIL-12 production. In this way, IL-10 inhibits the differentiation of naive CD4+ T cells into Th1 cells (D'Andrea et al. 1993; Hsieh et al. 1993).

Th1 cells produce IFNγ, which was first named as macrophage-activating factor because ofplaying an important role in macrophage stimulation. The activation of macrophages with IFNγ results in antimicrobial and antitumor effects (Pace et al. 1983). However, the primary cytokine produced by Th1 cells is IFNγ, and Th1 cells also produce IL-2 (Deng et al. 2014). IL-2 stimulates the proliferation of naive Th cells. IFN-gamma stimulates more IL-12 secretion from activated APCs, for the elevation of a Th1 response and suppression of any Th2 response and the activation of Tc (T cytotoxic) cells that kill infected cells.

HIV infection causes a shift in the Th1 subset response to a Th2 subset response. This Th2 response cannot control intracellular infections. So, this allows HIV persistence in CD4+T helpers (Osakwe et al. 2010; Klein et al. 1997). The significant cytokines produced by Th2 cells are IL-4, IL5, IL-13 and IL-9. These cytokines are especially associated with the allergic immune response. IL-4 and IL-2 are important stimulators for Th2 cell differentiation (Cote-Sierra et al. 2004; Walker and McKenzie 2018).

Th17 cells produce IL-17A, IL-17F, IL-22, and TNFα.IL6, IL21, IL23, and TGF-β are important stimulators for Th17 cell differentiation andIL-27 is a negative regulator for Th17 differentiation (Hirahara and Nakayama 2016; Luckheeram et al. 2012; Veldhoen et al. 2006). Th17 cells have a key task in mucosal immunity (Kolls and Khader 2010). Many studies have shown that both Th17 cells and Th17/Treg ratios play important roles. The possible correlations between these parameters and the HIV-specific antiviral T-cell adaptive response are remarkable. Unfortunately, some researches have shown that HIV infections causea selective depletion of Th17 cells in both the gut mucosa and blood that can result in microbial translocation and disease progression (Bixler and Mattapallil 2013; Falivene et al. 2015; Kanwar et al. 2010).

In the sigmoid colon mucosa of HIV-infected individuals, Th22 cell expression is dramatically absent and can be expressed after prolonged antiretroviral treatment (Kim et al. 2012). There is a small number of people who are not infected despite exposure to HIV. There is a study that includes these HIV-resistant people, HIV-infected sick people, and healthy people as a control group. In this study, Th22 cells were found to be significantly higher in HIV-resistant individuals (Oliveira et al. 2015). Th22 cells secrete IL-22.IL-22 can be considered as part of innate immunity (Missé et al. 2007). Both Th17 and Th22 cells are protective for mucosal tissues and both decrease during HIV infection. However, Th22 cell protection is stronger than that of Th17 cells. Besides, recombinant IL-22 can inhibit the demolition of epithelial cell integrity during HIV infection (Gong et al. 2021).

Tfh cells are found in the germinal centers within the lymph nodes and spleen. The generation of Tfh cells depends on the presence of IL-23, IL-12, and TGF-β (Fazilleau et al. 2009; Qin et al. 2018). IL-2 is the strongest inhibitor of Tfh cells (Ballesteros-Tato et al. 2012). Tfh cells produce IL-21, which is necessary for B-cell differentiation, and are associated with broad HIV neutralizing antibody responses (Moody et al. 2016). Also, Tfh cells express high levels of programmed cell death 1 (PDCD1; PD-1). Unfortunately, Tfh cells can be directly infected by HIV. Infected Tfh cells may cause an obstruction to curing HIV infection (Banga et al. 2016). Several researches have shown that Tfh cells are important reservoirs in HIV-infected individuals (Aid et al. 2018; Perreau et al. 2013).

Natural Treg (nTreg) gains functions during development in the thymus, and inducible Treg (iTreg) develops during peripheral naive CD4+ T-cell differentiation. The most important signal that activates Treg is transforming growth factor TGF-β (Chen et al. 2003; Shevach and Thornton 2014). Natural Treg cells border the violence of the effector immune response in order to limit tissue damage during infectious processes by producing IL-10 and TGF-β (Belkaid and Rouse 2005). Although Treg cells play a good role in the fight against HIV infection in terms of limiting the high immune activation, which is the cause of the progressive state of the disease, the HIV-specific immune response can be disrupted by its strong Treg cell effect. Therefore, the activity of Treg cells must be in balance (A Kinter et al. 2007; AL Kinter et al. 2007).

CD8+ T-Cell Cytokine Response to HIV/AIDS

The human immunodeficiency virus (HIV) causes severe immunodeficiency, but stimulates a strong immune response via cytotoxic T lymphocytes (CTL) in infected individuals. In the acute phase of infection, the CTL response first occurs to increase the viral load in blood, and when this response peaks, the viral levels decrease. There is then an inverse relationship between the CTL response and the viral load (Ogg et al. 1998).

The results of several researches have shown that virus-specific CTLs may have functional defects and their killing skills may be less efficient than expected in HIV-infected individuals (Kalams and Walker 1998; Zajac et al. 1998). In early HIV infection, CD4+ Tcells may help the CD8+ T-cell response and the first CD8+ T-cell response may be similar toother viruses. The troubles may start later. CD4+ T-cell help is important for maturing the CD8+ T-cell function and the CD8+ T-cell memory. HIV can disrupt all of these interactions. Besides, HIV can directly infect dendritic cells and disturb their function (McMichael and Rowland-Jones 2001).

Some *in-vitro* studies show that CD8+ T cells can suppress HIV replication in infected CD4+ T cells as a nonlytic function, and this is one of the most potent immune responses to HIV (Levy et al. 1996; Mackewicz and Levy 1992). HIV-specific CTL sproduce IFN-γ, MIP-1α, MIP-1β, and RANTES chemokines which can suppress HIV replication. Also HIV-specific CTLs produce TNF-α, which can increase HIV replication (McMichael and Rowland-Jones 2001)

NK Cells, NKT Cells, and γδ T-Cell-Related Cytokines in HIV/AIDS

NK cells, NKT cells and γδ T cells are important innate killer cells which can inhibit HIV replication by direct or indirect cytolytic effects or noncytolytic ways. Unfortunately, these cell functions are dysregulated and played out in chronic HIV infection. Common γ chain cytokines (IL-2, IL-7, IL-15 and IL-21) can stimulate these cells (Poonia 2013).

NK cell functions in HIV infection are not restricted to cytotoxic effects. Activated NK cells secrete IFN-γ and MIP-1β, which suppress HIV replication *in vitro* by inhibiting HIV entry to target cells. NK cells secrete IL-22, that induces epithelial cells for the production of antimicrobial molecules and IL-10. NK cells interact with dendritic cells (DCs) and regulate the maturation and function of DCs by a crosstalk with them. Also, NK cells set the induction of antibodies through the elimination of Tfh. Tfh supports HIV-1 replication which may limit the viral reservoir size (Flórez-Álvarez et al. 2018). IL-2, IL-12, IL-15, IL-18, IL-21, and type I interferons effect the maturation, survival and activation of NK cells (Zwirner and Domaica 2010).

Dendritic Cells, and Monocyte and Macrophage Related Cytokines in HIV/AIDS

Dendritic cells (DCs) are professional antigen-presenting cells that link innate and adaptive immunity. . DCs are activated by HIV and produce some cytokines (IL-12, IL-15, and type I IFN) supporting NK cell proliferation and cytotoxicity. Activated NK cells produce IFNα that supports DC maturation and Th1-type immune responses. In addition, NK cells eliminate immature DCs (Barroca et al. 2014).

Monocytes and macrophages have key roles in the inflammatory component of the cellular immune response and, through cytokine secretion, they interact with all phases of the immune system. One of the important functions of monocytes is cytokine secretion such as tumor necrosis factor a (TNF-a), interleukin-1 beta, and interleukin-6 (IL-6) (Lathey et al. 1994).

Neutrophil-Related Cytokines in HIV/AIDS

Neutrophils play an important role in primary defense against infections by phagocytosis and secreting enzymes and toxic molecules. It has been reported that human peripheral blood neutrophils can be infected by HIV because they express CD4 (Biswas et al. 2003). They can secrete a large variety of cytokines, including chemotactic cytokines: IL-1α, IL-1 receptor antagonist, IL-6, IL-8, tumor necrosis factor-alpha (TNF-α), interferon-alpha (IFN-α), granulocyte-macrophage CSF (GM-CSF), macrophage colony-stimulating factor (M-CSF), macrophage inflammatory protein-1α (MIP-1α) and IL-12. Studies have shown dysregulation in neutrophil cytokine production especially IL-12 during HIV infection. Therefore, HIV-infected individuals also have difficulties in combating other infections (Vecchiarelli et al. 2000).

Effect of Cytokines on HIV Replication and Progression into AIDS

Let's focus more on a few cytokines whose effects on HIV/AIDS have been more researched.

Tumor Necrosis Factor Alpha (TNF-α)

Tumor necrosis factor alpha (TNF-α) is a cytokine with a wide variety of effects on various cell types. TNF-α is the main regulator of inflammatory responses. It plays an active role in most phases of the immune system, but if it is produced in large quantities, it causes more damage than benefits. TNF-α plays an importantrole in the development of autoimmune diseases, cancer, and chronic inflammation. TNF-α also stimulates the release of other proinflammatory cytokines such as IL-1b, IL-6 and IL-8 (Bahia and Silakari 2010; Kedzierska and Crowe 2001; Pasquereau et al. 2017).

TNF-α plasma levels, like other proinflammatory cytokines, have been found to be high at all stages of HIV infection, and this increase is higher in untreated HIV-1-infected individuals (Devadas et al. 2004; Folks et al. 1989; Merrill et al. 1989; Guido Poli et al. 1990). In addition, the plasma level of TNF-α is positively correlated with HIV replication, which reveals the important role of TNF-α in HIV-1 pathogenesis (Kumar et al. 2016; Norris et al. 2006).

Even in the latency period, which is the low viremia period of the infection, and in patients receiving combination antiretroviral therapy, TNF-α levels are higher than in the general population, and these individuals may still have complications due to immune activation (Castillo-Mancilla et al. 2016; Sereti et al. 2017). New methods that also control TNF-α production during the treatment period may reduce immune activation (Pasquereau et al. 2017). In addition, some studies with anti-TNF-α have shown that it can reduce the HIV viral load and can be used in the treatment of autoimmune diseases caused by HIV (Freeman et al. 2016; Pasquereau et al. 2017). However, care should be taken against opportunistic infections that may occur during anti-TNF-α therapy (Freeman et al. 2016; Kumar et al. 2016)

IL-1

IL-1 is a proinflammatory cytokine released against infections and inflammation by endothelial cells and fibroblasts, especially macrophages and monocytes (Kedzierska and Crowe 2001; Kreuzer et al. 1997). IL-1, like other proinflammatory cytokines, makes an important contribution to the immune response, especially in the acute phase of inflammation. However, in the case of chronic inflammation, it can cause tissue damage and morbidity together with other proinflammatory cytokines (Baumann and Gauldie 1994; Lukens et al. 2012). As a result, it can cause autoimmune diseases, allergic diseases and even cancer development (Bendtzen et al. 1986; Brennan and Feldmann 1996; Dinarello 2018; Nambu and Nakae 2010). IL-1-beta, especially with TNF-α, activates the cytotoxic effect of neutrophils and macrophages, causes fever due to prostaglandin production, increases IL-2 production and increases antigen-specific CD4+ T-cell expansion (Merrill et al. 1989).

Although IL-1 is increased in all phases of HIV infection, it increases more especially in the virus replication phase. The IL-1 level correlates positively with the stage of the disease (Merrill et al. 1989). IL-1 induces both proliferation and apoptosis of CD4+ cells, and CD4+ cells are depleted as a result of many rounds of division (Freeman et al. 2016; Shive et al. 2014).

IL-1 and TNF-α are responsible for AIDS-related cachexia and dementia resulting from microglia activation (Chang et al. 1998; Cheung et al. 2008; Merrill et al. 1989).

IL-2

IL-2 is released by neutrophils, monocytes, NK cells and especially T cells (Freeman et al. 2016; Smith 1988) IL-2 induces the proliferation of activated CD4+ cells, increases the cytotoxic activity of CD8+ and NK cells, also activates the function of B cells and induces IGg release. Thus, it plays an important role in the elimination of intracellular pathogens (Alfano and Poli 2005; Freeman et al. 2016; Smith 1988). However, IL-2 also causes increased HIV replication (Vandergeeten et al. 2012). While the IL-2 level increases in the early phase of HIV infection, the IL-2 level decreases in the chronic phase. One of the functional defects detected in HIV-infected individuals during the AIDS period is the loss of CD4+ T cells due to IL-2 reduction (Hong et al. 1998; Orsilles et al. 2006). Based on this, it has been suggested that therapeutic administration of IL-2 may enhance systemic immune responses and improve CD4+ T-cell counts in HIV-infected persons receiving antiretroviral therapy (Freeman et al. 2016; Kinter and Fauci 1996; Alfano and Poli 2005). IL-2 administration induces CD4+ and CD8+ T-cell activation, proliferation and apoptosis, with a significant expansion in the number of circulating CD4+ T cells (Freeman et al. 2016). However, phase III trials on this subject have shown that these increases have no clinical benefit (Catalfamo et al. 2012; Vandergeeten et al. 2012).

IL-6

IL-6 is a pleotropic cytokine secreted by hematopoietic cells, fibroblasts, keratinocytes, mesangial cells and vascular endothelial cells against tissue damage and infections (Velazquez-Salinas et al. 2019). Il-6, like other proinflammatory cytokines (TNF-α, IL-1), has important effects on the cellular repair of infections and the acute phase of tissue damage, and also induces fever and the production of acute phase proteins (Velazquez-Salinas et al. 2019; Baumann and Gauldie 1994). As with other proinflammatory cytokines, it is responsible for morbidity due to its high and continuous secretion during chronic inflammation (Freeman et al. 2016).

IL-6 inhibits virus eradication by playing a role in polyclonal B-lymphocyte activation, one of the earliest immunological abnormalities of HIV infection (Emilie et al. 1994). IL-6 increases B-cell IgG production by regulating the expression of IL-21. IL-6 regulates the differentiation of monocytes into macrophages through having an effect on macrophage colony-stimulating factor expression. IL-6 plays a role in the negative regulation of dendritic cell maturation. Moreover, IL-6 promotes the Th2 response by inhibiting Th1 polarization by stimulating CD4 T cells to secrete IL-4 and direct the response to Th2, and effecting the secretion of IFNγ (Velazquez-Salinas et al. 2019).

IL-6 can induce HIV-1 replication. HIV envelope proteins, gp41 and gp120, can increase IL-6 stimulation by macrophages (Devadas et al. 2004; Takeshita et al. 1995). During HIV infection, IL-6 levels increase and correlate positively with the progression of HIV disease. This increase occurs more in the AIDS period (Honda et al. 1990; Kreuzer et al. 1997; G. Poli et al. 1994). Just like IL-1, IL-6 decreases IL-7 activity and the apoptosis of CD4+ T cells increases (Shive et al. 2014). During HIV infection, thymic atrophy and fibrosis in lymph nodes occur due to IL-6, causing the CD4+ T cells in these tissues to become insensitive to IL-7 (Fielding et al. 2014; Lynch et al. 2009; Schacker et al. 2006; Zeng et al. 2011). As a result of all these, the turnover of CD4+ cells increases and cell depletion occurs (Freeman et al. 2016). In addition, IL-6 is responsible for cachexia, Kaposi's sarcoma, encephalitis and lymphomas, especially during the AIDS period (Emilie et al. 1994).

IL-7

IL-7 is a cytokine that is produced by stromal and endothelial cells, especially in the thymus and lymph nodes, supports the proliferation and survival of mature T cells and plays a role in thymopoiesis (Freeman et al. 2016; Nunnari and Pomerantz 2005). By increasing BCL-2 expression, IL-7 inhibits T-cell apoptosis and increases especially CD4+ cell survival. It increases the number of CD4+ and CD8+ T cells by stimulating the thymus and stem cells, and can also increase the cytolytic activity of CD8+ T cells (Carini and Essex 1994).

IL-7 also stimulates the expression of the HIV co-receptor chemokine receptor CXCR4 in chronic stages of the disease and increases the sensitivity of T cells to HIV. Also, IL-7 increases HIV replication. IL-7 may indirectly increase HIV persistence by promoting the proliferation of infected cells (Alfano & Poli 2005; Catalfamo et al. 2012; Freeman et al. 2016). Although an increase in IL-7 levels has been found in the chronic stage, insensitivity to IL-7 develops due to the decrease in its receptor (CD127) (Catalfamo et al. 2012; Freeman et al. 2016). The effect of IL-1 and IL-6 is important in the reduction of IL-7 receptors (Shive et al. 2014).

Therapeutic administration of IL-7 in HIV-infected patients receiving antiretroviral therapy resulted in an increase in CD4+ T cells. There is insufficient information as to how this increase affects the immune function (Catalfamo et al. 2012; Freeman et al. 2016).

IL-10

IL-10 is an anti-inflammatory cytokine secreted mainly by Th2 and DC cells, and also by B cells, monocytes, and NK cells (Banchereau et al. 2003; Moore et al. 2001; Stylianou et al. 1999). IL-10 inhibits the secretion of proinflammatory cytokines. It decreases T-cell proliferation and macrophage and antigen presenting cell activation, and increases B-cell proliferation and activation (Moore et al. 2001). As a result, the T-cell response decreases and the humoral response increases (Moore et al. 2001).

IL-10 production increases due to the level ofviral replication in HIV infection(Norris et al. 2006). Different results have been found in studies on the effects of IL-10 on HIV infection. IL-10 enhances the entry of the virus by increasing the expression of CCR5 on monocytes (Moore et al. 2001; Sozzani et al. 1998). But IL-10 can prevent HIV replication by directly activating monocytes (Brockman et al. 2009). In the early stage of HIV infection, IL-10 enhances viral replication due to reduced cellular immunity. In the chronic period, it can limit HIV replication by reducing immune hyperactivation (Naicker et al. 2009).

IFN-1

IFN-α and IFN-β are the best characterized IFN-I cytokines. Almost all cell types secrete IFN-I but plasmacytoid DCs secrete rather than other cell types. Immunoregulatory and antiviral effects are both important for the control of acute stage viral infections. Plasma IFN-α levels are also increased in an untreated infection. But IFN-I expression may be detrimental for the host during chronic uncontrolled infection. IFN-α inhibits IL-7 induced signaling and the proliferation of T cells. Plasma IFN-α levels are correlated with HIV replication levels and inversely correlated with circulating CD4+ T-cell counts. IFN-α decreases during ART (Freeman et al. 2016).

IL-12 and IFN-γ

IL-12is a master switch cytokine that is secreted bydendritic cells and phagocytes. It supports the Th1 pathway ofCD4+ T cells and also activates NK cells (Villinger and Ansari 2010). It induces NK, T and NKT cell cytotoxicity, and supports macrophage activity (Egilmez et al. 2011; Trinchieri 2003). The pathway is inhibited by IL-10 (Villinger and Ansari 2010).

IL-12 production requires the presence of IFN-γ (Louis et al. 2010). HIV progression is caused to decrease IFN-γ (Louis et al. 2010). So, IL-12 concentration decreases. This is a risk for increasing opportunistic infections.

Importance of Cytokine-Based Therapies for HIV/AIDS Cure

The sign of an immunodeficiency level in HIV-infected individuals is a reduction in the CD4+ T-cell count. Low CD4+ T-cell counts are associated with a high frequency of opportunistic infections. Antiretroviral treatment (ART) increases the CD4+ T-cell count. But, HIV-infected individuals treated with ART have incomplete therapy of the immune system. HIV-infected individuals are also characterized by a polyclonal activation of T cells and B cells, which increases HIV replication and results in the destruction of CD4+ T cells. Various researches are being done in order to find cytokine-based strategies that reduce immune activation. (Allende and Lane 2001).

Conclusion

HIV infection, both untreated and ART-controlled, is characterized by the dysregulation of a number of bioactive cytokines. To understand the pathogenesis of HIV/AIDS and to develop treatment modalities that can provide a complete cure, it is necessary to understand this complex immunological network and cytokines, which are important elements of this network. There are still many unknowns that need to be clarified.

References

Aid, M., Dupuy, F. P., Moysi, E., et al. (2018). Follicular CD4 T Helper Cells as a Major HIV Reservoir Compartment: A Molecular Perspective. *Front Immunol*, *9*, 895. https://doi.org/10.3389/fimmu.2018.00895.

Alfano, M., and Poli, G. (2005). Role of cytokines and chemokines in the regulation of innate immunity and HIV infection. *Mol Immunol*, *42*(2) 161-182. https://doi.org/10.1016/j.molimm.2004.06.016.

Allende, M. C., and Lane, H. C. (2001) Cytokine-based therapies for HIV infection. *Aids*, *15* (Suppl 5), S183-191. https://doi.org/10.1097/00002030-200100005-00022.

Bahia, M. S., and Silakari, O. (2010). Tumor necrosis factor alpha converting enzyme: an encouraging target for various inflammatory disorders. *Chem Biol Drug Des*, *75*(5), 415-443. https://doi.org/10.1111/j.1747-0285.2010.00950.x.

Ballesteros-Tato, A., León, B., Graf, B. A., et al. (2012). Interleukin-2 inhibits germinal center formation by limiting T follicular helper cell differentiation. *Immunity*, *36*(5), 847-856. https://doi.org/10.1016/j.immuni.2012.02.012.

Banchereau, J., Paczesny, S., Blanco, P., et al. (2003). Dendritic cells: controllers of the immune system and a new promise for immunotherapy. *Ann N Y Acad Sci*, *987*, 180-187. https://doi.org/10.1111/j.1749-6632.2003.tb06047.x.

Banga, R., Procopio, F. A., Noto, A., et al. (2016). PD-1(+) and follicular helper T cells are responsible for persistent HIV-1 transcription in treated aviremic individuals. *Nat Med*, *22*(7), 754-761. https://doi.org/10.1038/nm.4113.

Barroca, P., Calado, M., and Azevedo-Pereira, J. M. (2014). HIV/dendritic cell interaction: consequences in the pathogenesis of HIV infection. AIDS Rev, 16(4), 223-235.

Baumann, H., and Gauldie, J. (1994). The acute phase response. *Immunol Today*, *15*(2), 74-80. https://doi.org/10.1016/0167-5699(94)90137-6.

Belkaid, Y., and Rouse, B. T. (2005). Natural regulatory T cells in infectious disease. *Nat Immunol*, *6*(4), 353-360. https://doi.org/10.1038/ni1181.

Bendtzen, K., Mandrup-Poulsen, T., Nerup, J., et al. (1986). Cytotoxicity of human pI 7 interleukin-1 for pancreatic islets of Langerhans. *Science*, *232*(4757), 1545-1547.

Biswas, P., Mantelli, B., Sica, A., et al. (2003). Expression of CD4 on human peripheral blood neutrophils. *Blood*, *101*(11), 4452-4456. https://doi.org/10.1182/blood-2002-10-3056.

Bixler, S. L., and Mattapallil, J. J. (2013). Loss and dysregulation of Th17 cells during HIV infection. *Clin Dev Immunol*, *2013*, 852418. https://doi.org/10.1155/2013/852418.

Brennan, F. M., and Feldmann, M. (1996). Cytokines in autoimmunity. *Curr Opin Immunol*, *8*(6), 872-877. https://doi.org/10.1016/s0952-7915(96)80018-5.

Brockman, M. A., Kwon, D. S., Tighe, D. P., et al. (2009). IL-10 is up-regulated in multiple cell types during viremic HIV infection and reversibly inhibits virus-specific T cells. *Blood*, 114(2), 346-356. https://doi.org/10.1182/blood-2008-12-191296.

Carini, C., and Essex, M. (1994). Interleukin 2-independent interleukin 7 activity enhances cytotoxic immune response of HIV-1-infected individuals. *AIDS Res Hum Retroviruses*, *10*(2), 121-130. https://doi.org/10.1089/aid.1994.10.121.

Castillo-Mancilla, J. R., Brown, T. T., Erlandson, K. M., et al. (2016). Suboptimal Adherence to Combination Antiretroviral Therapy is Associated with Higher Levels of Inflammation Despite HIV Suppression. *Clin Infect Dis*, *63*(12), 1661-1667. https://doi.org/10.1093/cid/ciw650.

Catalfamo, M., Le Saout, C., and Lane, H. C. (2012). The role of cytokines in the pathogenesis and treatment of HIV infection. *Cytokine Growth Factor Rev*, *23*(4-5), 207-214. https://doi.org/10.1016/j.cytogfr.2012.05.007.

Chang, H. R., Dulloo, A. G., and Bistrian, B. R. (1998). Role of cytokines in AIDS wasting. *Nutrition*, *14*(11-12), 853-863. https://doi.org/10.1016/s0899-9007(98)00108-7.

Chatzileontiadou, D. S. M., Sloane, H., Nguyen, A. T., et al. (2020). The Many Faces of CD4(+) T Cells: Immunological and Structural Characteristics. *Int J Mol Sci*, *22*(1), 73. https://doi.org/10.3390/ijms22010073.

Chen, W., Jin, W., Hardegen, N., et al. (2003). Conversion of peripheral CD4+CD25- naive T cells to CD4+CD25+ regulatory T cells by TGF-beta induction of transcription factor Foxp3. *J Exp Med*, *198*(12), 1875-1886. https://doi.org/10.1084/jem.20030152.

Cheung, R., Ravyn, V., Wang, L., et al. (2008). Signaling mechanism of HIV-1 gp120 and virion-induced IL-1beta release in primary human macrophages. *J Immunol*, *180*(10), 6675-6684. https://doi.org/10.4049/jimmunol.180.10.6675.

Cote-Sierra, J., Foucras, G., Guo, L., et al. (2004). Interleukin 2 plays a central role in Th2 differentiation. *Proc Natl Acad Sci USA*, *101*(11), 3880-3885. https://doi.org/10.1073/pnas.0400339101.

D'Andrea, A., Aste-Amezaga, M., Valiante, N. M., et al. (1993). Interleukin 10 (IL-10) inhibits human lymphocyte interferon gamma-production by suppressing natural killer cell stimulatory factor/IL-12 synthesis in accessory cells. *J Exp Med*, *178*(3), 1041-1048. https://doi.org/10.1084/jem.178.3.1041.

Deng, N., Weaver, J. M., and Mosmann, T. R. (2014). Cytokine diversity in the Th1-dominated human anti-influenza response caused by variable cytokine expression by Th1 cells, and a minor population of uncommitted IL-2+IFNγ- Thpp cells. *PLoS One*, *9*(5), e95986. https://doi.org/10.1371/journal.pone.0095986.

Devadas, K., Hardegen, N. J., Wahl, L. M., et al. (2004). Mechanisms for macrophage-mediated HIV-1 induction. *J Immunol*, *173*(11), 6735-6744. https://doi.org/10.4049/jimmunol.173.11.6735.

Dinarello, C. A. (2018). Overview of the IL-1 family in innate inflammation and acquired immunity. Immiunol *Rev*, *281*(1), 8-27. https://doi.org/10.1111/imr.12621.

Egilmez, N. K., Harden, J. L., Virtuoso, L. P., et al. (2011). Nitric oxide short-circuits interleukin-12-mediated tumor regression. *Cancer Immunol Immunother*, *60*(6), 839-845. https://doi.org/10.1007/s00262-011-0998-2.

Emilie, D., Fior, R., Jarrousse, B., et al. (1994) Cytokines in HIV infection. *Int J Immunopharmacol*, *16*(5-6), 391-396. https://doi.org/10.1016/0192-0561(94)90026-4.

Falivene, J., Ghiglione, Y., Laufer, N., et al. (2015). Th17 and Th17/Treg ratio at early HIV infection associate with protective HIV-specific CD8(+) T-cell responses and disease progression. *Sci Rep*, *5*, 11511. https://doi.org/10.1038/srep11511.

Fazilleau, N., Mark, L., McHeyzer-Williams, L. J., et al. (2009). Follicular helper T cells: lineage and location. *Immunity*, *30*(3), 324-335. https://doi.org/10.1016/j.immuni.2009.03.003.

Fielding, C.A., Jones, G. W., McLoughlin, R. M., et al. (2014). Interleukin-6 signaling drives fibrosis in unresolved inflammation. *Immunity*, *40*(1), 40-50. https://doi.org/10.1016/j.immuni.2013.10.022.

Flórez-Álvarez, L., Hernandez, J. C., and Zapata, W. (2018). NK cells in HIV-1 infection: from basic science to vaccine strategies. *Front Immunol*, *9*, 2290.

Folks, T. M., Clouse, K. A., Justement, J., et al. (1989). Tumor necrosis factor alpha induces expression of human immunodeficiency virus in a chronically infected T-cell clone. *Proc Natl Acad Sci USA*, *86*(7), 2365-2368. https://doi.org/10.1073/pnas.86.7.2365.

Freeman, M. L., Shive, C. L., Nguyen, T. P., et al. (2016). Cytokines and T-Cell Homeostasis in HIV Infection. *J Infect Dis*, *214*(Suppl 2), S51-57. https://doi.org/10.1093/infdis/jiw287.

Gong, J., Zhan, H., Liang, Y., et al. (2021). Role of Th22 Cells in Human Viral Diseases. *Front Med (Lausanne)*, *8*, 708140. https://doi.org/10.3389/fmed.2021.708140.

Hirahara, K., and Nakayama, T. (2016). CD4+ T-cell subsets in inflammatory diseases: beyond the Th1/Th2 paradigm. *Int Immunol*, *28*(4), 163-171. https://doi.org/10.1093/intimm/dxw006.

Hokello, J., Sharma, A. L., Dimri, M., et al. (2019). Insights into the HIV Latency and the Role of Cytokines. *Pathogens*, *8*(3), 137. https://doi.org/10.3390/pathogens8030137.

Honda, M., Kitamura, K., Mizutani, Y., et al. (1990). Quantitative analysis of serum IL-6 and its correlation with increased levels of serum IL-2R in HIV-induced diseases. *J Immunol*, *145*(12), 4059-4064.

Hong, M. A., Wakim, V. L., Salomão, S. J., et al. (1998). IL-2 and IFN-gamma, but not IL-4 secretion by peripheral blood mononuclear cells (PBMC) are related to CD4+ T cells and clinical status in Brazilian HIV-1-infected subjects. *Rev Inst Med Trop Sao Paulo*, *40*(6), 351-354. https://doi.org/10.1590/s0036-46651998000600003.

Hsieh, C. S., Macatonia, S. E., Tripp, C. S., et al. (1993). Development of TH1 CD4+ T cells through IL-12 produced by Listeria-induced macrophages. *Science*, *260*(5107), 547-549. https://doi.org/10.1126/science.8097338.

Kalams, S. A., and Walker, B. D. (1998). The critical need for CD4 help in maintaining effective cytotoxic T lymphocyte responses. *J Exp Med*, *188*(12), 2199-2204. https://doi.org/10.1084/jem.188.12.2199.

Kanwar, B., Favre, D., and McCune, J. M., (2010)/ Th17 and regulatory T cells: implications for AIDS pathogenesis. *CurrOpin HIV AIDS*, *5*(2), 151-157. https://doi.org/10.1097/COH.0b013e328335c0c1.

Kedzierska, K., and Crowe, S. M. (2001). Cytokines and HIV-1: interactions and clinical implications. *Antivir Chem Chemother*, *12*(3), 133-150. https://doi.org/10.1177/095632020101200301.

Kim, C. J., Nazli, A., Rojas, O. L., et al. (2012). A role for mucosal IL-22 production and Th22 cells in HIV-associated mucosal immunopathogenesis. *Mucosal Immunol*, *5*(6), 670-680. https://doi.org/10.1038/mi.2012.72.

Kinter, A., and Fauci, A. S. (1996). Interleukin-2 and human immunodeficiency virus infection: pathogenic mechanisms and potential for immunologic enhancement. *Immunol Res*, 15(1), 1-15. https://doi.org/10.1007/bf02918280.

Kinter, A., McNally, J., Riggin, L., et al. (2007). Suppression of HIV-specific T cell activity by lymph node CD25+ regulatory T cells from HIV-infected individuals. *Proc Natl Acad Sci USA*, *104*(9), 3390-3395. https://doi.org/10.1073/pnas.0611423104.

Kinter, A. L., Horak, R., Sion, M., et al. (2007). CD25+ regulatory T cells isolated from HIV-infected individuals suppress the cytolytic and nonlytic antiviral activity of HIV-specific CD8+ T cells *in vitro*. *AIDS Res Hum Retroviruses*, *23*(3), 438-450. https://doi.org/10.1089/aid.2006.0162.

Klein, S. A., Dobmeyer, J. M., Dobmeyer, T. S., et al. (1997), Demonstration of the Th1 to Th2 cytokine shift during the course of HIV-1 infection using cytoplasmic cytokine detection on single cell level by flow cytometry. Aids, 11(9), 1111-1118. https://doi.org/10.1097/00002030-199709000-00005.

Kolls, J. K., and Khader, S. A. (2010). The role of Th17 cytokines in primary mucosal immunity. *Cytokine Growth Factor Rev*, *21*(6), 443-448. https://doi.org/10.1016/j.cytogfr.2010.11.002.

Kreuzer, K. A., Dayer, J. M., Rockstroh, J. K., et al. (1997). The IL-1 system in HIV infection: peripheral concentrations of IL-1beta, IL-1 receptor antagonist and soluble IL-1 receptor type II. *Clin Exp Immunol*, *109*(1), 54-58. https://doi.org/10.1046/j.1365-2249.1997.4181315.

Kumar, A., Coquard, L., and Herbein, G. (2016). Targeting TNF-Alpha in HIV-1 Infection. *Curr Drug Targets*, *17*(1), 15-22. https://doi.org/10.2174/1573399811666150615145824.

Lathey, J. L., Kanangat, S., Rouse, B. T. et al. (1994). Dysregulation of cytokine expression in monocytes from HIV-positive individuals. *Journal of leukocyte biology*, *56*(3), 347-352.

Levy, J. A., Mackewicz, C. E., and Barker, E. (1996). Controlling HIV pathogenesis: the role of the noncytotoxic anti-HIV response of CD8+ T cells. *Immunol Today*, *17*(5), 217-224. https://doi.org/10.1016/0167-5699(96)10011-6.

Louis, S., Dutertre, C. A., Vimeux, L., et al. (2010). IL-23 and IL-12p70 production by monocytes and dendritic cells in primary HIV-1 infection. *J Leukoc Biol*, *87*(4), 645-653. https://doi.org/10.1189/jlb.1009684.

Luckheeram, R. V., Zhou, R., Verma, A. D., et al. (2012). $CD4^{+}$T cells: differentiation and functions. *Clin Dev Immunol*, 2012, 925135. https://doi.org/10.1155/2012/925135.

Lukens, J. R., Gross, J. M., and Kanneganti, T. D. (2012). IL-1 family cytokines trigger sterile inflammatory disease. *Front Immunol*, *3*, 315. https://doi.org/10.3389/fimmu.2012.00315.

Lynch, H. E., Goldberg, G. L., Chidgey, A., et al. (2009). Thymic involution and immune reconstitution. *Trends Immunol*, *30*(7), 366-373. https://doi.org/10.1016/j.it.2009.04.003.

Mackewicz, C., and Levy, J. A. (1992). CD8+ cell anti-HIV activity: nonlytic suppression of virus replication. *AIDS Res Hum Retroviruses*, *8*(6), 1039-1050. https://doi.org/10.1089/aid.1992.8.1039.

McMichael, A. J., and Rowland-Jones, S. L. (2001). Cellular immune responses to HIV. *Nature*, *410*(6831), 980-987. https://doi.org/10.1038/35073658.

Merrill, J. E., Koyanagi, Y., and Chen, I. (1989). Interleukin-1 and tumor necrosis factor alpha can be induced from mononuclear phagocytes by human immunodeficiency virus type 1 binding to the CD4 receptor. *Journal of virology*, *63*(10), 4404-4408.

Missé, D., Yssel, H., Trabattoni, D., et al. (2007). IL-22 participates in an innate anti-HIV-1 host-resistance network through acute-phase protein induction. *J Immunol*, *178*(1), 407-415. https://doi.org/10.4049/jimmunol.178.1.407.

Moody, M. A., Pedroza-Pacheco, I., Vandergrift, N. A., et al. (2016). Immune perturbations in HIV-1-infected individuals who make broadly neutralizing antibodies. *Sci Immunol*, *1*(1), aag0851. https://doi.org/10.1126/sciimmunol.aag0851.

Moore, K. W., de Waal Malefyt, R., Coffman, R. L., et al. (2001). Interleukin-10 and the interleukin-10 receptor. *Annu Rev Immunol*, *19*, 683-765. https://doi.org/10.1146/annurev.immunol.19.1.683.

Naicker, D. D., Werner, L., Kormuth, E., et al. (2009). Interleukin-10 promoter polymorphisms influence HIV-1 susceptibility and primary HIV-1 pathogenesis. *J Infect Dis*, 200(3), 448-452. https://doi.org/10.1086/600072.

Nambu, A., and Nakae, S. (2010). IL-1 and Allergy. *Allergol Int*, *59*(2), 125-135. https://doi.org/10.2332/allergolint.10-RAI-0190.

Norris, P. J., Pappalardo, B. L., Custer, B., et al. (2006). Elevations in IL-10, TNF-alpha, and IFN-gamma from the earliest point of HIV Type 1 infection. *AIDS Res Hum Retroviruses*, *22*(8), 757-762. https://doi.org/10.1089/aid.2006.22.757.

Nunnari, G., and Pomerantz, R. J. (2005). IL-7 as a potential therapy for HIV-1-infected individuals. *Expert Opin Biol Ther*, *5*(11), 1421-1426. https://doi.org/10.1517/14712598.5.11.1421.

Nyamweya, S., Hegedus, A., Jaye, A., et al. (2013). Comparing HIV-1 and HIV-2 infection: Lessons for viral immunopathogenesis. *Rev Med Virol*, *23*(4), 221-240. https://doi.org/10.1002/rmv.1739.

Ogg, G. S., Jin, X., Bonhoeffer, S., et al. (1998). Quantitation of HIV-1-specific cytotoxic T lymphocytes and plasma load of viral RNA. *Science*, *279*(5359), 2103-2106. https://doi.org/10.1126/science.279.5359.2103.

Oliveira, L. M., Lima, J. F., Cervantes, C. A., et al. (2015). Increased frequency of circulating Tc22/Th22 cells and polyfunctional CD38(-) T cells in HIV-exposed uninfected subjects. *Sci Rep*, *5*, 13883. https://doi.org/10.1038/srep13883.

Orsilles, M. A., Pieri, E., Cooke, P., et al. (2006). IL-2 and IL-10 serum levels in HIV-1-infected patients with or without active antiretroviral therapy. *Apmis*, *114*(1), 55-60. https://doi.org/10.1111/j.1600-0463.2006.apm_108.x.

Osakwe, C. E., Bleotu, C., Chifiriuc, M. C., et al. (2010). TH1/TH2 cytokine levels as an indicator for disease progression in human immunodeficiency virus type 1 infection and response to antiretroviral therapy. *Roum Arch Microbiol Immunol*, *69*(1), 24-34.

Pace, J. L., Russell, S. W., Schreiber, R. D., et al. (1983). Macrophage activation: priming activity from a T-cell hybridoma is attributable to interferon-gamma. *Proc Natl Acad Sci USA*, *80*(12), 3782-3786. https://doi.org/10.1073/pnas.80.12.3782.

Parkin, J., and Cohen, B. (2001). An overview of the immune system. *Lancet*, *357*(9270), 1777-1789. https://doi.org/10.1016/s0140-6736(00)04904-7.

Pasquereau, S., Kumar, A., and Herbein, G. (2017). Targeting TNF and TNF Receptor Pathway in HIV-1 Infection: from Immune Activation to Viral Reservoirs. *Viruses*, *9*(4), 64. https://doi.org/10.3390/v9040064.

Perreau, M., Savoye, A. L., De Crignis, E., et al. (2013). Follicular helper T cells serve as the major CD4 T cell compartment for HIV-1 infection, replication, and production. *J Exp Med*, *210*(1), 143-156. https://doi.org/10.1084/jem.20121932.

Poli, G., Kinter, A., Justement, J. S., et al. (1990). Tumor necrosis factor alpha functions in an autocrine manner in the induction of human immunodeficiency virus expression. *Proceedings of the National Academy of Sciences*, *87*(2), 782-785.

Poli, G., Kinter, A. L., and Fauci, A. S. (1994). Interleukin 1 induces expression of the human immunodeficiency virus alone and in synergy with interleukin 6 in chronically infected U1 cells: inhibition of inductive effects by the interleukin 1 receptor antagonist. *Proc Natl Acad Sci USA*, *91*(1), 108-112. https://doi.org/10.1073/pnas.91.1.108.

Poonia, B. (2013). Immunotherapy in HIV infection. Journal of Infectious Diseases and Therapy, 1(1) 1-5

Qin, L., Waseem, T. C., Sahoo, A., et al. (2018). Insights into the Molecular Mechanisms of T Follicular Helper-Mediated Immunity and Pathology. *Front Immunol*, *9*, 1884. https://doi.org/10.3389/fimmu.2018.01884.

Reuter, M. A., Pombo, C., and Betts, M. R. (2012) Cytokine production and dysregulation in HIV pathogenesis: lessons for development of therapeutics and vaccines. *Cytokine Growth Factor Rev*, *23*(4-5), 181-191. https://doi.org/10.1016/j.cytogfr.2012.05.005.

Schacker, T. W., Brenchley, J. M., Beilman, G. J. et al. (2006). Lymphatic tissue fibrosis is associated with reduced numbers of naive CD4+ T cells in human immunodeficiency virus type 1 infection. *Clin Vaccine Immunol*, *13*(5), 556-560. https://doi.org/10.1128/cvi.13.5.556-560.2006.

Sereti, I., Krebs, S. J., Phanuphak, N., et al. (2017). Persistent, Albeit Reduced, Chronic Inflammation in Persons Starting Antiretroviral Therapy in Acute HIV Infection. *Clin Infect Dis*, *64*(2), 124-131. https://doi.org/10.1093/cid/ciw683.

Shevach, E. M., and Thornton, A. M. (2014). tTregs, pTregs, and iTregs: similarities and differences. Immunol Rev, 259(1), 88-102. https://doi.org/10.1111/imr.12160.

Shive, C. L., Mudd, J. C., Funderburg, N. T., et al. (2014). Inflammatory cytokines drive CD4+ T-cell cycling and impaired responsiveness to interleukin 7: implications for immune failure in HIV disease. *J Infect Dis*, *210*(4), 619-629. https://doi.org/10.1093/infdis/jiu125.

Smith, K. A. (1988). Interleukin-2: inception, impact, and implications. *Science*, *240*(4856), 1169-1176. https://doi.org/10.1126/science.3131876.

Sozzani, S., Ghezzi, S., Iannolo, G., et al. (1998). Interleukin 10 increases CCR5 expression and HIV infection in human monocytes. *J Exp Med*, *187*(3), 439-444. https://doi.org/10.1084/jem.187.3.439

Stylianou, E., Aukrust, P., Kvale, D., et al. (1999). IL-10 in HIV infection: increasing serum IL-10 levels with disease progression--down-regulatory effect of potent anti-retroviral therapy. *Clin Exp Immunol*, *116*(1), 115-120. https://doi.org/10.1046/j.1365-2249.1999.00865.x.

Takeshita, S., Breen, E. C., Ivashchenko, M., et al. (1995). Induction of IL-6 and IL-10 production by recombinant HIV-1 envelope glycoprotein 41 (gp41) in the THP-1 human monocytic cell line. *Cell Immunol*, *165*(2), 234-242. https://doi.org/10.1006/cimm.1995.1210.

Trinchieri, G. (2003) Interleukin-12 and the regulation of innate resistance and adaptive immunity. *Nat Rev Immunol*, *3*(2), 133-146. https://doi.org/10.1038/nri1001.

Vandergeeten, C., Fromentin, R., and Chomont, N. (2012). The role of cytokines in the establishment, persistence and eradication of the HIV reservoir. *Cytokine Growth Factor Rev*, *23*(4-5), 143-149. https://doi.org/10.1016/j.cytogfr.2012.05.001.

Vecchiarelli, A., Monari, C., Palazzetti, B., et al. (2000). Dysregulation in IL-12 secretion by neutrophils from HIV-infected patients. *Clin Exp Immunol*, *121*(2), 311-319. https://doi.org/10.1046/j.1365-2249.2000.01278.x.

Velazquez-Salinas, L., Verdugo-Rodriguez, A., Rodriguez, L. L., et al. (2019). The Role of Interleukin 6 During Viral Infections. *Front Microbiol*, *10*, 1057. https://doi.org/10.3389/fmicb.2019.01057

Veldhoen, M., Hocking, R. J., Atkins, C. J., et al. (2006). TGFbeta in the context of an inflammatory cytokine milieu supports de novo differentiation of IL-17-producing T cells. *Immunity*, *24*(2), 179-189. https://doi.org/10.1016/j.immuni.2006.01.001.

Villinger, F., and Ansari, A. A. (2010). Role of IL-12 in HIV infection and vaccine. *Eur Cytokine Netw*, *21*(3), 215-218. https://doi.org/10.1684/ecn.2010.0206.

Walker, J. A., and McKenzie, A. N. J. (2018). T(H)2 cell development and function. *Nat Rev Immunol*, *18*(2), 121-133. https://doi.org/10.1038/nri.2017.118.

Zajac, A. J., Blattman, J. N., Murali-Krishna, K., et al. (1998). Viral immune evasion due to persistence of activated T cells without effector function. *J Exp Med*, *188*(12), 2205-2213. https://doi.org/10.1084/jem.188.12.2205.

Zeng, M., Smith, A. J., Wietgrefe, S. W., et al. (2011). Cumulative mechanisms of lymphoid tissue fibrosis and T cell depletion in HIV-1 and SIV infections. *J Clin Invest*, *121*(3), 998-1008. https://doi.org/10.1172/jci45157.

Zwirner, N. W., and Domaica, C. I. (2010). Cytokine regulation of natural killer cell effector functions. *Biofactors*, *36*(4), 274-288. https://doi.org/10.1002/biof.107.

Chapter 15

Cytokines and Insulin Resistance

Özerhan Özer*, MD

Department of Internal Medicine, Turhal State Hospital, Tokat, Turkey

Abstract

Insulin is one of the main metabolism-regulating hormones. Insulin resistance has a complex pathogenesis which is still not fully elucidated. Insulin resistance accompanies the pathogenesis of many diseases such as non-alcoholic fatty liver disease, type 2 diabetes (T2D), metabolic syndrome and atherosclerosis. Insulin resistance, one of the underlying causes of T2D, is thought to be "environmental" and a less obvious contributor than aging and genetics, a sedentary lifestyle, related to overeating, and the resulting overweight and obesity. In recent studies, it is also said that inflammatory and metabolic factors are effective in reducing the effects of insulin.

Keywords: insulin resistance, inflammation, diabetes, metabolic syndrome, cytokine, obesity

Introduction

Insulin is one of the main metabolism-regulating hormones. Insulin stimulates glucose uptake into tissues, and its ability to do so varies between individuals. Insulin resistance was coined as a term in 1922 to describe patients with diabetes who, several years after the initiation of insulin therapy, required increasing doses of insulin to control hyperglycemia. Most of these patients develop antibodies to both non-human and impure therapeutic insulin. Insulin resistance developed secondary to these antibodies (Kahn et al., 1979). The ability of tissues to respond to insulin action decreases with insulin resistance. Insulin secreted from the pancreas increases to compensate for the resistance. Therefore, people who are insulin resistant have high plasma insulin levels. The cluster of abnormalities associated with insulin resistance and consequent compensatory hyperinsulinemia was first termed as syndrome x by Reaven (Reaven 1988). It is also called by other names like metabolic syndrome and insulin resistance syndrome (Einhorn et al., 2003). Normally, when the blood glucose concentration increases, insulin secretion from pancreatic β cells is stimulated, while the release of the anti-insulin hormone glucagon is

* Corresponding Author's Email: dr.ozerhanozer@gmail.com.

In: Cytokines and Diseases
Editors: Kenan Demir, Selim Görgün and Bahar Uslu
ISBN: 979-8-88697-214-6

suppressed (LeRoith 2002). This increases glucose uptake in the liver, adipose tissues and muscle while suppressing hepatogluconeogenesis. The insulin resistance state, defined as β-cell dysfunction, occurs when there is a loss of first-phase insulin secretion or a sudden absence of insulin release in response to a glucose load. Postprandial hyperglycemia occurs due to acute insulin secretion deficiency. An exaggerated second-phase insulin response occurs to correct this glucose excess. Subsequent chronic hyperinsulinemia impairs the insulin action by downregulating insulin receptors (Del Prato et al., 1994; Roth et al., 2004). In fact, this phenomenon has been demonstrated through experiments with transgenic mice. In these mice, overexpression occurs in multiple copies of the human insulin gene. As a result of overexpression, a two-to-four-fold increase in serum insulin levels is seen. Despite the increased circulating insulin, mice remain hyperglycemic. In this study conducted in mice, it was shown that the insulin receptor was downregulated as a result of hyperinsulinemia, resulting in an insulin resistant state. Therefore, hyperinsulinemia can be observed both as a cause and as a consequence of insulin resistance (Marban et al., 1996).

Insulin resistance accompanies the pathogenesis of many diseases such as Non-alcoholic fatty liver disease, type 2 diabetes (T2D), metabolic syndrome and atherosclerosis. Insulin resistance, which is one of the underlying causes of T2D, is thought to be environmental and a less obvious contributor than aging and genetics, a sedentary lifestyle, related to overeating, and the resulting overweight and obesity. In other words, we can define insulin resistance when there is a lower glucose response to endogenous and/or exogenous insulin compared to normal. It most commonly occurs with obesity, but can also be caused by many other underlying causes (Table 1) (Semple et al., 2011). In addition, hyperglycemia itself can cause pancreatic β-cell dysfunction. As a result, insulin resistance can be exacerbated, leading to a vicious cycle of hyperglycemia that worsens the metabolic status (Kahn 1994; Robertson 1995).

Table 1. Major causes of insulin resistance (UpToDate 2021)

Inherited states
Insulin-receptor mutations
Leprechaunism (Abnormal facial appearance, early life growth retardation)
Rabson-Mendenhall syndrome (Dental and nail abnormalities, skin lesions)
Type A syndrome of insulin resistance
Some lipodystrophies
Secondary insulin resistance
Obesity
Inactivity
Anti-insulinemic hormones (cortisol, catecholamines, growth hormone, glucagon)
Pregnancy (placental lactogen)
Medications (e.g., glucocorticoids, oral contraceptives)
Immune mediated (anti-insulin antibodies, anti-insulin receptor antibodies)
Consequences of insulin resistance
Most cases of type 2 diabetes mellitus
Metabolic syndrome
Hypertension, cardiovascular disease
Polycystic ovary syndrome
Obesity-related cancers

Insulin resistance alone is not a reliable predictor of T2D (Beck-Nielsen et al., 1994; Stumvoll et al., 2005). For example, it is possible for insulin resistance to become more severe with age and weight gain, resulting in impaired beta-cell function, impaired glucose tolerance and ultimately hyperglycemia in susceptible individuals. Hyperglycemia itself may cause a worsening of hyperglycemia, possibly by reducing insulin gene expression, leading to glucotoxicity on beta cells (Hull et al., 2004).

In recent studies, it is also said that inflammatory and metabolic factors are effective in reducing the effects of insulin. The term metabolic inflammation is used for low-grade chronic inflammation conditions observed in various metabolic disorders such as obesity and diabetes (Hotamisligil 2006). Adipose tissue plays an important role in the initiation of the inflammatory response. Adipose tissue does not only serve as a place where excess calories are stored. It also actively releases fatty acids and secretes various adipocytokines that affect metabolic and endocrine functions (Rajala et al., 2003).

Clinical Features

Insulin resistance may present in various ways depending on the underlying etiology.

The following conditions can be seen in obesity-related insulin resistance;

Impaired fasting glucose, impaired glucose tolerance, and increased insulin requirements in type 1 diabetes and type 2 diabetes;

Polycystic ovary syndrome (PCOS);

Coronary artery disease;

Non-alcoholic fatty liver disease;

Metabolic syndrome;

Certain malignancies related to obesity (e.g., endometrial cancer).

Insulin resistance may accompany genetic syndromes and severe clinical manifestations may occur in this group. Although clinical features are associated with obesity and similar to other forms of insulin resistance, patients with genetic syndrome typically have extreme insulin resistance and thus more severe phenotypes (Table 2) (Mantzoros 2021).

The exact basis of the relationship between insulin resistance and clinical findings has not yet been determined. It is likely that serum insulin concentrations increased in response to greatly increased glucose levels, affecting glucose transport and, to a lesser extent, overstimulation of the insulin-responsive pathways (Mantzoros 2021).

Insulin Resistance and Cytokine Relationship

Many studies show the role of inflammation as a common mediator in associating the pathogenesis of both atherosclerosis and diabetes with obesity (Luna et al., 2001; Hovi et al., 2007). Individuals with insulin resistance and diabetes have been shown to have elevated levels of markers of inflammation, including tumor necrosis factor alpha (TNF-α), interleukin (IL)-6, C-reactive protein, chemokines (chemotactic proinflammatory cytokines), plasminogen activator inhibitor 1 (PAI-1) and white cell count (Henderson et al., 2000; Henderson 2001; Gianfrancesco et al., 2002; Officers et al., 2002; American Diabetes Association et al., 2004; Lipscombe et al., 2009; Jain et al., 2017; Quandt et al., 2020). Cytokines secreted from adipose tissue, called adipokine or adipocytokine, stimulate inflammatory activity associated with insulin resistance (Kostis et al., 2005). In addition, TNF-α levels are elevated in the blood and adipose tissue of obese rodents. Neutralization of TNF-α also increased insulin sensitivity in these animals (Hotamisligil et al., 1993). It has been shown that inflammation markers decrease after lifestyle interventions (Carlsen et al., 1990).

Table 2. Clinical manifestations of insulin resistance (UpToDate 2021)

Glucose homeostasis	Linear growth
Overt diabetes, impaired glucose tolerance, and hypoglycemia	Normal, impaired, increased
Cutaneous	Adipose tissue
Acanthosis nigricans	Normal, lipoatrophy, lipohypertrophy, obesity
Skin tags	*Musculoskeletal*
Alopecia	Normal, cramps, muscle hypertrophy, pseudoacromegaly
Reproductive	Lipid metabolism
Hirsutism	Normal or hypertriglyceridemia
Virilization	Autoimmunity
Amenorrhea	Some immune phenotypes of type B syndrome
Infertility (in women)	

C-Reactive Protein (CRP)

CRP is an acute phase reactant produced in response to IL-6 and synthesized in the liver. Circulating CRP concentrations are markers to indicate risk for cardiovascular diseases. It is also thought to be associated with insulin resistance (Pannacciulli et al., 2001; Müller et al., 2002; Festa et al., 2006). In addition, CRP levels were found to be higher in insulin-resistant obese individuals. In these individuals, the CRP level decreases with weight loss and an improvement of insulin sensitivity (McLaughlin et al., 2002; Kopp et al., 2003). Circulating CRP levels may decrease after bariatric surgery and during treatment with thiazolidinediones (TZD) (Kopp et al., 2003; Mohanty et al., 2004; Vázquez et al., 2005; Hung et al., 2006; Schernthaner et al., 2006). Debate continues as to whether CRP is a potential marker in cardiovascular disease and insulin resistance.

Tumor Necrosis Factor α (TNF-α)

TNF-α is a proinflammatory cytokine secreted by both immune cells and adipocytes. It is thought to be responsible for insulin resistance developing in adipose tissue (Hotamisligil et al., 1993). TNF-α mRNA levels in the adipose tissue of mice with genetically associated insulin resistance were significantly increased compared to wild-type controls (Hotamisligil et al., 1995). Obese individuals and lean human subjects were compared and it was shown that mRNA and TNF-α protein levels in the adipose tissue of obese individuals also increased. This situation also showed a positive correlation with plasma insulin levels (Hotamisligil et al., 1995). Although there are studies reporting that serum TNF-α levels are increased in insulin-resistant human subjects, studies suggesting the opposite have also been reported (Müller et al., 2002; Bruun et al., 2003). Importantly, studies in humans have failed to show that neutralizing anti-TNF antibodies help to improve insulin sensitivity (Ofei et al., 1996; Bernstein et al., 2006). Although it has been reported that TNF-α levels can be altered by TZD treatment, conflicting results have been reported (Mohanty et al., 2004; Di Gregorio et al., 2005). Bariatric surgery lowers circulating TNF-αR2 levels (Vázquez et al., 2005).

Interleukins

Interleukin 1α and 1β (IL-1α and IL-1β)

IL-1 is one of the major proinflammatory cytokines acting through the IL-1 receptor. IL-1 is a group of cytokines with 11 members. IL-1β is one of the most prominent mediators of inflammation that results in fever and immune activation by acting on the IL-1 receptor 1, and it is the best characterized member of IL-1. Although many studies have shown the relationship between insulin resistance and TNF-α, much less is known about whether there is a relationship between insulin sensitivity and IL-1 (Hotamisligil 2006). Böni-Schnetzler and colleagues reported in their study that IL-1 production was altered in the pancreatic islets of diabetic patients (Böni-Schnetzler et al., 2008). IL-1β levels were found to be high in non-diabetic children of individuals with diabetes. This condition has been found to be associated with metabolic syndrome (Salmenniemi et al., 2004). Increased concentrations of IL-1 with IL-6 are reported to better predict T2D risk in humans than cytokines alone (Spranger et al., 2003). Finally, both receptor expression and IL-1β levels are increased in the visceral adipose tissue of obese individuals (Juge-Aubry et al., 2004).

Interleukin 6 (IL-6)

IL-6 is a multifunctional cytokine that regulates the immune response, hematopoiesis and inflammation. It is also referred to as a B-cell differentiation factor. It is one of the first cytokines to be included as a determinant or pathogenic mediator of cardiovascular disease and insulin resistance. IL-6 levels are elevated in the circulation of patients with T2D (Pickup et al., 1997; Müller et al., 2002). A decrease in circulating IL-6 levels is observed as a result of polymorphism in the IL-6 gene. This polymorphism is associated with increased insulin sensitivity (Fernández-Real et al., 2000). The circulating IL-6 concentration is reduced in patients undergoing bariatric surgery. This was associated with an improvement of insulin resistance and weight loss (Kopp et al., 2003). When the abdominal adipose tissue and subcutaneous adipose tissue were compared, the level of IL-6 produced in the abdominal adipose tissue was found to be 3 times higher. An increased IL-6 level in the abdominal adipose tissue indicates that it may be one of the high risk factors for the development of insulin resistance (Fried et al., 1998). In addition, IL-6 may have an important role in the development of hepatic insulin resistance. Dietary obese mice treated with IL-6 antibodies have increased insulin sensitivity, which is thought to be due to improved hepatic insulin resistance (Klover et al., 2005). The diminished hepatic and skeletal muscle insulin action accompanying IL-6 treatment can be reversed by co-treatment with the anti-inflammatory cytokine IL-10 (Kim et al., 2004). However, IL-6-deficient mice show insulin resistance and these mice are diabetic (Wallenius et al., 2002).

Interleukin 8 (IL-8)

Phagocytes and a wide variety of tissue cells secrete IL-8 when exposed to inflammatory stimuli. IL-8 is a chemokine required for inflammation and angiogenesis. IL-8 is known to attract polymorphonuclear leukocytes to sites of inflammation and activate monocytes. Although it has been shown that IL-8 levels increase in insulin-resistant male individuals due to obesity, it has been reported that IL-8 levels do not decrease with increased insulin sensitivity and weight loss (Bruun et al., 2003).

Interleukin 10 (IL-10)

IL-10 family cytokines are mainly secreted from epithelial cells. These cytokines, secreted during various infections, stimulate host defense mechanisms. The IL-10 family of cytokines is essential for maintaining homeostasis and the integrity of tissue epithelial layers. These cytokines may facilitate tissue healing in damage caused by infection or inflammation. The plasma levels of IL-10 are positively associated with insulin sensitivity, and a correlation has been found between the decrease in plasma levels of IL-10 and the development of T2D (van Exel et al., 2002; Straczkowski et al., 2006). One study showed that IL-10 is expressed in adipose tissue-derived macrophages and the IL-10 receptor is expressed in adipocytes. However, it is not synthesized in immune or endothelial cells in fat (Lumeng et al., 2007).

Plasminogen Activator Inhibitor 1 (PAI-1)

PAI-1 is the structure that inhibits plasminogen activators, which convert inactive plasminogen to plasmin during fibrinolytic activity. One of the cardiovascular risk factors is considered to be PAI-1. However, peripheral insulin resistance and PAI-1 concentrations were correlated in obese type 2 diabetic patients (Potter van Loon et al., 1993; Festa et al., 2006). Wild type mice fed a high-fat diet developed hyperglycemia and hyperinsulinemia. An approximately 2.5-fold increase in PAI-1 levels and PAI-1 mRNA expression was detected in the plasma and adipose tissue of these mice compared to the control mice fed diet (Ma et al., 2004). Positive effects are seen in insulin resistance with TZD treatment and bariatric surgery. Parallel to this, circulating PAI-1 levels have also been shown to decrease (Primrose et al., 1992; Vázquez et al., 2005).

Adiponectins (Adipocytokines)

Leptin

Leptin is an adipose tissue-specific adipocytokine which is released in proportion to the adipocyte mass. This cytokine regulates body weight, food intake, neuroendocrine functions and energy expenditure. It plays a role in carbohydrate and lipid metabolism, the reproductive system, and inflammatory and immune reactions (Mantzoros 2021). Studies in animals and humans have shown that leptin resistance and leptin deficiency are associated with insulin resistance and obesity (Kwon et al., 2013).

Adiponectin

Adiponectin is the adipocytokine that is secreted in the highest amount from adipose tissue. This cytokine plays an essential role in energy, insulin sensitivity and homeostasis. It increases insulin sensitivity by increasing the beta oxidation of fatty acids and decreasing free fatty acids and triglyceride levels (Mantzoros et al., 2005). In addition to this effect, it also has anti-inflammatory and antiatherogenic effects. It is detected at low levels in type 2 diabetes, obesity, insulin resistance, cardiovascular diseases and dyslipidemia. It has been shown that adiponectin levels increase with weight loss in obese patients (Bulcão et al., 2006). In addition, adiponectin was inversely associated with diabetes risk in non-diabetic populations (Weyer et al., 2001; Kadowaki et al., 2006; Li et al., 2009).

Resistin

This is an adipocytokine secreted from adipose tissue, which acts as a metabolic mediator between inflammation and atherosclerosis. Resistin increases with inflammation and increases insulin resistance. Resistin impairs insulin sensitivity by suppressing insulin-mediated signaling in adipocytes (Kwon et al., 2013). In the neutralization of resistin, insulin-mediated glucose uptake by adipocytes increases (Steppan et al., 2001). The hypothalamic administration of resistin also increases glucose production independent of changes in glucoregulatory hormones (Muse et al., 2007). Therefore, resistin may be a hormone that links obesity to diabetes (Emamalipour et al., 2019).

Retinol-Binding Protein 4 (RBP-4)

RBP-4 is an adipocytokine synthesized in adipocytes. RBP-4 is associated with impaired glucose tolerance or obesity in patients with T2D, as well as the degree of insulin resistance in normal weight subjects with or without a family history of T2D (Graham et al., 2006; Gavi et al., 2007). Mice lacking adipocyte glucose transporter 4 (GLUT4) have been shown in a mouse model to have increased levels of RBP4 and insulin resistance occurs in the mouse muscle and liver (Yang et al., 2005). A human study showed an inverse relationship between serum RBP-

4 and GLUT4 in adipocytes (Graham et al., 2006). Whether RBP4 causes or is associated with insulin resistance in humans remains to be determined.

Obestatin

Obestatin is a hormone that suppresses the effect of ghrelin on food intake and is encoded by the ghrelin gene. It was first isolated from the rat stomach. Circulating obestatin concentrations are increased in individuals with normal glucose tolerance compared to individuals with diabetes and impaired glucose tolerance (Qi et al., 2007). In obesity-associated type 2 diabetes, the expression of the obestatin receptor in adipose tissue is down-regulated, whereas it is not up-regulated in normoglycemic subjects who have obesity. Therefore, independent of obesity, obestatin is thought to play a role in T2D development and glucose regulation (Catalán et al., 2007; Green et al., 2018).

Conclusion

It is important to clarify the pathogenesis of insulin resistance and to better understand its mechanisms, especially in terms of developing diagnosis and treatment methods. However, with their newly discovered roles, cytokines will play an important role both in our understanding of the mechanism and in improving treatment.

References

American Diabetes Association, American Psychiatric Association, American Association of Clinical Endocrinologists, Obesity NaaFTSO (2004) Consensus Development Conference on Antipsychotic Drugs and Obesity and Diabetes. *Diabetes Care* 27:596-601.

Beck-Nielsen H, Groop LC (1994) Metabolic and genetic characterization of prediabetic states. Sequence of events leading to non-insulin-dependent diabetes mellitus. *The Journal of clinical investigation* 94:1714-1721.

Bernstein LE, Berry J, Kim S, Canavan B, Grinspoon SK (2006) Effects of etanercept in patients with the metabolic syndrome. *Archives of internal medicine* 166:902-908.

Böni-Schnetzler M, Thorne J, Parnaud G, Marselli L, Ehses J A, Kerr-Conte J, Pattou F, Halban P A, Weir G C, Donath M Y (2008) Increased interleukin (IL)-1beta messenger ribonucleic acid expression in beta - cells of individuals with type 2 diabetes and regulation of IL-1beta in human islets by glucose and autostimulation. *The Journal of clinical endocrinology and metabolism* 93:4065-4074.

Bruun J M, Verdich C, Toubro S, Astrup A, Richelsen B (2003) Association between measures of insulin sensitivity and circulating levels of interleukin-8, interleukin-6 and tumor necrosis factor-alpha. Effect of weight loss in obese men. *Eur. J. Endocrinol.* 148:535-542.

Bulcão C, Ferreira S R, Giuffrida F M, Ribeiro-Filho F F (2006) The new adipose tissue and adipocytokines. *Curr. Diabetes Rev.* 2:19-28.

Carlsen J E, Køber L, Torp-Pedersen C, Johansen P (1990) Relation between dose of bendrofluazide, antihypertensive effect, and adverse biochemical effects. *Bmj* 300:975-978.

Catalán V, Gómez-Ambrosi J, Rotellar F, Silva C, Gil M J, Rodríguez A, Cienfuegos J A, Salvador J, Frühbeck G (2007) The obestatin receptor (GPR39) is expressed in human adipose tissue and is down-regulated in obesity-associated type 2 diabetes mellitus. *Clinical endocrinology* 66:598-601.

Del Prato S, Leonetti F, Simonson D C, Sheehan P, Matsuda M, Defronzo R A (1994) Effect of sustained physiologic hyperinsulinaemia and hyperglycaemia on insulin secretion and insulin sensitivity in man. *Diabetologia* 37:1025-1035.

Di Gregorio G B, Yao-Borengasser A, Rasouli N, Varma V, Lu T, Miles LM, Ranganathan G, Peterson C A, Mcgehee RE, Kern PA (2005) Expression of CD68 and macrophage chemoattractant protein-1 genes in human adipose and muscle tissues: association with cytokine expression, insulin resistance, and reduction by pioglitazone. *Diabetes* 54:2305-2313.

Einhorn D, Reaven G M, Cobin R H, Ford E, Ganda O P, Handelsman Y, Hellman R, Jellinger P S, Kendall D, Krauss R M, Neufeld N D, Petak S M, Rodbard H W, Seibel J A, Smith D A, Wilson P W (2003) American College of Endocrinology position statement on the insulin resistance syndrome. *Endocr. Pract.* 9:237-252.

Emamalipour M, Seidi K, Jahanban-Esfahlan A, Jahanban-Esfahlan R (2019) Implications of resistin in type 2 diabetes mellitus and coronary artery disease: Impairing insulin function and inducing pro-inflammatory cytokines. *J. Cell Physiol.* 234:21758-21769.

Fernández-Real J M, Broch M, Vendrell J, Gutiérrez C, Casamitjana R, Pugeat M, Richart C, Ricart W (2000) Interleukin-6 gene polymorphism and insulin sensitivity. *Diabetes* 49:517-520.

Festa A, Williams K, Tracy R P, Wagenknecht L E, Haffner S M (2006) Progression of plasminogen activator inhibitor-1 and fibrinogen levels in relation to incident type 2 diabetes. *Circulation* 113:1753-1759.

Fried SK, Bunkin D A, Greenberg AS (1998) Omental and subcutaneous adipose tissues of obese subjects release interleukin-6: depot difference and regulation by glucocorticoid. *The Journal of clinical endocrinology and metabolism* 83:847-850.

Gavi S, Stuart LM, Kelly P, Melendez M M, Mynarcik D C, Gelato M C, Mcnurlan M A (2007) Retinol-binding protein 4 is associated with insulin resistance and body fat distribution in nonobese subjects without type 2 diabetes. *The Journal of clinical endocrinology and metabolism* 92:1886-1890.

Gianfrancesco F D, Grogg A L, Mahmoud R A, Wang R H, Nasrallah H A (2002) Differential effects of risperidone, olanzapine, clozapine, and conventional antipsychotics on type 2 diabetes: findings from a large health plan database. *J. Clin. Psychiatry* 63:920-930.

Graham T E, Yang Q, Blüher M, Hammarstedt A, Ciaraldi T P, Henry R R, Wason C J, Oberbach A, Jansson P A, Smith U, Kahn B B (2006) Retinol-binding protein 4 and insulin resistance in lean, obese, and diabetic subjects. *The New England journal of medicine* 354:2552-2563.

Green B D, Grieve D J (2018) Biochemical properties and biological actions of obestatin and its relevence in type 2 diabetes. *Peptides* 100:249-259.

Henderson D C, Cagliero E, Gray C, Nasrallah RA, Hayden D L, Schoenfeld D A, Goff DC (2000) Clozapine, diabetes mellitus, weight gain, and lipid abnormalities: A five-year naturalistic study. *Am. J. Psychiatry* 157:975-981.

Henderson D C (2001) Clozapine: diabetes mellitus, weight gain, and lipid abnormalities. *J. Clin. Psychiatry* 62 (Suppl 23):39-44.

Hotamisligil G S, Shargill N S, Spiegelman B M (1993) Adipose expression of tumor necrosis factor-alpha: direct role in obesity-linked insulin resistance. *Science* 259:87-91.

Hotamisligil G S, Arner P, Caro J F, Atkinson R L, Spiegelman B M (1995) Increased adipose tissue expression of tumor necrosis factor-alpha in human obesity and insulin resistance. *The Journal of clinical investigation* 95:2409-2415.

Hotamisligil G S (2006) Inflammation and metabolic disorders. *Nature* 444:860-867.

Hovi P, Andersson S, Eriksson J G, Järvenpää A L, Strang-Karlsson S, Mäkitie O, Kajantie E (2007) Glucose regulation in young adults with very low birth weight. *The New England journal of medicine* 356:2053-2063.

Hull R L, Westermark G T, Westermark P, Kahn S E (2004) Islet amyloid: a critical entity in the pathogenesis of type 2 diabetes. *The Journal of clinical endocrinology and metabolism* 89:3629-3643.

Hung Y J, Lin S H, Pei D, Kuo S W, Hsieh C H, He CT, Hsing Lee C, Fan SC, Sheu WH (2006) Rosiglitazone improves insulin sensitivity in nonobese subjects with impaired glucose tolerance: the role of adiponectin and C-reactive protein. *Metabolism: clinical and experimental* 55:439-444.

Jain V, Patel RK, Kapadia Z, Galiveeti S, Banerji M, Hope L (2017) Drugs and hyperglycemia: A practical guide. *Maturitas* 104:80-83.

Juge-Aubry CE, Somm E, Chicheportiche R, Burger D, Pernin A, Cuénod-Pittet B, Quinodoz P, Giusti V, Dayer JM, Meier CA (2004) Regulatory effects of interleukin (IL)-1, interferon-beta, and IL-4 on the production of IL-1 receptor antagonist by human adipose tissue. *The Journal of clinical endocrinology and metabolism* 89:2652-2658.

Kadowaki T, Yamauchi T, Kubota N, Hara K, Ueki K, Tobe K (2006) Adiponectin and adiponectin receptors in insulin resistance, diabetes, and the metabolic syndrome. *The Journal of clinical investigation* 116:1784-1792.

Kahn C R, Rosenthal A S (1979) Immunologic reactions to insulin: insulin allergy, insulin resistance, and the autoimmune insulin syndrome. *Diabetes Care* 2:283-295.

Kahn C R (1994) Banting Lecture. Insulin action, diabetogenes, and the cause of type II diabetes. *Diabetes* 43:1066-1084.

Kim H J, Higashimori T, Park S Y, Choi H, Dong J, Kim Y J, Noh H L, Cho Y R, Cline G, Kim Y B, Kim K J (2004) Differential effects of interleukin-6 and -10 on skeletal muscle and liver insulin action in vivo. *Diabetes* 53:1060–1067.

Klover P J, Clementi A H, Mooney R A (2005) Interleukin-6 depletion selectively improves hepatic insulin action in obesity. *Endocrinology* 146:3417-3427.

Kopp H P, Kopp C W, Festa A, Krzyzanowska K, Kriwanek S, Minar E, Roka R, Schernthaner G (2003) Impact of weight loss on inflammatory proteins and their association with the insulin resistance syndrome in morbidly obese patients. *Arterioscler. Thromb. Vasc. Biol*. 23:1042-1047.

Kostis J B, Wilson A C, Freudenberger R S, Cosgrove NM, Pressel S L, Davis BR (2005) Long-term effect of diuretic-based therapy on fatal outcomes in subjects with isolated systolic hypertension with and without diabetes. *The American journal of cardiology* 95:29-35.

Kwon H, Pessin J E (2013) Adipokines mediate inflammation and insulin resistance. *Front. Endocrinol.* (Lausanne) 4:71.

Leroith D (2002) Beta-cell dysfunction and insulin resistance in type 2 diabetes: role of metabolic and genetic abnormalities. Am J Med 113 Suppl 6A:3s-11s.

Li S, Shin H J, Ding E L, Van Dam R M (2009) Adiponectin levels and risk of type 2 diabetes: a systematic review and meta-analysis. *Jama* 302:179-188.

Lipscombe L L, Lévesque L, Gruneir A, Fischer H D, Juurlink DN, Gill S S, Herrmann N, Hux J E, Anderson GM, Rochon PA (2009) Antipsychotic drugs and hyperglycemia in older patients with diabetes. *Archives of internal medicine* 169:1282-1289.

Lumeng C N, Bodzin J L, Saltiel A R (2007) Obesity induces a phenotypic switch in adipose tissue macrophage polarization. *The Journal of clinical investigation* 117:175-184.

Luna B, Feinglos M N (2001) Drug-induced hyperglycemia. Jama 286:1945-1948.

Ma L J, Mao S L, Taylor K L, Kanjanabuch T, Guan Y, Zhang Y, Brown NJ, Swift LL, Mcguinness OP, Wasserman DH, Vaughan DE, Fogo AB (2004) Prevention of obesity and insulin resistance in mice lacking plasminogen activator inhibitor 1. *Diabetes* 53:336-346.

Mantzoros C (2021) Lipodystrophic syndromes. Avaible via https://www.uptodate.com/contents/ lipodystrophic-syndromes.

Mantzoros C (2021) In: *Pi-Sunyer FX (ed). UpToDate*. Avaible via https://www.uptodate.com/.

Mantzoros C S, Li T, Manson J E, Meigs J B, Hu F B (2005) Circulating adiponectin levels are associated with better glycemic control, more favorable lipid profile, and reduced inflammation in women with type 2 diabetes. *The Journal of clinical endocrinology and metabolism* 90:4542-4548.

Marban S L, Roth J (1996) In: Shafrir E (ed) Lessons from animal diabetes IV. *Birkhauser*, p 201-224.

Mclaughlin T, Abbasi F, Lamendola C, Liang L, Reaven G, Schaaf P, Reaven P (2002) Differentiation between obesity and insulin resistance in the association with C-reactive protein. *Circulation* 106:2908-2912.

Mohanty P, Aljada A, Ghanim H, Hofmeyer D, Tripathy D, Syed T, Al-Haddad W, Dhindsa S, Dandona P (2004) Evidence for a potent antiinflammatory effect of rosiglitazone. *The Journal of clinical endocrinology and metabolism* 89:2728-2735.

Muse E D, Lam T K, Scherer P E, Rossetti L (2007) Hypothalamic resistin induces hepatic insulin resistance. *The Journal of clinical investigation* 117:1670-1678.

Müller S, Martin S, Koenig W, Hanifi-Moghaddam P, Rathmann W, Haastert B, Giani G, Illig T, Thorand B, Kolb H (2002) Impaired glucose tolerance is associated with increased serum concentrations of interleukin 6 and co-regulated acute-phase proteins but not TNF-alpha or its receptors. *Diabetologia* 45:805-812.

Ofei F, Hurel S, Newkirk J, Sopwith M, Taylor R (1996) Effects of an engineered human anti-TNF-alpha antibody (CDP571) on insulin sensitivity and glycemic control in patients with NIDDM. *Diabetes* 45:881-885.

Officers T A, Group CFTaCR (2002) Major Outcomes in High-Risk Hypertensive Patients Randomized to Angiotensin-Converting Enzyme Inhibitor or Calcium Channel Blocker vs DiureticThe Antihypertensive and Lipid-Lowering Treatment to Prevent Heart Attack Trial (ALLHAT). *Jama* 288:2981-2997.

Pannacciulli N, Cantatore F P, Minenna A, Bellacicco M, Giorgino R, De Pergola G (2001) C-reactive protein is independently associated with total body fat, central fat, and insulin resistance in adult women. International journal of obesity and related metabolic disorders : *journal of the International Association for the Study of Obesity* 25:1416-1420.

Pickup J C, Mattock M B, Chusney G D, Burt D (1997) NIDDM as a disease of the innate immune system: association of acute-phase reactants and interleukin-6 with metabolic syndrome X. *Diabetologia* 40:1286-1292.

Potter Van Loon B J, Kluft C, Radder J K, Blankenstein M A, Meinders A E (1993) The cardiovascular risk factor plasminogen activator inhibitor type 1 is related to insulin resistance. *Metabolism: clinical and experimental* 42:945-949.

Primrose J N, Davies J A, Prentice C R, Hughes R, Johnston D (1992) Reduction in factor VII, fibrinogen and plasminogen activator inhibitor-1 activity after surgical treatment of morbid obesity. *Thromb Haemost.* 68:396-399.

Qi X, Li L, Yang G, Liu J, Li K, Tang Y, Liou H, Boden G (2007) Circulating obestatin levels in normal subjects and in patients with impaired glucose regulation and type 2 diabetes mellitus. *Clinical endocrinology* 66:593-597.

Quandt Z, Young A, Anderson M (2020) Immune checkpoint inhibitor diabetes mellitus: a novel form of autoimmune diabetes. *Clinical and experimental immunology* 200:131-140.

Rajala MW, Scherer PE (2003) Minireview: The adipocyte--at the crossroads of energy homeostasis, inflammation, and atherosclerosis. *Endocrinology* 144:3765-3773.

Reaven GM (1988) Banting lecture 1988. Role of insulin resistance in human disease. Diabetes 37:1595-1607.

Robertson RP (1995) Antagonist: diabetes and insulin resistance--philosophy, science, and the multiplier hypothesis. *J. Lab. Clin. Med.* 125:560-565.

Roth J, Qiang X, Marbán SL, Redelt H, Lowell BC (2004) The obesity pandemic: where have we been and where are we going? *Obes. Res.* 12(Suppl 2):88s-101s.

Salmenniemi U, Ruotsalainen E, Pihlajamäki J, Vauhkonen I, Kainulainen S, Punnonen K, Vanninen E, Laakso M (2004) Multiple abnormalities in glucose and energy metabolism and coordinated changes in levels of adiponectin, cytokines, and adhesion molecules in subjects with metabolic syndrome. *Circulation* 110:3842-3848.

Schernthaner GH, Kopp HP, Krzyzanowska K, Kriwanek S, Koppensteiner R, Schernthaner G (2006) Soluble CD40L in patients with morbid obesity: significant reduction after bariatric surgery. *European journal of clinical investigation* 36:395-401.

Semple RK, Savage DB, Cochran EK, Gorden P, O'rahilly S (2011) Genetic syndromes of severe insulin resistance. *Endocr. Rev.* 32:498-514.

Spranger J, Kroke A, Möhlig M, Hoffmann K, Bergmann MM, Ristow M, Boeing H, Pfeiffer AF (2003) Inflammatory cytokines and the risk to develop type 2 diabetes: results of the prospective population-based European Prospective Investigation into Cancer and Nutrition (EPIC)-Potsdam Study. *Diabetes* 52:812-817.

Steppan C M, Bailey S T, Bhat S, Brown E J, Banerjee R R, Wright C M, Patel H R, Ahima R S, Lazar M A (2001) The hormone resistin links obesity to diabetes. *Nature* 409:307-312.

Straczkowski M, Kowalska I, Nikolajuk A, Adamska A, Karolczuk-Zarachowicz M, Karczewska-Kupczewska M, Kozlowska A, Gorska M (2006) Plasma levels of soluble tumor necrosis factor-α receptors are related to total and LDL-cholesterol in lean, but not in obese subjects. *Cardiovascular Diabetology* 5:14.

Stumvoll M, Goldstein B J, Van Haeften T W (2005) Type 2 diabetes: principles of pathogenesis and therapy. *Lancet* 365:1333-1346.

Van Exel E, Gussekloo J, De Craen A J, Frölich M, Bootsma-Van Der Wiel A, Westendorp RG (2002) Low production capacity of interleukin-10 associates with the metabolic syndrome and type 2 diabetes: the Leiden 85-Plus Study. *Diabetes* 51:1088-1092.

VáZquez L A, Pazos F, Berrazueta J R N, FernáNdez-Escalante C, García-Unzueta MaT, Freijanes J, Amado JA (2005) Effects of Changes in Body Weight and Insulin Resistance on Inflammation and Endothelial Function in Morbid Obesity after Bariatric Surgery. *The Journal of Clinical Endocrinology, Metabolism* 90:316-322.

Wallenius V, Wallenius K, Ahrén B, Rudling M, Carlsten H, Dickson SL, Ohlsson C, Jansson JO (2002) Interleukin-6-deficient mice develop mature-onset obesity. *Nature medicine* 8:75-79.

Weyer C, Funahashi T, Tanaka S, Hotta K, Matsuzawa Y, Pratley RE, Tataranni PA (2001) Hypoadiponectinemia in obesity and type 2 diabetes: close association with insulin resistance and hyperinsulinemia. *The Journal of clinical endocrinology and metabolism* 86:1930-1935.

Yang Q, Graham T E, Mody N, Preitner F, Peroni O D, Zabolotny J M, Kotani K, Quadro L, Kahn B B (2005) Serum retinol binding protein 4 contributes to insulin resistance in besity and type 2 diabetes. *Nature* 436:356-362.

Chapter 16

Cytokines and Inflammation

Yusuf Muhammed Durna[1] and Taner Daştan[2,*]
[1]Department of Otolaryngology and Head and Neck Surgery, Medipol University, Faculty of Medicine, Istanbul, Turkey
[2]Department of Biochemistry, Sivas Cumhuriyet University, Faculty of Science, Sivas, Turkey

Abstract

Cytokines are polymer compounds produced by cells, and these molecules act as molecular messengers between cells. In many diseases, cytokine molecules regulate different inflammatory conditions. As part of the immune system, cytokine molecules regulate and control organisms' response to disorders, inflammation, environmental conditions and infection, as well as mediate normal cellular processes in living organisms.

Keywords: cytokines, inflammation, immunity, inflammation mediators

Introduction

The concept of inflammation predates humanity as the earliest evidences of inflammatory processes were discovered from dinosaur fossils. Even before humans had a scientific understanding of inflammation, ancient cultures devised healing approaches to then-unknown inflammatory diseases (Cavaillon 2018). In the current times, humanity discovered a wide array of mechanisms, pathways, and mediators of inflammation (Cavaillon 2018). Back in 1930, an interaction was identified between a serum component and a carbohydrate extract called the C-fraction of *S. pneumoniae* in rabbits. This is the discovery of CRP, today's recognized inflammatory biomarker (Tillet and Francis 1930). CRP is today the most widely acknowledged biomarker for the presence of an inflammatory response. Prostaglandins were later distinguished in 1935. In Switzerland, Tadeusz Reichstein obtained various substances from adrenal glands and a few of them were found to be biologically reactive. He started desoxycorticosterone production in 1937

* Corresponding Author's Email: tdastan@cumhuriyet.edu.tr.

In: Cytokines and Diseases
Editors: Kenan Demir, Selim Görgün and Bahar Uslu
ISBN: 979-8-88697-214-6

together with the first clinical trials (Steiger and Reichstein 1937). The first endogenous pyrogen was distinguished in 1953 which was then followed by the identification of interferons. The British researcher Alick Isaacs and the Swiss researcher Jean Lindenmann published a report three years later and proposed the term "interferon" in their article, and thus, they are recognized as the discoverers of interferons (Steiger and Reichstein 1937; Cavaillon 2018).

The term known today as MIF was distinguished as a novel cytokine by Bloom and Bennet in 1966 by showing that T-cell supernatants have the capacity to prevent macrophage migration in delayed type hypersensitivity reactions (Bloom and Bennet 1966). MIF was also the driving force to lead Stanley Cohen to devise the "cytokine" terminology in 1974 (Cohen et al. 1974). Even though lymphokine and monokine were frequently used terms back then, the discovery of the MIF release from virus-infected fibroblasts by Cohen resulted in acknowledging that the mediators are universal for all cells of the organism instead of limited to the immune system. Between the years 1953 and 1981, various mediator molecules were distinguished and later understood to be different aspects of a single molecule that is Interleukin-1, which is then divided into IL-1α and IL-1β that are also members of a large 11-molecule family including the agonist and antagonist molecules (Dinarello 2010). Then in 1986, the existence of TNF in the plasma was distinguished (Waage et al. 1986). Over time, all of the other inflammatory cytokines were discovered from the plasma of patients with various septic and aseptic systemic inflammation. Such research pointed out that the concept known as "cytokine storm" is present in severe inflammatory conditions, yet this was not all of it (Cavaillon et al. 1992). One particularly striking statement about the cytokines and their relationship in inflammation was made by William Osler back in 1904, which is "Except on a few occasions, the patient appears to die from the body's response to infection rather than from it" (Cavaillon 2018).

Cytokines and Inflammatory Cells

Monocytes, Macrophages and Cytokines

In addition to their immune functions as the forefront host defense, monocytes and macrophages also have functions in developmental biology, particularly in organogenesis (Shalova et al. 2018; Ginhoux et al. 2016). Consequently, they have a wide array of functions, namely; inflammation triggering, the killing of pathogens, tissue repair and remodeling, and control of the immune responses (Wynn et al. 2013). Therefore, understanding how these molecules recognize and act according to the micro-environmental changes, and in cases of abnormal behavior, how they cause pathogenic outcomes is crucially important (Shalova et al. 2018).

Both monocytes and macrophages can act on their perceived stimuli from the milieu by recognizing the stimulating phenotype, which triggers them to neutralize or destroy the perceived threat. More often than not, these cells provide finely tailored immune responses to perceived stimuli, e.g., bacteria from Gram (-) strains or bacterial fractions like lipopolysaccharides (LPSs) have an inducing effect on macrophages, which in turn triggers the secretion of cytokine molecules about the inflammatory process and antimicrobial substances that would result in the total destruction of the pathogen through the inflammatory process

(Shalova et al. 2018; Wynn et al. 2013). Considering the diversity and flow levels of the micro-environmental variables, it is only natural for these cells to have a quite diverse phenotype and an ability to dynamically switch between different phenotypes. All in all, the defining characteristics for both monocytes and macrophages are diversity and plasticity (Shalova et al. 2018; Biswas and Mantovani 2010; Gordon and Taylor 2005).

That being said, initial research revealed two encompassing activation phenotypes of macrophages despite their having diverse phenotypes for functions. These two activation phenotypes are named as the (1) classical activation, and (2) alternative activation phenotypes. The classical activation phenotype of macrophages is triggered by the stimulation of inflammatory steps, which in return trigger the release of RNI and ROI intermediaries from macrophages that would raise the regulatory T-helper-1 (Th-1) response to mediate either antimicrobial or anti-tumor effects (Shalova et al. 2018; Adams and Hamilton 1984; Van Epps 2005). However, in the alternative activation, the trigger is from the anti-inflammatory cytokines of IL-4 or IL-13 that would inhibit the ability of macrophages to express proinflammatory cytokines, occurring through arginine conversion to ornithine by arginase-1 (Arg-1) enzyme expression, and consequently resulting in an increase in scavenger receptor expression and phagocytic activities (Stein et al. 1992; Loke et al. 2002). Two different mice strains, C57/B6 for Th-1 and BALB/c for Th-2, were reported by Mills et al. to express dissimilar nitrogen metabolism actions (Mills et al. 2000). From the results, the researchers postulated contrasting metabolism actions similar to the Th-1 vs. Th-2 response. Later on, Mantovani et al. elaborated on the results and reported that macrophages directed to LPS-like inducers and Th-1 cytokines like INFγ; and to Th-2 anti-inflammatory cytokine stimulation, therefore, pointed to the similarity to the established Th-1 and Th-2 denomination (Shalova et al. 2018; Mantovani et al. 2002).

Against the infectious agents both circulating monocytes and tissue embedded macrophages provide the initial step of immune response, which is possible through the PRRs on their cell surfaces that enable them to correctly recognize pathogens and pathogenic products (also PAMPs). As an example, TLRs, which are one of the major PRRs of these cells, have the ability to recognize a wide array of microbial elements that would activate intracellular signaling pathways to selectively activate transcriptional factors (Bonizzi and Karin 2004), which in turn trigger the expression of proinflammation cytokines, and antimicrobial mediators, e.g., RNI and ROI. These released proinflammatory cytokines result in fully developed immunity through the activation of other cellular elements like T and B cells. Consequently, the infectious microbial agent is ultimately destroyed by the immune-mediated inflammatory response. Since cytokines are instrumental in the immune-mediated inflammatory response, their quantity and persistence are possible drawbacks if the condition turns into a "cytokine storm" that would develop into septic shock and systemic failure of the organism (Beutler 1999). Researchers provided results showing that monocytes stimulate proinflammatory gene expression in cases of sepsis (Shalova et al. 2015; Biswas and Lopez-Collazo 2009). In the case of chronic inflammation, e.g., obesity and cancer, an increase in the tissue infiltration of macrophages is more pronounced. In the case of obesity, activated adipose tissue macrophage (ATM) infiltration that has a significant expression of TNFα and iNOS was reported (Nguyen et al. 2007; Lumeng et al. 2007). Studies on cancerous tissues revealed the retrieval of monocytes and macrophages in the tissue that would release IL-1β, IL-6, and TNF inflammatory cytokines, resulting in cancer-mediated inflammation progression and tumoral growth processes (Mantovani et al. 2008). Due to the damaging potential of inflammatory cytokines to encircling tissues, they are strictly regulated in their mechanisms, which is possible through the simultaneous ability to express IL-10 and IL-1RA anti-inflammatory cytokines, by the monocytes and macrophages. The gradual inhibition of an inflammatory response provided by macrophages over the inflammatory process is reported thoroughly (Lawrence and Gilroy 2007).

Additionally, both monocytes and macrophages have their effects in the control of immunity (Mosser and Edwards 2008; Lawrence et al. 2001). During the resolution phase of the inflammation, macrophages devour apoptotic cells to carry out waste disposal and at the same time shift into an appropriate phenotype for the promotion of resolving, anti-fibrosis, and tissue repair, which is seen as having an elevated expression profile for TGFβ, IL-10, and lipoxin, but having a repressed profile for proinflammatory cytokine expressions (Serhan et al. 2009; 2007). Continuous research in mice also revealed the presence of variant macrophages of $CD11b^{hi}$ and $CD11b^{lo}$ during the resolution of the inflammation (Schif-Zuck et al. 2011). Of these variants, the $CD11b^{hi}$ phenotype was revealed to express significant M2 markers (Arg-1), have high phagocytic activity, and a mild to mediocre expression profile for inflammatory markers, e.g., NOS2, COX-2, MMP-9, and 12/15-Lipoxygenase (Stables et al. 2011). On the other hand, the $CD11b^{lo}$ variant was revealed to have no Arg-1 expression and no phagocytic activity, and also a lower expression profile for inflammatory markers, but elevated levels of TNFβ. This phenotype variant is proposed to take part in anti-fibrosis and immune regulation functions (Ariel and Serhan 2012). In a recent study, three different macrophage populations with immunoregulatory functions were reported in the case of polarization of macrophages having TLR ligands that are coupled with prostaglandin E2 (PGE2) or adenosine (Fleming et al. 2015). These three different macrophage populations have the shared traits of having significant expression profiles for angiogenic factors, growth factors, and IL-10; and decreased expression profiles for inflammatory cytokines. Nevertheless, more *in-vivo* research is necessary to further evaluate the relevance of these macrophages.

Endotoxin-tolerant macrophages are another variation in macrophages with immune regulation functions. In the case of sepsis, monocytes and macrophages are turned into endotoxin-tolerant phenotypes by the overexposure to inflammatory cytokines, making them unable to respond to further exposure to endotoxins (Biswas and Lopez-Collazo 2009; Cavaillon et al. 2003). An M2-like activation phenotype is suggested for endotoxin-tolerant variants due to their having pronounced expression for anti-inflammatory cytokines, and repressed expression for proinflammatory cytokines, and also increased phagocytic activity and tissue remodeling capabilities (Porta et al. 2009; Pena et al. 2011). Isolated monocytes obtained from sepsis patients are revealed to have this particular phenotype (Shalova et al. 2015). It can be postulated that this particular phenotype is a result of adaptation for protection from an excessive inflammatory reaction. Another variant of macrophages, tumor-associated macrophages (TAMs), also has regulatory functions in the immune response as these macrophages have traits promoting immune suppression and tissue remodeling, which are vital for concepts of cancer immune evasion, tumoral angiogenesis, and metastasis (Mantovani et al. 2008; Qian and Pollard 2010). The immunoregulatory and tissue remodeling functions of macrophages can also be clearly observed in developmental processes in tissue-embedded macrophages and embryonic macrophages (Pollard 2009).

Cytokines and Neutrophils

The nuclear form and granules of neutrophils contribute to their morphological traits (Cuzzocrea 2018). The nucleus is known to have 3 to 5 lobules. Not only do neutrophils synthesize cytokines de novo, they also release cytokines from preliminary stores at a basal level (Cuzzocrea 2018). An autoregulatory pathway mostly directs the proinflammatory functions of different proinflammatory cytokines and chemokines. Cytokines, chemokines, and different growth factors like granulocyte and monocyte colony stimulating factors (G and G/M – CSFs) mainly target neutrophils. The affecting agonist differentiates the cytokine production pattern by the neutrophils, and the pattern also has the potential of modulation by the effects of immunomodulatory cytokines, e.g., IL-4/IL-10, IFN-ɣ, and IL-13, which suggest an influence on cytokine secretion from neutrophils by the Th-1 and Th-2 cells (Cuzzocrea 2018). TNF-α is a member of the membrane-bound and soluble cytokine superfamily which is a pleiotropic cytokine and has significant roles in T-cell-mediated immune functions. TNF-α is mainly known for its primary effects in tumor cell inhibition and normal cell proliferation, but it also has roles in other conditions such as septic shock, autoimmunity processes, and other inflammatory diseases. The potency of TNF-α in the proinflammatory process is attributed to its enhancing effects in the expression of the endothelial cell adhesion molecules, resulting in the increased recruitment of neutrophils into the vessel endothelia. The mNAs for IL-1α and IL-1β are expressed by neutrophils, and therefore, IL-1 proteins are released from neutrophils (Cuzzocrea 2018). However, it is seen that the amount of IL-1β is greater than those of IL-1α. The inhibitory effects of neutrophil-derivated cytokines on IL-1 production from neutrophils were demonstrated by the essential release of the IL-1 receptor antagonist (IL-1Ra) in the case of the presence of G/M-CSF and TNF-α as agonists (Cuzzocrea 2018; Brinkman and Zychlinsky 2015; Tiku et al. 1986). It is supposed that the microbiocidal effectiveness of neutrophils is enhanced by the effects of proinflammatory cytokines, and they are being evaluated as additional options for potential immunomodulatory agents for humans to address either severe or persistent infections (Hubel et al. 2002). Both positive and negative regulation of cytokine expression profiles of neutrophils can be achieved by the presence of T-cell-derivated cytokines, e.g., positive regulation by Th-1 derivated INF-ɣ and negative regulation by Th-2 derivated IL-13, IL-10, and IL-4 (Cassatella 1999). INF-ɣ is known to enhance IL-1Ra production and results in IL-1Ra mRNA accumulation. IL-10 is known to particularly inhibit the production of IL-1β, IL-8, and TNF-α (Cuzzocrea 2018). IL-4 also has an enhancing effect on IL-1Ra production from neutrophils, and also demonstrated that IL-4 primes TNF-α and IL-8 production from neutrophils when induced by LPS.

Cytokines and Mast Cells

Mast cells have their innate traits to make them effective players in immune responses. First among these is their strategic localization in host to environment intersections where external stimuli first engage, which enables them to respond to an external threat by releasing reserve mediators and/or by synthesizing necessary mediators on the spot. This trait of the mast cells is used in vaccination protocols to enhance immune responses (Ang and Abraham 2018). Mast cells are prevalent in the body, mostly localized in the connective tissue; however, they are tightly concentrated in the skin, gastrointestinal tract, and respiratory pathway where the external stimuli are first encountered (Abraham and St John 2010). Their close proximity to circulation (blood and lymph vessels) and neural fibers is an indication of their capacity to signal about the pathogen by releasing appropriate mediators in the close vicinity (Ang and Abraham 2018; Cheng et al. 2013). PAMPs are specifically recognized by the PRRs expressed by the mast cells, which include TLRs, C-type lectins, and other surface molecules like CD14 (Ang and Abraham 2018). The majority of TLRs of mast cells are defined in the transcriptional level, and they are either essential or hotspot according to the perceived stimulus (Ang and Abraham 2018). The pattern of TLR ligation either as singles or coupled with different receptors results in distinct outcomes with different cytokine releases, e.g., TLR2 activated by bacterial peptidoglycan results in both degranulation and synthesis, but TLR4 activated by LPS only results in cytokine release (Ang and Abraham 2018). There is still no definitive consensus about which TLR activation results in degranulation or cytokine synthesis. In any event, TLRs can couple with other receptors to stimulate cytokine release like FceRI (Qiao et al. 2006), which is further complicating the TLR-mediated immune responses. Contrariwise, TLR signaling has the capacity to alter mast cell phenotypes through downregulation, e.g., FcRI, granular protease differentiation, and the regulation of cytokine secretion (Ang and Abraham 2018). Mast cells have the potential to produce too many of the attracting chemicals and cytokines, i.e., signaling leucocytes to infection cores for either pathogen clearance or inflammation amplification via proinflammatory cytokines. Of these, TNF-α is prominent in its function of signaling neutrophils to cores where mast cells are activated, and it therefore contributes to bacterial clearance (Ang and Abraham 2018).

Cytokines and Dendritic Cells

Both the initiation and controlling of T-cell immunity are essentially depended DCs, which are specifically antigen-presenting cells (Banchereau and Steinman 1998). These cells scale the immune balance between tolerance and immunity through the connection of innate and adaptive immunity. Present knowledge about DCs describes them as specialized cells with the ability to recruit antigens and convert them to small molecules for a demonstration to naive T cells in an immunogenic way coupled with T-cell co-stimulators, e.g., CD80, CD86, and other cytokines like IL-12 (Lambrecht et al. 2018; Otsuka et al. 2013; Hammad and Lambrecht 2015; Lambrecht and Galli 2015; Lambrecht and Hammad 2015). DCs have the capacity to secrete diverse cytokine receptors through autocrine and paracrine ways, which then induce activation. Recent findings indicate that the majority of known allergens have the potential of activating distinct PRR classes; however, it is implied that the precise T-helper cell response is actually related to the nature of the allergen, which complicates the mechanism of action (Gregory and Lloyd 2011; Wills-Karp 2010). TGF-β, IL-6, IL-12, and IL-23 are cytokines taking roles in Th-1 and Th-17 differentiation and the situation is different in this case. Recent postulation indicates that Th2 differentiation is a default pathway but this changes to Th1 or Th17 differentiation when DCs release polarizing cytokines. In the absence of such polarizing cytokines from DCs, ligand attachment to notch receptors defaults to the Th2 differentiation pathway (Lambrecht et al. 2018).

Cytokines and Natural Killer (NK) Cells

Recent understanding about the NK cells implies that they are functioning both as immune respondents against infectious agents, e.g., viruses, bacteria, and parasites, and as immune modulators in the course of autoimmunity and chronic inflammatory processes (Vosshenrich and Di Santo 2018; Horowitz et al. 2012; Serafini et al. 2015). NK cells can pass on either activating or inhibiting signals when ligands bind to their distinct surface receptors, which are all defined in the germline. The NK cells remain tolerant to normal cells in this way, but retain their optimum reactivity to infected or otherwise altered cells. The dominant actions of the NK cells are cytokine secretion and cytotoxicity (Colucci et al. 2003). IFN-γ is known to be significantly produced by the NK cells, and it is known that it has pleiotropic effects on targets, hematopoietic (myeloids, macrophages), and non-hematopoietic (epithelium, stromae) cells. Cytotoxicity functions of the NK cells primarily depend on cellular contact between the NK and the target, and its mediation is done either through granules or through TNF-mediated pathways, e.g., FasL, and TRAIL. Of particular note is the stimulation of the NK cells in the absence of cellular contact when cytokine stimulation is enough to induce activation. Such cytokines include IL-2, IL-18, IL-21, IL-12, and INF-I. In the absence of cellular contact, IL-12 coupled with any of the aforementioned cytokines is enough to activate NK cells. Overall, the NK cells are generally activated by the released cytokines/chemokines from the sentinels (epithelium, macrophages, and DCs) when they detect pathogens (Vosshenrich and Di Santo 2018).

Cytokines and Innate Lymphoid Cells

ILCs, which are a family of uncommon effector lymphocytes, were defined as cells closely associated to inflammatory processes (Serafini and Di Santo 2018). While ILCs share the overall morphological traits of other lymphoid cells, they have marked differences as they lack organized antigen receptors like T- or B-cell receptors and other myeloid-associated markers, and also granulocytes. However, ILCs uniquely express surface markers, transcription factors (Tfs) expressed by T helper or NK cells, and therefore, ILCs have the capacity to quickly respond to environmental changes by the significant production of various proinflammatory and immunomodulatory molecules. ILCs can effectively and rapidly influence the immune outcome following the inflammation or infection. The expression profiles of specific TFs define the effector functions of ILCs, resulting in three different subsets (Serafini and Di Santo 2018). The ILC1 (Group 1 ILC) population contains NK cells and other IFN-γ-producing ILCs, and they require a TF known as eomesodermin (EOMES). ILC2 (Group 2 ILC) contains cytokine-producing ILCs that are associated with the Th-2 pathway, and they require both GATA-3 and RORα as TFs. ILC3 (Group 3 ILC) includes ILCs that are producing IL-17A and IL-22, which are T-helper 17 associated cytokines, and the ILC3 population both expresses and requires

RORɣt as a TF. At first, the ILC2 population was defined with different names like natural helper cells, innate helper 2 cells, and nuocytes (Serafini and Di Santo 2018). The ILC2 population was shown to express IL-33R, IL-7Rα, TSLP-R, and IL-25R to respond to changes by the significant secretion of type 2 cytokines, which include IL-13, IL-4, IL-9, IL-5 and amphiregulin, which is an EGFR ligand (Serafini and Di Santo 2018).

Cytokines and T-helper (Th) Cells

When excited with antigens, T cells are known to secrete specific and transmittable cytokine subsets. T cells are divided into Th-1 cells, which secrete INF-ɣ, IL-2, and lymphotoxin, and Th-2 cells, which secrete IL-4, IL-5, and IL-10. It is defining for T cells to secrete specified cytokine subsets which leads to their functional division. Specialized Th functions require the activation of the genes responsible for cytokines and their receptors, and Th cells can express the required TFs for these genes (Ulrich et al. 2018). Th-9 cells are defined as the IL-9-secreting Th subset, and they are differentiated by the effects of IL-2, IL-4, and TGF-β, which was discovered more than 20 years ago (Ulrich et al. 2018). The aforementioned cytokines are able to activate distinct pathways to induce the transcription factors for IL-9 production and Th-9 development. Again, the functions of these cytokines also depend on their ability to promote IL-9 production. IL-25, which is a part of the IL-17 family, can promote IL-9 production, and IL-9 is required for IL-25 induced allergy (Ulrich et al. 2018). Of particular note is the highest IL-25R transcripts found in Th-9 cells (Ulrich et al. 2018). Th-9 cells also have their roles in tumor immunity by producing IL3, which increases the survival rates of DCs. T-helper 17 cells are known to produce a major proinflammatory cytokine, i.e., IL-17, which is known to take part in defense against extracellular pathogens and fungi (Noack and Miossec 2018; Miossec et al. 2009). Again, it is documented that the excessive reaction of T-helper 17 cells leads to autoimmunity and inflammation (Noack and Miossec 2018; Miossec et al. 2009; Maddur et al. 2012). While Th-17 cells show certain markers with other T-helper subsets, they require their specific cytokines and associated TFs to differentiate (Korn et al. 2009). The proinflammatory and pathogenic nature of Th-17 cells makes them favorable targets for treatment strategies as they start the development and chronicity of various autoimmune inflammations, which are formed from proinflammatory cytokines produced by Th-17 cells (Noack and Miossec 2018; Miossec et al. 2009; Korn et al. 2009; Maddur et al. 2012). Among these products, IL-17, IL-21, IL-22, and CCL20 are the foremost (Ouyang et al. 2008). These cytokines are also responsible for Th-17 regulation, e.g., constant exposure to TGF-β1 and IL-6 leads to the production of both IL-10 and IL-17 (Noack and Miossec 2018). As implied, IL-10 is associated with a pathogen Th-17 phenotype (Morrison et al. 2011). IL-23 is offset by the effects of IL-27 through negative regulation, and is responsible in INF-ɣ induction (Noack and Miossec 2018). It is stated that IL-27 suppresses the immune response during chronic inflammation with its anti-inflammatory functions.

Cytokines and Platelets

The platelets of mammalian organisms are primarily responsible for the continuation of the hemostatic mechanisms by supporting vessel integrity and blood coagulation (Levin 2018).

However, they do have some potential in inflammation with their elemental bactericidal and phagocytosis-like activities (Zander and Klinger 2009; Youssefian et al. 2002). In this regard, ultrastructural research on particle interactions revealed that platelets are not proper phagocytes and bacterial intake involves the mechanisms associated with open canalicular system (OCS) channels (White 2005). Nevertheless, findings indicate meaningful contributions of platelets in inflammatory processes. Platelet microparticles (PMPs) formed from platelets are primarily pro-coagulant structures and are observed in different stages of inflammation (Nurden 2011; Reid and Webster 2012). Being rich in IL-1 content, PMPs are implied in inflammation enhancement (Boilard et al. 2010; Brown and McIntyre 2011). The TLRs present on platelets and monocytes enable cellular interactions to enable mechanisms to recruit platelets into immune pathways (Levin 2018; Bruserud 2013). A wide array of different surface receptors of platelets enables them to process biochemical signals to inflammatory pathways which include platelets (Vieira-de-Abreu et al. 2012). It is known that thrombin induction of human platelets results in the releasing of inflammatory mediators and antibacterials through degranulation, which also leads to the aggregation of platelets and monocytes (Levin 2018; Vieira-de-Abreu et al. 2012; Kasirer-Friede 2007).

Epithelial Cells, Endothelial Cells and Cytokines

Epithelial cells are tightened cells to excessively cover the organ and lumen surfaces of the body, and they also contribute to the formation of glands and vessels (Hoffman and Pothoulakis 2018). An intact barrier of epithelial cells serves to limit and control substance trafficking while also preventing the introduction of pathogenic agents such as viruses, bacteria, and fungi. Aside from this, epithelial cells have the capacity and functioning of immune coordination, cellular signalization between different targets, and initiation of regeneration (Hoffman and Pothoulakis 2018). While the precise involvement of epithelial cells is not known in chronic intestinal inflammatory conditions, it is speculated that their contribution is formed by the immune responses towards commensal gut microbiota from defective epithelium (Podolsky 2002), which then leads to the activation of both innate and acquired immunity, and ends in proinflammatory cytokine release coupled with alterations in barrier functions. Both proinflammatory cytokines and antimicrobial polypeptides are released from neutrophils on the inflammation site, leading to the reshaping of localized innate immunity. Cathelicidins are function-wise similar to defensins, having antimicrobial effects, and are released from both neutrophils and epithelial cells (Hoffman and Pothoulakis 2018). The activation of TLRs directly with the bacteria or associated molecules, e.g., short-chain fatty acids, results in cathelicidin release. This is related to the increase in mucous secretion and to the decrease in apoptosis of intestinal epithelia. They are also known to promote epithelial integrity and tissue repair (Hoffman and Pothoulakis 2018). Various cells, namely, Paneth cells, enterocytes, and neutrophils, are known to secrete cathelicidin-like molecules named alpha-defensins (Cunliffe 2003). Alpha-defensins have the ability of altering the cytokine release patterns of epithelia, which suggests another linkage between innate and acquired immunity (Hoffman and Pothoulakis 2018). The NF-KB pathway partially regulates proinflammatory cytokine release, and by the prevention of phosphorylation of the p65 subunit of NF-KB via beta-defensin intervention, the cytokine release is inhibited, which is consistent with the anti-inflammatory functions of these proteins. Beta-defensin molecules are also involved in the acute phase of inflammation with their increasing effect in protein and mucin expressions, and decreasing effect in intestinal epithelia apoptosis rates (Hoffman and Pothoulakis 2018). Overall, immune responses provided by the endothelia are short-term protective measures; however, they can develop into pathological severity in cases of overloaded inflammatory processes, which might lead to tissue necrosis, visceral dysfunctions, and even to death. Leukocyte to endothelia adhesion is a well-known mechanism in the inflammation response, and is finely observed in post-capillary venules where inflammation elements are recruited to the hot-spot (Alexander et al. 2018). It should be noted that endothelia have their distinct role in inflammation modulation by their ability to control the trafficking of inflammatory elements between the inflammation site and the circulation. Also, their ability to finetune the blood flow in vessels enables coagulation activation and deposition. Endothelia also contribute to the formation of new vessels. Each one of the stated functions of endothelia has related pathological connections that can be attributed to the end results of tissue/organ damage and increased mortality from inflammation.

Cytokines and Inflammatory Mediators

IL Superfamily Mediators

It is known that there are eleven IL-1 cytokines, and ten IL-1 receptors. More than anything, IL-1 cytokines are associated with damage causing inflammation, but they are also associated with elevated non-specific resistance against infections and immune response development against foreign substances (Dinarello 2018). There are also members of the IL-1 family that suppress inflammation, namely, IL-1Ra, IL-37, and IL-36Ra. IL-38, the last of the IL-1 family, is stated to be able to non-specifically restrain inflammation and inhibit innate immune responses (Dinarello 2018; Boraschi and Tagliabue 2013). IL-1R1 has the capacity to attach to IL-1α, IL-1β, and IL-1Ra, but it can bind to either IL-1α or IL-1β. For IL-1β, there is a blind receptor that is IL-1R2. IL-1R3 has a wide range of attachable cytokines, namely, IL-1α, IL-1β, IL-33, IL-36a, IL-36β, and IL-36γ, due to its co-receptor structure, and can be found in both integral and soluble forms. IL-1 receptors also contain receptors for anti-inflammation effects (Garlanda et al. 2013), which are IL-1R8, IL-1R9, and IL-1R10. IL-1α is known as a "dual function" cytokine due to its DNA-binding, and receptor-binding duality. When it binds to receptors, it is responsible for biochemical signaling. IL-1α has a nuclear localization sequence, which enables it to act as a TF (Dinarello 2018). IL-18, which is similar to IL-1β, requires a signal peptide for activation, and from the similarities between IL-18 and IL-37 precursors, and their genetic make-up, it is implied that both genes of IL-18 and IL-37 are closely related. IL-18 precursors are essentially secreted throughout the gastrointestinal tract from the intestinal epithelia, along with endothelia and keratinocytes. Activated IL-18 is primarily released from macrophages and DCs, while IL-18 precursors remain in the mesenchymal cells. Again, IL-18 precursors are released from apoptotic cells, similar to IL-1α and IL-33, and released precursors are targeted by proteases from neutrophils, e.g., proteinase-3 (Dinarello 2018). If IL-18 activity is inhibited, the severity of the inflammation is generally reduced. IL-33 is particularly located in endothelia and epithelia, along with the brain, but also present in all normal cells as in the precursor form. Particularly in microglias, astrocytes, and in oligodendroglias, IL-33 is present in the precursor form. There are treatment approaches involving IL-33 blockage, which in turn reduces Th-2 cytokines. IL-33 blockage is a rational approach since IL-33 is upstream to Th-2 cytokines.

TNF Superfamily Mediators

There are 19 ligands and 29 receptors present in the TNF superfamily. Examples of ligands include FasL, CD95L, TNFS6-10-12-13B-14, TNFRSF4-18, etc. while receptors include TL1A, Fas, CD95, LIGHT, TRAIL, TWEAK, BAFF, etc. (Cuzzocrea 2018; Aggarwal et al. 2012). Immunity, inflammation, and the cell cycle are essentially controlled by this superfamily. Members of this superfamily are mostly in immune cells, and have their functions in balancing T-cell-mediated immunity by controlling T-cell regulation, contracting effector T-cell reserves, and maintaining memory T cells (Cuzzocrea 2018). Therefore, members of this superfamily are directly responsible in T-cell associated autoimmune disorders, which include asthma, diabetes, and arthritis (Croft 2009). Of particular note is the ability of TNF-α production from macrophages and monocytes, which controls and regulates diverse biosignals, to induce either apoptosis or necrosis of targets.

Interleukin-17 Mediators

The IL-17 family contains six cytokine molecules like IL-17A/IL-17B/IL-17C/IL-17D/IL-17E/IL-17F, which have shared protein structures that are highly conserved in four particular cysteine residues (Korn et al. 2009). Among these members, IL-17E is also called IL-25. Generally, the IL-17 family primarily takes part in the immune response against extracellular pathogens and in autoimmunity development. IL-17A is the chief one among the members and is a hallmark of the activated CD4+ Th cells, also known as T-helper 17 cells. IL-17A is a glycoprotein of 155 amino acid residues (Ivanov et al. 2006; Korn et al. 2007; Monteleone et al. 2008). Paneth cells can also synthesize IL-17A and IL-17F, and IL-17A can be secreted by mesenchymal stem cells (Yang et al. 2013). The IL-17A/F can enhance proinflammatory cytokine production to induce certain inflammatory pathways to sustain pathologies (Monteleone et al. 2018).

IL-6 Superfamily Mediators

IL-6 is unique in that it has both pleiotropy and redundancy. Either the infection hot spot or the damaged tissue area is responsible for IL-6 secretion. IL-6 secretion induces acute phase proteins like CRP and fibrinogen (Tanaka et al. 2018). IL-6 is also important in acquired immunity. It is also implied in the prolonged survival of plasma blast cells (Tanaka et al. 2018). IL-6 is also known to promote Th 17 from naive T-cells, and to suppress Treg cell action

(Kimura and Kishimoto 2010). Certain non-immune cells are differentiated by IL-6 promotion, including cardiac myocytes, neuronal cells, hematopoietic cells, and endothelia. It is supposed that IL-25 and IL-35 might be evolved from the IL-6 family as these two are analogous to the IL-6/IL-6R complex, and they have soluble receptors. For these reasons, both IL-27 and IL-35 are counted in the IL-6 family, which currently includes IL-6, CNTF, IL-11, LIF, CT-1, OSM, CLCF1, IL-27, and IL-35. Members of this family share gp130 as a common signal transducer, and show some redundancy in biological activities. Research conducted on the signal transduction pathways and biological activities of IL-6 family members revealed possible clinical approaches for a variety of diseases that might include IL-6 members as targets.

Cytokine Networks in Inflammation

The microenvironments of the tissue and the inflammation site are equally important in the signal transductions of cytokines. Cytokine functioning may greatly differ between different environments; for example, cytokines may function in a proinflammatory way in one site, while the same cytokines may act as anti-inflammatory in another. This environment-based differentiation is particularly important in the context of lineage-specific cytokine expressions, e.g., macrophages activated by classical or alternative ways. The same cytokine that prompts proinflammation such as INF-γ in M1/Th-1 can be considered as prompting anti-inflammation in a contrasting context, as in M2/Th-2. As a term, inflammation is an overall expression to define the intricate mechanism of immunity against distinct classes of pathogens, e.g., immunity against viruses includes disparate pathways as opposed to pathways for parasites. Therefore, specific cytokine functions should be investigated in regard to their position in the grander picture of immunity. All in all, cytokines are essential for the optimum development of inflammatory response against the specific pathogens in question by stimulating through signaling the specific leukocytes and directing their effector functions toward immunity. They are then essential in inflammation clearance and the induction of regeneration, which will lead to homeostasis (Carson and Kunkel 2018).

Conclusion

Rigorous research of cytokines in recent years has revealed enormous amounts of data on the ontogeny, activation, functions, and producing mechanisms. The discoveries have distinguished the functional roles of cytokines in a wide spectrum of many diseases, e.g., obesity, cancer, allergy, inflammation diseases, autoimmune diseases, etc. Consequently, therapeutic strategies utilizing the modulation of cytokines, are taken into clinical trials (Shalova et al. 2018). Cytokines are basically soluble proteins to act as signal transducers to traffic biosignals between cells and targets with either paracrine (adjacent cells) or autocrine (identical cells) secretion. Both cytokine-binding and signal-transducing receptors are in use by cytokines for intracellular induction, collectively termed as multicomponent receptor systems. The ability of the target to interact with the given cytokine is dependent on having the cytokine-specific binding receptor which leads to dimer formations with signal receptors to activate intracellular signaling pathways (Tanaka et al. 2018). With the increased research on the molecular biology of cytokines, the functions of specific cytokines in particular inflammatory conditions will be revealed in more detail.

References

Abraham, S. N., and St John, A. L. (2010). Mast cell-orchestrated immunity to pathogens. *Nat Rev Immunol, 10*, 440-452.

Adams, D. O., and Hamilton, T. A. (1984). The cell biology of macrophage activation. *Annu Rev Immunol, 2*, 283-318.

Aggarwal, B. B., Gupta, S. C., and Kim, J. H. (2012). Historical perspectives on tumor necrosis factor and its superfamily, 25 years later, a golden journey. *Blood, 119*,651-665.

Alexander, J. S., Granger, D. N., and Harris, N. R. (2018). Inflammation: The Role of Endothelial Cells. In: Cavaillon JM and Singer M (eds). *Inflammation from molecular and cellular mechanisms to the clinic*, vol 1-4. Wiley-VCH, 457-477.

Ang, W. X. G., and Abraham, S. N. (2018). Mast Cells: Master Drivers of Immune Responses against Pathogens. In: Cavaillon JM and Singer M (eds). *Inflammation from molecular and cellular mechanisms to the clinic*, vol 1-4. Wiley-VCH, 273-288.

Ariel, A., and Serhan, C. N. (2012). New lives given by cell death: macrophage differentiation following their encounter with apoptotic leukocytes during the resolution of inflammation. *Front Immunol, 3*(4), 1-6.

Banchereau, J., and Steinman, R. M. (1998). Dendritic cells and the control of immunity. *Nature, 392*, 245-252.

Beutler, B. A. (1999). The role of tumor necrosis factor in health and disease. *J Rheumatol Suppl, 57*,16-21.

Biswas, S. K., and Lopez-Collazo, E. (2009). Endotoxin tolerance: new mechanisms, molecules and clinical significance. *Trends Immunol*, 30,475-487.

Biswas, S. K., and Mantovani, A. (2010). Macrophage plasticity and interaction with lymphocyte subsets: cancer as a paradigm. *Nat Immunol, 11*, 889-896.

Bloom, B. R., and Bennet, B. (1966). Mechanism of a reaction *in vitro* associated with delayed-type hypersensitivity. *Science, 153*, 80-82.

Boilard, E., Nigrovic, P. A., Larabee, K., Watts, G. F., Coblyn, J. S., Weinblatt, M. E., Massarotti, E. M., Remold-O'Donnell, E., Farndale, R. W., Ware, J., and Lee, D. M. (2010). Platelets amplify inflammation in arthritis via collagendependent microparticle production. *Science, 327*,580-583.

Bonizzi, G, and Karin, M (2004). The two NF-kappaB activation pathways and their role in innate and adaptive immunity. *Trends Immunol, 25*, 280-288.

Boraschi, D, and Tagliabue, A (2013). The interleukin-1 receptor family. *Semin Immunol, 25*,394-407.

Brinkmann, V, and Zychlinsky, A (2012). Neutrophil extracellular traps: is immunity the second function of chromatin? *J Cell Biol*, 198(5),773-783

Brown, G. T., and McIntyre, T. M. (2011). Lipopolysaccharide signaling without a nucleus: kinase cascades stimulate platelet shedding of proinflammatory IL-1b-rich microparticles. *J Immunol, 186*, 5489-5496.

Bruserud, O. (2013). Bidirectional crosstalk between platelets and monocytes initiated by Toll-like receptor: an important step in the early defense against fungal infections? *Platelets, 24*, 85-97.

Carson, W. F., and Kunkel, S. L. (2018). Type I and II Cytokine Superfamilies in Inflammatory Responses. In: Cavaillon JM and Singer M (eds) *Inflammation from molecular and cellular mechanisms to the clinic*, vol 1-4. Wiley-VCH, 587-617.

Cassatella, M. A. (1999). Neutrophil-derived proteins: selling cytokines by the pound. *Adv Immunol, 73*,369-509.

Cavaillon, J. M. (2018). Inflammation through the Ages: A Historical Perspective In: Cavaillon JM and Singer M (eds) *Inflammation from molecular and cellular mechanisms to the clinic*, vol 1-4. Wiley-VCH, 1-15 .

Cavaillon, J. M., Adrie, C., Fitting, C., and Adib-Conquy, M. (2003). Endotoxin tolerance: is there a clinical relevance? *J Endotoxin Res, 9*,101-107.

Cavaillon, J. M., Muñoz, C., Fitting C., Misset, B., and Carlet, J. (1992). Circulating cytokines: the tip of the iceberg? *Circ. Shock, 38*,145-152

Cheng, L. E., Hartmann, K., Roers, A., Krummel, M. F., and Locksley, R. M. (2013). Perivascular mast cells dynamically probe cutaneous blood vessels to capture immunoglobulin E. *Immunity*, *38*,166-175

Cohen, S., Bigazzi, P. E., and Yoshida, T. (1974). Commentary. Similarities of T cell function in cell-mediated immunity and antibody production. *Cell Immunol*, *12*,150-159

Colucci, F., Caligiuri, M. A., and Di Santo, J. P. (2003). What does it take to make a natural killer? *Nat Rev Immunol*, *3*, 413-425.

Croft, M. (2009). The role of TNF superfamily members in T-cell function and diseases. *Nat Rev Immunol*, 9, 271-285.

Cunliffe, R. N. (2003). Alpha-defensins in the gastrointestinal tract. *Mol Immunol*, 40(7), 463-467.

Cuzzocrea, S. (2018). Neutrophils. In: Cavaillon JM and Singer M (eds) *Inflammation from molecular and cellular mechanisms to the clinic*, vol 1-4. Wiley-VCH, 253-272.

Cuzzocrea, S. (2018). TNF Superfamily. In: Cavaillon JM and Singer M (eds) *Inflammation from molecular and cellular mechanisms to the clinic*, vol 1-4. Wiley-VCH, 529-547.

Dinarello, C. A. (2010). IL-1, discoveries, controversies and future direction. *Eur J Immunol*, *40*, 595-653.

Dinarello, C. A. (2018). IL-1 Superfamily and Inflammasome. In: Cavaillon JM and Singer M (eds). *Inflammation from molecular and cellular mechanisms to the clinic*, vol 1-4. Wiley-VCH, p 479-527.

Fleming, B. D., Chandrasekaran, P., Dillon, L. A., Dalby, E., Suresh, R., Sarkar, A., El-Sayed, N. M., and Mosser, D. M. (2015). The generation of macrophages with anti-inflammatory activity in the absence of STAT6 signaling. *J Leukoc Biol*, *98*, 395-407

Garlanda, C., Riva, F., Bonavita, E., and Mantovani, A. (2013). Negative regulatory receptors of the IL-1 family. *Semin Immunol*, *25*, 4087-4415.

Ginhoux, F., Schultze, J. L., Murray, P. J., Ochando, J., and Biswas, S. K. (2016). New insights into the multidimensional concept of macrophage ontogeny, activation and function. *Nat Immunol*, *17*, 34-40.

Gordon, S., and Taylor, P. R. (2005). Monocyte and macrophage heterogeneity. *Nat Rev Immunol*, *5*, 953-964.

Gregory, L. G., and Lloyd, C. M. (2011). Orchestrating house dust mite-associated allergy in the lung. *Trends Immunol*, *32*, 402-411.

Hammad, H., and Lambrecht, B. N. (2015). Barrier epithelial cells the control of type 2 immunity. *Immunity*, *43*, 29-40.

Hoffman, J. M., and Pothoulakis, C. (2018). Epithelial Cells. In: Cavaillon JM and Singer M (eds) *Inflammation from molecular and cellular mechanisms to the clinic*, vol 1-4. Wiley-VCH, p 437-455

Horowitz, A., Stegmann, K. A., and Riley, E. M. (2012). Activation of natural killer cells during microbial infections. *Front NK Cell Biol*, *2*, 88.

Hubel, K., Dale, D. C., and Liles, W. C. (2002). Therapeutic use of cytokines to modulate phagocyte function for the treatment of infectious diseases: current status of granulocyte colony-stimulating factor, granulocyte-macrophage colony-stimulating factor, macrophage colony-stimulating factor, and interferon-gamma. *J Infect Dis*, *185*(10),1490-1501.

Ivanov, II, McKenzie, B. S., Zhou, L., Tadokoro, C. E., Lepelley, A., Lafaille, J. J., Cua, D. J., and Littman, D. R. (2006). The orphan nuclear receptor RORγt directs the differentiation program of proinflammatory IL-17+ T helper cells. *Cell*, *126* 6),1121-1133.

Kasirer-Friede, A., Kahn, M. L., and Shattil, S. J. (2007). Platelet integrins and immunoreceptors. *Immunol Rev*, *218*, 247-264.

Kimura, A., and Kishimoto, T. (2010). IL-6: regulator of Treg/Th17 balance. Eur *J Immunol*, *40*(7), 1830-1835.

Korn, T., Bettelli, E., Gao, W., Awasthi, A., Jager, A., Strom, T. B., Oukka, M., and Kuchroo, V. K. (2007). IL-21 initiates an alternative pathway to induce proinflammatory T(H) 17 cells. *Nature*, *448*(7152),484-487.

Korn, T., Bettelli, E., Oukka, M., and Kuchroo, V. K. (2009). IL-17 and Th17 Cells. *Annu Rev Immunol*, 27,485-517.

Korn, T., Bettelli E., Oukka M., and Kuchroo, V. K. (2009). IL-17 and Th17 Cells. *Annu Rev Immunol*, *27*,485-517.

Lambrecht, B. N., and Galli, S. J. (2015). SnapShot: integrated type 2 immune responses. *Immunity*, 43,408-408: e401.

Lambrecht, B. N., Guilliams, M., and Hammad, H. (2018). Dendritic Cells in Inflammatory Disease, In: Cavaillon JM and Singer M (eds) *Inflammation from molecular and cellular mechanisms to the clinic*, vol 1-4. Wiley-VCH, p 289-313.

Lambrecht, B. N., and Hammad, H. (2015). The immunology of asthma. *Nat Immunol, 16*,45-56.

Lawrence, T., and Gilroy, D. W. (2007). Chronic inflammation, a failure of resolution? *Int J Exp Pathol, 88*, 85-94.

Lawrence, T., Gilroy, D. W., Colville-Nash, P. R., and Willoughby, D. A. (2001). Possible new role for NF-kappaB in the resolution of inflammation. *Nat Med, 7*, 1291-1297.

Levin, J (2018). *Platelets*. In: Cavaillon JM and Singer M (eds) *Inflammation from molecular and cellular mechanisms to the clinic*, vol 1-4. Wiley-VCH, p 419-435.

Loke, P., Nair, M. G., Parkinson, J., Guiliano, D., Blaxter, M., and Allen, J. E. (2002). IL-4 dependent alternatively-activated macrophages have a distinctive *in vivo* gene expression phenotype. *BMC Immunol, 3*, 7

Lumeng, C. N., Bodzin, J. L., and Saltiel, A. R. (2007). Obesity induces a phenotypic switch in adipose tissue macrophage polarization. *J Clin Invest, 117*,175-184.

Maddur, M. S., Miossec, P., Kaveri, S. V., and Bayry, J. (2012). Th17 cells: biology, pathogenesis of autoimmune and inflammatory diseases, and therapeutic strategies. *Am J Pathol, 181*, 8-18.

Mantovani, A., Allavena, P., Sica, A., and Balkwill, F. (2008). Cancer-related inflammation. *Nature, 454*, 436-444.

Mantovani, A., Sozzani, S., Locati, M., Allavena, P., and Sica A. (2002). Macrophage polarization: tumor-associated macrophages as a paradigm for polarized M2 mononuclear phagocytes. *Trends Immunol, 23*, 549-555.

Mills, C. D., Kincaid, K., Alt, J. M., Heilman, M. J., and Hill, A. M. (2000). M-1/ M-2 macrophages and the Th1/Th2 paradigm. *J Immunol, 164*, 6166-6173.

Miossec, P., Korn, T., and Kuchroo, V. K. (2009). Interleukin-17 and type 17 helper T cells. *N Engl J Med, 361*, 888-898.

Monteleone, G., Marafini, I., and Troncone, E. (2018). Interleukin-17 A-E. In: Cavaillon JM and Singer M (eds). *Inflammation from molecular and cellular mechanisms to the clinic*, vol 1-4. Wiley-VCH, 549-571.

Morrison, P. J., Ballantyne, S. J., and Kullberg, M. C. (2011). Interleukin-23 and T helper 17-type responses in intestinal inflammation: from cytokines to T-cell plasticity. *Immunology, 133*, 397–408.

Mosser, D. M., and Edwards, J. P. (2008). Exploring the full spectrum of macrophage activation. *Nat Rev Immunol, 8*, 958-969.

Nguyen, M. T., Favelyukis, S., Nguyen, A. K., Reichart, D., Scott, P. A., Jenn, A., Liu-Bryan, R., Glass, C. K., Neels, J. G., and Olefsky, J. M. (2007). A subpopulation of macrophages infiltrates hypertrophic adipose tissue and is activated by free fatty acids via Toll-like receptors 2 and 4 and JNK-dependent pathways. *J Biol Chem, 282*, 35279-35292.

Noack, M., and Miossec, P. (2018). Th17 Cells. In: Cavaillon JM and Singer M (eds) *Inflammation from molecular and cellular mechanisms to the clinic*, vol 1-4. Wiley-VCH, 395-417.

Nurden, A. T. (2011). *Platelets*, inflammation and tissue regeneration. *Thromb Haemost, 105*(Suppl 1),13-23.

Otsuka, A., Nakajima, S., Kubo, M, Egawa, G, Honda, T, Kitoh, A., Nomura, T., Hanakawa, S., Sagita Moniaga, C., Kim, B., Matsuoka, S., Watanabe, T., Miyachi, Y., and Kabashima, K. (2013). Basophils are required for the induction of Th2 *immunity* to haptens and peptide antigens. *Nat Commun, 4*, 1739.

Ouyang, W., Kolls, J. K., and Zheng, Y. (2008). The biological functions of T helper 17 cell effector cytokines in inflammation. *Immunity, 28*, 454-467.

Pena, O. M., Pistolic, J., Raj, D., Fjell, C. D., and Hancock, R. E. (2011). Endotoxin tolerance represents a distinctive state of alternative polarization (M2) in human mononuclear cells. *J Immunol,186*, 7243-7254.

Podolsky, D. K. (2002). Inflammatory bowel disease. *N Engl J Med, 347*(6). 417-429.

Pollard, J. W. (2009). Trophic macrophages in development and disease. *Nat Rev Immunol, 9*, 259-270.

Porta, C., Rimoldi, M., Raes, G., Brys, L., Ghezzi, P., Di Liberto, D., Dieli, F., Ghisletti, S., Natoli, G., De Baetselier, P., Mantovani, A., and Sica, A. (2009). Tolerance and M2 (alternative). macrophage polarization are related processes orchestrated by p50 nuclear factor kappaB. *Proc Natl Acad Sci USA, 106*, 14978-14983.

Qian, B. Z., and Pollard, J. W. (2010). Macrophage diversity enhances tumor progression, metastasis. *Cell*, *141*, 39-51.

Qiao, H., Andrade, M. V., Lisboa, F. A., Morgan, K., and Beaven, M. A. (2006). FcepsilonR1 and toll-like receptors mediate synergistic signals to markedly augment production of inflammatory cytokines in murine mast cells. *Blood, 107*, 610-618.

Reid, V. L., and Webster, N. R. (2012). Role of microparticles in sepsis. *Brit J Anaesth*, *109*, 503-513.

Schif-Zuck, S., Gross, N., Assi, S., Rostoker, R., Serhan, C. N., and Ariel, A. (2011). Saturated-efferocytosis generates pro-resolving CD11b low macrophages: modulation by resolvins glucocorticoids. *Eur J Immunol*, *41*, 366-379.

Serafini, N., and Di Santo, J. P. (2018). Group 2 and 3 Innate Lymphoid Cells: New Actors in *Immunity* and Inflammation. In: Cavaillon JM and Singer M (eds) *Inflammation from molecular and cellular mechanisms to the clinic*, vol 1-4. Wiley-VCH, 341-363.

Serafini, N., Vosshenrich, C. A. J., and Di Santo, J. P. (2015). Transcriptional regulation of innate lymphoid cell fate. *Nat Rev Immunol*, *15*(7), 415-428.

Serhan, C. N., Brain, S. D., Buckley, C. D., Gilroy, D. W., Haslett, C., O'Neill, L. A., Perretti, M., Rossi, A. G., and Wallace, J. L. (2007). Resolution of inflammation: state of the art, definitions and terms. *FASEB J*, *21*, 325-332.

Serhan, C. N., Yang, R., Martinod, K., Kasuga, K., Pillai, P. S., Porter, T. F., Oh, S. F., and Spite, M. (2009). Maresins: novel macrophage mediators with potent antiinflammatory and proresolving actions. *J Exp Med*, *206*, 15-23.

Shalova, I. N., Lim, J. Y., Chittezhath, M., Zinkernagel, A. S., Beasley, F., Hernandez-Jimenez, E., Toledano, V., Cubillos-Zapata, C., Rapisarda, A., Chen, J., Duan, K., Yang, H., Poidinger, M., Melillo, G., Nizet, V., Arnalich F., Lopez-Collazo, E., and Biswas, S. K. (2015). Human monocytes undergo functional reprogramming during sepsis mediated hypoxia-inducible factor-1alpha. *Immunity*, *42*, 484-498.

Shalova, I. N., Lim, J. Y., Chittezhath, M., Zinkernagel, A. S., Beasley, F., Hernandez-Jimenez, E., Toledano, V, Cubillos-Zapata, C., Rapisarda, A., Chen, J., Duan, K., Yang, H, Poidinger, M., Melillo, G., Nizet, V., Arnalich, F., Lopez-Collazo, E., and Biswas, S. K. (2015). Human monocytes undergo functional reprogramming during sepsis mediated by hypoxia-inducible factor-1alpha. *Immunity*, *42*, 484-498.

Shalova, I. N., Saha, S., and Biswas, S. K. (2018). Monocytes and Macrophages. In: Cavaillon JM and Singer M (eds) *Inflammation from molecular and cellular mechanisms to the clinic*, vol 1-4. Wiley-VCH, p 219-251.

Stables, M. J., Shah, S., Camon, E. B., Lovering, R. C., Newson, J., Bystrom, J., Farrow, S., and Gilroy D. W. (2011). Transcriptomic analyses of murine resolution-phase macrophages. *Blood*, *118*, e192-e208.

Steiger, M., and Reichstein, T. (1937). Desoxy-cortico-steron (21-oxyprogesteron) aus Δ (-3-oxy-atio-cholensaure). *Helv Chim Acta*, *20*, 1164-1179.

Stein, M., Keshav, S., Harris, N., and Gordon, S. (1992). Interleukin 4 potently enhances murine macrophage mannose receptor activity: a marker of alternative immunologic macrophage activation. *J Exp Med*, *176*, 287-292.

Tanaka, T., Narazaki, M., and Kishimoto, T. (2018). IL-6 Superfamily. In: Cavaillon JM and Singer M (eds) *Inflammation from molecular and cellular mechanisms to the clinic*, vol 1-4. Wiley-VCH, p 573-586

Tiku, K., Tiku, M. L., and Skosey, J. L. (1986). Interleukin 1 production by human polymorphonuclear neutrophils. *J Immunol*, *136*(10), 3677-3685.

Tillet, W. S., and Francis, T. (1930). Serological reactions in pneumonia with a non-protein somatic fraction of pneumococcus. *J Exp Med*, *52*, 561-571.

Ulrich, B. J., Hufford, M. M., and Kaplan, M. H. (2018). Th9 Cells: From the Bench to the Bedside and Back Again. In: Cavaillon JM and Singer M (eds) *Inflammation from molecular and cellular mechanisms to the clinic*, vol 1-4. Wiley-VCH, 365-394.

Van Epps, H. L. (2005). Macrophage activation unveiled. *J Exp Med*, *202*, 884.

Vieira-de-Abreu, A., Campbell, R. A., Weyrich, A. S., and Zimmerman, G. A. (2012). Platelets: versatile effector cells in hemostasis, inflammation, and the immune continuum. *Sem Immunopathol*, *34*, 5-30.

Vosshenrich, C. A. J., and Di Santo, J. P. (2018). Roles for NK Cells and ILC1 in Inflammation and Infection. In: Cavaillon JM and Singer M (eds) *Inflammation from molecular and cellular mechanisms to the clinic*, vol 1-4. Wiley-VCH, 315-340.

Waage, A., Espevik, T., and Lamvik, J. (1986). Detection of tumour necrosis factor-like cytotoxicity in serum from patients with septicaemia but not from untreated cancer patients. *Scand J Immunol*, *24*, 739-743.

White, J. G. (2005). *Platelets* are covercytes, not phagocytes: uptake of bacteria involves channels of the open canalicular system. *Platelets*, *16*, 121-131.

Wills-Karp, M. (2010). Allergen-specific pattern recognition receptor pathways. *Curr Opin Immunol*, *22*, 777-782.

Wynn, T. A., Chawla, A., and Pollard, J. W. (2013). Macrophage biology in development, homeostasis and disease. *Nature*, *496*, 445-455.

Yang, R., Liu, Y., Kelk, P., Qu, C., Akiyama, K., Chen, C., Atsuta, I., Chen, W., Zhou, Y., and Shi, S. (2013). A subset of IL-17(+) mesenchymal stem cells possesses anti-Candida albicans effect. *Cell Res*, *23*(1), 107-121.

Youssefian, T., Drouin, A., Masse, J. M., Guichard, J., and Cramer, E. M. (2002). Host defense role of *platelets*: engulfment of HIV and *Staphylococcus aureus* occurs in a specific subcellular compartment and is enhanced by platelet activation. *Blood*, *99*, 4021-4029.

Zander, D. M. W., and Klinger, M. H. F. (2009). The *blood platelets* contribution to innate host defense: what they have learned from their big brothers. *Biotechnol J*, *4*, 914-926.

Chapter 17

Cytokines and Tissue

Kadir Gem[*]**, MD**
Ministry of Health Alaşehir State Hospital Orthopedics and Traumatology, Manisa, Turkey

Abstract

Cytokines, which are polypeptides that different cell types produce and secrete, ensure the regulation of the immune and inflammatory events involving a systemic response to inflammation, cell growth and healing, and injury. As an endocrine organ, adipose tissue receives information from other metabolic tissues, e.g., the muscles, liver, and brain, and also transmits soluble signals with specific cytokines called "adipokines" with local and systemic effects in order to regulate the nutritional balance. It also has a structure containing the cells of the innate and acquired immune systems. Leukocytes that infiltrate the connective tissue generate soluble cellular mediators or cytokines, triggering the proliferation of capillary cells, smooth muscle cells, and fibroblasts. Bone morphogenetic protein(s) (BMPs) represent very potent cytokines that cause the bone and cartilage to be formed. Osteoblast and chondrocyte differentiation is also stimulated by BMPs. Bone morphogenetic protein(s) (BMPs), BMP2 and BMP4 in particular, represent potent growth factors that cause the cartilage and bone to be formed as a result of stimulating osteoblast and chondrocyte differentiation. BMPs belong to the TGF-β family, which has been indicated to stimulate osteoblast differentiation.

Keywords: adipokine, insulin resistance, growth factors, cytokines, arthrosis

Introduction

Cytokines, which are polypeptides that different cell types produce and secrete, ensure the regulation of the immune and inflammatory events involving a systemic response to inflammation, cell growth and healing, and injury. Cytokines are similar to hormones. However, they are not exactly hormones (Nororiha et al., 1995).

Cells secrete cytokines in a fairly short time when stimulated, but they are not stored. They are also produced de novo in response to an immune stimulus.

---

[*] Corresponding Author's Email: kadirgem.ege@hotmail.com.

In: Cytokines and Diseases
Editors: Kenan Demir, Selim Görgün and Bahar Uslu
ISBN: 979-8-88697-214-6

They have agonist and antagonist effects on each other. Cytokines act via binding to specific receptors on the target cell, as in polypeptide hormones (Utexas 2006).

Many cytokines have both proinflammatory and anti-inflammatory potential. They identify these effects based on the cellular source and target and the phase of the immune response (Borish and Steinke 2003).

Cytokines Secreted from Adipose Tissue

As an endocrine organ, adipose tissue receives information from other metabolic tissues, e.g., the muscles, liver, and brain and also transmits soluble signals with specific cytokines called "adipokines" with local and systemic effects in order to regulate the nutritional balance. Furthermore, it also has a structure containing the cells of the innate and acquired immune systems (DiSpirito and Mathis 2015).

The immune cells found in adipose tissue actively secrete pro- and anti-inflammatory cytokines. Changes take place in the metabolism with the restructuring of adipose tissue, alterations in adipocyte size, and reversible alterations in the composition of immune cells, leading to changes in adipocyte functions (Choe et al., 2016).

Adipose tissue macrophages are classified into two as M1 (classically activated) and M2 (alternatively activated). While type M1 macrophages express inducible nitric oxide synthase (iNOS), CD11c on the cell surface, and proinflammatory cytokines including TNF-α and IL-1β, M2 macrophages express arginase, IL-10, and macrophage surface antibody Ym-1. Type M1 macrophages in adipose tissue have been reported to be the type of macrophage that mainly contributes to the inflammation of adipose tissue and insulin resistance in obesity. Moreover, it has been shown that insulin resistance and adipose tissue inflammation are mild in the case of dietary obesity in mice transplanted with bone marrow with reduced CD11c-positive cells (Choe et al., 2016).

M2 macrophages secrete IL-10, an anti-inflammatory cytokine (Choe et al., 2016). It is indicated to treat adipocytes with IL-10 to improve TNF-α-mediated insulin resistance (Lumeng et al., 2007).

It was found that in the case of the increased level of IL-10, TNF-α expression was reduced and insulin resistance and glucose intolerance were improved. It was determined to have positive effects by stimulating STAT3 phosphorylation in neurons secreting proopiomelanocortin in cases of obesity and hyperphagia (Nakata et al., 2016).

It has recently been determined that natural killer T (iNKT) cells in adipose tissue have beneficial effects in the inflammation of adipose tissue and insulin sensitivity. These cells have been reported to be related to the secretion of anti-inflammatory cytokines, including IL-4 and IL-10 (Choe et al., 2016). Recent studies have shown that maximal preadipocyte proliferation early in life requires IL-4Rα pathway signaling and that the injection of the IL-4 complex is adequate to stimulate the white preadipocyte proliferation (Lee et al., 2015). Furthermore, IL-4 and IL-33 have been revealed to lead to the differentiation of white adipocytes (Lee et al., 2015; Brestoff et al., 2015).

TNF-α was reported to be the first white adipose tissue-derived cytokine affecting insulin resistance, and it was found that the majority of its source was macrophages in adipose tissue. The circulating level of TNF-α, which is found in high amounts in the adipose tissue and plasma of obese people, decreases with weight loss (Makki et al., 2013). It was found that TNF-α directly reduced insulin signaling and insulin secretion in tissues sensitive to insulin (Dunmore and Brown 2013). In addition to TNF-α's direct negative effect on insulin signaling, it provides the indirect stimulation of insulin resistance by changing adipocyte lipid metabolism and adipocyte differentiation. Furthermore, it is also known that it initiates lipolysis and the release of free fatty acids, which will make a contribution to increased glucose formation in the liver. It leads to the potential enlargement of the adipose tissue mass by inhibiting the conversion of preadipocytes into mature adipocytes. TNF-α also has adverse effects on the generation of adiponectin, which affects lipid and glucose homeostasis. It acts by contributing to the increased synthesis of other cytokines, e.g., IL-6, instead of directly affecting the immune responses (Makki et al., 2013).

IL-6 represents a cytokine with multifaceted effects in regulating hematopoiesis, inflammation, the defense mechanism, and immune responses (Dunmore and Brown 2013). One-third of IL-6 in the circulation of healthy subjects is derived from adipose tissue. While a part of the IL-6 secreted from adipose tissue is secreted from adipocytes, a part of it is secreted from other cells, especially macrophages (Pricola et al., 2009). The occurrence of IL-6 increases in relation to an increase in waist circumference, body mass, and free fatty acids, as in TNF-α (Dunmore and Brown 2013). IL-6 may have varying effects depending on tissue and metabolic conditions. Along with its anti-inflammatory effect during exercise, while IL-6 increases the intake of glucose in a way to direct fatty acid oxidation, skeletal muscle mass hypertrophy, and myogenesis, it increases insulin resistance in the liver and adipose tissue and also increases proinflammatory activities (Makki et al., 2013). Furthermore, IL-6 causes the fatty acid metabolism to be imbalanced in white adipose tissue by increasing the proliferation of mesenchymal stem cells and inhibiting the differentiation of cells (chondrogenic and adipogenic) and adipogenesis (Pricola et al., 2009). Lipolysis in humans is stimulated by IL-6, which increases the concentration of free fatty acids and whole-body fat oxidation but does not cause hypertriglyceridemia (Sopasakis et al., 2004). Apart from the other markers of adipocyte differentiation, IL-6 reduces the secretion and expression of adiponectin from adipocytes in humans (Tack et al., 2012).

IL-1β represents a proinflammatory cytokine secreted by both immune cells and adipose tissue. IL-1β is reported to decrease fat accumulation and adipocyte differentiation by decreasing the expression of PPAR-γ, adiponectin and GLUT 4, which are effective in insulin sensitivity, during adipocyte differentiation (Van Hall et al., 2003).

Insulin resistance or sensitivity is determined by the secretion of proinflammatory and anti-inflammatory cytokines from adipose tissue.

Cytokines Secreted from the Connective Tissue

Connective tissue is a component that is present in all parts of an organism. It consists of proteins and proteoglycans with or without collagen (Krieg et al., 1988). The roles of cytokines in the control of the connective tissue metabolism in the course of wound healing and fibrosis have been gradually addressed more (Kovacs et al., 1994). Leukocytes that infiltrate the connective tissue generate soluble cellular mediators or cytokines, triggering the proliferation of fibroblasts, capillary cells, and smooth muscle cells (Kovacs et al., 1994).

It was demonstrated that epidermal growth factor (EGF), platelet-derived growth factor (PDGF), fibroblast growth factor (FGF), and transforming growth factor-β (TGF-β) are various growth factors that increase wound healing (Pierce et al., 1992). TGF-β and PDGF represent powerful growth factors. They stimulate the repair of soft tissue in animal models (Ksander et al., 1989; Lynch et al., 1989; Lynch et al., 1987; Mustoe et al., 1987). In fibroblasts, glycosaminoglycan (GAG), fibronectin, and hyaluronic acid synthesis are selectively stimulated by PDGF (Allen-Hoffman et al., 1990; Blatti et al., 1988; Heldin et al., 1989). On the contrary, TGF-β triggers the synthesis of fibronectin, GAG, and procollagen type I (Bassols and Massague 1988; Ignotz and Massague 1986; Keska-Oja et al., 1988). In-vivo repair is accelerated by TGF-β and PDGF through significantly variable mechanisms. However, the synthesis of collagen, which is crucial for normal healing, is accelerated by both growth factors (Peacock 1984; Ross 1968). It was demonstrated that TGF-β had direct effects on fibroblasts in order to accelerate the synthesis of collagen, while PDGF strengthened the acute inflammatory response by recruiting and activating wound macrophages in a specific manner at the beginning of the repair process (Pierce et al., 1992). PDGF, EGF, and TGF-β function as chemoattractants for fibroblasts (Graves et al., 1983; Kang 1978). Growth factors may also activate the biosynthesis of collagen and other connective tissue components (Pierce et al., 1992).

TGF-β leads to the quick creation of granulation tissue and then an increase in matrix proteins. While these events partially result from the increased migration and proliferation of fibroblasts, they also result from an increase in collagen synthesis (Roberts et al., 1986). TGF-β stimulates collagen and fibronectin gene expression (Raghow et al., 1987; Rossi et al., 1988; Varga et al., 1987). With the use of different collagen promoter constructs, it was found that collagen gene expression up to ten-fold could be induced by TGF-β, acting through the nuclear factor-1 (NF1) region in the promoter region (Rossi et al., 1988). It was demonstrated that TGF-β stimulated the collagen and fibronectin gene expression and also the production and secretion of ECM proteins (Sporn and Roberts 1988).

TNF-α represents a cytokine, primarily generated by macrophages and inhibiting the collagen gene transcription of dermal fibroblasts (Scharffetter et al., 1989; Takeda et al., 1993). TNF-α and IL-8 lead to a significant decrease in angiogenesis by blocking the biological activity (by adding an anti-cytokine antibody) (Kovacs et al., 1994).

It was demonstrated that PDGF, TGF-β, and TNF-α, which are fibrinogenic cytokines, might directly act to affect fibroblast proliferation under certain conditions (Thorton et al., 1990; Kahari et al., 1990). It was reported that both TNF-α and TGF-β acted as the inducers and inhibitors of fibroblast growth, although PDGF is fibroproliferative (Thorton et al., 1990). Low concentrations of TNF-α stimulate the proliferation of a number of fibroblast cell lines and block growth at a more significant dose. Nevertheless, it directly inhibits proliferation in some cells (Thorton et al., 1990). The proliferative impacts of TNF-α and TGF-β on fibroblasts partially depend on the generation of the PDGF-A chain by target cells (Battegay et al., 1990).

The above-mentioned findings indicate that specific cytokines taking part in angiogenesis and tissue repair and even cell types can be different according to the repair site.

Cytokines Secreted from the Cartilage and Bone Tissue

Bone morphogenetic protein(s) (BMPs) represent potent cytokines causing the creation of cartilage and bone. The differentiation of osteoblasts and chondrocytes is also stimulated by BMPs (Nishimura et al., 2011). Bone morphogenetic protein(s) (BMP), particularly BMP2 and BMP4, represent potent growth factors causing cartilage and bone creation as a result of stimulating osteoblast and chondrocyte differentiation (Nishimura et al., 2008). BMPs belong to the TGF-β family, which has been stated to stimulate the differentiation of osteoblasts (Miyazono et al., 2004; ten Dijke et al., 2000).

Multifunctional regulators of cell growth, differentiation, and apoptosis are the transforming growth factor-β (TGF-β) superfamily members. They represent powerful inducers and regulators of chondrogenesis and osteogenesis. In addition to TGF-β, the majority of the BMPs (bone morphogenetic proteins), inhibins, activins, particular growth and differentiation factors (GDFs), and some other proteins are included in this family (Massague 1998; Zwijsen et al., 2003). The osteoblast differentiation of mesenchymal cells is robustly inhibited by TGF-β (S Maeda et al., 2004). It was demonstrated that TGF-β stimulated the correlation between the TGF-β receptor complex and the parathyroid hormone (PTH) receptor and affected the phosphorylation of the PTH receptor (Qiu et al., 2010). TGF-β is present in very high amounts in the articular cartilage, and biglycan, decorin, and fibromodulin, the small leucine-rich proteoglycans of the cartilage, are capable of regulating TGF-β activity by sequestering it (Hildebrand et al., 1994).

RANKL, known as a TNF family member, together with M-CSF, is essential for the differentiation of osteoclasts (Yasuda et al., 1998). Inflammatory cytokines, including IL-1, IL-6, IL-17, and TNF-α, induce excessive RANKL on the membranes of synovial fibroblasts or osteoblasts. The receptor activator of the nuclear factor kappa B (RANK)/RANKL pathway is activated by the direct cell-to-cell contact between osteoblasts and osteoclast progenitors, eventually supporting the differentiation of osteoclasts (Yasuda et al., 1998; Braun and Zwerina 2011). The occurrence of pannus can be shown as a pathological example of this activity. Pannus is composed of synovial fibroblasts, T cells, and macrophages, generating inflammatory cytokines, e.g., interleukin-1 (IL-1), IL-6, IL-17, and tumor necrosis factor (TNF)-α. The said inflammatory cytokines lead to the destruction of bones by activating the osteoclasts. There are subsets in T helper (Th) cells, e.g., Th1, Th2, and Th17 cells. The differentiation of naive T cells into Th17 cells occurs via transforming growth factor-β (TGF-β), IL-1β, IL-6, and IL-21. Th17 cells generate IL-17, activating inflammation by functioning on different immune cells and causing osteoclast activation by the receptor induction. Nuclear factor kappa B (RANKL) can also be activated by synovial fibroblasts. The differentiation of osteoclasts is regulated by IFN-γ, IL-4, and cytotoxic T-lymphocyte associated protein-4 (CTLA-4) generated by Th1, Th2, and Treg, respectively. The destruction of the cartilage is induced by matrix metalloproteinase (MMP) and a disintegrin and metalloproteinase with thrombospondin motifs (ADAMTS) generated by synovial fibroblasts, synovial macrophages, and chondrocytes (Daisuke et al., 2019).

Conclusion

In conclusion, cytokines regulate both anabolic and catabolic processes on the tissue via various intracellular pathways through their specific receptors. The balance of cytokine activity is of critical importance for the continuation of normal function on tissues. As explained in detail above, impairments in this balance may trigger pathological processes. We obtain new information about the effects of cytokines on tissues every day, which sheds light on our understanding of the pathophysiology of diseases. Thus, it can contribute to establishing new treatment protocols for chronic diseases. However, many studies are needed.

References

Allen-Hoffman B. L., Schlosser S. J., Brondyk W. H., Fahl W. E. (1990) Fibronectin levels are enhanced in human fibroblasts overexpressing the c-sis protooncogene. *J Biol Chem* 265:5219-5225.

Bassols A., Massague J. (1988) Transforming growth factor regulates the expression and structure of extracellular matrix chondroitan/dermatan sulfate proteoglycans. *J Biot Chem* 263:3039-3045.

Battegay E. J., Raines E. W., Seifer R. A., Bowen-Pope D. F., Ross R. (1990) TGF-β induces bimodal proliferation of connective tissue cells via complex control of an autocrine PDGF loop. *Cell* 63:515-524.

Blatti S. P., Foster D. N., Ranganathan G., Moses H. L., Getz M. J. (1988) Induction of fibronectin gene transcription and MRNA is a primary response to growth-factor stimulation of AKR-2B cells. *Proc Natl Acad Sci USA* 85:1119-1123.

Borish L. C., Steinke J. W. (2003) Cytokines and chemokines. *J Allergy Clin Immunol* 111(2 Suppl):S460-475.

Braun T., Zwerina J. (2011) Positive regulators of osteoclastogenesis and bone resorption in rheumatoid arthritis. *Arthritis Res Ther* 13:235.

Brestoff J. R., Kim B. S., Saenz S. A., Rachel R. Stine, Laurel A. Monticelli, Gregory F. Sonnenberg, Joseph J. Thome, Donna L. Farber, Kabirullah Lutfy, Patrick Seale, David Artis (2015) Group 2 innate lymphoid cells promote beiging of white adipose tissue and limit obesity. *Nature* 519:242-246.

Choe S. S., Huh J. Y., Hwang I. J., Jong In Kim, Jae Bum Kim (2016) Adipose tissue remodeling: Its role in energy metabolism and metabolic disorders. *Front Endocrinol* (Lausanne) 7:30.

Daisuke T., Hideki Y. and Takashi K. (2019) Cartilage and Bone Destruction in Arthritis: Pathogenesis and Treatment Strategy: A Literature Review. *Cells* 8(8):818.

DiSpirito J. R., Mathis D. (2015) Immunological contributions to adipose tissue homeostasis. *Semin. Immunol* 27:315-321.

Dunmore S. J., Brown J. E. P. (2013) The role of adipokines in beta-cell failure of type 2 diabetes. *J Endocrinol* 216: T37-45.

Graves P. N., Wess I. K., Perlish J. S., Fleischmajer R. (1983) Increased procollagen mRNA levels in scleroderma skin fibroblasts. *J Int Rheumatol* 80:130-132.

Heldin P., Laurent T. C., Heidin H. C. (1989) Effect of growth factors on hyaluronan synthesis in cultured human fibroblasts. *Biochem J* 258:919-922.

Hildebrand A., Romaris M., Rasmussen L. M., D. Heinegård, D. R. Twardzik, W. A. Border, E. Ruoslahti (1994) Interaction of the small interstitial proteoglycans biglycan, decorin and fibromodulin with transforming growth factor beta. *Biochem J* 302:527-534.

Ignotz R. A., Massague J. (1986) Transforming growth factor-~ stimulates the expression of fibronectin and collagen and their incorporation into the extracellular matrix. *J Biol Chem* 261:4337-4345.

Kahari V. M., Chen Y. Q., Su M. W., Ramirez, F., Uitto J. (1990) TNFa and IFN-y suppress the activation of human type I collagen gene expression by transforming growth factorfi. *J Clin Invest* 86:1489-149.

Kang A. H. (1978) Fibroblast activation. *J Lab Clin Med* 92:1-4.

Keska-Oja J., Raghow R., Sawdey M., Loskutoff D. J., Postlethwaite S. E., Kang A. H., Moses H. L. (1988) Regulation of the mRNAs for type I plasminogen activator inhibitor, fibronectin, and type I procollagen by transforming growth factor-~. *J Biol Chem* 263:3111-3115.

Kovacs E. J., DiPietro L. A. (1994) Fibrogenic cytokines and connective tissue production *FASEB J* 8(11):854-61.

Krieg T. H., Hein R., Hatamochi A., Aumailley M. (1988) Molecular and clinical aspects of connective tissue. *Eur J Clin Invest* 18:105-123.

Ksander G. A., Ogawa Y., Chu G. H., McMullin H., Rosenblatt J. S., McPherson J. M. (1989) Exogenous transforming growth factorbeta 2 enhances connective tissue formation and wound strength in guinea pig derma wounds healing by secondary intent. *Ann Surg* 211:288-294.

Lee M. W., Odegaard J. I., Mukundan L., Yifu Qiu, Ari B. Molofsky, Jesse C. Nussbaum, Karen Yun, Richard M. Locksley, Ajay Chawla (2015) Activated Type 2 Innate Lymphoid Cells Regulate Beige Fat Biogenesis. *Cell* 160:74-87.

Lumeng C. N., Bodzin J. L., Saltiel A. R. (2007) Obesity induces a phenotypic switch in adipose tissue macrophage polarization. *J Clin Invest* 117:175-184.

Lynch S. E., Colvin R. B., Antoniades N. H. (1989) Growth factors in wound healing. *J Clin Invest* 84:640-646.

Lynch S. E., Nixon J. C., Colvin R. B., Antoniades H. N. (1987) Role of platelet-derived growth factor in wound healing: synergistic effects with other growth factors. *Proc Natl Acad Sci USA* 84:7696-7700.

Maeda S., Hayashi M., Komiya S., Imamura T., Miyazono K. (2004) Endogenous TGF-beta signaling suppresses maturation of osteoblastic mesenchymal cells. *EMBO J* 23:552563.

Makki K., Froguel P., Wolowczuk I. (2013) Adipose tissue in obesity-related inflammation and insulin resistance: cells, cytokines, and chemokines. *ISRN Inflamm* 2013:139239.

Massague J. (1998) TGF-beta signal transduction. *Annu Rev Biochem* 67:753-91.

Miyazono K., Maeda S., Imamura T. (2004) Coordinate regulation of cell growth and differentiation by TGF-beta superfamily and Runx proteins. *Oncogene* 23:42324237.

Mustoe T. A., Pierce G. F., Thomason A., Gramates P., Sporn M. B., Deuel T. F. (1987) Accelerated healing of incisional wounds in rats induced by transforming growth factor-J3. *Science* 237:1333-1335.

Nakata M., Yamamoto S., Okada T. D., Gantulga, H. Okano, K. Ozawa & T. Yada (2016) IL-10 gene transfer upregulates arcuate POMC and ameliorates hyperphagia, obesity and diabetes by substituting for leptin. *Int J Obes* 40:425-433.

Nishimura R., Hata K., Ikeda F., Ichida F., Shimoyama A., Matsubara T., Wada M., Amano K., and Yoneda T. (2008) Signal transduction and transcriptional regulation during mesenchymal cell differentiation. *J Bone Miner Metab* 26:203212.

Nishimura R., Hata K., Matsubara T., Wakabayashi M., Yoneda T. (2012) Regulation of bone and cartilage development by network between BMP signalling and transcription factors. *J Biochem* 151(3):247-254.

Nororiha I. L., Niemir Z., Stein H., Waldher R. (1995) Cytokines and growth factors in renal disease: *Nephrol Dial Transplant* 10:775-786.

Peacock E. E. Jr. (1984) *Wound repair*, 2nd edn. W. B. Saunders, Philadelphia.

Pierce G. F., Tarpley J. E., Yanagihara D., Mustoe T. A., Fox G. M., Thomason A. (1992) Platelet-derived growth factor (BBhomodimer), transforming growth factor--~31, and basic fibroblast growth factor in dermal wound healing. *Am J Pathol* 140:1375-1388.

Pricola K. L., Kuhn N. Z., Haleem-Smith H., Yingjie Song, Rocky S. Tuan (2009) Interleukin-6 maintains bone marrowderived mesenchymal stem cell stemness by an ERK1/2-dependent mechanism. *J Cell Biochem* 108:577-588.

Qiu T., Wu X., Zhang F., Clemens T. L., Wan M., Cao X. (2010) TGF-beta type II receptor phosphorylates PTH receptor to integrate bone remodelling signalling. *Nat Cell Biol* 12:224234.

Raghow R., Postlethwaite A. E., Keski-Oja J., Moses H. L., Kang A. H. (1987) Transforming growth factor-beta increases steady state levels of type I procollagen and fibronectin messenger RNA's posttranslationally in cultured human dermal fibroblasts. *J Clin Invest* 79:1285-1288.

Roberts A. B., Sporn M. B., Assoian R. K., Smith J. M., Roche N. S., Wakefield L. M., Heine U. I., Liotta L. A., Falanga V., Kehrl J. H., Fanci A. S. (1986) Transforming growth factor type beta:rapid induction of fibrosis and angiogenesis in vivo and stimulation of collagen formation in vitro. *Proc Natl Acad Sci USA* 83:4167-4171.

Ross R. (1968) The fibroblast and wound repair. *Biol Rev Camb Philos Soc* 43:51-96.

Rossi P., Karsenty G., Roberts A. B., Roche N. S., Sporn M. B., de Crombrugghe B. (1988) A nuclear factor 1 binding site mediates the transcriptional activation of a type I collagen promoter by transforming growth factor. *Cell* 52(3):405-414.

Scharffetter K., Heckmann M., Hatamochi A., Mauch C., Stein B., Riethmtiller G., Ziegler-Heitbrock J., Krieg T. (1989) Synergistic effect of tumor necrosis factor-alpha and interferon-gamma on collagen synthesis of human skin fibroblasts in vitrol *Exp Cell Res* 181:409-419.

Sopasakis V. R., Sandqvist M., Gustafson B., ve ark. 2004. High local concentrations and effects on differentiation implicate interleukin-6 as a paracrine regulator. *Obes Res* 12:454-460.

Sporn, M. B., Roberts, A. B. (1988) Peptide growth factors are mul-tifunctional. *Nature* (London) 332:217-21.

Tack C. J., Stienstra R., Joosten L. A. B., Mihai G Netea (2012) Inflammation links excess fat to insulin resistance: The role of the interleukin-1 family. *Immunol Rev* 249:239-252.

Takeda K., Hatamochi A., Arakawa M., Ueki H. (1993) Effects of tumor necrosis factor-c~ on connective tissue metabolism in normal and scleroderma fibroblast cultures. *Arch Dermatol Res* 284:440-444.

ten Dijke P., Miyazono K., Heldin C. H. (2000) Signaling inputs converge on nuclear effectors in TGF-beta signaling. *Trends Biochem Sci* 25:6470.

Thorton S. C., Pot S. B., Walsh B. J., Penny R., Breit S. N. (1990) Interaction of immune and connective tissue cells: the effects of lymphokines and monokines on fibroblast growth. *J Leukocyte Blot* 47:312-320.

Utexas (2006) *Properties of cytokines.* Avaible via http://www.sbs.utexas.edu/sanders/Bio347/Lectures/2006/Lecture%2014%202006.htm.

Van Hall G., Steensberg A., Sacchetti M., Christian Fischer, Charlotte Keller, Peter Schjerling, Natalie Hiscock, Kirsten Møller, Bengt Saltin, Mark A. Febbraio, Bente K. Pedersen (2003) Interleukin-6 stimulates lipolysis and fat oxidation in humans. *J Clin Endocrinol Metab* 88:3005-3010.

Varga J., Rosenbloom J., Jimenez S. A. (1987) Transforming growth factor beta (TGF-[3) causes a persistant increase in steady-state amounts of type I and type III collagen and fibronectin mRNA's in normal human dermal fibroblasts. *Biochem J* 297:597-604.

Yasuda H., Shima N., Nakagawa N., Yamaguchi K., Kinosaki M., Mochizuki S., Tomoyasu A., Yano K., Goto M., Murakami A., E. Tsuda, T. Morinaga, K. Higashio, N. Udagawa, N. Takahashi, T. Suda (1998) Osteoclast differentiation factor is a ligand for osteoprotegerin/osteoclastogenesis-inhibitory factor and is identical to TRANCE/RANKL. *Proc Natl Acad Sci USA* 95:3597-3602.

Zwijsen A., Verschueren K., Huylebroeck D. (2003) New intracellular components of bone morphogenetic protein/Smad signaling cascades. *FEBS Lett* 546:133-139.

Chapter 18

Psoriasis and Cytokines

Gökhan Şahin[1,*], MD and Seda Koç Şahin[2], MD

[1]Ondokuz Mayis University, Department of Dermatology, Samsun, Turkey

[2]Health Sciences University, Samsun Training and Research Hospital, Department of Pathology, Samsun, Turkey

Abstract

Psoriasis is an immune-mediated inflammatory skin disease characterized by erythematous scaly plaques on the skin that occurs in genetically susceptible individuals. In individuals with a genetic predisposition, for an unknown reason, proinflammatory cytokines (such as TNF α, IL-17, IL-12 and IL-23) are secreted from Th1 and Th17 cells in the skin. These cytokines cause hyperproliferation in the skin. In the past, the focus was on keratinocyte hyperproliferation in the pathogenesis of psoriasis. Today, however, it is believed that the dysregulation of the immune system plays a key role in the pathogenesis, and treatments are being developed in this direction. Psoriasis can occur in many different clinical forms and extracutaneous involvement can be seen. Plaque psoriasis is the most common clinical form of psoriasis and is also known as psoriasis vulgaris. Psoriasis can be triggered by external factors such as trauma, infections, burns and medications. Both innate and adaptive immune responses contribute to the inflammation that occurs in psoriasis. While conventional treatments have a non-selective effect in the treatment of psoriasis, anti-cytokine treatments selectively suppress inflammation, increase efficacy and decrease side effects.

Keywords: psoriasis, pathogenesis, cytokines, TNF-α inhibitors, IL-17 inhibitors, IL-23 inhibitors

Introduction

Psoriasis is an immune-mediated inflammatory skin disease characterized by erythematous scaly plaques on the skin that occurs in genetically susceptible individuals. Psoriatic arthritis is a common comorbidity that should be investigated in all psoriasis patients. Psoriasis is also

---

* Corresponding Author's Email: sgokhan55@hotmail.com.

In: Cytokines and Diseases
Editors: Kenan Demir, Selim Görgün and Bahar Uslu
ISBN: 979-8-88697-214-6

thought to be associated with obesity, metabolic syndrome, hypertension, diabetes and atherosclerotic diseases. In the past, the focus was on keratinocyte hyperproliferation in the pathogenesis of psoriasis; however, it is believed that the dysregulation of the immune system plays a key role in the pathogenesis, and treatments are being developed in this direction.

In this chapter, after briefly describing the epidemiological, histopathological and clinical features of psoriasis, the role of cytokines in the pathogenesis of psoriasis will be emphasized, and anti-cytokine treatments in psoriasis will be discussed.

Epidemiology

The prevalence of psoriasis varies according to countries and ethnic groups throughout the world. In a review of 76 studies, it was reported that the prevalence of psoriasis in adults ranged from 0.51 to 11.43%, and from 0 to 1.37% in children (Michalek et al., 2018). There is no consensus on whether the prevalence of psoriasis shows a gender difference, but it can be accepted that it is seen with a similar frequency. Psoriasis can occur at any age, but peaks between the ages of 30-39 and 50-69 (Parisi et al., 2013).

Genetic

In one study, it was stated that if both parents have psoriasis, the risk of developing psoriasis in the child is 41%, and if only one parent has it, the risk is 14% (Andressen and Henseler 1982). Monozygotic twins have a 2-3 times higher risk of developing psoriasis compared to dizygotic twins, and the distribution, severity and age of onset of psoriasis lesions in monozygotic twins are similar, suggesting that genetic factors play a role in the occurrence and clinical course of psoriasis (Van de Kerkhov and Nestlé 2018).

Histopathology

The histopathology of psoriasis includes regular epidermal hyperplasia, parakeratosis, neutrophils in the stratum corneum and epidermis, granular layer thinning/loss, thinning of suprapapillary dermal plaques and enlarged dermal papillary vessels (Van de Kerkhov and Nestlé 2018).

Clinical Presentation

Psoriasis can occur in many different clinical forms and extracutaneous involvement can be seen. The onset of psoriasis lesions may be sudden (as in guttate psoriasis), and a slowly progressive course may also be observed. Elementary lesions of psoriasis are erythema, scaling, and skin thickening. The size of a lesion can range from a punctuated papule to a plaque 20 cm in diameter. Psoriasis is a Koebner positive disease, and erythematous scaly lesions appear on the traumatized skin. Plaque psoriasis is the most common clinical form of psoriasis and it is also known as psoriasis vulgaris.

The erythematous scaly lesions are sharply separated from the normal skin and distributed relatively symmetrically. Involvement of the scalp, knee, elbow and lumbosacral region is common. Psoriasis severity is evaluated with the psoriasis area and severity index (PASI). In the PASI scoring, a total score of 0-72 is given to the scalp, trunk, and upper and lower extremity lesions according to erythema, induration, lesion thickness and involvement rate. The PASI score is used to determine the severity of the disease and to evaluate the effectiveness of the treatment given.

Guttate psoriasis is characterized by widespread erythematous lesions that are scaly and papular (guttate) which usually occur after upper respiratory tract infection in children and adolescents.

Patients with erythrodermic psoriasis have widespread erythema and scaly lesions throughout the body. Characteristic nail changes, the presence of previous psoriasis lesions, and histopathology suggest that erythroderma may be caused by psoriasis.

Pregnancy, rebound due to corticosteroid withdrawal, hypocalcemia and infections may cause generalized pustular psoriasis. It is characterized by millimetric pustular lesions over generalized erythema throughout the body.

Erythematous scaly lesions on the palms of the hands and soles of the feet are considered to be the palmoplantar form of psoriasis, plaque psoriasis lesions may accompany, and are not expected to be generalized.

Acrodermatitis continua of Hallopeau is usually characterized by pustules that occur on the distal of the fingers and sometimes the toes. Pustules can also form in the nail bed, which can lead to destruction of the nail plates.

Scalp involvement is also common in psoriasis. It can be difficult to differentiate from seborrheic dermatitis, unlike seborrheic dermatitis, psoriasis lesions can spread to the retroauricular region and neck.

In inverse (flexural) psoriasis, there are lesions in the flexural areas (such as the retroauricular region, intergluteal area, inguinal fold, and axilla, and under the breast). The lesions are bright pink in color, in thin plaques, with relatively little scaling.

Psoriasis affects the nail matrix and nail bed. Small parakeratotic foci in the proximal part of the nail matrix cause pitting in the nails (Van de Kerkhov and Nestlé 2018).

Pathogenesis of Psoriasis

Psoriasis can be triggered by external factors such as trauma, infections, burns and medications (Mahler et al., 2014). Interactions between dendritic cells, T cells, keratinocytes, and neutrophils and cytokines released from immune cells cause the initiation and maintenance of cutaneous inflammation (Yan et al., 2021). Both innate and adaptive immune responses contribute to the resulting inflammation.

Epithelial tissue is the producer and promoter of anti-inflammatory cytokines. Keratinocytes produce interleukin 10 (IL-10), which inhibits the T helper 1 (Th1) response, while Langerhans cells produce IL-4, which promotes the Th2 response. Fibroblasts are producers of transforming growth factor β (TGF-β), which controls cell growth and proliferation. In the peripheral blood immunophenotyping of patients with psoriasis, an increase in Th1/Th17 cells and a relative decrease in Th2/Regulatory T cells (T-reg cells) were observed when compared to healthy controls (de Alcantara et al., 2021).

Innate Immune Responses – Cell Components

Cells that contribute to the innate immune response in pathogenesis are dendritic cells (plasmacytoid and myeloid), macrophages, and neutrophils.

Dendritic Cells

Plasmacytoid dendritic cells are the primary producers of interferon α (IFN-α). IFN-α production is increased in early lesions of psoriasis, and plasmacytoid dendritic cells are the cells that increase in number in early lesions of psoriasis (Wollenberg et al., 2002). Myeloid dendritic cells are potent antigen presenting cells that produce proinflammatory cytokines (such as TNF-α, IL-23, IL-12) that activate T cells (Martini et al., 2017).

Macrophages

It is believed that macrophages may be a greater source of IL-23 than myeloid dendritic cells in psoriatic skin. It is thought that they may contribute to inflammation and angiogenesis because they are cells that produce tumor necrosis factor α (TNF-α) and vascular endothelial growth factor (VEGF) (Mehta et al., 2021).

Neutrophils

Neutrophils concentrate in Munro microabscesses in the epidermis and contribute to inflammation.

Innate Immune Responses – Cytokines

Interferon A and Interferon Γ (IFN-A and IFN-Γ)

In early lesions of psoriasis, type 1 IFN levels are upregulated. IFN-α released from plasmacytoid dendritic cells and IFN-γ released from both keratinocytes and plasmacytoid dendritic cells activate the maturation of myeloid dendritic cells (de Alcantara et al., 2021). The fact that INF-α treatments can exacerbate psoriasis and that imiquimod, which increases local IFN-α production, can cause psoriasis, is evidence that IFNs have an important role in the pathogenesis of psoriasis (Patel et al., 2011).

Interleukin 1β (IL-1β)

The IL-1β level is high in psoriatic skin, while blood serum levels are similar to those of normal humans (Dowlatshahi et al., 2013). Interleukin 36 receptor antagonist (IL-36Ra); IL-36α blocks the proinflammatory signals of IL-36β and IL-36γ and is a member of the IL-1 cytokine family. A mutation in the gene encoding IL-36Rα (IL-36RN gene) may be associated with severe pustular psoriasis, a condition called a "deficiency of interleukin 36 receptor antagonist" (DITRA) (Marrakchi et al., 2011).

Tumor Necrosis Factor α (TNF-α)

This is a proinflammatory cytokine that plays an important role in many inflammatory diseases. Macrophages, dendritic cells, Th1 and Th7 cells and keratinocytes produce TNF-α. TNF-α increases the IL-23 production of dendritic cells, and synergistically with IL-17 increases the proinflammatory mediator production of keratinocytes (de Alcantara et al., 2021).

Interleukin 23 (IL-23)

This is the cytokine responsible for the proliferation and survival of Th17 and Tc17 (cytotoxic T cell 17) cells, which are important T-cell subgroups in many autoimmune diseases such as psoriasis and Crohn's disease. It is produced by dendritic cells and macrophages (Blauvelt 2008).

Interleukin 12 (IL-12)

Produced by myeloid dendritic cells such as IL-23, this contributes to the differentiation of Th1 cells. It is thought that IL-12 has a regulatory role in the inactivation of the IL-23/Th17 immunological pathway (Kulig et al., 2016).

Adaptive Immune Responses – Cell Components

T lymphocytes, one of the most important cells of the adaptive immune system, and especially Th17 cells, a subgroup of T lymphocytes, are the most critical cells in the pathogenesis of psoriasis.

CD4+ T Cells

The Th17 subset of CD4+ T cells and, to a lesser extent, Th1 and Th22 cells contributes to the formation of psoriasis lesions. While previously Th1 cells were thought to play a key role in the pathogenesis of psoriasis, recent studies indicate that the contribution of Th17 cells is more critical.

Epidermal dendritic cells encounter an autoantigen and present this antigen to naive Tregs in the adjacent lymph node. Naive Tregs differentiate into Th17, which produces more IL-17 in the skin, with the effect of IL-1β, IL-6 and TGF-β being released from keratinocytes. The activation of Th17 cells by IL-23 causes the release of IL-17, TNF-α and IL-22, increased inflammation and keratinocyte hyperplasia (Rizzo et al., 2011).

T helper 1 cells produce proinflammatory cytokines such as IFN-γ, IL-2 and TNF-α. IL-12 promotes the differentiation of Th1 cells (Kulig et al., 2016).

CD8+ Cytotoxic T cells

Cytotoxic T cells, especially Tc17, produce cytolytic enzymes, but in psoriasis they exert their main effects by functionally affecting the cells that produce IL-17 (Rizzo et al., 2011).

Adaptive Immune Responses – Cytokines

Interleukin 17 (IL-17)

This is a cytokine produced by Th17 and Tc17 cells. IL-17 activates keratinocytes and increases chemokine production from keratinocytes. It increases the production of TNF-α, IL-1, IL-6 and IL-23 (Albanesi et al., 2000).

Interleukin 22 (IL-22)

This is secreted by Th17, Tc17 and Th22 cells. In keratinocytes, IL-22 plays a role in tissue repair and wound healing. It stimulates the hyperproliferation of keratinocytes, reduces keratinocyte differentiation, and increases the production of chemokines and chemoattractants. Despite the role of IL-22 in the pathophysiology of psoriasis, the efficacy of IL-22 inhibitors in the treatment of psoriasis has not yet been demonstrated (de Alcantara et al., 2021).

Other Cytokines

Interleukin 8 (IL-8)

This is secreted by macrophages and endothelial cells. It acts as a chemoattractant for neutrophils in inflammatory reactions. In pustular psoriasis, there is the presence of neutrophils that respond to IL-8. Narrowband ultraviolet therapy (nbUVB) can improve patients with psoriasis by reducing plasma IL-8 levels (Chen et al., 2016).

Interleukin 10 (IL-10)

This is a type 2 cytokine that inhibits the formation of type 1 proinflammatory cytokines and has an effect on immunoregulation. Compared with other inflammatory dermatoses, there is a relative deficiency in cutaneous IL-10 mRNA expression in psoriasis. An objective clinical improvement was reported as a result of the subcutaneous administration of IL-10 for 10 days in 3 patients with psoriasis (Asadullah et al., 1998).

Transforming Growth Factor β (TGF-β)

Psoriasis may occur as a result of the insufficient inhibitory effect of TGF-β. There are studies that suggest TGF-β may be associated with increased PASI (Zaher et al., 2009). In addition, psoriatic skin may be associated with decreased levels of TGF-β and TGF-β receptors compared to intact skin (Doi et al., 2003).

Adiponectin

This is a cytokine produced by adipocytes. While it increases IL-10 expression, it regulates IL-2, IL-6, TNF-α and IFN-γ secretion. In obesity patients, the inflammatory response mediated by TNF-α and IL-6 inhibits adiponectin production. Although it is thought that there is a relationship between low adiponectin levels and psoriasis, there is no relationship between adiponectin levels and the severity of psoriasis (Gerdes et al., 2020).

Anti-Cytokine Treatments in Psoriasis

The aim of treatment in psoriasis is to heal the lesions, control the symptoms and improve the patient's quality of life. When choosing a treatment for a patient with psoriasis, a decision should be made by considering the type of psoriasis, the severity of the disease and the patient's expectations. While topical treatment is recommended for patients with mild psoriasis, phototherapy and systemic treatments are recommended for patients with moderate-to-severe psoriasis. Conventional systemic treatments used in psoriasis are methotrexate, acitretin and cyclosporine. Acitretin, which is one of the conventional treatments used in the treatment of psoriasis for many years, has anti-inflammatory and immunomodulatory effects on reducing keratinocyte hyperproliferation, while methotrexate is a dihydrofolate reductase inhibitor which has an immunosuppressive effect by suppressing lymphocyte proliferation and cytokine production. Cyclosporine suppresses T lymphocytes (both helper T cells and suppressor T cells) by inhibiting calcineurin. In other words, conventional treatments in psoriasis show a non-selective effect to suppress inflammation.

If the lesions of the patient with psoriasis are resistant to conventional systemic treatments or if conventional systemic treatments are contraindicated for the patient, biological (anti-cytokine) treatments are recommended to the patient. Anti-cytokine therapies used in the treatment of psoriasis are TNF-α inhibitors, IL-17 inhibitors and IL-23 inhibitors.

Tumor Necrosis Factor α Inhibitors

Etanercept

This is the first approved TNF-α inhibitor anti-cytokine drug for the treatment of psoriasis. It has the capacity to bind both free TNF and membrane-bound TNF. The recommended dose of etanercept in patients with moderate-to-severe psoriasis is 50 mg subcutaneously twice a week for the first 12 weeks, followed by 50 mg once a week thereafter. In the pediatric population, 0.8 mg/kg (maximum 50 mg) once a week is recommended for ages 4-17 years (Segaert 2009). Etanercept is effective and safe in psoriatic arthritis (Sterry et al., 2010). Etanercept is a pregnancy category B drug. However, there are not enough data to recommend its safe use in pregnant patients. It carries a lower risk for serious infections compared to other TNF inhibitors, so it may be considered as a better option for those at high risk of immunosuppression. The advantages of etanercept are its short half-life, its effectiveness in intermittent therapy, and the availability of high-dose options. Since the efficacy of etanercept has been found to be relatively low in recent biologic treatments with different mechanisms of action, it is included as a second-line treatment option in some treatment guidelines (Shah et al., 2018).

Infliximab

This is a chimeric immunoglobulin G1 (IgG1) monoclonal antibody produced in recombinant cell culture. It is administered at a dose of 5 mg/kg at 0, 2 and 6 weeks and every 8 weeks (Smith et al., 2017). Infliximab is a good treatment option, especially in patients with severe psoriasis, due to its rapid onset and high efficacy. Its efficacy in psoriatic arthritis has been demonstrated in randomized controlled studies (Antoni et al., 2005). Serious infections and infusion reactions may occur in patients receiving infliximab therapy. Anti-infliximab antibody formation has been reported in patients with psoriasis using infliximab. It is thought that adding an immunosuppressive drug to infliximab treatment may reduce antibody formation (Hsu et al., 2014). It is a pregnancy category B drug. Although it is relatively safe to use in the early stages of pregnancy, it may remain in the blood of babies exposed to the drug especially in the late intrauterine period, leading to the risk of immunosuppression (Smith et al., 2017). Although there are case studies showing that infliximab is effective in pediatric patients, it is not approved under the age of 18.

Adalimumab

This is a human monoclonal IgG1 antibody that specifically binds TNF-α. In the treatment of psoriasis, 80 mg is administered subcutaneously at week 0, 40 mg after 1 week and 40 mg every 2 weeks thereafter (Nast et al., 2015). It was first used in the treatment of rheumatoid arthritis and psoriatic arthritis, then it was approved for the treatment of psoriasis. Like etanercept and infliximab, the pregnancy category is B, but it is recommended that female patients do not become pregnant for up to 6 months after discontinuation of therapy. In 2015, the European Medicines Agency approved its use in pediatric patients aged 4 years and older who are unresponsive to topical treatments and phototherapy (Wu and Valdecantos 2017).

Certolizumab Pegol

This is a combination of two polyethylene glycol molecules with the fragment antigen binding (Fab) part of the monoclonal antibody that binds and neutralizes TNF-α. It can be administered both intravenously and subcutaneously. The recommended use in psoriasis is 200 mg every 2 weeks for patients with ≤90 kg, and 400 mg every 2 weeks for patients with >90 kg, following an induction dose of 2 x 400 mg at weeks 0, 2, and 4 (Campanati et al., 2017). It has been used for a longer time in psoriatic arthritis. Since certolizumab does not bind to the neonatal Fc receptor due to the absence of the Fc region in the pegol, it crosses the placenta by passive diffusion, so placental transmission is minimal. It is considered to be the first-choice anti-cytokine treatment option in female patients of childbearing potential (Mariette et al., 2018).

Interleukin 17 (IL-17) Inhibitors

Secukinumab

Secukinumab is a humanized monoclonal antibody to IL-17A. In psoriasis, 300 mg is administered subcutaneously at 0, 1, 2, 3 and 4 weeks and then every 4 weeks. It is also effective in psoriatic arthritis. Although TNF-α inhibitors are recommended in inflammatory bowel diseases, it has been reported that IL-17 inhibitors may trigger new attacks and have a paradoxical effect in these patients (Fauny et al., 2020). It has been reported that, unlike TNF-α inhibitors, it specifically affects IL-17A, resulting in fewer infections (such as tuberculosis, disseminated herpes) and better efficacy in the treatment of psoriasis (greater PASI 90-PASI 100 response) (Sawyer et al., 2019).

Ixekizumab

This is a humanized Ig G4 monoclonal antibody that acts by neutralizing IL-17A. While it specifically binds to IL-17A, it does not bind to 5 other members of the IL-17 cytokine family (IL-17B, IL-17C, IL-17D, IL-17E, IL-17F) or IL-22 (Liu et al., 2016). The recommended treatment for psoriasis is an initial dose of 160 mg followed by a subcutaneous injection of 80 mg at weeks 2, 4, 6, 8, 10, and 12, and every 4 weeks thereafter. A paradoxical increase in inflammatory bowel disease may occur with the use of ixekizumab, as with secukinumab (Fauny et al., 2020).

Brodalumab

Brodalumab inhibits IL-17-mediated signaling by binding to IL-17 receptor A. The dosing schedule for brodalumab is 210 mg at weeks 0, 1, and 2, and every 2 weeks thereafter. While ixekizumab and secukinumab target IL-17A, brodalumab inhibits other subgroups of the IL-17 family as it inhibits the IL-17 receptor. Although there is information that brodalumab may increase suicidal ideation, this is controversial (Chiricozzi et al., 2016). Warnings regarding the use of IL-17 inhibitors in inflammatory bowel diseases are also valid for brodalumab.

Interleukin 23 (IL-23) Inhibitors

Ustekinumab

This is a human monoclonal antibody to p40 that is present as a subunit in both IL-12 and IL-23. The recommended dose of ustekinumab is the subcutaneous administration of 45 mg under 100 kg and 90 mg over 100 kg at 0, 4, and then every 12 weeks. The advantage of ustekinumab is that dose selection can be made according to weight and the injection frequency is relatively low compared to other biologic treatments. It is also approved for use in pediatric patients aged 6 years and older (Yang et al., 2021). Ustekinumab is also effective in the treatment of psoriatic arthritis and Crohn's disease (Feagan et al., 2016).

Guselkumab

This is a human IgG1 λ monoclonal antibody that binds to the p19 subunit of IL-23. The recommended dose is a 100 mg subcutaneous administration at 0, 4 and every 8 weeks. Treatment discontinuation should be considered in patients who do not respond to treatment at the end of the 16th week. It is also thought to be effective for psoriatic arthritis. There is no information that it can exacerbate inflammatory bowel diseases like IL-17 inhibitors (Langley et al., 2018).

Risankizumab

This is a humanized IgG1 monoclonal antibody that selectively binds to the p19 subunit of the IL-23 cytokine. The recommended dose is a subcutaneous injection of 150 mg every 0, 4, and then every 12 weeks. There are insufficient data to recommend it in psoriatic arthritis (Yang et al., 2021).

Tildrakizumab

This is an IgG1κ antibody targeting the p19 subunit of IL-23. The recommended dose is a 100 mg subcutaneous administration at 0, 4 and every 12 weeks. Like risankizumab, there are not yet sufficient data to recommend it in psoriatic arthritis (Yang et al., 2021).

While ustekinumab is in pregnancy category B, more studies are needed to recommend guselkumab, risankizumab and tildrakizumab to pregnant women. There are insufficient data in the literature to recommend guselkumab, risankizumab and tildrakizumab to pediatric patients (Yang et al., 2021).

The interactions between cells and cytokines in the pathogenesis of psoriasis and the mechanisms of action of anti-cytokine treatments are summarized in Figure 1.

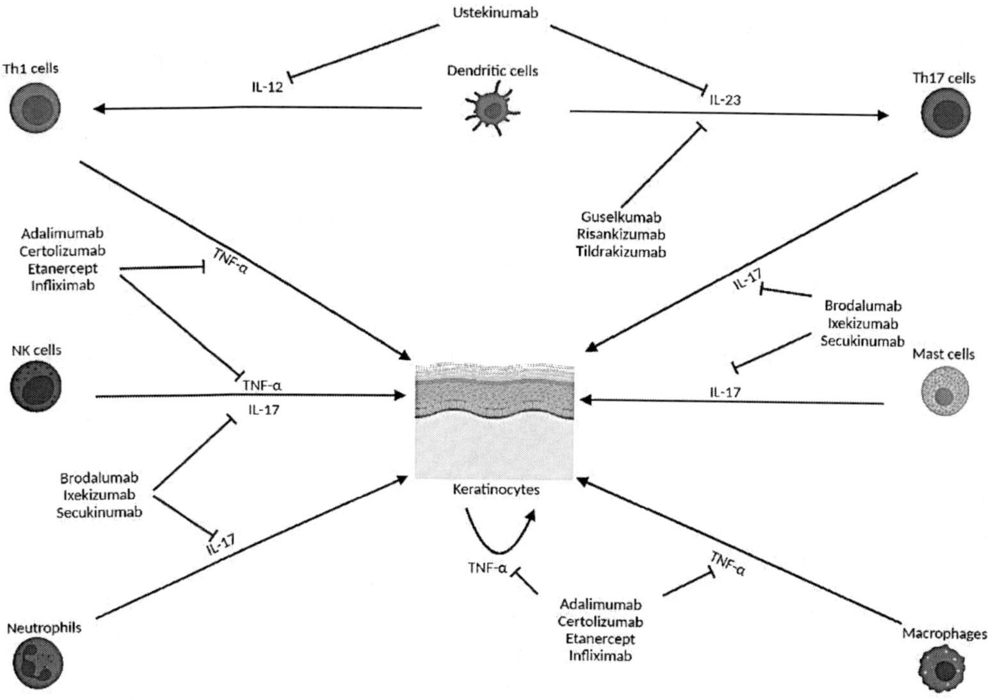

Figure 1. The interactions between cells and cytokines in the pathogenesis of psoriasis and the mechanisms of action of anti-cytokine treatments.

Conclusion

Psoriasis is a chronic inflammatory skin disease that can affect any part of the body, including joint involvement. It is thought that the innate and adaptive immune response plays a role in its etiopathogenesis. Environmental factors, T cells, dendritic cells, multiple cytokines and genetic predisposition are responsible for inflammation in psoriasis. In individuals with a genetic predisposition to psoriasis, for an unknown reason, proinflammatory cytokines (such as TNF α, IL-17, IL-12 and IL-23) are secreted from Th1 and Th17 cells in the skin. These cytokines cause keratinocyte hyperproliferation and the clinical presentation of psoriasis.

As the pathogenesis of psoriasis is understood, it is thought that selectively suppressing the inflammation in psoriasis may both increase the efficiency of and cause less immunosuppression as inflammation is selectively blocked. In the studies conducted, the data give results in parallel with this hypothesis, while a 50% reduction in the PASI score is accepted as a successful result in conventional treatments, the expectation is a 90-100% decrease in the PASI score, especially with the latest biological treatments.

Psoriatic arthritis may precede psoriasis, but it usually occurs after psoriasis lesions. It is thought that this situation may be caused by the inability to stop the inflammation that plays a role in psoriasis. Therefore, studies are continuing on the idea that anti-cytokine treatments that can be recommended instead of conventional treatments at the beginning of treatment can stop the progression of psoriasis to psoriatic arthritis.

In conclusion, suppressing the inflammation caused by cytokines in the pathogenesis of psoriasis with targeted anti-cytokine therapies has revolutionized the treatment of psoriasis.

References

Albanesi C, Scarponi C, Cavani A, et al. (2000) Interleukin-17 is produced by both Th1 and Th2 lymphocytes, and modulates interferon-gamma- and interleukin-4-induced activation of human keratinocytes. *The Journal of investigative dermatology* 115(1):81–87 https://doi.org/10.1046/j.1523-1747.2000.00041.x.

Andressen C, Henseler T (1982) Erblichkeit der Psoriasis. Eine Analyse von 2035 Familienanamnesen [Inheritance of psoriasis. Analysis of 2035 family histories]. *Der Hautarzt; Zeitschrift fur Dermatologie, Venerologie, und verwandte Gebiete [The Dermatologist; Journal of Dermatology, Venereology, and Related Fields*] 33(4):214–217.

Antoni C E, Kavanaugh A, Kirkham B, et al. (2005) Sustained benefits of infliximab therapy for dermatologic and articular manifestations of psoriatic arthritis: results from the infliximab multinational psoriatic arthritis controlled trial (IMPACT). *Arthritis and rheumatism* 52(4):1227–1236. https://doi.org/10.1002/art.20967.

Asadullah K, Sterry W, Stephanek K, et al. (1998) IL-10 is a key cytokine in psoriasis. Proof of principle by IL-10 therapy: a new therapeutic approach. *The Journal of clinical investigation* 101(4):783–794. https://doi.org/10.1172/JCI1476.

Blauvelt A (2008) T-helper 17 cells in psoriatic plaques and additional genetic links between IL-23 and psoriasis. *The Journal of investigative dermatology* 128(5):1064–1067. https://doi.org/10.1038/jid.2008.85.

Campanati A, Benfaremo D, Luchetti M M, et al. (2017) Certolizumab pegol for the treatment of psoriasis. *Expert opinion on biological therapy* 17(3):387–394. https://doi.org/10.1080/14712598.2017.1283401.

Chen H Q, Li X, Tang R (2016) Effects of Narrow Band Ultraviolet B on Serum Levels of Vascular Endothelial Growth Factor and Interleukin-8 in Patients with Psoriasis. *American journal of therapeutics* 23(3):e655–e662. https://doi.org/10.1097/MJT.0000000000000330.

Chiricozzi A, Romanelli M, Saraceno R, Torres T (2016) No meaningful association between suicidal behavior and the use of IL-17A-neutralizing or IL-17RA-blocking agents. *Expert opinion on drug safety* 15(12):1653–1659. https://doi.org/10.1080/14740338.2016.1228872.

de Alcantara C C, Reiche E, Simão A (2021) Cytokines in psoriasis. *Advances in clinical chemistry* 100:171–204. https://doi.org/10.1016/bs.acc.2020.04.004.

Doi H, Shibata M A, Kiyokane K, Otsuki Y (2003) Downregulation of TGFbeta isoforms and their receptors contributes to keratinocyte hyperproliferation in psoriasis vulgaris. *Journal of dermatological science* 33(1):7–16. https://doi.org/10.1016/s0923-1811(03)00107-5.

Dowlatshahi E A, van der Voort E A, Arends L R, Nijsten T (2013) Markers of systemic inflammation in psoriasis: a systematic review and meta-analysis. *The British journal of dermatology* 169(2):266–282. https://doi.org/10.1111/bjd.12355.

Fauny M, Moulin D, D'Amico F, et al. (2020) Paradoxical gastrointestinal effects of interleukin-17 blockers. Annals of the rheumatic diseases 79(9):1132–1138. https://doi.org/10.1136/annrheumdis-2020-217927.

Feagan BG, Sandborn WJ, Gasink C, et al; UNITI–IM-UNITI Study Group (2016) Ustekinumab as Induction and Maintenance Therapy for Crohn's Disease. *The New England journal of medicine* 375(20):1946–1960. https://doi.org/10.1056/NEJMoa1602773.

Gerdes S, Pinter A, Biermann M, et al. (2020) Adiponectin levels in a large pooled plaque psoriasis study population. *The Journal of dermatological treatment* 31(5):531–534. https://doi.org/10.1080/09546634.2019.1621979.

Hsu L, Snodgrass B T, Armstrong AW (2014) Antidrug antibodies in psoriasis: a systematic review. *The British journal of dermatology* 170(2):261–273. https://doi.org/10.1111/bjd.12654.

Kulig P, Musiol S, Freiberger SN, et al. (2016) IL-12 protects from psoriasiform skin inflammation. *Nature communications* 7:13466. https://doi.org/10.1038/ncomms13466.

Langley R G, Tsai T F, Flavin S, et al. (2018) Efficacy and safety of guselkumab in patients with psoriasis who have an inadequate response to ustekinumab: results of the randomized, double-blind, phase III NAVIGATE trial. The British journal of dermatology 178(1):114–123. https://doi.org/10.1111/bjd.15750.

Liu L, Lu J, Allan BW, et al. (2016) Generation and characterization of ixekizumab, a humanized monoclonal antibody that neutralizes interleukin-17A. *Journal of inflammation research* 9:39–50. https://doi.org/10.2147/JIR.S100940.

Mahler V, Diepgen T, Skudlik C, et al. Work Group "Assessment of allergens in occupational disease (BK) 5101" of the Study Group Occupational and Environmental Dermatology (ABD), & German Contact Dermatitis Group (DKG) of the German Dermatological Society (2014) Psoriasis predisposition and occupational triggering factors in the appraisal of occupational medical expertises. *Journal der Deutschen Dermatologischen Gesellschaft* [*Journal of the German Society of Dermatology (JDDG)*] 12(6):519–529. https://doi.org/10.1111/ddg.12262.

Mariette X, Förger F, Abraham B, et al. (2018) Lack of placental transfer of certolizumab pegol during pregnancy: results from CRIB, a prospective, postmarketing, pharmacokinetic study. *Annals of the rheumatic diseases* 77(2):228–233. https://doi.org/10.1136/annrheumdis-2017-212196.

Marrakchi S, Guigue P, Renshaw B R, et al. (2011) Interleukin-36-receptor antagonist deficiency and generalized pustular psoriasis. *The New England journal of medicine* 365(7):620–628. https://doi.org/10.1056/NEJMoa1013068.

Martini E, Wikén M, Cheuk S, et al. (2017) Dynamic Changes in Resident and Infiltrating Epidermal Dendritic Cells in Active and Resolved Psoriasis. *The Journal of investigative dermatology* 137(4):865–873. https://doi.org/10.1016/j.jid.2016.11.033.

Mehta H, Mashiko S, Angsana J, et al. (2021) Differential Changes in Inflammatory Mononuclear Phagocyte and T-Cell Profiles within Psoriatic Skin during Treatment with Guselkumab vs. Secukinumab. *The Journal of investigative dermatology* 141(7):1707–1718. https://doi.org/10.1016/j.jid.2021.01.005.

Michalek I M, Loring B, John S M (2017) A systematic review of worldwide epidemiology of psoriasis. *J. Eur. Acad. Dermatol. Venereol.* 31(2):205–212. https://doi.org/10.1111/jdv.13854.

Nast A, Gisondi P, Ormerod A D, et al. (2015) European S3-Guidelines on the systemic treatment of psoriasis vulgaris--Update 2015--Short version--EDF in cooperation with EADV and IPC. *Journal of the European Academy of Dermatology and Venereology (JEADV)* 29(12):2277–2294. https://doi.org/10.1111/jdv.13354.

Parisi R, Symmons D P, Griffiths C E, Ashcroft D M; Identification and Management of Psoriasis and Associated ComorbidiTy (IMPACT) project team (2013) Global epidemiology of psoriasis: a systematic review of incidence and prevalence. *The Journal of investigative dermatology* 133(2):377–385. https://doi.org/10.1038/jid.2012.339.

Patel U, Mark N M, Machler B C, Levine V J (2011) Imiquimod 5% cream induced psoriasis: a case report, summary of the literature and mechanism. *The British journal of dermatology* 164(3):670–672. https://doi.org/10.1111/j.1365-2133.2010.10124.x.

Rizzo H L, Kagami S, Phillips K G, et al. (2011) IL-23-mediated psoriasis-like epidermal hyperplasia is dependent on IL-17A. *Journal of immunology* (Baltimore, Md.: 1950) 186(3):1495–1502. https://doi.org/10.4049/jimmunol.1001001.

Sawyer L M, Malottki K, Sabry-Grant C, et al. (2019) Assessing the relative efficacy of interleukin-17 and interleukin-23 targeted treatments for moderate-to-severe plaque psoriasis: A systematic review and network meta-analysis of PASI response. *PloS one* 14(8):e0220868. https://doi.org/10.1371/journal.pone.0220868.

Segaert S (2009) Etanercept, improved dosage schedules and combinations in the treatment of psoriasis: an update. *Journal of inflammation research* 2:29–36. https://doi.org/10.2147/jir.s4405.

Shah V V, Lee E B, Reddy S, et al. (2018) Comparison of guidelines for the use of TNF inhibitors for psoriasis in the United States, Canada, Europe and the United Kingdom: a critical appraisal and comprehensive review. *The Journal of dermatological treatment* 29(6):586–592. https://doi.org/10.1080/09546634.2018.1428723.

Smith C H, Jabbar-Lopez Z K, Yiu Z Z, et al. (2017) British Association of Dermatologists guidelines for biologic therapy for psoriasis 2017. *The British journal of dermatology* 177(3):628–636. https://doi.org/10.1111/ bjd.15665.

Sterry W, Ortonne J P, Kirkham B, et al. (2010) Comparison of two etanercept regimens for treatment of psoriasis and psoriatic arthritis: PRESTA randomised double blind multicentre trial. *BMJ* (Clinical research ed.) 340:c147. https://doi.org/10.1136/bmj.c147.

Van de Kerkhov P C M, Nestlé F O (2018) Psoriasis. In: Bolognia J L, Schaffer J V, Cerroni L (eds) *Dermatology*, Fourth edn. Elsevier Limited, p. 138-160.

Wollenberg A, Wagner M, Günther S, et al. (2002) Plasmacytoid dendritic cells: a new cutaneous dendritic cell subset with distinct role in inflammatory skin diseases. *The Journal of investigative dermatology* 119(5):1096–1102. https://doi.org/10.1046/j.1523-1747.2002.19515.x.

Wu J J, Valdecantos W C (2017) Adalimumab in Chronic Plaque Psoriasis: A Clinical Guide. *Journal of drugs in dermatology (JDD)* 16(8):779–790.

Yan D, Gudjonsson J E, Le S, et al. (2021) New Frontiers in Psoriatic Disease Research, Part I: Genetics, Environmental Triggers, Immunology, Pathophysiology, and Precision Medicine. *The Journal of investigative dermatology* 141(9):2112–2122.e3. https://doi.org/10.1016/j.jid.2021.02.764.

Yang K, Oak A, Elewski B E (2021) Use of IL-23 Inhibitors for the Treatment of Plaque Psoriasis and Psoriatic Arthritis: A Comprehensive Review. *American journal of clinical dermatology* 22(2):173–192. https://doi.org/10.1007/s40257-020-00578-0.

Zaher H, Shaker O G, EL-Komy M H, et al. (2009) Serum and tissue expression of transforming growth factor beta 1 in psoriasis. *Journal of the European Academy of Dermatology and Venereology (JEADV)* 23(4):406–409. https://doi.org/10.1111/j.1468-3083.2008.03064.x.

Chapter 19

Cytokines Profile in Inflammatory Skin Disorders

Gabriela Turcu*, MD, Roxana Ioana Nedelcu, MD and Alice Brinzea, MD

"Carol Davila" University of Medicine and Pharmacy Bucharest, Romania

Abstract

The skin is the host of complex interaction between resident and nonresident immune and nonimmune cells. It accommodates classical immune cells, but keratinocytes, fibroblasts, adipocytes, melanocytes, and endothelial cells are also involved in the local immune response. The inflammatory profile of each disease is difficult to define precisely, because it is dynamic during the evolution of a disease and can vary significantly on different skin regions, and according to the commensal flora and immune defense, but K. Eyerich and S. Eyerich defined six immune response models based on the predominant subset of lymphocytes and the response after interaction with keratinocytes: psoriatic, lichenoid, bullous, fibrogenic, and granulomatous. Recent studies on immunopathogenesis changed the clinical approach in common dermatological disorders (revealing the fact that circulating cytokines have systemic consequences) and identified useful targets for new therapies.

Keywords: inflammatory skin disorders, metabolic disorders, IL-23, IL-17

Introduction

The skin is the largest organ in the body in surface area and weight. One of the main functions of the skin is to protect the body through its intact structures and the complex interaction of resident and nonresident immune and nonimmune cells. The skin contains myeloid and lymphoid cells. The basal epidermal layer contains basal keratinocytes, melanocytes, and immune cells (Langerhans cells, T cells). The cellular component of the dermal layer includes fibroblasts, myofibroblasts, and immune cells (macrophages, lymphocytes, innate lymphoid cells, mast cells, and dendritic cells) (Nguyen & Soulika 2019).

* Corresponding Author's Email: dr.gabriela.turcu@gmail.com.

In: Cytokines and Diseases
Editors: Kenan Demir, Selim Görgün and Bahar Uslu
ISBN: 979-8-88697-214-6

In addition to classical immune cells, keratinocytes, fibroblasts, adipocytes, melanocytes, and endothelial cells are involved in the local immune response. They express pattern recognition receptors (PRR) and their activation results in the production of cytokines and chemokines that modulate the inflammatory infiltrate (Chen & Dipietro 2017).

Inflammatory skin diseases include autoimmune and autoinflammatory disorders, characterized by a high level of pro-inflammatory cytokines produced by the activated innate and adaptive immune system (De Sá & Festa Neto 2016). All chronic inflammatory skin diseases have a genetic background and environmental factors endow their phenotype.

The inflammatory profile of a disease is difficult to be precisely defined because it is dynamic and can vary significantly during the evolution of a disease and because there are regional particularities of the skin, in regard to anatomy, commensal flora, and immune defense (Werfel 2009; Chang et al. 2002).

K. Eyerich and S. Eyerich defined six immune response models based on the predominant subset of lymphocytes and the response after interaction with keratinocytes: psoriatic (accelerated epidermal turnover and neutrophilic infiltrate), eczematous (in defective skin barrier with a low level of antimicrobial peptides and eosinophilic infiltrate), lichenoid (secondary to a cytotoxic reaction), bullous (antibody deposits with secondary blistering), fibrogenic (reduced cellularity and extracellular matrix deposits) and granulomatous (granuloma formation) (Eyerich & Eyerich 2018).

Since cytokines play an essential role in immunopathogenesis, researchers have tried to identify the patterns most commonly associated with inflammatory skin disorders, with the final goal of finding useful targets for therapy.

In this chapter, we will focus on the cytokine profile of the most common inflammatory skin disorders: atopic dermatitis, lupus erythemathosus, lichen planus, acne, and hidradenitis suppurativa. Psoriasis, a common skin disease recently defined as a chronic multisystemic inflammatory disorder, will be discussed in a different chapter.

Atopic Dermatitis

Atopic dermatitis (AD) is one of the most common, heterogeneous, often relapsing, chronic inflammatory skin diseases, affecting 5% to 20% of children and adults from different populations (DaVeiga 2012). Clinically, patients present with itch, xerosis, and eczematous lesions and frequently associate an elevated serum level of immunoglobulin E (IgE) and a personal or family history of atopy (eczema, asthma, or allergic rhinitis) (Spergel 2010; Eichenfield et al. 2014).

It appears to result from a combination of genetic and environmental factors that induce skin barrier dysfunctions, skin and systemic immune dysfunctions, and alteration of the skin microbiome (Weston & Howe, 2021). They are strongly interconnected and influence each other to initiate and aggravate DA (Weston & Howe; 2021).

AD appears to be driven by Th2 (IL-4/IL-13/IL-25) and Th22 (IL22), with variable activation of Th1 and Th17 (Guttman-Yassky et al. 2011a; Guttman-Yassky et al. 2011b).

Interleukin-4 and IL-13 are pivotal cytokines involved in the generation of allergic diseases (Brunner et al. 2017).

IL-4 and IL-13 modify the integrity of the skin barrier: significantly decrease the expression of main structural proteins (such as filaggrin, filaggrin 2, loricrin, involucrin, keratin 1, keratin 10), modify the lipid composition, decrease AMP production by keratinocytes, and alter the microbioma (Berdyshev et al. 2018; Howell et al. 2006; Kim et al. 2008; O'Reilly et al. 2016; Totsuka et al. 2017).

Recent data shows that IL-4 has more central roles, related to humoral immunity, including IgE production, while IL-13 has more roles at the tissue level, in the periphery, in both epidermal integrity and immune response (Bao & Reinhardt 2015; Bieber 2020).

Immune responses Th-22 and Th-17 contribute to tissue remodeling and dermal thickening from chronic skin lesions of AD (Liu et al. 2020). Epidermal hyperplasia and immune abnormalities of lesional atopic skin can be seen in psoriasis, but patients with AD also exhibit immunological anomalies on nonlesional skin and blood (Guttman-Yassky et al. 2011a; Guttman-Yassky et al. 2011b; Leung & Guttman-Yassky 2014; Suárez-Fariñas et al. 2011; Tang et al. 2012).

Studies of the effects of anti-IL-17 anti-IL-12/23 (successfully used in psoriasis) in AD proved that IL-17 and IL-12/23 are not central cytokines in the pathogenesis of AD (Ungar et al. 2021; Pan et al. 2018). Whereas psoriatic changes are mainly caused by Th17/IL-23, AD has a more heterogeneous inflammatory profile (Esaki et al. 2016; Suárez-Fariñas et al. 2011).

Lupus Erythematous (LE)

LE is a multifactorial disease, incompletely defined, in which genetic polymorphisms, environmental factors (especially UV radiation) and hormonal changes induce immune dysregulation and loss of self-immunological tolerance (Schur & Bevra 2021).

Cutaneous lupus erythematosus (CLE) with its three subcategories (acute (ACLE), subacute (SCLE) and chronic (CCLE)) can occur in association with systemic lupus erythematosus (SLE) or independently (Schur & Bevra 2021; Merola 2021).

Studies on the cytokine profile in SLE have shown increased levels of cytokines associated with Th1, Th17 and Tregs and low levels of Th2 cytokines, such as IL-4 (Guimarães et al. 2017).

UV radiation affects DNA integrity and causes keratinocyte apoptosis and necrosis, with the release of pro-inflammatory cytokines (TNF-α, IL-1α and IL-1β, IL-6 and interferon (IFN) α,κ,λ that attract and activate neutrophils, macrophages, lymphocytes, and plasmacytoid dendritic cells) and autoantigens (activating T and B cells) (Achtman & Werth 2015). Therefore, assaulted keratinocytes act as part of the innate immune system and activate the adaptive immune system to the injured site.

TNFβ gene polymorphisms influence the outcome of SLE (Bettinotti et al. 1993).

One of the most important pro-inflammatory cytokines is type I IFN, which activates innate immune cells and modulates disease activity, making CCLE an interferonopathy with epidermal cells targeted by cytotoxic $CD8^+$ T cells (Sarkar et al. 2018; Zahn et al. 2014).

Other relevant cytokines for CLE pathogenesis appear to be IL-18, as it stimulates TNF-α release from keratinocytes and IL-12, found at high levels in CLE skin lesions of CLE(Dey-Rao et al. 2014; Wang et al. 2008).

Cytokine blocking offers the best results in autoimmune disease, but an efficient treatment – blocking either TNF-α, IFN-α, IL-17 or IL-12/23 has not yet been approved for CCLE (Little & Vesely 2020).

LE is a heterogeneous disease and there is still more to learn about its pathogenesis.

Lichen Planus

Lichen planus (LP) is a chronic inflammatory disease that affects 0.5-2% of the world's population.

The pathogenesis of LP is multifactorial and the inflammatory infiltrate suggests an autoimmune mechanism (Weber et al. 2017).

There are several clinical subtypes, cutaneous (CLP) and oral lichen planus (OLP) being the most common. Despite histopathological similarities, these two forms are different clinically, have different outcomes, and have a partially different cytokine pattern (Weber et al. 2017).

Immunohistochemical studies revealed that CD8 + T cells infiltrate the epidermis (probably responsible for basal keratinocyte apoptosis) and CD4+ and CD8+ in the dermis, distributed in a band-like manner (Ioannides et al. 2020).

B Weber and his group found a significantly higher number of CD4+ T lymphocytes CLP compared to OLP, and significantly higher numbers of cytotoxic CD8+ T lymphocytes in OLP that may explain the more frequent erosive and persistent forms of OLP (Weber et al. 2017). NK cells and plasmacytoid DC are also important players in the pathogenesis of LP (Carbone et al. 2010; Parolini et al. 2007).

The cytokine pattern identified in both CLP and OLP (high levels of TNF- α and IFN-γ, IL-23/IL-17, IL-22 and IL-9) suggested an autoimmune pathogenesis (Weber et al. 2017).

In CLP especially an overexpression of IL-22 was found, which may be responsible for acanthosis, as in psoriasis, where it was related to proliferation of undifferentiated keratinocytes (Ma et al. 2008).

The high levels of IL-17 found in OLP and CLP modulate not only immune cells but also keratinocytes and fibroblasts and may be produced by Th17 cells, but also by neutrophils, natural killer cells (NK), mast cells, and macrophages (Żychowska et al. 2020).

The serum level of IL-23 in OLP was significantly higher than in patients with CLP (Mardani et al. 2021). IL-23 activates Th17 cells that promote autoimmunity.

B Weber and his group have identified for the first time significantly higher IL-9 expressing cells in CLP compared to OLP, Th9 being also involved in psoriasis and other autoimmune diseases (Nalleweg et al. 2014).

The new studies on the immune pathogenesis of LP explain the observed differences between CLP and OLP and bring hope for the severe cases, for targeted therapies.

Suppurative Hidradenitis (SH)

SH is a chronic, relapsing, inflammatory disease characterized by inflamed nodules, suppurating sinus tracts, scarring, and secondary contracture affecting mostly flexural areas, with apocrine glands (Ingram 2021; Turcu et al. 2019).

Histopathologically, in early stages, we can see follicular hyperkeratosis, follicular plugging, follicular dilation, and lymphocytic perifolliculitis, and in chronic lesions, psoriasiform hyperplasia of the interfollicular epithelium or a dense mixed inflammatory infiltrate (von Laffert et al. 2011; Weedon 2010).

Bacterial growth inside the occluded follicle activates local immune cells (macrophages) and the production of IL-1β and TNF-α, that will continue to attract immune cells, neutrophils, B cells and Th1 and Th17 (Wolk et al. 2020). T cell infiltration in HS lesions is comparable to that found in psoriasis and is centered on Th1 and Th17 (Wolk et al. 2020).

Lesional, perilesional, and nonlesional skin of patients with HS expresses high levels of IL-17, IL-23, IL-1β, TNF-α, and IL-12. High levels of IL-17 are produced by neutrophils and Th17 cells (Kelly et al. 2015; Schlapbach et al. 2011). Matrix metalloproteinases (MMPs) are responsible for structural changes and the final fibrotic reorganization of tissue (Wolk et al. 2020).

Antimicrobial peptides are also highly expressed in hidradenitis suppurativa, as in psoriasis, and can be correlated with the reduced risk of infections in both diseases (Zouboulis et al. 2015).

The new information on the pathogenesis of HS offers the hope of new and efficient therapies that target key players.

Acne

Acne is the most common inflammatory dermatosis in the world, a disease of the pilosebaceous unit, that manifests clinically as papules, pustules, open and closed comedones, affecting mainly the face, with a significant social impact (Layton et al. 2016).

The main pathological mechanisms include microbiome changes, sebum alteration, follicular hyperkeratinization, and inflammation, but which is the first step, was not yet established (Bolognia et al. 2018).

Histopathologically, pustules are associated with a neutrophilic inflammatory response, whereas papules, nodules, and cysts are associated with helper T lymphocytes, giant foreign body cells and neutrophils.

Acne-associated strains of *Cutibacterium acnes* stimulate TH17 cells to produce IFN-γ and pro-inflammatory IL-17 and activate the innate immune system to produce pro-inflammatory IL-1 (Li et al. 2014; Qin et al. 2014).

Acne, HS, and pyoderma gangrenosum have several aspects in common: follicular centered, activation of the innate immune system, increased IL-1 production and skin neutrophilic inflammation, altered matrix metalloproteinase expression, and may be present in the same patient, as part of PASH syndrome (Nedelcu 2020).

Conclusion

Skin is a highly immunologically active organ and new data show that increased levels of IL-23 and IL-17 are linked to the pathogenesis of many autoimmune diseases, such as lupus erythematosus, systemic lupus erythematosus, psoriasis, chronic spontaneous urticaria, morphea, bullous pemphigoid, pemphigus vulgaris, and vitiligo (Atwa et al. 2014; Danczak-Pazdrowska et al. 2012; Jeon et al. 2017; Plée et al. 2015; Rana et al. 2012; Vaccaro et al. 2015; Xue et al. 2014).

Additionally, the high level of circulating cytokine (TNF-α, IL-6, IL-10, and IL-4) associated with some dermatological diseases such as psoriasis, alopecia areata, hidradenitis suppurativa, atopic dermatitis and vitiligo, lichen planus has systemic consequences and explains a high prevalence of metabolic syndrome in these cases, compared to the general population (Ataş & Gönül 2017; Lee et al. 2019; Phan et al. 2019; Rodríguez-Zúñiga & García-Perdomo 2017; Shalom et al. 2019; Ying et al. 2020).

The clinical aspect of the aforementioned diseases is very different and we have to consider the fact that the function of each cytokine can depend on many local and host-related particularities. The complex inflammatory network that defines each disease needs further studies.

Despite their different presentation, many autoimmune skin disorders (psoriasis, atopic dermatitis, lupus erythemathosus, lichen planus, acne, and hidradenitis suppurativa) are now associated with elevated levels of IL-23 and IL-17. Therefore, we have to consider the fact that the function of each cytokine can be dependent on many local and host-related particularities that still need to be deciphered.

References

Achtman JC, Werth VP (2015) Pathophysiology of cutaneous lupus erythematosus. *Arthritis Research and Therapy* 17(1):1-10. https://doi.org/10.1186/s13075-015-0706-2

Ataş H, Gönül M (2017) Increased risk of metabolic syndrome in patients with vitiligo. *Balkan Medical Journal* 34(3):219-225. https://doi.org/10.4274/balkanmedj.2016.1005

Atwa MA, Emara AS, Youssef N, Bayoumy NM (2014) Serum concentration of IL-17, IL-23 and TNF-α among patients with chronic spontaneous urticaria: Association with disease activity and autologous serum skin test. *Journal of the European Academy of Dermatology and Venereology* 28(4):469-474. https://doi.org/10.1111/jdv.12124

Austin LM, Ozawa M, Kikuchi T, Walters IB, Krueger JG (1999) The majority of epidermal T cells in psoriasis vulgaris lesions can produce type 1 cytokines, interferon-γ, interleukin-2, and tumor necrosis factor-α, defining TC1 (cytotoxic T lymphocyte) and TH1 effector populations: A type 1 differentiation bias is al. *Journal of Investigative Dermatology* 113(5):752-759. https://doi.org/10.1046/j.1523-1747.1999.00749.x

Bao K, Reinhardt RL (2015) The differential expression of IL-4 and IL-13 and its impact on type-2 immunity. *Cytokine* 75(1):25-37. https://doi.org/10.1016/j.cyto.2015.05.008

Berdyshev E, Goleva E, Bronova I, Dyjack N, Rios C, Jung J, … Leung DY (2018) Lipid abnormalities in atopic skin are driven by type 2 cytokines. *JCI Insight* 3(4):e98006. https://doi.org/10.1172/jci.insight.98006

Bettinotti MP, Hartung K, Deicher H, Messer G, Keller E, Weiss EH, Albert ED (1993) Polymorphism of the tumor necrosis factor beta gene in systemic lupus erythematosus: TNFB-MHC haplotypes. *Immunogenetics* 37(6):449-454. https://doi.org/10.1007/BF00222469

Bieber T (2020) Interleukin-13: Targeting an underestimated cytokine in atopic dermatitis. Allergy. *European Journal of Allergy and Clinical Immunology* 75(1):54-62. https://doi.org/10.1111/all.13954

Bolognia Jean L, Schaffer JV, Cerroni L (2018) *Dermatology - Acne Vulgaris,* 4th edn. Elsevier

Brunner PM, Silverberg JI, Guttman-Yassky E, Paller AS, Kabashima K, Amagai M, … Taieb A (2017) Increasing Comorbidities Suggest that Atopic Dermatitis Is a Systemic Disorder. J*ournal of Investigative Dermatology* 137(1):18-25. https://doi.org/10.1016/j.jid.2016.08.022

Carbone T, Nasorri F, Pennino D, Donnarumma M, Garcovich S, Eyerich K, … Cavani A (2010) CD56highCD16- NK cell involvement in cutaneous lichen planus. *European Journal of Dermatology* 20(6):724-730. https://doi.org/10.1684/ejd.2010.1096

Chang HY, Chi JT, Dudoit S, Bondre C, Van De Rijn M, Botstein D, Brown PO (2002) Diversity, topographic differentiation, and positional memory in human fibroblasts. *Proceedings of the National Academy of Sciences of the United States of America* 99(20):12877-12882. https://doi.org/10.1073/pnas.162488599

Chen L, Dipietro LA (2017) Toll-like receptor function in acute wounds. *Advances in Wound Care* 6(10):344-355. https://doi.org/10.1089/wound.2017.0734

Danczak-Pazdrowska A, Kowalczyk M, Szramka-Pawlak B, Gornowicz-Porowska J, Szewczyk A, Silny W, … Hrycaj P (2012) Interleukin-17A and interleukin-23 in morphea. *Archives of Medical Science* 8(6):1089. https://doi.org/10.5114/aoms.2012.32421

DaVeiga SP (2012) Epidemiology of atopic dermatitis: A review. *Allergy and Asthma Proceedings* 33(3):227-234. https://doi.org/10.2500/aap.2012.33.3569

De Sá DC, Festa Neto C (2016) Inflammasomes and dermatology. *Anais Brasileiros de Dermatologia* 91:566-578. https://doi.org/10.1590/abd1806-4841.20165577

Dey-Rao R, Smith JR, Chow S, Sinha AA (2014) Differential gene expression analysis in CCLE lesions provides new insights regarding the genetics basis of skin vs. Systemic disease. *Genomics* 104(2):144-155. https://doi.org/10.1016/j.ygeno.2014.06.003

Eichenfield LF, Tom WL, Chamlin SL, Feldman SR, Hanifin JM, Simpson EL, … Sidbury R (2014) Guidelines of care for the management of atopic dermatitis: Section 1. Diagnosis and assessment of atopic dermatitis Work Group. *Journal of the American Academy of Dermatology* 70(2):338-351. https://doi.org/10.1016/j.jaad.2013.10.010

Esaki H, Brunner PM, Czarnowicki T, Rodriguez G, Immaneni S, Renert-Yuval Y, … Guttman-Yassky E (2016) 039 Early onset pediatric atopic dermatitis skin phenotype is Th2, but also Th17-polarized. *Journal of Investigative Dermatology* 136(5):S7. https://doi.org/10.1016/j.jid.2016.02.064

Eyerich K, Eyerich S (2018) Immune response patterns in non-communicable inflammatory skin diseases. *Journal of the European Academy of Dermatology and Venereology* 32(5):692-703. https://doi.org/10.1111/jdv.14673

Gottlieb AB, Chamian F, Masud S, Cardinale I, Abello MV, Lowes MA, … Krueger JG (2005) TNF Inhibition Rapidly Down-Regulates Multiple Proinflammatory Pathways in Psoriasis Plaques. *The Journal of Immunology* 175(4):2721-2729. https://doi.org/10.4049/jimmunol.175.4.2721

Guimarães PM, Scavuzzi BM, Stadtlober NP, Franchi Santos LFDR, Lozovoy MAB, Iriyoda TV, … Simão ANC (2017) Cytokines in systemic lupus erythematosus: Far beyond Th1/Th2 dualism lupus: Cytokine profiles. *Immunology and Cell Biology* 95(9):824-831. https://doi.org/10.1038/icb.2017.53

Guttman-Yassky E, Nograles KE, Krueger JG (2011a) Contrasting pathogenesis of atopic dermatitis and psoriasis - Part I: Clinical and pathologic concepts. *Journal of Allergy and Clinical Immunology* 127(5):1110-1118. https://doi.org/10.1016/j.jaci.2011.01.053

Guttman-Yassky E, Nograles KE, Krueger JG (2011b) Contrasting pathogenesis of atopic dermatitis and psoriasis - Part II: Immune cell subsets and therapeutic concepts. *Journal of Allergy and Clinical Immunology* 127(6):142-32

Howell MD, Boguniewicz M, Pastore S, Novak N, Bieber T, Girolomoni G, Leung DYM (2006) Mechanism of HBD-3 deficiency in atopic dermatitis. *Clinical Immunology* 121(3):332-338. https://doi.org/10.1016/j.clim.2006.08.008

Ingram JR (2021) *Hidradenitis suppurativa: Pathogenesis, clinical features, and diagnosis.* Avaible via https://www.uptodate.com/contents/hidradenitis-suppurativa-pathogenesis-clinical-features-and-diagnosis

Ioannides D, Vakirlis E, Kemeny L, Marinovic B, Massone C, Murphy R, … Neumann M (2020) European S1 guidelines on the management of lichen planus: a cooperation of the European Dermatology Forum with the European Academy of Dermatology and Venereology. *Journal of the European Academy of Dermatology and Venereology* 34(7):1403-1414. https://doi.org/10.1111/jdv.16464

Jeon C, Sekhon S, Yan D, Afifi L, Nakamura M, Bhutani T (2017) Monoclonal antibodies inhibiting IL-12, -23, and -17 for the treatment of psoriasis. *Human Vaccines and Immunotherapeutics* 13(10):2247-2259. https://doi.org/10.1080/21645515.2017.1356498

Kelly G, Hughes R, McGarry T, Van Den Born M, Adamzik K, Fitzgerald R, … Kirby B (2015) Dysregulated cytokine expression in lesional and nonlesional skin in hidradenitis suppurativa. *British Journal of Dermatology* 173(6):1431–1439. https://doi.org/10.1111/bjd.14075

Kim BE, Leung DYM, Boguniewicz M, Howell MD (2008) Loricrin and involucrin expression is down-regulated by Th2 cytokines through STAT-6. *Clinical Immunology* 126(3):332-337. https://doi.org/10.1016/j.clim.2007.11.006

Layton AM, Eady AE, Zouboulis CC (2016) *Rook's Textbook of Dermatology*- Acne, 9th edn. Wiley-Blackwell

Lee S, Lee H, Lee CH, Lee WS (2019) Comorbidities in alopecia areata: A systematic review and meta-analysis. *Journal of the American Academy of Dermatology* 80(2):466-477. https://doi.org/10.1016/j.jaad.2018.07.013

Leung DYM, Guttman-Yassky E (2014) Deciphering the complexities of atopic dermatitis: Shifting paradigms in treatment approaches. *Journal of Allergy and Clinical Immunology* 134(4):769-779. https://doi.org/10.1016/j.jaci.2014.08.008

Li ZJ, Choi DK., Sohn KC, Seo MS, Lee HE, Lee Y, … Im M (2014) Propionibacterium acnes activates the NLRP3 inflammasome in human sebocytes. *Journal of Investigative Dermatology* 134(11):2747-2756. https://doi.org/10.1038/jid.2014.221

Little AJ, Vesely MD (2020) Cutaneous lupus erythematosus: Current and future pathogenesis-directed therapies. *Yale Journal of Biology and Medicine* 93(1):81-95

Liu T, Li S, Ying S, Tang S, Ding Y, Li Y, … Fang H (2020) The IL-23/IL-17 Pathway in Inflammatory Skin Diseases: From Bench to Bedside. *Frontiers in Immunology* 11:594735. https://doi.org/10.3389/fimmu.2020.594735

Lynde CW, Poulin Y, Vender R, Bourcier M, Khalil S (2014) Interleukin 17A: Toward a new understanding of psoriasis pathogenesis. *Journal of the American Academy of Dermatology* 71(1):141-50. https://doi.org/10.1016/j.jaad.2013.12.036

Ma HL, Liang S, Li J, Napierata L, Brown T, Benoit S, … Young DA (2008) IL-22 is required for Th17 cell-mediated pathology in a mouse model of psoriasis-like skin inflammation. *Journal of Clinical Investigation* 118(2):597-607. https://doi.org/10.1172/JCI33263

Mardani M, Mofidi H, Dastgheib L, Ranjbar S, Hamidizadeh N (2021) Elevated Serum Interleukin-23 Levels in Patients with Oral and Cutaneous Lichen Planus. *Mediators of Inflammation* 2021:5578568. https://doi.org/10.1155/2021/5578568

Merola JF (2021) *Overview of cutaneous lupus erythematosus.* Avaible via https://www.uptodate.com/contents/overview-of-cutaneous-lupus-erythematosus

Nalleweg N, Chiriac MT, Podstawa E, Lehmann C, Rau TT, Atreya R, … Mudter J (2014) IL-9 and its receptor are predominantly involved in the pathogenesis of UC. *Gut* 64(5):743-55. https://doi.org/10.1136/gutjnl-2013-305947

Nedelcu RI (2020) PASH Syndrome: Comparing Pathogenic Mechanism of Pyoderma Gangrenosum, Acne and Suppurative Hidradenitis. *American Journal of Biomedical Science Research* 11(1):64-70. https://doi.org/10.34297/ajbsr.2020.11.001587

Nestle FO, Turka LA, Nickoloff BJ (1994) Characterization of dermal dendritic cells in psoriasis. Autostimulation of T lymphocytes and induction of Th1 type cytokines. *Journal of Clinical Investigation* 94(1):202-9. https://doi.org/10.1172/jci117308

Nguyen AV, Soulika AM (2019) The dynamics of the skin's immune system. *International Journal of Molecular Sciences* 20(8):1811. https://doi.org/10.3390/ijms20081811

O'Reilly S, Ciechomska M, Fullard N, Przyborski S, Van Laar JM (2016) IL-13 mediates collagen deposition via STAT6 and microRNA-135b: A role for epigenetics. *Scientific Reports* 6:25066. https://doi.org/10.1038/srep25066

Ogawa E, Sato Y, Minagawa A, Okuyama R (2018) Pathogenesis of psoriasis and development of treatment. *Journal of Dermatology* 45(3):264-272. https://doi.org/10.1111/1346-8138.14139

Pan Y, Xu L, Qiao J, Fang H (2018) A systematic review of ustekinumab in the treatment of atopic dermatitis. *Journal of Dermatological Treatment* 29(6):539-541. https://doi.org/10.1080/09546634.2017.1406894

Parolini S, Santoro A, Marcenaro E, Luini W, Massardi L, Facchetti F, … Sozzani S (2007) The role of chemerin in the colocalization of NK and dendritic cell subsets into inflamed tissues. *Blood* 109(9):3625-32. https://doi.org/10.1182/blood-2006-08-038844

Phan K, Charlton O, Smith SD (2019) Hidradenitis suppurativa and metabolic syndrome – systematic review and adjusted meta-analysis. *International Journal of Dermatology* 58(10):1112-1117. https://doi.org/10.1111/ijd.14500

Plée J, Le Jan S, Giustiniani J, Barbe C, Joly, P., Bedane C, … Bernard P (2015) Integrating longitudinal serum IL-17 and IL-23 follow-up, along with autoantibodies variation, contributes to predict bullous pemphigoid outcome. *Scientific Reports* 5:18001. https://doi.org/10.1038/srep18001

Qin M, Pirouz A, Kim MH, Krutzik SR, Garbán HJ, Kim J (2014) Propionibacterium acnes induces IL-1β secretion via the NLRP3 inflammasome in human monocytes. *Journal of Investigative Dermatology* 134(2):381-388. https://doi.org/10.1038/jid.2013.309

Rana A, Minz RW, Aggarwal R, Anand S, Pasricha N, Singh S (2012) Gene expression of cytokines (TNF-α, IFN-γ), serum profiles of IL-17 and IL-23 in paediatric systemic lupus erythematosus. *Lupus* 21(10):1105-12. https://doi.org/10.1177/0961203312451200

Rodríguez-Zúñiga MJM, García-Perdomo HA (2017) Systematic review and meta-analysis of the association between psoriasis and metabolic syndrome. *Journal of the American Academy of Dermatology* 77(4):657-666. https://doi.org/10.1016/j.jaad.2017.04.1133

Sarkar MK, Hile GA, Tsoi LC, Xing X, Liu J, Liang Y, … Kahlenberg JM (2018) Photosensitivity and type i IFN responses in cutaneous lupus are driven by epidermal-derived interferon kappa. *Annals of the Rheumatic Diseases* 77(11):1653-1664. https://doi.org/10.1136/annrheumdis-2018-213197

Schlapbach C, Hänni T, Yawalkar N, Hunger RE (2011) Expression of the IL-23/Th17 pathway in lesions of hidradenitis suppurativa. *Journal of the American Academy of Dermatology,* 65(4), 790–798. https://doi.org/10.1016/j.jaad.2010.07.010

Schur PH, Bevra HH (2021) *Epidemiology and pathogenesis of systemic lupus erythematosus.* Avaible via https://www.uptodate.com/contents/epidemiology-and-pathogenesis-of-systemic-lupus-erythematosus

Shalom G, Dreiher J, Kridin K, Horev A, Khoury R, Battat E, … Cohen AD (2019) Atopic dermatitis and the metabolic syndrome: a cross-sectional study of 116 816 patients. *Journal of the European Academy of Dermatology and Venereology* 33(9):1762-1767. https://doi.org/10.1111/jdv.15642

Spergel JM (2010) From atopic dermatitis to asthma: The atopic march. *Annals of Allergy, Asthma and Immunology* 105(2):99-106 https://doi.org/10.1016/j.anai.2009.10.002

Suárez-Fariñas M, Tintle SJ, Shemer A, Chiricozzi A, Nograles K, Cardinale I, … Guttman-Yassky E (2011) Nonlesional atopic dermatitis skin is characterized by broad terminal differentiation defects and variable immune abnormalities. *Journal of Allergy and Clinical Immunology* 127(4):954-64. https://doi.org/10.1016/j.jaci.2010.12.1124

Tang TS, Bieber T, Williams HC (2012) Does "autoreactivity" play a role in atopic dermatitis? *Journal of Allergy and Clinical Immunology* 129(5):1209-1215. https://doi.org/10.1016/j.jaci.2012.02.002

Totsuka A, Omori-Miyake M, Kawashima M, Yagi J, Tsunemi Y (2017) Expression of keratin 1, keratin 10, desmoglein 1 and desmocollin 1 in the epidermis: Possible downregulation by interleukin-4 and interleukin-13 in atopic dermatitis. *European Journal of Dermatology* 27(3):247-253. https://doi.org/10.1684/ejd.2017.2985

Tsuruta D (2009) NF-kappaB Links Keratinocytes and Lymphocytes in the Pathogenesis of Psoriasis. *Recent Patents on Inflammation Allergy Drug Discovery* 3(1):40-8. https://doi.org/10.2174/187221309787158399

Turcu G, Nedelcu R, Nedelcu I, Hodorogea A, Balaban M, Brinzea A, … Andrei R (2019) Pyoderma gangrenosum and suppurative hidradenitis association, overlap or spectrum of the same disease? Case report and discussion. *Experimental and Therapeutic Medicine* 20(1):38-41. https://doi.org/10.3892/etm.2019.8150

Ungar B, Pavel AB, Li R, Kimmel G, Nia J, Hashim P, … Guttman-Yassky E (2021) Phase 2 randomized, double-blind study of IL-17 targeting with secukinumab in atopic dermatitis. *Journal of Allergy and Clinical Immunology* 147(1):394-397. https://doi.org/10.1016/j.jaci.2020.04.055

Vaccaro M, Cannavò SP, Imbesi S, Cristani M, Barbuzza O, Tigano V, Gangemi S (2015) Increased serum levels of interleukin-23 circulating in patients with non-segmental generalized vitiligo. *International Journal of Dermatology* 54(6):672-4. https://doi.org/10.1111/ijd.12392

von Laffert, M., Stadie, V., Wohlrab, J., Marsch, W. C. (2011) Hidradenitis suppurativa/acne inversa: bilocated epithelial hyperplasia with very different sequelae. *British Journal of Dermatology,* 164(2), 367–371. https://doi.org/10.1111/j.1365-2133.2010.10034.x

Wang D, Drenker M, Eiz-Vesper B, Werfel T, Wittmann M (2008) Evidence for a pathogenetic role of interleukin-18 in cutaneous lupus erythematosus. *Arthritis and Rheumatism* 58(10):3205-3215. https://doi.org/10.1002/art.23868

Weber B, Schlapbach C, Stuck M, Simon HU, Borradori L, Beltraminelli H, Simon D (2017) Distinct interferon-gamma and interleukin-9 expression in cutaneous and oral lichen planus. *Journal of the European Academy of Dermatology and Venereology* 31(5):880-886. https://doi.org/10.1111/jdv.13989

Weedon D (2010) Diseases of cutaneous appendages. In: *Skin Pathology.* Elsevier L, Edinburgh p 397

Werfel T (2009) The role of leukocytes, keratinocytes, and allergen-specific IgE in the development of atopic dermatitis. Journal of Investigative Dermatology 129(8):1878-1891. https://doi.org/10.1038/jid.2009.71

Weston WL, Howe W (2021) *Atopic dermatitis (eczema): Pathogenesis, clinical manifestations, and diagnosis.* Avaible via https://www.uptodate.com/contents/atopic-dermatitis-eczema-pathogenesis-clinical-manifestations-and-diagnosis

Wolk K, Join-Lambert O, Sabat R (2020) Aetiology and pathogenesis of hidradenitis suppurativa. *British Journal of Dermatology* 183(6):999-1010. https://doi.org/10.1111/bjd.19556

Wolk K, Haugen HS, Xu W, Witte E, Waggie K, Anderson M, … Sabat R (2009) IL-22 and IL-20 are key mediators of the epidermal alterations in psoriasis while IL-17 and IFN-γ are not. *Journal of Molecular Medicine* 87(5):523-536. https://doi.org/10.1007/s00109-009-0457-0

Xue J, Su W, Chen Z, Ke Y, Du X, Zhou Q (2014) Overexpression of interleukin-23 and interleukin-17 in the lesion of pemphigus vulgaris: A preliminary study. *Mediators of Inflammation* 2014:463928. https://doi.org/10.1155/2014/463928

Ying J, Xiang W, Qiu Y, Zeng X (2020) Risk of metabolic syndrome in patients with lichen planus: A systematic review and meta-analysis. P*LoS ONE* 15(8):e0238005. https://doi.org/10.1371/journal.pone.0238005

Zahn S, Graef M, Patsinakidis N, Landmann A, Surber C, Wenzel J, Kuhn A (2014) Ultraviolet light protection by a sunscreen prevents interferon-driven skin inflammation in cutaneous lupus erythematosus. *Experimental Dermatology* 23(7):516-518. https://doi.org/10.1111/exd.12428

Zouboulis CC, Desai N, Emtestam L, Hunger RE, Ioannides D, Juhász I, … Jemec GBE (2015) European S1 guideline for the treatment of hidradenitis suppurativa/acne inversa. *Journal of the European Academy of Dermatology and Venereology* 29(4):619–644. https://doi.org/10.1111/jdv.12966

Żychowska M, Batycka-Baran A, Baran W (2020) Increased Serum Level and High Tissue Immunoexpression of Interleukin 17 in Cutaneous Lichen Planus: A Novel Therapeutic Target for Recalcitrant Cases? *Disease Markers* 2020:6521274. https://doi.org/10.1155/2020/6521274

Chapter 20

Cytokines in Kidney Failure

Nezaket Kadı*, MD and Demet Yavuz[2], MD

[1] Samsun Training and Research Hospital, Department of Internal Medicine, Samsun, Turkey
[2] Samsun Training and Research Hospital, Department of Nephrology, Samsun,Turkey

Abstract

Kidney injury is divided into two types as acute injury and chronic injury according to the development period. While a quick decrease in kidney function, which develops in hours or days, and the accumulation of excreta, e.g., urea, characterize acute kidney injury (AKI), chronic kidney disease (CKD) may develop due to ongoing permanent inflammation, inappropriate repair, and interstitial fibrosis. This may result in the loss of functional kidney tissue, which may progress to a level that requires renal replacement therapy. In all these processes, immune cells and renal parenchyma cells play a regulatory role via the cytokines, chemokines and cellular proteins they release. Many studies have been conducted to determine the targets that could be therapeutic and assist us with a better understanding of the pathogenesis of AKI and CKD and developing agents for these targets. In this chapter, information about the part played by cytokines in kidney injury is shared from the studies on the pathogenesis of CKD and AKI.

Keywords: acute kidney injury, chronic kidney disease, cytokines, inflammation, cytokines in kidney failure

Introduction

Cytokines take a significant part in host defense against microorganisms. They induce local inflammation and systemic acute-phase responses and thus regulate natural immunity. Moreover, they play an essential role in initiating, strengthening, directing, and regulating acquired immunity. Cytokines represent potential therapeutic targets under the said conditions. Immune cells secrete soluble mediators, chemokines and cytokines, impairing the biological function and cellular structure of kidney cells. Apart from immune cells, kidney cells, including

* Corresponding Author's Email: nezaketkadi@icloud.com.

In: Cytokines and Diseases
Editors: Kenan Demir, Selim Görgün and Bahar Uslu
ISBN: 979-8-88697-214-6

podocytes, tubular cells, and mesangial cells, also secrete a lot of cytokines likely to cause kidney injury (Gabay and Kushner 1999).

Cytokines in Acute Kidney Injury

AKI is described as a clinical syndrome that is characterized by a quick reduction in kidney function and accumulation of excreta, e.g., urea. According to Acute Kidney Diseases and Disorders (KDIGO 2012), AKI refers to an increase of ≥0.3 mg/dL (≥26.5 μmoL/L) in serum creatinine (SCr) during 48 hours or an increase of ≥1.5 times the initial value in SCr during the last 7 days or a urine volume of <0.5 mL/kg/hour for 6 hours. It is possible to classify the etiology of AKI as prerenal, renal, and postrenal. Prerenal AKI is the most frequently observed cause and appears in the case of decreased blood flow to the kidney. Renal AKI indicates the injury of kidney structures, namely vascular, interstitial, glomerular, and tubular structures. Postrenal AKI generally results from urinary tract obstruction. Prerenal and postrenal AKI may turn into renal kidney disease in the end (Kidney Int Suppl 2011).

AKI usually occurs due to ischemia or nephrotoxicity. The proximal tubule is usually the area affected in AKI. In the early period of AKI, inflammatory cell infiltration and tubular necrosis are observed in the affected area (Ysebaert et al. 2000; Berger 2014). Inflammatory responses are initiated by necrotic tubular endothelial cells, leading to the infiltration of immune cells. Neutrophils that accumulate in the injury area in the early period of AKI adhere to the endothelium via P-selectin and intercellular adhesion molecule-1 (ICAM-1) and release the cytokines they contain. ICAM-1, interleukin-1 (IL-1) and tumor necrosis factor-alpha (TNF-α) levels increase in an hour following ischemia/reperfusion. Macrophages and monocytes, which follow neutrophils, migrate to the injury areas and clear away the damaged cells and neutrophil remnants (Awad et al. 2009). Moreover, dendritic cells and undifferentiated epithelial cells also clear away the cellular debris. Undamaged epithelial cells differentiate and proliferate for the replacement of damaged cells in order to restore the tubular epithelial cell layer's integrity (Jo et al. 2006; Kelly et al. 1996; Chaturvedi 2013).

There are two experimental models which help us understand the injury mechanisms in AKI: ischemia-reperfusion injury (IRI) and cisplatin-induced AKI. The above-mentioned models enable us to understand the roles of leukocytes and cytokines, which are mediators in injuries. Caspases represent a family of intracellular cysteine proteases with a cysteine residue in their active areas. Caspase-1 takes a significant part in activating interleukin-1 beta (IL-1β) and interleukin-18 (IL-18), which are proinflammatory cytokines (Fantuzzi et al. 1998). Caspase-3 is an important caspase in apoptotic cell death in vivo (Cheng et al. 1998). NLRPs (nod-like receptor pyrin domain containing proteins) form a complex in the cytoplasm called the NLRP inflammasome with apoptosis-associated speck-like protein containing a CARD (ASC) and inactive caspase-1. Previous studies have indicated that caspase-1 mediates ischemic AKI and cisplatin-induced AKI (Faubel et al. 2004; Melnikov et al. 2001). It has been revealed that the increased TNF-α level in the serum is prevented and protected against injury due to the inhibition of the degranulation of monocytic cells in cisplatin-induced AKI with disodium cromoglycate (Summers et al. 2011). The inhibition of TNF-α also protects against injury in AKI induced by endotoxin, cisplatin, and ischemia (Donnahoo et al. 1999; Akcay et al. 2009). IL-1 is involved in intensifying neutrophil infiltration in IRI-induced AKI (Burne et al. 2001). The NLRP3 inflammasome mediates ischemic AKI. However, it does not take any part in cisplatin-induced AKI. It has been demonstrated that NLRP3 inflammasome knockout (-/-) mice are protected against IRI-induced AKI. However, they are not protected against cisplatin-induced AKI (Kim et al. 2013). It has also been shown that caspase-1 (−/−) mice are protected against cisplatin-induced AKI, whereas IL-1 β (−/−) mice are not (Faubel et al. 2004; Faubel et al. 2007). The part that IL-6 takes in AKI is complicated. In ischemic AKI, IL-6 has an exacerbating effect on inflammation (Patel et al. 2005). On the other hand, IL-6 gives protective responses with different mechanisms in the mercury chloride ($HgCl_2$)-induced AKI model (Nechemia-Arbely et al. 2008).

Cytokines in Chronic Kidney Disease

In line with Kidney Diseases and Disorders (KDIGO 2021), CKD is described as the presence of kidney injury or a glomerular filtration rate (GFR) of <60 ml/min/1.73 m2 and its continuation for at least three months.

Inappropriate repair, interstitial fibrosis, and permanent inflammation characterize CKD. Severe or repetitive injury causes cell cycle arrest in tubular epithelial cells that cannot repair damaged kidney structures. The macrophage phenotype is significant for the continuity of repair in kidney diseases. The macrophage is phenotypically classified as M1 (proinflammatory) and M2 (anti-inflammatory). In the early phase of repair, there is the dominance of M1 macrophages for clearing away cellular debris. Macrophages switch from M1 to M2 to assist with tissue regeneration as a result of improving tubular cell proliferation in the late phase. Nevertheless, cells with cell cycle arrest lead to the macrophage remaining as the M1 phenotype as a result of the release of proinflammatory cytokines. Furthermore, glomerular mesangial cells gain the myofibroblast phenotype and are involved in renal fibrosis (Pannu et al. 2011; Grams et al. 2010; James et al. 2010). Yang et al. (2010) revealed that tubular epithelial cells at the G2/M phase in AKI models increased the expression of transforming growth factor beta-1 (TGF-β1), collagen-1 and collagen-4, which are fibrogenic factors, through the c-Jun N-terminal kinase (JNK) signaling pathway (Yang et al. 2010).

The local proliferation of tubular and interstitial cells, extracellular matrix synthesis, endothelial procoagulant activity, the formation of reactive oxygen radicals (ROS), and the increase in the expression of adhesion molecules and biologically active lipids are induced by cytokines (Rao et al. 2007; Klahr et al. 2003). The renin-angiotensin system (RAS) regulates the inflammatory response in connection with the progression of kidney disease and susceptibility to cardiovascular dysfunction by playing a central role in intracellular cytokine signaling processes (Eddy et al. 2005). Genetic polymorphisms of RAS and cytokines may specify the altered expression of inflammatory cytokines. This type of genetic variation may be responsible for differences observed in the progression of renal and cardiovascular dysfunctions in patients with CKD (Rao et al. 2007; Wong et al. 2008).

There are many factors leading to impaired immunity and inflammatory activation in CKD. These factors are primary disease, genetic and epigenetic causes. The uremic environment produces oxidative and carbonyl stress, which is extremely proinflammatory (Kim et al. 2010; Aveles et al. 2010). In CKD, another cause of inflammation is metabolic acidosis (Ori et al. 2013). Frequent infections and thrombotic events observed in CKD and particularly in dialysis patients result in additional inflammatory stimulation (Nassar 2013). Chronic periodontal inflammation is related to elevated inflammatory biomarkers in HD (hemodialysis) patients and negatively influences the survival of patients (Ruospo et al. 2014; Buhlin et al. 2007; Kshirsagar et al. 2009). It has been asserted that uremic toxins lead to intestinal dysbiosis and increase the circulation of intestinal flora bacteria and bacterial components in CKD, and systemic inflammation is activated as a result (Anders et al. 2013; Shi et al. 2014; Natarajan et al. 2014). In subjects with CKD and end-stage renal disease (ESRD), immune dysfunction related to vitamin D deficiency has been indicated among the causes of the inflammatory response observed in the mentioned population (Sterling et al. 2012). Not only lymphocytes but also different tissues, including adipose tissues, which become dysfunctional in CKD, produce inflammatory cytokines in CKD (Iglesias et al. 2010). Hemodialysis treatment has been shown to acutely increase the transcription of proinflammatory cytokines (Friedrich et al. 2006). Extracorporeal factors have been associated with inflammatory activation in dialysis subjects. These factors consist of the microbiological quality of dialysate, impurities in dialysis water, and bioincompatibility in the extracorporeal dialysis circuit (Santoro and Mancini 2014; Panichi et al. 2008).

In the chronic renal insufficiency cohort (CRIC) research, biomarkers of inflammation (IL-1β, IL-6, IL-1 receptor antagonist, CRP, TNF-α, and fibrinogen) were directly proportional to impaired kidney function and albuminuria (Gupta et al. 2012). A large multicenter international study including hemodialysis (HD) patients revealed that CRP determined mortality better in a comparative study conducted with CRP, albumin, increased ferritin, and white blood cell count (Bazeley et al. 2011). On the other hand, IL-6 is seen to predict all-cause and cardiovascular mortality in a better way compared to CRP and other cytokines, e.g., IL-1beta, TNF-alpha, and IL-18 (Honda et al. 2006; Tripepi et al. 2005).

Tumor necrosis factor-like weak inducer of apoptosis (TWEAK) has been observed to stimulate the expression of inflammatory cytokines locally in kidney cells and decrease the expression of Klotho in vivo and in vitro (Sanz et al. 2014). Soluble TWEAK levels were found to be related to the severity of coronary artery disease in subjects with stage 2-3 CKD (Azak et al. 2014).

In CKD, permanent inflammation is not only linked to cardiovascular disease, involving early atherosclerosis, it also plays a significant role in developing protein-energy wasting (PEW). In CKD and ESRD, this may lead to malnutrition-inflammation-cachexia syndrome (MICS) (Kalantar-Zadeh et al. 2005). There is a strong association of hypoalbuminemia with mortality in dialysis subjects. It is known that not only malnutrition but also inflammation, though partially, cause this relationship (Kalantar-Zadeh et al. 2005; De Mutsert et al. 2009). Proinflammatory cytokines can directly cause anorexia through their effects on the brain. Moreover, inflammatory markers, specifically IL-6, can lead to depression and eventually a decrease in food intake in CKD and ESRD (Taraz et al. 2014).

TNF-alpha is among the strongest inducers of the receptor activator of the NF-kB ligand (RANKL), which is the main trigger of osteoclast activation and bone resorption, and can be linked with fractures occurring in dialysis subjects (Panuccio et al. 2012). It has been demonstrated that IL-1 and IL-6 suppress PTH secretion. In a subgroup analysis of a study on dialysis patients, it was asserted that low PTH levels were likely to reflect MICS rather than low bone turnover disease (Feroze et al. 2011). In pediatric dialysis subjects, low 1, $25(OH)_2$ vitamin D levels have been found to be related to higher CRP (Shroff et al. 2008). The IL-2 level has been higher in HD subjects having uremic pruritus than in age-sex-matched controls not having pruritus (Fallahzadeh et al. 2011).

Cytokines in Kidney Failure

IL-1 (interleukin-1): Caspase-1 mediates IL-1β (interleukin-1beta) activation. Caspase-1 is linked with pyroptosis, which is a programmed lytic cell death that quickens tubular epithelial cell death and represents the most frequently observed cause of AKI (Zhang et al. 2018; Lorenz et al. 2013; Chung et al. 2012; Yang et al. 2013). The expression of IL-6 and IL-8 in kidney fibroblasts and mesangial cells is increased by IL-1β (Lovett et al. 1983; Lonnemann et al. 1995; Robson et al. 1995). The NLRP3 inflammasome may activate IL-18, related to the pathogenesis of many kidney diseases (Hutton et al. 2016; Wu et al. 2008; Bani-Hani et al. 2009; Kitching et al. 2005). Kidney functions and inflammation have been shown to improve in mice with nephrotoxic nephritis and IL-1β deficiency (Timoshanko et al. 2004; Lei et al. 2019). IL-1β is involved in developing diabetic nephropathy (DN). Faubel et al. observed an increase in the IL-1β level in mice with cisplatin-induced AKI. Shahzad et al. revealed that IL-1β increased in a gradual manner in mice with the progression to DN (db/db) (Shahzad et al. 2015). A critical point in kidney fibrosis is that IL-1β supports the differentiation of tubular epithelial cells into a fibroblast-like phenotype (Fan et al. 2001; Zhang et al. 2005). IL-1β increases SOR production and fibrotic factor expression. These fibrotic factors are comprised of TGF-β, collagen I, and fibronectin. The relation between plasma levels of IL-1 and IL-1Ra takes an essential part in the susceptibility to and severity of numerous diseases. Studies indicate that this relation predicts the progression of glomerulopathies and mortality in CKD (Arend 2002). In an animal model of CKD, administration of IL-1 antagonists has been demonstrated to inhibit tubulointerstitial fibrosis (Lan et al. 1995).

With the effect of some cytokines including IL-1β and TNF-α, kidney cells, e.g., tubular epithelial cells, mesangial cells, and podocytes, can generate interleukin-6 (IL-6). This shows its effects with different pathways via two different receptors (Moutabarrik et al. 1994; Boswell et al. 1994; Van den Dobbelsteen et al. 1993; Ruef et al. 1990). IL-6 participates in podocyte apoptosis by regulating the activation of caspase-3 and caspase-9. Moreover, it increases the production of p21 and p27 and leads to cell cycle arrest in podocytes (Kim et al. 2013). Improved renal function and decreased neutrophil infiltration have been observed in IRI-AKI and $HgCl_2$-induced AKI models with IL-6 deficiency. IL-6 induces factors such as collagen I and collagen IV and TGF-β and increases the fibrotic response in the IRI-AKI model (Nechemia-Arbely et al. 2008; Patel et al. 2005). In IRI-AKI mice, IL-6 blockage decreases IL-1β and TNF-α production and the expression of ICAM-1 and P-selectin that are important in neutrophil infiltration and reduces kidney inflammation. Tocilizumab (TCZ), an IL-6R antibody, suppresses NLRP3 inflammasome activation and decreases glomerular hypertrophy and albuminuria in mice with diabetes and lupus nephritis (Chen et al. 2019). These findings show that IL-6 increases kidney inflammation, decreases kidney functions and impairs the glomerular structure. According to some research, IL-6 also has anti-inflammatory impacts in kidney diseases. The administration of IL-6 has been observed to protect against nephrotoxic nephritis (Nechemia-Arbely et al. 2008; Karkar et al. 1997). IL-6 increases the differentiation of B lymphocytes into antibody-producing cells and the production of acute-phase proteins such as CRP and fibrinogen (Yvan-Charvet et al. 2009). Furthermore, this cytokine stimulates the proliferation of kidney mesangial cells and takes a significant part in mesangial proliferative glomerulopathy (Horii et al. 1993).

Interleukin-8 (IL-8): This is a chemotactic cytokine. It functions as a chemoattractant that directs neutrophils to inflammation areas by binding to C-X-C motif chemokine receptor 1 (CXCR1) and C-X-C motif chemokine receptor 2 (CXCR2). It stimulates ICAM-1 generation in proximal tubule cells via the p38 pathway. The expression of IL-8 in mesangial and proximal tubule cells is stimulated by IL-1 and TNF-α, which are proinflammatory cytokines (Brown et al. 1991; Abbott et al. 1991; Kusner et al. 1991; Li et al. 2009; Gerritsma et al. 1996). G31P, which is a CXCR1/CXCR2 inhibitor, heals sepsis-induced kidney injury by decreasing IL-6, IL-1β, and TNF-α expression, neutrophil infiltration, and renal cell apoptosis. Furthermore, similar findings have been confirmed in the cisplatin-induced AKI model (Li et al. 2014; Zhou et al. 2019). G31P reduces connective tissue growth factor (CTGF), TGF-β, and fibronectin expression and increases the expression of matrix metalloproteinases-2 (MMP-2) and matrix metalloproteinases-9 (MMP-9). Moreover, it decreases the phosphorylation of Janus kinase 2 (JAK2), signal transducer and activator of transcription 3 (STAT3) and extracellular signal regulated kinases 1/2 (ERK1/2) and inhibits high glucose-induced TNF-α and TGF-β expression in mesangial cells. It prevents renal inflammation as a result of decreasing IL-1β, IL-6, and TNF-α expression and macrophage infiltration. With G31P, changes in kidney structures such as glomerular basal membrane (GBM) thickening, collagen deposition, mesangial enlargement, and podocyte loss in diabetic mice have been observed to decrease (Cui et al. 2017). The urinary excretion of β2 microglobulin, IL-6 and IL-8/CXCL8 is linked with renal inflammatory activity in lupus nephritis. Urinary IL-8/CXCL8 has been found to rise in subjects having lupus nephritis or immunoglobulin A (IgA) nephropathy (Wada et al. 1994). Yokoyama et al. revealed that IL-8/CXCL8 increased in the acute phase of IgA nephropathy characterized by endocapillary proliferation. Urinary IL-8/CXCL8 has also been observed to increase in the early stages of diabetic nephropathy (Tashiro K. et al. 2002). There are clinical and experimental studies suggesting that the said chemokine influences glomerular permeability (Souto et al. 2008). Garin showed that IL-8/CXCL8 administration led to proteinuria in animals probably via increased glomerular permeability (Garin 2000).

Tumor necrosis factor-alpha (TNF-α): This stimulates ICAM-I expression as well as the expression of IL-8 and monocyte chemoattractant protein-1 (MCP-1) in tubular epithelial cells, mesangial cells, and podocytes for promoting monocyte and neutrophil infiltration. It increases the production of ROS in mesangial cells. It is linked with albumin excretion in the urine (Lampropoulou et al. 2014; Navarro et al. 2006; McCarthy et al. 1998). It leads to kidney injury by inducing apoptosis in tubular, epithelial, and mesangial cells (Peralta Soler et al. 1996; Meldrum et al. 2001; Guo et al. 1998). It causes loss of glomerular endothelial cell fenestration, reduction in GFR, and albuminuria. In the DN animal model, albuminuria was shown to decrease due to reduced levels of granulocyte-macrophage colony-stimulating factor (G-MCS), keratinocyte-derived cytokine (KC) and MCP-1 with TNF-α inhibition from macrophages (Awad et al. 2015). Various studies have revealed that systemic TNF-α inhibition reduces inflammation and improves kidney functions in many animal models of kidney disease (Gao et al. 2013; Wang et al. 2017; Karkar et al. 2001). TNF-α is a proinflammatory cytokine stimulated by angiotensin II (Ang II) and helps with the differentiation of myofibroblasts into interstitial fibrosis (Abbas et al. 2003). In an experimental model of glomerulopathy, glomerular lesion development was reduced with both genetic deficiency of TNF-α and pharmacological inhibition of this cytokine (Karkar et al. 2001). In children with nephrotic syndrome related to minimal change disease (MCD), an increase in the urinary excretion of TNF-α has been observed (Cho et al. 2003).

There are three isoforms of TGF-β (transforming growth factor-beta) in mammals: TGF-β1, TGF-β2, and TGF-β3. A large number of studies show that TGF-β1 participates in renal fibrosis and causes extracellular matrix (ECM) components to accumulate excessively in kidney cells by reducing matrix metalloproteinases (MMP) and increasing natural tissue inhibitors (TIMP). Fibroblast proliferation is induced by TGF-β1 through basic fibroblast growth factor (bFGF). Furthermore, TGF-β1 increases collagen I and osteopontin expression from fibroblasts in mice with unilateral obstruction (Strutz et al. 2001). Additionally, TGF-β1 participates in the epithelial-mesenchymal transition (EMT) and mediates its accumulation in the extracellular matrix (ECM) while mediating tubulointerstitial fibrosis by increasing macrophage infiltration (Yang and Liu 2001, Chung et al. 2018). TGF-β both promotes fibrosis and induces caspase-3-dependent podocyte apoptosis as a result of the mTOR pathway activation (Schiffer et al. 2001, Das et al. 2015). Based on the role of TGF-β1 in fibrogenesis, it has been proven that strategies developed to inhibit TGF-β1 effectively alleviate kidney fibrosis. Ziyadeh et al. (2000) revealed that TGF-β1 antibody therapy prevented kidney fibrosis in mice with diabetic nephropathy (Ziyadeh et al. 2000). Gewin et al. (2012) demonstrated that apoptosis was mild in the proximal tubule epithelial cells of mice with TGF-β1 receptor deficiency and $Hgcl_2$-induced AKI (Gewin et al. 2012). It interacts with Ang-II intracellular signaling pathways, which stimulate renal interstitial fibrosis and its progression to CKD (Ruiz-Ortega et al. 2001). In subjects having focal and segmental glomerulosclerosis (FSGS) and DN, an increase in the expression of the cytokine and in serum and urine levels was observed (Vasconcelos et al. 2011).

Conclusion

In light of clinical and experimental evidence, the role of inflammation in kidney failure is undebatable. Despite significant progress in the information about the pathophysiological mechanisms associated with kidney failure, it is still necessary to clarify many aspects. For this reason, considering the possibility of defining new prognostic markers and perhaps alternative and more effective therapeutic targets, it is essential to understand the impacts of chemokines and cytokines on the onset and progression of kidney injury.

References

Abbas AK, Lichtman AH (2003) Cytokines In: *Cellular and Molecular Immunology,* 5th edn. Saunders Elsevier Science, Philadelphia, p 243-74.

Abbott F, Ryan JJ, Ceska M, Matsushima K, Sarraf CE, Rees AJ (1991) Interleukin-1 stimulates human mesangial cells to synthesize and release interleukins-6 and-8. *Kidney Int.* 40:597–605. https://doi.org/10.1038/ki.1991.250.

Akcay A, Nguyen Q, Edelstein CL (2009) Mediators of inflammation in acute kidney injury. *Mediators Inflamm* 2009:137072.

Anders HJ, Andersen K, Stecher B (2013) The intestinal microbiota, a leaky gout, and abnormal immunity in kidney disease. *Kidney Int;* 83:1010-1016.

Arend WP (2002) The balance between IL-1 and IL-1Ra in disease. *Cytokine Growth Factor Rev* 13:323-40.

Aveles PR, Criminacio CR, Goncalves S, Bignelli AT, Claro LM, Siqueira SS, Nakao LS, Pecoits-Filho R (2010) Association between biomarkers of carbonyl stress with increased systemic inflammatory response in different stages of chronic kidney disease and after renal transplantation. *Nephron Clin Pract* 116:c294-c299.

Awad AS, Rouse M, Huang L, Vergis AL, Reutershan J, Cathro HP, Linden J, Okusa MD (2009) Compartmentalization of neutrophils in the kidney and lung following acute ischemic kidney injury. *Kidney Int* 75:689–698. https://doi.org/10.1038/ki.2008.648.

Awad AS, You H, Gao T, Cooper TK, Nedospasov SA, Vacher J, Wilkinson PF, Farrell FX, Brian Reeves W (2015) Macrophage-derived tumor necrosis factor-α mediates diabetic renal injury. *Kidney Int* 88:722–733. https://doi.org/10.1038/ki.2015.162.

Azak A, Akdogan MF, Denizli N, Huddam B, Kocak G, Gucun M, Tatlisu MA, Demirci R, Yilmaz B, Dikec M, Bakirtas M, Akdag I, Duranay M (2014) Soluble TWEAK levels are independently associated with coronary artery disease severity in patients with stage 2-3 kidney disease. *Int Urol Nephrol* 46:411-415.

Bani-Hani AH, Leslie JA, Asanuma H, Dinarello CA, Campbell MT, Meldrum DR, Zhang H, Hile K, Meldrum KK (2009) IL-18 neutralization ameliorates obstruction-induced epithelial–mesenchymal transition and renal fibrosis. *Kidney Int* 76:500–511. https://doi.org/10.1038/ki.2009.216.

Bazeley J, Bieber B, Li Y, Morgenstern H, de Sequera P, Combe C, Yamamoto H, Gallagher M, Port FK, Robinson BM (2011) C-reactive protein and prediction of 1-year mortality in prevalent hemodialysis patients. *Clin J Am Soc Nephrol* 6:2452-2461.

Berger K, Moeller MJ (2014) Mechanisms of Epithelial Repair and Regeneration after Acute Kidney Injury. *Semin Nephrol* 34:394–403. https://doi.org/10.1016/j.semnephrol.2014.06.006.

Boswell RN, Yard BA, Schrama E, van Es LA, Daha MR, van der Woude FJ (1994) Interleukin 6 production by human proximal tubular epithelial cells in vitro: Analysis of the effects of interleukin-1α (IL-1α) and other cytokines. *Nephrol Dial Transplant* 9:599–606. https://doi.org/10.1093/ndt/9.6.599.

Brown Z, Strieter RM, Chensue SW, Ceska M, Lindley I, Neild GH, Kunkel SL, Westwick J (1991) Cytokine-activated human mesangial cells generate the neutrophil chemoattractant, interleukin 8. *Kidney Int* 40:86–90. https://doi.org/10.1038/ki.1991.184.

Buhlin K, Barany P, Heimburger O, Stenvinkel P, Gustafsson A (2007) Oral health and pro-inflammatory status in end-stage renal disease patients. *Oral Health Prev Dent* 2007; 5: 235-244.

Burne MJ, Elghandour A, Haq M, Saba SR, Norman J, Condon T, Bennett F, Rabb H (2001) IL-1 and TNF independent pathways mediate ICAM-1/VCAM-1 up-regulation in ischemia reperfusion injury. *J Leukoc Biol* 70:192–198.

Chaturvedi S, Yuen DA, Bajwa A, Huang YW, Sokollik C, Huang L, Lam GY, Tole S, Liu GY, Pan J, et al. (2013) Slit2 prevents neutrophil recruitment and renal ischemia-reperfusion injury. *J Am Soc Nephrol* 24:1274–1287. https://doi.org/10.1681/ASN.2012090890.

Chen W, Yuan H, Cao W, Wang T, Chen W, Yu H, Fu Y, Jiang B, Zhou H, Guo H, et al. (2009) Blocking interleukin-6 trans-signaling protects against renal fibrosis by suppressing STAT3 activation. *Theranostics* 9:3980–3991. https://doi.org/10.7150/thno.32352.

Cheng Y et al. (1998) Caspase inhibitor affords neuroprotection with delayed administration in a rat model of neonatal hypoxic-ischemic brain injury. *J Clin Invest* 101:1992–1999.

Cho MH, Lee HS, Choe BH, Kwon SH, Chung KY, Koo JH, et al. (2003) Interleukin-8 and tumor necrosis factor-alpha are increased in minimal change disease but do not alter albumin permeability. *Am J Nephrol* 23:260-6.

Chung S, Overstreet JM, Li Y, Wang Y, Niu A, Wang S, Fan X, Sasaki K, Jin G-N, Khodo SN, et al. (2018) TGF-β promotes fibrosis after severe acute kidney injury by enhancing renal macrophage infiltration. *JCI Insight* 3:e123563. https://doi.org/10. 1172/ jci. insight.123563.

Chung SD, Lai TY, Chien CT, Yu HJ (2012) Activating Nrf-2 signaling depresses unilateral ureteral obstruction-evoked mitochondrial stress-related autophagy, apoptosis and pyroptosis in kidney. *PLoS ONE* 7:e47299. https://doi.org/10.1371/journal.pone.0047299.

Cui S, Zhu Y, Du J, Khan MN, Wang B, Wei J, Cheng J-W, Gordon JR, Mu Y, Li F (2017) CXCL8 Antagonist Improves Diabetic Nephropathy in Male Mice with Diabetes and Attenuates High Glucose–Induced Mesangial Injury. *Endocrinology* 158:1671–1684. https://doi.org/10. 1210/en.2016-1781.

Das R, Xu S, Nguyen TT, Quan X, Choi S-K, Kim S-J, Lee EY, Cha S-K, Park K-S (2015) Transforming Growth Factor β1-induced Apoptosis in Podocytes via the Extracellular Signal-regulated Kinase-

Mammalian Target of Rapamycin Complex 1-NADPH Oxidase 4 Axis. *J Biol Chem* 290:30830–30842. https://doi.org/10. 1074/ jbc.M115.703116.

De Mutsert R, Grootendorst DC, Indemans F, Boeschoten EW, Krediet RT, Dekker FW (2009) Association between serum albumin and mortality in dialysis patients is partly explained by inflammation, and not by malnutrition. *J Ren Nutr* 19:127-135.

Donnahoo KK, Meng X, Ayala A, Cain MP, Harken AH, Meldrum DR (1999) Early kidney TNF-alpha expression mediates neutrophil infiltration and injury after renal ischemia-reperfusion. *Am J Physiol* 277:R922–R929.

Eddy AA (2005) Progression in chronic kidney disease. *Adv Chronic Kidney Dis* 12:353-65.

Fallahzadeh MK, Roozbeh J, Geramizadeh B, Namazi MRI (2011) Interleukin-2 serum levels are elevated in patients with uremic pruritus: a novel finding with practical implications. *Nephrol Dial Transplant* 26:3338-3344.

Fan J-M, Huang X-R, Ng Y-Y, Nikolic-Paterson DJ, Mu W, Atkins RC, Lan HY (2001) Interleukin-1 induces tubular epithelial-myofibroblast transdifferentiation through a transformational growth factor-β1-dependent mechanism in vitro. *Cunt J Kidney Dis* 37:820–831. https://doi.org/10.1016/S0272-6386(01)80132-3.

Fantuzzi G, Puren AJ, Harding MW, Livingston DJ, Dinarello CA (1998) Interleukin-18 regulation of interferon gamma production and cell proliferation as shown in interleukin-1 beta-converting enzyme (caspase-1)-deficient mice. *Blood* 91:2118–2125.

Faubel S, Lewis EC, Reznikov L, Ljubanovic D, Hoke TS, Somerset H, Oh DJ, Lu L, Klein CL, Dinarello CA, Edelstein CL (2007) Cisplatin-induced acute renal failure is associated with an increase in the cytokines interleukin (IL)-1beta, IL-18, IL-6, and neutrophil infiltration in the kidney. *J Pharmacol Exp Ther* 322:8–15.

Faubel SG, Ljubanovic D, Reznikov LL, Somerset H, Dinarello CA, Edelstein CL (2004) Caspase-1-deficient mice are protected against cisplatin-induced apoptosis and acute tubular necrosis. *Kidney Int* 66:2202–2213.

Feroze U, Molnar MZ, Dukkipati R, Kovesdy CP, Kalantar-Zadeh K (2011) Insights into nutritional and inflammatory aspects of low parathyroid hormone in dialysis patients. *J Ren Nutr* 21:100-104.

Friedrich B, Alexander D, Janessa A, Haring HU, Lang F, Risler T (2006) Acute effects of hemodialysis on cytokine transcription profiles: evidence for C-reactive protein-dependency of mediator induction. *Kidney Int* 70:2124-2130.

Gabay C, Kushner I (1999) Acute-phase proteins and other systemic responses to inflammation. *N Engl J Med* 340:448–454.

Gao G, Zhang B, Ramesh G, Betterly D, Tadagavadi RK, Wang W, Reeves WB (2013) TNF-α mediates increased susceptibility to ischemic AKI in diabetes. *Am J Physiol Ren Physiol* 304:F515–F521. https://doi.org/10.1152/ajprenal.00533.2012.

Garin EH (2000) Circulating mediators of proteinuria in idiopathic minimal lesion nephrotic syndrome. *Pediatr Nephrol* 14:872-8.

Gerritsma JS, Hiemstra PS, Gerritsen AF, Prodjosudjadi W, Verweij CL, Van Es LA, Daha MR (1996) Regulation and production of IL-8 by human proximal tubular epithelial cells in vitro. *Clin Exp Immunol* 103:289–294. https://doi.org/10.1046/j.1365-2249. 1996.d01-617.x.

Gewin L, Vadivelu S, Neelisetty S, Srichai MB, Paueksakon P, Pozzi A, Harris RC, Zent R (2012) Deleting the TGF-β receptor attenuates acute proximal tubule injury. *J Am Soc Nephrol* 23:2001–2011. https://doi.org/10. 1681/ASN.2012020139.

Grams ME, Astor BC, Bash LD, Matsushita K, Wang Y, Coresh J (2010) Albuminuria and estimated glomerular filtration rate independently associate with acute kidney injury. *J. Am Soc Nephrol* 21:1757–1764. https://doi.org/10.1681/ASN.20100128.

Guo Y-L, Baysal K, Kang B, Yang L-J, Williamson JR (1998) Correlation between Sustained c-Jun N-terminal Protein Kinase Activation and Apoptosis Induced by Tumor Necrosis Factor-α in Rat Mesangial Cells. *J Biol Chem* 273:4027–4034. https://doi.org/10. 1074/jbc.273.7.4027.

Gupta J, Mitra N, Kanetsky PA, Devaney J, Wing MR, Reilly M, Shah VO, Balakrishnan VS, Guzman NJ, Girndt M, Periera BG, Feldman HI, Kusek JW, Joffe MM, Raj DS (2012) Association between albuminuria, kidney function, and inflammatory biomarker profile in CKD in CRIC. *Clin J Am Soc Nephrol* 7:1938-1946.

Honda H, Qureshi AR, Heimburger O, Barany P, Wang K, Pecoits-Filho R, Stenvinkel P, Lindholm B (2006) Serum albumin, C-reactive protein, interleukin 6, and fetuin a as predictors of malnutrition, cardiovascular disease, and mortality in patients with ESRD. *Am J Kidney Dis* 47:139-148.

Horii Y, Iwano M, Hirata E, Shiiki M, Fujii Y, Dohi K, et al. (1993) Role of interleukin-6 in the progression of mesangial proliferative glomerulonephritis. *Kidney Int Suppl* 39(Supp l):S71-75.

Hutton HL, Ooi JD, Holdsworth SR, Kitching AR (2016) The NLRP3 inflammasome in kidney disease and autoimmunity. *Nephrology* 21:736–744. https://doi.org/10.1111/nep.12785.

Iglesias P, Diez JJ (2010) Adipose tissue in renal disease: clinical significance and prognostic implications. *Nephrol Dial Transplant* 25:2066-2077.

James M, Hemmelgarn B, Wiebe N, Pannu N, Manns B, Klarenbach S, Tonelli M (2010) Glomerular filtration rate, proteinuria, and the incidence and consequences of acute kidney injury: A cohort study. *Lancet* 376:2096–2103. https://doi.org/10.1016/S0140-6736(10)61271.

Jo SK, Sung SA, Cho WY, Go KJ, Kim HK (2006) Macrophages contribute to the initiation of ischaemic acute renal failure in rats. *Nephrol Dial Transplant* 21:1231–1239. https://doi.org/10.1093/ndt/gfk047.

Kalantar-Zadeh K (2005) Recent advances in understanding the malnutrition-inflammation-cachexia syndrome in chronic kidney disease patients: what is next? *Semin Dial* 18:365-369.

Kalantar-Zadeh K, Kilpatrick RD, Kuwae N, McAllister CJ, Alcorn H Jr, Kopple JD, Greenland S (2005) Revisiting mortality predictability of serum albumin in the dialysis population: time dependency, longitudinal changes and population-attributable fraction. *Nephrol Dial Transplant* 20:1880-1888.

Karkar AM, Smith J, Pusey CD (2001) Prevention and treatment of experimental crescentic glomerulonephritis by blocking tumour necrosis factor-α Nephrol. *Dial. Transplant.* 16:518–524. https://doi.org/10.1093/ndt/16.3.518.

Karkar AM, Smith J, Pusey CD (2001) Prevention and treatment of experimental crescentic glomerulonephritis by blocking tumour necrosis factor-alpha. *Nephrol Dial Transplant* 16:518-24.

Karkar AM, Smith J, Tam FWK, Pusey CD, Rees AJ (1997) Abrogation of glomerular injury in nephrotoxic nephritis by continuous infusion of interleukin-6. *Kidney Int* 52:1313–1320. https://doi.org/10.1038/ki.1997.456.

Kelly KJ, Williams WW Jr, Colvin RB, Meehan SM, Springer TA, Gutierrez-Ramos JC, Bonventre JV (1996) Intercellular adhesion molecule-1-deficient mice are protected against ischemic renal injury. *J Clin Investig* 97:1056–1063. https://doi.org/10.1172/JCI118498.

Kidney Int. Suppl. (2011) Section 2: AKI Definition. 2(1):19–36. https://doi.org/10.1038/kisup.2011.32.

Kim DI, Park SH (2013) Sequential signaling cascade of IL-6 and PGC-1α is involved in high glucose-induced podocyte loss and growth arrest. *Biochem Biophys Res Commun* 435:702–707. https://doi.org/10.1016/j.bbrc.2013.05.046.

Kim HJ, Lee DW, Ravichandran K, O Keys D, Akcay A, Nguyen Q, He Z, Jani A, Ljubanovic D, Edelstein CL (2013) NLRP3 inflammasome knockout mice are protected against ischemic but not cisplatin-induced acute kidney injury. *J Pharmacol Exp Ther* 346:465–472.

Kim HJ, Vaziri ND (2010) Contribution of impaired Nrf2-Keap1 pathway to oxidative stress and inflammation in chronic renal failure. *Am J Physiol Renal Physiol* 298:F662-F671.

Kitching AR, Turner AL, Wilson GRA, Semple T, Odobasic D, Timoshanko JR, O'Sullivan KM, Tipping PG, Takeda K, Akira S et al. (2005) IL-12p40 and IL-18 in Crescentic Glomerulonephritis: IL-12p40 is the Key Th1-Defining Cytokine Chain, Whereas IL-18 Promotes Local Inflammation and Leukocyte Recruitment. *J Am Soc Nephrol* 16:2023. https://doi.org/10.1681/ASN.2004121075.

Klahr S, Morrissey J (2003) Progression of chronic renal disease. *Am J Kidney Dis* 41: 3-7.

Kshirsagar AV, Craig RG, Moss KL, Beck JD, Offenbacher S, Kotanko P, Klemmer PJ, Yoshino M, Levin NW, Yip JK, Almas K, Lupovici EM, Usvyat LA, Falk RJ (2009) Periodontal disease adversely affects the survival of patients with end-stage renal disease. *Kidney Int* 75:746-751.

Kusner DJ, Luebbers EL, Nowinski RJ, Konieczkowski M, King CH, Sedor JR (1991) Cytokine- and LPS-induced synthesis of interleukin-8 from human mesangial cells. *Kidney Int* 39:1240–1248. https://doi.org/10. 1038/ki.1991.157.

Lampropoulou I-T, Stangou M, Papagianni A, Didangelos T, Iliadis F, Efstratiadis G (2014) TNF-α and Microalbuminuria in Patients with Type 2 Diabetes Mellitus. *J Diabetes Res* 2014:7. https://doi.org/10.1155/2014/394206.

Lan HY, Nikolic-Paterson DJ, Mu W, Vannice JL, Atkins RC (1995) Interleukin-1 receptor antagonist halts the progression of established crescentic glomerulonephritis in the rat. *Kidney Int* 47: 1303-9.

Lei Y, Devarapu SK, Motrapu M, Cohen CD, Lindenmeyer MT, Moll S, Kumar SV, Anders H-J (2019) Interleukin-1β Inhibition for Chronic Kidney Disease in Obese Mice with Type 2 Diabetes. *Front Immunol* 10:1223. https://doi.org/10.3389/fimmu.2019.01223.

Li H, Nord EP (2009) IL-8 amplifies CD40/CD154-mediated ICAM-1 production via the CXCR-1 receptor and p38-MAPK pathway in human renal proximal tubule cells. *Am J Physiol Ren Physiol* 296:F438–F445. https://doi.org/10.1152/ajprenal. 90214.2008.

Li L, Khan N, Li Q, Chen X, Wei J, Wang B, Cheng J-W, Gordon J, Li F (2014) G31P, CXCR1/2 inhibitor, with cisplatin inhibits the growth of mice hepatocellular carcinoma and mitigates high-dose cisplatin-induced nephrotoxicity. *Oncol Rep* 33:751–757. https://doi.org/10. 3892/or. 2014.3659.

Lonnemann G, Engler-Blum G, Müller GA, Koch KM, Dubarello CA (1995) Cytokines in human renal interstitial fibrosis. II. Intrinsic interleukin (IL)-1 synthesis and IL-1-dependent production of IL-6 and IL-8 by cultured kidney fibroblasts. *Kidney Int* 47:845–854. https://doi.org/10.1038/ki.1995.127.

Lorenz G, Darisipudi MN, Anders H-J (2013) Canonical and non-canonical effects of the NLRP3 inflammation in kidney inflammation and fibrosis. *Nephrol Dial It's a transplant* 29: 41–48. https://doi.org/10.1093/ndt/gft332.

Lovett DH, Ryan JL, Sterzel RB (1983) Stimulation of rat mesangial cell proliferation by macrophage interleukin 1. *J Immunol* 131:2830.

McCarthy ET, Sharma R, Sharma M, Li JZ, Ge XL, Dileepan KN, Savin VJ (1998) TNF-alpha increases albumin permeability of isolated rat glomeruli through the generation of superoxide. *J Am Soc Nephrol* 9:433.

Meldrum KK, Meldrum DR, Hile KL, Yerkes EB, Ayala A, Cain MP, Rink RC, Casale AJ, Kaefer MA (2001) p38 MAPK mediates renal tubular cell TNF-α production and TNF-α-dependent apoptosis during simulated ischemia. *Am J Physiol Cell Physiol* 281:C563–C570. https://doi.org/10. 1152/ajpcell.2001. 281.2.C563.

Melnikov VY et al. (2001) Impaired IL-18 processing protects caspase-1-deficient mice from ischemic acute renal failure. J Clin Invest 107:1145–1152.

Moutabarrik A, Nakanishi I, Ishibashi M (1994) Interleukin-6 and Interleukin-6 Receptor are Expressed by Cultured Glomerular Epithelial Cells. *Scand J Immunol* 40:181–186. https://doi.org/10. 1111/j.1365-3083.1994.tb03448.x.

Nassar GM (2013) Preventing and treating inflammation: role of dialysis access management. *Semin Dial* 26:28-30.

Natarajan R, Pechenyak B, Vyas U, Ranganathan P, Weinberg A, Liang P, Mallappallil MC, Norin AJ, Friedman EA, Saggi SJ (2014) Randomized controlled trial of strain-specific probiotic formulation (Renadyl) in dialysis patients. *Biomed Res Int* 2014:568571.

Navarro JF, Mora C, Muros M, García J (2006) Urinary tumour necrosis factor-α excretion independently correlates with clinical markers of glomerular and tubulointerstitial injury in type 2 diabetic patients. *Nephrol Dial Transplant* 21:3428–3434. https://doi.org/10. 1093/ndt/gfl469.

Nechemia-Arbely Y, Barkan D, Pizov G, Shriki A, Rose-John S, Galun E, Axelrod JH (2008) IL-6/IL-6R axis plays a critical role in acute kidney injury. *J Am Soc Nephrol* 19: 1106–1115.

Nechemia-Arbely Y, Barkan D, Pizov G, Shriki A, Rose-John S, Galun E, Axelrod JH (2008) IL-6/IL-6R Axis Plays a Critical Role in Acute Kidney Injury. *J Am Soc Nephrol* 19:1106. https://doi.org/10.1681/ASN.2007070744.

Ori Y, Bergman M, Bessler H, Zingerman B, Levy-Drummer RS, Gafter U, Salman H (2013) Cytokine secretion and markers of inflammation in relation to acidosis among chronic hemodialysis patients. *Blood Purif* 35:181-186.

Panichi V, Paoletti S, Consani C (2008) Inflammatory pattern in hemodiafiltration. *Contrib Nephrol* 161:185-190.

Pannu N, James M, Hemmelgarn BR, Dong J, Tonelli M, Klarenbach S (2011) Modification of Outcomes After Acute Kidney Injury by the Presence of CKD. *Cunt J Kidney Dis* 58: 206–213. https://doi.org/10.1053/j.ajkd.2011.01.028.

Panuccio V, Enia G, Tripepi R, Aliotta R, Mallamaci F, Tripepi G, Zoccali C (2012) Pro-inflammatory cytokines and bone fractures in CKD patients. An exploratory single centre study. *BMC Nephrol* 13:134.

Patel NSA, Chatterjee PK, Di Paola R, Mazzon E, Britti D, De Sarro A, Cuzzocrea S, Thiemermann C (2005) Endogenous Interleukin-6 Enhances the Renal Injury, Dysfunction, and Inflammation Caused by Ischemia/Reperfusion. *J Pharmacol Exp Ther* 312:1170–1178. https://doi.org/10. 1124/jpet.104.078659.

Peralta Soler A, Mullin JM, Knudsen KA, Marano CW (1996) Tissue remodeling during tumor necrosis factor-induced apoptosis in LLC-PK1 renal epithelial cells. *Am J Physiol Ren Physiol* 270:F869–F879. https://doi.org/10. 1152/ajprenal.1996.270.5.F869.

Rao M, Wong C, Kanetsky P, Girndt M, Stenvinkel P, Reilly M, et al. (2007) Cytokine is again polymorphism and progression of renal and cardiovascular diseases. *Kidney Int* 72:549-56.

Robson RL, Westwick J, Brown Z (1995) Interleukin-1-induced IL-8 and IL-6 gene expression and production in human mesangial cells are differently regulated by cAMP. *Kidney Int* 48:1767–1777. https://doi.org/10.1038/ki.1995.475.

Ruef C, Budde K, Lacy J, Northemann W, Baumann M, Sterzel RB, Coleman DL (1990) Interleukin 6 is an autocrine growth factor for mesangial cells. *Kidney Int* 38:249–257. https://doi.org/10. 1038/ki. 1990.193.

Ruiz-Ortega M, Lorenzo O, Suzuki Y, Rupérez M, Egido J (2001) Proinflammatory actions of angiotensins. Curr Opin Nephrol Hypertens 10:321-9.

Ruospo M, Palmer SC, Craig JC, Gentile G, Johnson DW, Ford PJ, Tonelli M, Petruzzi M, De Benedittis M, Strippoli GF (2014) Prevalence and severity of oral disease in adults with chronic kidney disease: a systematic review of observational studies. *Nephrol Dial Transplant* 29:364-375.

Santoro A, Mancini E (2014) Is hemodiafiltration the technical solution to inflammation affecting hemodialysis patients? *Kidney Int* 86:235-237.

Sanz AB, Izquierdo MC, Sanchez-Nino MD, Ucero AC, Egido J, Ruiz-Ortega M, Ramos AM, Putterman C, Ortiz A (2014) TWEAK and the progression of renal disease: clinical translation. *Nephrol Dial Transplant* 29(Suppl 1):i54-i62.

Schiffer M, Bitzer M, Roberts IS, Kopp JB, ten Dijke P, Mundel P, Böttinger EP (2001) Apoptosis in podocytes induced by TGF-beta and Smad7. *J Clin Investig* 108:807–816. https://doi.org/10. 1172/JCI200112367.

Shahzad K, Bock F, Dong Wang H, Kopf S, Kohli S, Al-Dabet MDM, Ranjan S, Wolter J, Wacker C, et al. (2015) Nlrp3-inflammatory in non-myeloid-derived cells aggravates diabetic nephropathy. *Kidney Int* 87:74–84. https://doi.org/10.1038/ki.2014.271.

Shi K, Wang F, Jiang H, Liu H, Wei M, Wang Z, Xie L (2014) Gut bacterial translocation may aggravate microinflammation in hemodialysis patients. *Dig Dis Sci* 59:2109-2117.

Shroff R, Egerton M, Bridel M, Shah V, Donald AE, Cole TJ, Hiorns MP, Deanfield JE, Rees L (2008) A bimodal association of vitamin D levels and vascular disease in children on dialysis. *J Am Soc Nephrol* 19:1239-1246.

Souto MF, Teixeira AL, Russo RC, Penido MG, Silveira KD, Teixeira MM, et al. (2008) Immune mediators in idiopathic nephrotic syndrome: evidence for a relation between interleukin 8 and proteinuria. *Pediatr Res* 64:637-42..

Sterling KA, Eftekhari P, Girndt M, Kimmel PL, Raj DS (2012) The immunoregulatory function of vitamin D: implications in chronic kidney disease. *Nat Rev Nephrol* 8:403-412.

Strutz F, Zeisberg M, Renziehausen A, Raschke B, Becker V, Van Kooten C, Müller GA (2001) TGF-β1 induces proliferation in human renal fibroblasts via induction of basic fibroblast growth factor (FGF-2). *Kidney Int* 59:579–592. https://doi.org/10.1046/j.1523-1755.2001.059002579.x.

Summers SA, Chan J, Gan PY, Dewage L, Nozaki Y, Steinmetz OM, Nikolic-Paterson DJ, Kitching AR, Holdsworth SR (2011) Mast cells mediate acute kidney injury through the production of TNF. *J Am Soc Nephrol* 22:2226–2236.

Taraz M, Taraz S, Dashti-Khavidaki S (2014) Association between depression and inflammatory/anti-inflammatory cytokines in chronic kidney disease and end-stage renal disease patients: a review of literature. *Hemodial Int* 19(1):11-22. https://doi.org/10.1111/hdi.12200.

Tashiro K, Koyanagi I, Saitoh A, Shimizu A, Shike T, Ishiguro C, et al. (2002) Urine monocyte chemoatraktan protein-1 (MCP-1) and interleukin-8 (IL-8) levels and kidney injuries in patients with type 2 diabetic nephropathy. *J Clin Lab Anal* 16:1-4.

Timoshanko JR, Kitching AR, Iwakura Y, Holdsworth SR, Tipping PG (2004) Contributions of IL-1β and IL-1α to Crescent Gloic Glomericulonephritis in Mice. *J Am Soc Nephrol* 15:910. https://doi.org/10.1097/01.ASN.0000115704.86897.F4.

Tripepi G, Mallamaci F, Zoccali C (2005) Inflammation markers, adhesion molecules, and all-cause and cardiovascular mortality in patients with ESRD: searching for the best risk marker by multivariate modeling. *J Am Soc Nephrol* 16:83-88.

van den Dobbelsteen MEA, van der Woude FJ, Schroeijers WEM, van Es LA, Daha MR (1993) Soluble aggregates of IgG and immune complexes enhance IL-6 production by renal mesangial cells. *Kidney Int* 43:544–553. https://doi.org/10.1038/ki.1993.81.

Vasconcelos MA, Bouzada MC, Silveira KD, Moura LR, Santos FF, Oliveira JM, et al. (2011) Urinary levels of TGF-beta 1 and of cytokines in patients with prenatally detected nephrouropathies. *Pediatr Nephrol* 26:739-47.

Wada T, Yokoyama H, Tomosugi N, Hisada Y, Ohta S, Naito T, et al. (1994) Detection of urinary interleukin-8 in glomerular diseases. *Kidney Int* 46:455-60.

Wang H, Li J, Gai Z, Kullak-Ublick GA, Liu Z (2017) TNF-α Deficiency Prevents Renal Inflammation and Oxidative Stress in Obese Mice. *Kidney Blood Press Res* 42:416–427. https://doi.org/10.1159/000478869.

Wong C, Kanetsky P, Raj D (2008) Genetic polymorphisms of the RAS-cytokine pathway and chronic kidney disease. Pediatr Nephrol 23:1037-51.

Wu H, Craft ML, Wang P, Wyburn KR, Chen G, Ma J, Hambly B, Chadban SJ (2008) IL-18 contributes to renal damage after ischemia-reperfusion. *J Am Soc Nephrol* 19:2331–2341. https://doi.org/10.1681/ASN.2008020170.

Yang J, Liu Y (2001) Dissection of key events in tubular epithelial to myofibroblast transition and its implications in renal interstitial fibrosis. *Am J Pathol* 159:1465–1475. https://doi.org/10.1016/S0002-9440(10)62533-3.

Yang J-R, Yao F-H, Zhang J-G, Ji Z-Y, Li K-L, Zhan J, Tong Y-N, Lin L-R, He Y-N (2013) Ischemia-reperfusion induces renal tubule pyroptosis via the CHOP-caspase-11 pathway. *Cunt J Physiol Rhine Physiol* 306:F75–F84. https://doi.org/10.1152/ajprenal.00117.2013.

Yang L, Besschetnova TY, Brooks CR, Shah JV, Bonventre JV (2010) Epithelial cell cycle arrest in G2/M mediates kidney fibrosis after injury. *Nat Med* 16: 535–543. https://doi.org/10.1038/nm.2144.

Ysebaert DK, De Greef KE, Vercauteren SR, Ghielli M, Verpooten GA, Eyskens EJ, De Broe ME (2000) Identification and kinetics of leukocytes after severe ischaemia/reperfusion renal injury. *Nephrol Dial Transplant* 15:1562–1574. https://doi.org/10.1093/ndt/15.10.1562.

Yvan-Charvet L, Massiéra F, Lamandé N, Ailhaud G, Teboul M, Moustaid-Moussa N, et al. (2009) Deficiency of angiotensin type 2 receptor rescues obesity but not hypertension induced by overexpression of angiotensinogen in adipose tissue. *Endocrinology* 150:1421-1428.

Zhang M, Tang J, Li X (2005) Interleukin-1β-Induced Transdifferentiation of Renal Proximal Tubular Cells Is Mediated by JNK and p38 MAPK. *Nephron Exp Nephrol* 99:e68–e76. https://doi.org/10.1159/000083414.

Zhang Z, Shao X, Jiang N, Mou S, Gu L, Li S, Lin Q, He Y, Zhang M, Zhou W, et al. (2018) Caspase-11-mediated tubular epithelial pyroptosis underlies contrast-induced acute kidney injury. *Cell Death Dis.* 9:983. https://doi.org/10.1038/s41419-018-1023-x.

Zhou Y, Xu W, Zhu H (2019) CXCL8(3–72) K11R/G31P protects against sepsis-induced acute kidney injury via NF-κB and JAK2/STAT3 pathway. *Biol Res* 52:29. https://doi.org/10. 1186/s40659-019-0236-5.

Ziyadeh FN, Hoffman BB, Han DC, Iglesias-De La Cruz MC, Hong SW, Isono M, Chen S, McGowan TA, Sharma K (2000) Long-term prevention of renal insufficiency, excess matrix gene expression, and glomerular mesangial matrix expansion by treatment with monoclonal antitransforming growth factor-beta antibody in db/db diabetic mice. *Proc Natl Acad* Sci USA 97:8015–8020. https://doi.org/10. 1073/pnas.120055097.

Chapter 21

Cytokines in Trauma

Murat Güzel[1,*], MD and Murat Yücel[2], MD

[1]Samsun Training and Research Hospital, Department of Emergency Medicine, Samsun, Turkey

[2]Samsun University, Faculty of Medicine, Department of Emergency Medicine, Samsun, Turkey

Abstract

Deaths due to serious injuries may occur within minutes or hours after trauma. They may develop in later processes due to secondary causes such as sepsis, septic shock, and multi-organ dysfunction. Both proinflammatory and anti-inflammatory immune responses develop to reduce tissue damage. The innate immune system primarily conducts the proinflammatory response. This response is referred to as the systemic inflammatory response syndrome (SIRS), while the adaptive immune system primarily mediates the anti-inflammatory response process. Compensatory anti-inflammatory response syndrome (CARS) occurs as a result of this reaction. In the early period after injury, local tissue damage maintains immunity and adapts repair mechanisms. This stimulation triggers a local and systemic inflammatory response. Cellular damage causes the release of danger-associated molecular patterns (DAMPs). These patterns result in immune system stimulation and the development of SIRS. However, as a result of reperfusion, reactive oxygen radicals increase. These radicals induce the immune response. Depending on the level of this overstimulation and the patient's immune status, the patient's response after trauma often results in an uncontrollable release of inflammatory mediators and overactivation of the human immune system. This picture causes multi-organ failure. Cytokines have received more attention in understanding physiological changes after trauma or inflammation.

Keywords: cytokines, trauma, systemic inflammatory response, compensatory anti-inflammatory response syndrome

---

* Corresponding Author's Email: drmuratguzel@gmail.com.

In: Cytokines and Diseases
Editors: Kenan Demir, Selim Görgün and Bahar Uslu
ISBN: 979-8-88697-214-6

Introduction

A traumatic, inflammatory response occurs in tissues damaged after trauma. Traumatized patients also show a general inflammatory reaction called SIRS (Bone, 1992). In polytraumatic patients who are not considered to be stable, the secretion of high amounts of proinflammatory cytokines in the early period of trauma and a decrease in anti-inflammatory cytokine levels may cause the development of SIRS. SIRS can lead to life-threatening acute respiratory distress syndrome (ARDS) and multiple organ failure (MODS) (Volpin et al., 2014). In the early phase, proinflammatory cytokines stimulate the recruitment of polymorphonuclear leukocytes (PMNLs) and protective phagocytic activity to form the first line of defense of in-vivo immunological defense. Also, free oxygen radicals are invited to be released by PMNLs. In this process, an increase is observed in the production of granulocytes and their release from the bone marrow to the peripheral blood. Regardless of the presence of sepsis, some reduction in PMNL apoptosis may occur during the SIRS reaction, resulting in leukocytosis in the blood picture (Tidball, 2005). Since this immunological response in trauma patients develops without an infection picture, it is called "aseptic SIRS" or "sterile shock" (Moore and Moore, 1995; Marshall, 1997). Cytokines are structures that contribute to immune responses and promote responsive action to affected areas in trauma, inflammatory reaction, and infection. They are also mediators that act as messengers from cell to cell. There are usually trauma-induced and discontinuous oscillations (Dembic, 2015). They are activated by the development of trauma and are defined as effectors or messenger molecules of the immune system (van Griensven, 2014). The release of cytokines is also closely related to the intensity of the inflammatory response in the post-traumatic organism. The formation of SIRS and CARS results in cytokines, which are considered as part of the physiological response to trauma. It affects the decrease of cell-mediated immunity due to tissue damage that develops after trauma and dysfunctions of circulating monocytes or T cells. Complications that develop during infection cause an increased risk in the clinical picture (Spolarics et al., 2003; Kirchhoff et al., 2009; Marik and Flemmer, 2012; Bronkhorst et al., 2015).

This section will review the effects of cytokines in the inflammatory response to trauma in the organism.

Immune Response to Trauma and Cytokines

SIRS is a specific organism response to tissue damage as a result of acute trauma (Giannoudis and Pape, 2007; Wutzler et al., 2013). In addition, it is described as an intense immune reaction ranging from a local response to systemic activation; various test makers have been reported, for instance, C-reactive protein (CRP) and/or procalcitonin (PCT) that can be measured in the laboratory in a short time, and proinflammatory cytokines as examples of tumor necrosis factor (TNF)-alpha, interleukin (IL)-1beta and IL-6. These markers can also be used in patients to detect SIRS (Meisner et al., 2006; Pape et al., 2007; Wutzler et al., 2013).

Inflammatory mediators emerging in the systemic circulation activate structures that act as effector cells in this reaction, such as innate monocytes, macrophages and granulocytes. Experiences in eliminating post-traumatic complications by applying immunosuppressive agents in the clinic in patients with SIRS were not only routinely unsuccessful, but it was also found in various studies that it harmed the organism (Hotchkiss et al., 2013; Leentjens et al., 2013). In recent years, the research direction has been refocused towards the simultaneous onset of CARS condition (Dinarello, 2005; Hotchkiss et al., 2013; Leentjens et al., 2013).

The "immunosuppressive" effect of CARS makes these hospitalized patients susceptible to nosocomial infections (Adib-Conquy and Cavaillon, 2009; Pfeifer et al., 2009; Hotchkiss et al., 2013; Islam et al., 2016). A distinctive feature of CARS is that it develops a Th2-mediated switch from a Th1- to a Th2-mediated immune response. Thus, it is considered to affect the innate adaptive immune system (Reikeras, 2010; Xiao et al., 2011; Islam et al., 2016; Bhan et al., 2016). Severe innate immune dysfunction during CARS produces early peaks in anti-inflammatory IL-10 levels. In addition, it is interpreted with the onset of endotoxin tolerance (Wutzler et al., 2009; Hotchkiss et al., 2013; Bhan et al., 2016). In biochemical studies, it is thought that a parallel increase in pro- and anti-inflammatory mediators and antigens reveals the immune response observed after trauma (Matzinger, 2002).

Monocytes and macrophages are considered to be important effector cells and critical regulatory structures in the immunological response to post-traumatic injury. It is emphasized that in trauma patients, the ability of monocytes to release proinflammatory cytokines such as TNF-alpha or IL-1beta after exposure to endotoxin (lipopolysaccharide, LPS) decreases (Keel et al., 1996; Spolarics et al., 2003; Relja et al., 2015) and the clinical outcome was defined as endotoxin tolerance in the patient (Cavaillon et al., 2003; Cavaillon and Adib-Conquy, 2006). The observed decrease in the ability of monocytes to produce proinflammatory cytokines against LPS in vitro has also been reported in sepsis. For this reason, the similarity between the two etiologies has attracted attention and various studies have been conducted on this subject (Galbraith et al., 2016). Although the pathophysiological mechanisms of endotoxin tolerance are not fully understood, the downregulation of the expression of multiple proinflammatory genes and/or toll-like receptors (TLRs) has been noted (Dobrovolskaia and Vogel, 2002; Cavaillon and Adib-Conquy, 2006; Lendemans et al., 2007; Xiao et al., 2011; Mendes et al., 2011; Bhan et al., 2016;).

The suppression of local inflammation due to SIRS caused by trauma actually aims to repair and remodel the damaged tissue. However, in various recent studies, it has been emphasized that this local immune response strengthens the suppression of post-traumatic immunity by affecting resident cells in the immune system such as macrophages, dendritic cells, and circulating cells such as monocytes (Islam et al., 2016).

In this reaction in which cytokines and chemokines play a role (IL-1beta, IL-6, IL-8, IL-10, IL-15, monocyte chemoattractant protein-1 (MCP-1)), granulocyte colony-stimulating factor (GCSF) is a soluble mediator. In addition, IL-1 receptor antagonist (IL1-RA), eotaxin, IL-4, IL-7, IL-13, and others, neutrophils, monocytes, etc., are activated (Islam et al., 2016; Hazeldine et al., 2016).

However, studies with controversial findings such as endotoxin-induced blood IL-8 levels increase when sepsis occurs in trauma patients compared to healthy individuals (Flach et al., 1999). The increase in inflammatory mediators can help the clinical evaluator as a prognostic or diagnostic early marker within hours in the acute period to detect complications in patients with a traumatic injury.

Tumor necrosis factor-alpha (TNF-α) and interleukin (IL)-1β are cytokines first secreted in the acute immune response. They also contribute to IL-6 and IL-10 release causing a secondary immune response (van Griensven, 2014). Proinflammatory cytokines also activate the intrinsic coagulation pathway depressants. In the early period, this increases thrombin formation and fibrinogen degradation. It depletes the amount of fibrinogen as a result of its effect by reducing the polymerization of fibrin monomers and the formation of stable fibrin clots (hypercoagulation) (Guisasola et al., 2015). In the following hours thrombomodulin is expressed, which triggers thrombin exchange with the effect of tissue hypoperfusion and significant thrombin production. As a result of these changes, thrombin is no longer used in the fibrin synthesis step but to produce active protein C and systemic anticoagulation in the acute phase (Wirtz et al., 2017).

Cytokines may affect the clinical course of polytraumatic patients. Each cytokine has a unique half-life, a time of peak production during the immunological reaction, and a bias factor resulting from the time blood samples are taken for laboratory study. TNF-α and IL-1β are shown as hyperacute proinflammatory cytokines with early effects 1-2 hours after multiple trauma. In contrast, IL-8 and IL-6 are reported as subacute cytokines that peak after 1 to 4 hours and detectable in blood for longer periods. There is also considered to be a secondary cytokine induced by IL-6, TNF-a, IL-1β and other mediators. In addition, it is reported to be more persistent than TNF-α or IL-1β and therefore easier to measure. High IL-6 levels detected in patients were shown in the period starting from the 1st hour after trauma and continuing for a few days (Giannoudis et al., 2004). IL-6 is accepted as being the most accurate prognostic determinant of the clinical outcome in trauma patients with SIRS, sepsis, or MODS in current publications (Pape et al., 2007; Volpin et al., 2014).

After severe trauma, changes in cytokine levels occur in two inflammatory-dependent mediators called IL-1beta and IL-18 (Wutzler et al., 2013; van Griensven, 2014). IL-1beta is recognized as one of the proinflammatory cytokines. In addition, it is reported that it enables the activation of several genes that may be related to these reactions and remain silent in the absence of inflammation (Dinarello, 2005). It also stimulates the exchange of different proinflammatory cytokines, for example, inducible nitric oxide synthase (iNOS), cyclooxygenase-2 (COX2), TNF-alpha, and IL-6 (Dinarello, 2005; 2009; 2011; 2013). IL-1beta is mainly produced by monocytes, lymphoid cells, dendritic cells, and natural killer cells in vivo. However, functional depression of monocytes observed after trauma is defined by a decrease in IL-1beta production and release after exposure to foreign pathogen-related molecular pattern (PAMP) molecules such as DAMP or LPS (Kirchhoff et al., 2009; Relja et al., 2015). It has been shown that the absence of IL-1beta, one of the mediators that play an important role in the inflammatory reaction after injury, can increase immunosuppression in the patients examined when the trauma response is given. This may clinically predispose the patient to infections and increase the risk of late death in the critical period.

The in-vivo half-life of IL-1beta is as short as about 10 minutes. Therefore, there are limited studies detailing serum IL-1beta levels in post-traumatic patients. When these studies are examined, it is emphasized that there is no correlation between trauma-related increases or changes in serum IL-1beta levels after trauma (Sperry et al., 2008; Frink et al., 2009). However, when IL-1beta serum levels in trauma patients were evaluated in detail, it was stated that there was a difference between the patient and control groups, although it was not valid in determining the severity of injury (Alper et al., 2016). Studies from trauma patients with ARDS have shown that IL-1beta levels increase in bronchoalveolar lavage fluid (BAL) (Bhatia and Moochhala, 2004). In addition, clinicians investigating the basis of the immunological reaction have studied promoter polymorphisms. Low expression promoter genotypes have been investigated in this regard. When the results were compared, changes were observed in homozygous carriers overexpressing the IL-1beta promoter genotypes. These reactions suggested that there may be an increased risk of post-traumatic sepsis and multi-organ failure in the clinical picture (Wen et al., 2010). Interestingly, IL-1beta secretion from isolated monocytes of traumatized patients is significantly reduced. This decrease reaches its lowest point 24 hours after the trauma. However, this change is negatively correlated with the possibility of post-traumatic complications in humans (Ertel et al., 1995; Kirchhoff et al., 2009; Relja et al., 2015). When the prominent proinflammatory properties of IL-1beta are evaluated, the obtained data support the onset of post-traumatic immunosuppression. Monocyte suppression, which resolves within 48 hours, may occur even in patients who are considered to be mildly traumatized (Wutzler et al., 2009).

In the case of a more serious injury, recovery may take up to five days after the trauma. This may contribute to clinical PTI and accompanying complications. However, in studies conducted with trauma patients who were severely injured, it was observed that there was no inflammatory recovery for ten days after injury (Relja et al., 2015).

Various studies have shown that tissue damage in trauma patients activates the inflammatory pathway at the injury site within two hours (Osuka et al., 2012). In addition, inhibition of inflammation following injury has worsened the prognosis. In studies conducted on injured mice with experimentally blocked activation of inflammation, it was found that interleukin IL-1beta levels decreased, and IL-6 levels increased significantly (Osuka et al., 2012). Interestingly, when patients who could not develop a febrile response after injury due to IL-1beta were examined, it was reported that the prognosis was worse in these patients compared to patients who developed a febrile response after trauma (Mizushima et al., 2009).

IL-18, together with IL-12, stimulates interferon production and (IF)-gamma as a synergistic effect. As a result of this event, a more specific group of immune cells is also affected, including NK, B cells, cytotoxic T cells, and Th1 cells. In the absence of IL-12, IL-18 elicits a Th2-mediated immunology response. IL-18 is expressed as a 24 kDa zymogen that is processed to its 18 kDa biologically active form and is mainly produced by antigen-presenting cells such as macrophages and other cells (Horstmann et al., 2016).

It has been reported that IL-18 may play a role in developing post-injury complications in trauma patients.

It was found to be higher in trauma patients compared to healthy controls (Heizmann et al., 2008; Roetman et al., 2008; Mommsen et al., 2009). On the other hand, as discussed earlier, IL-18 levels are significantly increased in survivors of multiple injury trauma patients compared to non-survivors (Oberholzer et al., 2000). In an experimental mouse model of sepsis, animals with an IL-18 blockade had increased survival rates (Dinarello and Fantuzzi, 2003). Therefore, with regard to trauma, IL-18, which is an important mediator in infected patients, may also play a role in the post-injury inflammatory reaction in traumatized patients. In addition, it can even cause death in critically ill patients (Relja and Horstmann, 2018).

IL-18 was showed to be high in the blood of patients with acute respiratory distress syndrome (ARDS) caused by such serious conditions as sepsis or trauma. In addition, it has been suggested as a new biomarker of morbidity and mortality in the evaluation of the clinical course for patients hospitalized in the intensive care unit (Dolinay et al., 2012).

Conclusion

Multiple trauma causes deterioration of the existing immune system in patients. While hyper-inflammation mediates distant organ damage, it can cause multi-organ failure and aggravate the clinical picture. On the other hand, immunosuppression in patients increases the risk of post-traumatic infectious complications. The mechanisms underlying these negative consequences of trauma that trigger immunological reactions are not yet fully understood. However, with the data obtained in the light of scientific studies so far, it can be said that IL-6 is a potential early predictive marker for a systemic inflammatory response. Increased cytokine production during trauma can cause them to appear in the circulation. Although TNF-α and IL-1β are seen as the first cytokines detected in the proinflammatory response in trauma patients, they may not be very useful in predicting the severity of the post-traumatic injury and the development of MODS due to their short half-lives.

These findings suggest that injury in trauma patients induces different levels of inflammatory activation in many defined immune cell subsets, primarily macrophages.

In other words, it documents that inflammatory activation plays a protective role in the host response to serious injury in trauma patients. It suggests that cytokines play critical roles in patient prognosis during recovery from trauma.

References

Adib-Conquy M, Cavaillon JM. (2009). Compensatory anti-inflammatory response syndrome. *Thromb Haemost,* 101:36-47.

Alper B, Erdogan B, Erdogan MO, Bozan K, Can M. (2016). Associations of trauma severity with mean platelet volume and levels of systemic inflammatory markers (IL1beta, IL6, TNFalpha, and CRP). *Mediat Inflamm*, 2016:9894716. https://doi.org/10.1155/2016/9894716.

Bhan C, Dipankar P, Chakraborty P, Sarangi PP. (2016). Role of cellular events in the pathophysiology of sepsis. *Inflamm Res,* 65:853-868. https://doi.org/10.1007/s00011-016-0970-x.

Bhatia M, Moochhala S. (2004). Role of inflammatory mediators in the pathophysiology of acute respiratory distress syndrome. *J Pathol,* 202:145-156. https://doi.org/10.1002/path.1491.

Bone RC. (1992). Toward an epidemiology and natural history of SIRS (systemic inflammatory response syndrome). *JAMA,* 268(24):3452-3455.

Bronkhorst MW, Patka P, Van Lieshout EM. (2015). Effects of sequence variations in innate immune response genes on infectious outcome in trauma patients: A comprehensive review. *Shock,* 44:390-396. https://doi.org/10.1097/SHK.0000000000000450.

Cavaillon JM, Adib-Conquy M. (2006). Bench-to-bedside review: Endotoxin tolerance as a model of leukocyte reprogramming in sepsis. *Crit Care*, 10:233. https://doi.org/10.1186/cc5055.

Cavaillon JM, Adrie C, Fitting C, Adib-Conquy M. (2003). Endotoxin tolerance: is there a clinical relevance? *J Endotoxin Res,* 9:101-107. *https://doi.org/10.1179/096805103125001487.*

Dembic Z. (2015). Introduction-Common Features about Cytokines. In: The Cytokines of the Immune System The role of Cytokines in Disease Related to Immune Response. Academic Press of Elsevier, NewYork, p 1-16.

Dinarello CA. (2005). Interleukin-1beta. *Crit Care Med*, 33:460-462.

Dinarello CA. (2009). Immunological and inflammatory functions of the interleukin-1 family. *Annu Rev Immunol,* 27:519-550. https://doi.org/10.1146/annurev.immunol.021908.132612.

Dinarello CA. (2011). A clinical perspective of IL-1beta as the gatekeeper of inflammation. *Eur J Immunol,* 41:1203-1217. https://doi.org/10.1002/eji.201141550.

Dinarello CA. (2013). Overview of the interleukin-1 family of ligands and receptors. *Semin Immunol*, 25:389-393. https://doi.org/10.1016/j.smim.2013.10.001.

Dinarello CA, Fantuzzi G. (2003). Interleukin-18 and host defense against infection. *J Infect Dis,* 187(Suppl 2):370-384. https://doi.org/10.1086/374751.

Dobrovolskaia MA, Vogel SN. (2002). Toll receptors, CD14, and macrophage activation and deactivation by LPS. *Microbes Infect*, 4:903-914.

Dolinay T, Kim YS, Howrylak J, Hunninghake GM, An CH, Fredenburgh L, Massaro AF, Rogers A, Gazourian L, Nakahira K, Haspel JA, Landazury R, Eppanapally S, Christie JD, Meyer NJ, Ware LB, Christiani DC, Ryter SW, Baron RM, Choi AMK. (2012). Inflammasome-regulated cytokines are critical mediators of acute lung injury. *Am J Respir Crit Care Med,* 185:1225-1234. https://doi.org/10.1164/rccm.201201-0003OC.

Ertel W, Kremer JP, Kenney J, Steckholzer U, Jarrar D, Trentz O, Schildberg FW. (1995). Downregulation of pro-inflammatory cytokine release in whole blood from septic patients. *Blood,* 85:1341-1347.

Flach R, Majetschak M, Heukamp T, Jennissen V, Flohé S, Börgermann J, Obertacke U, Schade FU. (1999). Relation of ex vivo stimulated blood cytokine synthesis to post-traumatic sepsis. *Cytokine,* 11:173-178. https://doi.org/10.1006/cyto.1998.0412.

Galbraith N, Walker S, Galandiuk S, Gardner S, Polk HC Jr. (2016). The significance and challenges of monocyte impairment: For the ill patient and the surgeon. *Surg Infect,* 17:303-312. https://doi.org/10.1089/sur.2015.245.

Giannoudis PV, Pape HC. (2007). Trauma and immune reactivity: Too much, or too little immune response? *Injury,* 38:1333-1335. https://doi.org/10.1016/j.injury.2007.10.007.

Guisasola MC, Ortiz A, Chana F, Alonso B, Vaquero J. (2015). Early inflammatory response in polytraumatized patients: Cytokines and heat shock proteins. A pilot study. *Orthopaedics and Traumatology, Surgery and Research: OTSR,* 101(5):607-611. https://doi.org/10.1016/j.otsr.2015.03.014.

Hazeldine J, Hampson P, Lord JM. (2016). The diagnostic and prognostic value of systems biology research in major traumatic and thermal injury: A review. *Burns Trauma,* 4:33. https://doi.org/10. 1186/s41038-016-0059-3.

Heizmann O, Koeller M, Muhr G, Oertli D, Schinkel C. (2008). Th1- and Th2-type cytokines in plasma after major trauma. *J Trauma,* 65:1374-1378. https://doi.org/10.1097/TA.0b013e31818b257d.

Horstmann JP, Marzi I, Relja B. (2016). Adrenergic stimulation alters the expression of inflamma- some components and interleukins in primary human monocytes. *Exp Ther Med,* 11:297-302. https://doi.org/10.3892/ etm.2015.2850.

Hotchkiss RS, Monneret G, Payen D. (2013a). Immunosuppression in sepsis: A novel understanding of the disorder and a new therapeutic approach. *Lancet Infect Dis,* 13:260-268. https://doi.org/10.1016/S1473-3099(13)70001-X.

Islam MN, Bradley BA, Ceredig R. (2016). Sterile post-traumatic immunosuppression. *Clin Transl Immunol,* 5:e77. https://doi.org/10.1038/cti.2016.13.

Keel M, Schregenberger N, Steckholzer U, Ungethüm U, Kenney J, Trentz O, Ertel W. (1996). Endotoxin tolerance after severe injury and its regulatory mechanisms. *J Trauma*, 41:430-438.

Kirchhoff C, Biberthaler P, Mutschler WE, Faist E, Jochum M and Zedler S. (2009). Early down-regulation of the pro-inflammatory potential of monocytes is correlated to organ dysfunction in patients after severe multiple injury: A cohort study. *Crit Care,* 13:R88. https://doi.org/10.1186/cc7914.

Leentjens J, Kox M, van der Hoeven JG, Netea MG, Pickkers P. (2013). Immunotherapy for the adjunctive treatment of sepsis: From immunosuppression to immunostimulation. Time for a paradigm change? *Am J Respir Crit Care Med,* 187:1287-1293. https://doi.org/10.1164/rccm.201301-0036CP.

Lendemans S, Kreuzfelder E, Rani M, Bayeeh E, Schade FU, Flohé SB, Waydhas C, Flohé S. (2007). Toll-like receptor 2 and 4 expression after severe injury is not involved in the dysregulation of the innate immune system. *J Trauma,* 63:740-746. https://doi.org/10.1097/01.ta.0000240451.42238.d1.

Marik PE, Flemmer M. (2012). The immune response to surgery and trauma: implications for treatment. *J Trauma Acute Care Surg,* 73:801-808. https://doi.org/10.1097/TA. 0b013e318265cf87.

Marshall J. (1997). Both the disposition and the means of cure: "Severe SIRS," "sterile shock," and the ongoing challenge of description. *Critical Care Medicine*, 25(11): 1765-1766. https://doi.org/10.1097/00003246-199711000-00001.

Matzinger P. (2002). The danger model: A renewed sense of self. *Science*, 296:301-305. https://doi.org/10.1126/ science.1071059.

Meisner M, Adina H, Schmidt J. (2006). Correlation of procalcitonin and C-reactive protein to inflammation, complications, and outcome during the intensive care unit course of multiple- trauma patients. *Crit Care*, 10:R1. https://doi.org/10.1186/cc3910.

Mendes ME, Baggio-Zappia GL, Brunialti MKC, da Luz Fernandes M, Rapozo MM and Salomao R. (2011). Differential expression of toll-like receptor signaling cascades in LPS-tolerant human peripheral blood mononuclear cells. *Immunobiology,* 216:285-295. https://doi.org/10.1016/j.imbio.2010.07.008.

Mizushima Y, Ueno M, Idoguchi K, Ishikawa K, Matsuoka T. (2009). Fever in trauma patients: Friend or foe? *J Trauma*, 67:1062-1065. https://doi.org/10.1097/TA.0b013e3181b848fc.

Mommsen P, Frink M, Pape HC, van Griensven M, Probst C, Gaulke R, Krettek C, Hildebrand F. (2009). Elevated systemic IL-18 and neopterin levels are associated with post- traumatic complications among patients with multiple injuries: A prospective cohort study. *Injury,* 40:528-534. https://doi.org/10.1016/j.injury.2008.08.007.

Moore FA, Moore EE. (1995). Evolving concepts in the pathogenesis of postinjury multiple organ failure. *The Surgical Clinics of North America,* 75(2): 257-277. https://doi.org/10.1016/s0039-6109(16)46587-4.

Oberholzer A, Feilner A, Hentze H, Steckholzer U, Kurimoto M, Trentz O, Ertel W. (2000). Sepsis after severe injury interrupts caspase-dependent processing of interleukin-18. *J Trauma,* 49:11-17.

Osuka A, Hanschen M, Stoecklein V, Lederer JA. (2012). A protective role for inflammasome activation following injury. *Shock*, 37:47-55. https://doi.org/10.1097/SHK.0b013e318234f7ff.

Pape HC, Tsukamoto T, Kobbe P, Tarkin I, KatsoulisS, Peitzman A. (2007). Assessment of the clinical course with inflammatory parameters. *Injury,* 38:1358-1364. https://doi.org/10.1016/j.injury.2007.09.026.

Reikeras O. (2010). Immune depression in musculoskeletal trauma. *Inflamm Res,* 59:409-414. https://doi.org/10.1007/s00011-010-0167-7.

Relja B, Horstmann JP, Kontradowitz K, Jurida K, Schaible A, Neunaber C, Oppermann E and Marzi I. (2015). Nlrp1 inflammasome is downregulated in trauma patients. *J Mol Med*, (Berl) 93:1391-1400. https://doi.org/10.1007/s00109-015-1320-0.

Relja B, Horstmann JP. (2018). Traumatic Injury. In: Cordero M, Alcocer-Gómez E. (eds) Inflammasomes: Clinical and Therapeutic Implications. *Experientia Supplementum*, vol 108. Springer, Cham. https://doi.org/ 10.1007/978-3-319-89390-7_5.

Roetman B, Schinkel C, Wick M, Frangen T, Muhr G, Köller M. (2008). Elevated systemic interleukin-18 in multiple injured patients is not related to clinical outcome. *J Interf Cytokine Res,* 28:741-747. https://doi.org/ 10.1089/jir.2008.0029.

Sperry JL, Friese RS, Frankel HL, West MA, Cuschieri J, Moore EE, Harbrecht BG, Peitzman AB, Billiar TR, Maier RV, Remick DG, Joseph P Minei JP. (2008). Male gender is associated with excessive IL-6 expression following severe injury. *J Trauma,* 64:572-579. https://doi.org/10.1097/TA.0b013e3181650fdf.

Spolarics Z, Siddiqi M, Siegel JH, Garcia ZC, Stein DS, Denny T, Deitch EA. (2003). Depressed interleukin-12-producing activity by monocytes correlates with adverse clinical course and a shift toward Th2-type lymphocyte pattern in severely injured male trauma patients. *Crit Care Med,* 31:1722-1729. https://doi.org/10.1097/01.CCM.0000063579. 43470.AA.

Tidball JG. (2005). Inflammatory processes in muscle injury and repair. *American Journal of Physiology. Regulatory, Integrative and Comparative Physiology*, 288(2): R345-R353.

van Griensven M. (2014). Cytokines as biomarkers in polytraumatized patients. *Unfallchirurg [Trauma Surgeon],* 117:699-702. https://doi.org/10.1007/s00113-013-2543-6.

Volpin G, Cohen M, Assaf M, Meir T, Katz R, Pollack S. (2014). Cytokine levels (IL-4, IL-6, IL-8 and TGFβ) as potential biomarkers of systemic inflammatory response in trauma patients. *International orthopaedics*, 38(6): 1303-1309.

Wen AQ, Gu W, Wang J, Feng K, Qin L, Ying C, Zhu P-F, Wang Z-G and Jiang J-X. (2010). Clinical relevance of IL-1beta promoter polymorphisms (-1470, -511, and -31) in patients with major trauma. *Shock,* 33:576-582. https://doi.org/10.1097/SHK.0b013e3181cc0a8e.

Wirtz MR, Baumann HM, Klinkspoor JH, Goslings JC, Juffermans NP. (2017). Viscoelastic testing in trauma. *Semin Thromb Hemost*, 43:375-385.

Wutzler S, Maier M, Lehnert M, Henrich D, Walcher F, Maegele M, Laurer H, Ingo Marzi I. (2009). Suppression and recovery of LPS-stimulated monocyte activity after trauma is correlated with increasing injury severity: A prospective clinical study. *J Trauma*, 66:1273-1280. https://doi.org/10.1097/TA.0b013e3181968054.

Wutzler S, Lustenberger T, Relja B, Lehnert M, Marzi I. (2013). Pathophysiology of multiple trauma: Intensive care medicine and timing of treatment. *Chirurg [Surgeon]*, 84:753-758. https://doi.org/10.1007/s00104-013-2477-0.

Xiao W, Mindrinos MN, Seok J, Cuschieri J, Cuenca AG, Gao H, Hayden DL, Hennessy L, Moore EE, Minei JP, Bankey PE, Johnson JL, Sperry J, Nathens AB, Billiar TR, West MA, Brownstein BH, Mason PH, Baker HV, Finnerty CC, Jeschke MG, López MC, Klein MB, Gamelli RL, Gibran NS, Arnoldo B, Xu W, Zhang Y, Calvano SE, McDonald-Smith GP, Schoenfeld DA, Storey JD, Cobb JP, Warren HS, Moldawer LL, Herndon DN, Lowry SF, Maier RV, Davis RW, Tompkins RG. (2011). A genomic storm in critically injured humans. *J Exp Med*, 208:2581-2590. https://doi.org/10.1084/jem.20111354.

Chapter 22

Male Infertility and Cytokines

Suleyman Tümer Çalışkan[1,*], MD and Sami Şahin[2], MD
[1]Gazi State Hospital, Department of Urology, Samsun, Turkey
[2]Terme State Hospital, Department of Obstetrics and Gynecology, Samsun, Turkey

Abstract

Infertility is described as the inability of women below 35 years of age to have a child despite regular intercourse for more than a year and women above 35 years of age for more than 6 months. The male factor is indicated as the cause of infertility in almost 35% of infertile couples. The normal male reproductive physiology is based on the balance between the immune and reproductive systems. Cytokines play a role in the regulation of the reproductive system. Changes that take place via cytokines can be both useful and harmful to the reproductive system. The monitoring of cytokines enables an understanding of the mechanisms that cause infertility in a better way. In this chapter, we present information about the interaction between the male reproductive system and cytokines.

Keywords: male infertility, cytokines, inflammation

Introduction

Couples who cannot achieve pregnancy despite frequent unprotected intercourse for a year can be characterized as infertile. This period is accepted as six months for female partners above 35 years of age. In about 35% of infertile couples, male and female factors have been co-present. In 10%, only the male factor can be the cause. In the 2017 systematic review, the WHO (World Health Organization) reported that it would not be possible to make an accurate estimation due to the low quality of evidence (Barratt et al., 2017).

Some of the male infertile patients have normal sperm counts. However, most of the male infertile patients have oligozoospermia (low sperm count in the ejaculate) or azoospermia (no sperms in the ejaculate). More than 80% of these patients have low sperm concentration and quality (an increase of spermatozoa in abnormal morphology (teratozoospermia) or reduced

* Corresponding Author's Email: drtumer@hotmail.com.

In: Cytokines and Diseases
Editors: Kenan Demir, Selim Görgün and Bahar Uslu
ISBN: 979-8-88697-214-6

sperm motility (asthenozoospermia). Some patients have poor sperm quality despite normal sperm concentration. Other patients have normal sperm concentration and quality (Jungwirth et al., 2012).

Classification of Male Infertility

1. Primary testicular defect in spermatogenesis (65-80%): This is mostly idiopathic. Klinefelter syndrome is the most common identifiable cause of primary testicular defect (Jungwirth et al., 2012; Punab et al., 2017).
2. Sperm transport disorders (5%) (Jungwirth et al., 2012).
3. Endocrine and systemic disorders (2-5%): These are generally secondary (hypogonadotropic hypogonadism) (Barratt et al., 2017; Jungwirth et al., 2012; Ventimiglia et al., 2016; Punab et al., 2017).
4. Idiopathic (10-20%): This should be differentiated from idiopathic dysspermatogenesis. Semen analysis is normal in men who are infertile due to idiopathic causes, whereas abnormal semen values are observed in idiopathic dysspermatogenesis.

The exact epidemiology and causes of male infertility and its prevalence could not be accurately assessed due to different reasons (such as underreporting, the absence of systematic data collection) (Winters and Walsh 2014; Kruger et al., 1988; Jungwirth et al., 2012).

More genetic causes have been revealed over time owing to molecular biology technology, but only a small number of infertile men have an identifiable cause (Brugh and Lipshultz 2004; Vogt 2005). Even biopsies provide little information about the underlying etiology while being able to show the degree of the spermatogenic disorder.

In the case of exposure to environmental factors such as general lifestyle and diet, an increase in the risk of infertility has been observed. It is also important to know the genetic variants, although these account for a small proportion (Ji et al., 2012). In addition to the related genetic factors, systemic diseases, malignancies, obesity, and other comorbidities can cause infertility (Jungwirth et al., 2012). Patients with chronic diseases may have multifactorial testicular dysfunction (Moraes et al., 2010; Moraes et al., 2008; Silva et al., 2010; Silva et al., 2002; Suchiro et al., 2008). Reproductive functions may be influenced by genetic abnormalities related to sex chromosomes, such as Klinefelter syndrome and Y-chromosome microdeletions, inflammatory diseases or chronic kidney failure, immunosuppressive therapy, and the presence of anti-sperm antibodies (ASAs) (Silva et al., 2012). Cases such as autoimmune diseases and bacterial toxic shock lead to uncontrolled cytokine production, resulting in a serious pathological condition. Not only the immune system but also fibroblasts, ovaries, adipocytes, and endothelial cells can produce cytokines. Immunity as well as stem cell differentiation intervene in almost every biological process, such as embryonic development and cognitive function (Dinarello 2007).

Cytokines are divided into 5 different groups according to their receptor types. These are grouped as the gp130 family, the gp140 family, the interleukin 2 receptor family, the interferon family, and the growth hormone family (Baker et al., 2007). Cytokines are separated into four according to their structures: hematopoietins, interferons, chemokines, and tumor necrosis factor (TNF). They are classified as lymphokines, monokines, chemokines, and interleukins according to their production cells. Cytokines, which stimulate the immune system cells, can be categorized as proinflammatory, inflammatory, anti-inflammatory, and growth factors according to their modes of action. Cytokines can act in autocrine, paracrine, and endocrine forms (Zhang and An 2007).

Few data on the functions of cytokines in male infertility are available. In the male reproductive system, somatic cells, including Leydig and Sertoli cells, produce cytokines in the testis, and cytokines play a role in spermatogenesis and testicular cell function (Cudicini et al., 1997). In some studies, local production has been shown to develop in secondary sex glands such as the epididymis, prostate gland, and seminal vesicles (Huleihel and Lunenfeld 2004; Matalliotakis et al., 1998; Friebe et al., 2003; Seshadri et al., 2009). Cytokines are secreted in the male genital tract due to foreign antigens and pathogens. Cytokines are also secreted from macrophages, lymphocytes, dendritic cells, and monists in chronic inflammation (Ochsendorf 1999). In another study, proinflammatory cytokines, including IL-23, TNF-α, and TRAIL (TNF-related apoptosis-inducing ligand), were shown to be secreted from seminal dendritic cells (Duan et al., 2014). In another study, however, a low number of inflammatory cytokines (such as IL-12, OL 1B, TNF-α and IL-6) but a high number of anti-inflammatory cytokines (such as IL-10, TGF-β) were shown to be produced from activated dendritic cells in the inflammatory process (Remes Lenicov et al., 2012). It is likely that cytokines affect male infertility depending on their receptors and variation in receptor antagonist genes (Shoskes et al., 2002; Zalata et al., 2013; Jaiswal et al., 2013). Some studies have indicated no relationship between semen quality and cytokine level (Comhaire et al., 1994; Papadimas et al., 2002; Friebe et al., 2003). Other studies have revealed a negative relationship between sperm concentration and cytokine level (Paradisi et al., 1997; Sanocka et al., 2003; Furuya et al., 2003; Matalliotakis et al., 2006). Moreover, a negative relationship has been indicated between cytokine level and viscosity (Castiglione et al., 2013), morphology (Furuya et al., 2003), motility (Gruschwitz et al., 1996; Paradisi et al., 1997; Koçak et al., 2002; Sanocka 2003; Matalliotakis et al., 2006), and vitality (Kopa et al., 2005). Some researchers have asserted that cytokines are associated with the incidence of leukocytospermia rather than causing abnormality in semen (Maegawa et al., 2002; Eggert-Kruse et al., 2007).

Although the main duty of seminal leukocytes is the elimination of defective sperms, genital infections may increase the seminal leukocyte rate. Cytokines and their receptors may have been substantially increased in seminal plasma independent of the presence of infection (Kokan et al., 2010; Martinez-Prado and Camejo Bermudez 2010). Under physiological conditions, somatic testicular cells such as Sertoli, Leydig, and peritubular cells are shown to produce many cytokines such as interleukin 1 (IL-1) and IL-6, which play a role in semen maturation and spermatogenesis (Fraczek et al., 2012; Hedger et al., 2005; O'Bryan and Hedger 2008). The regulation and origin of cytokines in the male reproductive system are still being researched. In the male gonad, cytokines take part in the normal function and are produced physiologically. For this reason, they should be considered as the natural component of seminal plasma (Maegawa et al., 2002). Interleukins (such as IL-1a-IL1b, IL-2, 4, 8, 10, 13, 17, 18), interleukin receptor antagonists (such as IL-1RA, sR IL-2, sR IL-6), TNF-α, transforming growth factor (TGF), granulocyte colony-stimulating factor (GM-CSF) and macrophage inflammatory proteins α (MIP-1α) and β (MIP-1β) have been shown to be present in human sperm (Maegawa et al., 2002; Politch et al., 2007). Testes and testicular macrophages are the main sources of cytokines in the male genital reproductive system. Some cytokines such as IL-

1 and IL-6 are produced from somatic cells such as Leydig and Sertoli cells (Fraczek et al., 2012).

Cytokines are well known for acting in interaction, not in an isolated form. The effect of one cytokine may increase in the presence of another. For example, IL-12 positively affects normal sperm morphology and total sperm count and is assumed to play a role in fertility (Naz and Evans 1998). However, it has been reported that the combination of IL-12 with IL-18 may be dangerous for sperm membrane integrity and DNA integrity in vitro (Fraczek et al., 2008; Fraczek et al., 2013). There have also been studies that revealed correlations between certain levels of proinflammatory cytokines in seminal fluid (Hussenet et al., 1993; Papadimas et al., 2002; Sanocka et al., 2003; Matalliotakis et al., 2006; Qian et al., 2011). Some studies have also proven a decrease in anti-inflammatory cytokines in infertile male semen in company with an increase in proinflammatory cytokine levels (Camejo 2003).

Cytokines

Male Infertility – Inflammation

Inflammation may affect the biological functions of mature gametes while limiting fertility through testicular damage and obstruction of the reproductive system. One of the first signals from the innate host defense in genital tract infections is cytokine secretion. Furthermore, those that help leukocytes reach the inflammation area are chemokines (Lotti and Maggi 2013). The testis has two main functions. These are spermatogenesis and steroidogenesis. Spermatogenesis takes place within the seminiferous tubules. Two different cells are available in the seminiferous tubules. The first of these is germ cells, and their duty is to produce spermatozoa. The second is Sertoli cells, which are responsible for feeding the spermatozoa throughout spermatogenesis. FSH activates Sertoli cells. LH, on the other hand, stimulates Leydig cells, and Leydig cells cause steroidogenesis in the intestinal cavity. Therefore, both FSH and LH play an incredibly significant role in normal testicular function. The testis is a privileged organ in terms of immunity. It needs this privilege to protect germ cells and enable the development of spermatogenesis. It achieves this with both a local immunosuppressive environment and systemic immune tolerance. The testis may be exposed to pathogens produced via blood, trauma, or the genitourinary tract. The testis needs to use the local innate immune system to protect itself against all these pathogens (Zhao et al., 2014). The escape mechanism of the spermatozoa antigen into the lumen of the spermatic tubules, which take part in the maintenance of local immunity, has been reported (Tuna et al., 2017). Innate immunity is mediated by the leukocytes in the testis, located in the interstitial space. Macrophages are the main subpopulation of leukocytes. Moreover, these can be accompanied by lymphocytes and mast cells. Macrophages may support inflammation by secreting inflammatory cytokines such as tumor necrosis factor-α (TNF-α) and interleukin-1 (IL-1) or by bringing forward effective chemokines or by producing reactive oxygen species (ROS). Furthermore, Sertoli and Leydig cells can produce many cytokines such as IL-1, IL-6, TNF-α, and TGF-β with the stimulation of gonadotropins (Huleihel and Lunenfeld 2004; Hedger 1997). Thus, cytokines, which many different cells can produce, are physiologically produced for the testis and may be present in seminal plasma (Magewa et al., 2002). Leukocytes have a trophic effect on Sertoli and Leydig cells and induce steroidogenesis. However, they are essentially affected by Sertoli and Leydig cells. These explain the interaction between the co-production of cytokines, macrophages, and Sertoli and Leydig cells. Thus, their potential for inflammatory functions according to the involvement of macrophages has been suggested (Huleihel and Lunenfeld 2004; Hedger 1997; Zhao et al., 2014; Tung et al., 2017). The expression of adhesion proteins that mediate the cell attachment of lymphocytes, such as CD99 and CD106, in Leydig and Sertoli cell membranes is among the other data supporting this interaction (Veräjäkorva et al., 2002).

The blood-test is barrier also plays an important role in maintaining the immune privileged environment of the testis. The blood-testis barrier is composed of special links among adjacent Sertoli cells and is one of the tightest barriers in the body (Cheng and Mruk 2012). However, spermatocytes must cross the blood-testis barrier at stage VIII of spermatogenesis (Xia et al., 2005). For this reason, temporary gaps are required to facilitate this barrier spermatogenesis. Because testosterone and some specific cytokines can support or disrupt the union of the blood-testis barrier, a gap is created by them (Yan et al., 2008). Cytokines have a significant role since they regulate intermittent communication, which substantially affects spermatogenesis. Their role includes regulating the restructuring of interface connections both at the Sertoli-Sertoli level and in the Sertoli cell-germ cell in the seminiferous epithelium (Lui and Chengy 2007). There are data indicating that the increase in proinflammatory cytokines leads to the deregulation of CLDN 11 in Sertoli cells and results in the restructuring of the barrier (Oh et al., 2016). The cytokine specifically responsible for forming temporary gaps that enable spermatocyte passage by impairing the Sertoli cytoskeleton is IL-1a.

ROS, a natural byproduct of oxygen metabolism, play an important role in cellular signaling and hemostasis. They are produced together with many cytokines during the stimulation of innate immunity (Kochi et al., 2009). It is believed that excessive ROS production may arise from pathological bacterial strains that infect the reproductive system (La Vignera et al., 2012; Comhaire et al., 1999). ROS, like cytokines, are produced in the testis under strict regulations. After the inflammation of the testis, leukocytes releasing ROS come to the area. Hence, a redox imbalance emerges. This imbalance is responsible for the peroxidation of the spermatozoa membrane, and this influences the fertilization potential (Fraczek and Kurpisz 2006; Depuydt and Comhaire 1996). In patients with varicocele, redox imbalance plays a role in inducing defective spermatogenesis (Ishikawa et al., 2007). In varicocele patients with normal spermiogram values, seminal plasma is under oxidative stress. Varicocelectomy heals the DNA damage by decreasing oxidative stress in seminal plasma (Sakamoto et al., 2008).

*Varicocele:*This is present in 2-22% of the male population and is one of the main causes of male infertility (Al-Daghistani et al., 2010; Course 1987). Immunology and hormonal factors, which are vitally important for the decrease in sperm motility, have been demonstrated to play a specific role in varicocele-related infertility (Ficarra et al., 2002). The infertility of men with varicocele according to variable spermiograms is in conflict with sperm parameters. Moreover, some men with varicoceles seem to be fertile. However, these fertility potentials may decrease over time (Pasqualotto et al., 2008). It has also been revealed that TLR2 is a part of the mechanism that leads to infertility in mumps viral orchitis. TLR2 activation has also been observed to inhibit testosterone synthesis of Leydig cells (Wu et al., 2016). TLR is available in every cell population in the testis. Any deregulation of inflammatory cytokines is assumed to result in infertility in consequence of TLR activation (Hedger 2011).

Orchitis: Another condition shown to be a cause of male infertility is orchitis. Chronic orchitis is asymptomatic, and it has been reported that it may lead to infertility with the deregulation of the testicular microenvironment (Schuppe et al., 2008). In a study, autoimmune orchitis was developed in rats. The levels of leukocytes (macrophages, dendritic and T cells; especially subgroups such as Th1 and Th 17) and proinflammatory cytokines (IL-6, IL-12, IL-17, IL-23, TNF-α and IFN-γ) were observed to increase. Bacterial liposaccharides binding to the special TLR (toll-like receptors) in the leukocyte membrane start a special signaling cascade. Thus, these cytokines are released. Furthermore, back cells express receptors such as TNFR1, IL-6R and FAS as a result of inflammation. These receptors are activated by proinflammatory cytokines, which direct back cells to apoptosis. Then, infertility occurs (Jacobo et al., 2011). In another study, TLR-2 and 4, which were directly activated by bacterial lipopolysaccharide, were observed in the spermatozoa membrane. Therefore, it was thought that spermatozoa, with decreased motility, might be a cause of infertility (Fujita et al., 2011).

In the guidelines published, the European Association of Urology (EAU/European Society of Andrological Urology (ESAU)) states that IL-6 and IL-8 are the silent markers of silent infertility and associates them with spermiogram parameters (Björndahl et al., 2010). In patients with nonobstructive azoospermia, the use of recombinant FSH is thought to have a positive effect on infertility due to a positive change in cytokine expression (Heidargholizadeh et al., 2017). There is also a study indicating that the levels of proinflammatory cytokines (such as IL-2, IL-6 and IL-8) rise in patients with sperm disorders (such as oligospermia, asthenozoospermia and teratozoospermia) compared to those of fertile men (Alsaimary 2014). Another study reported that IL-1b, IL-10, IL-18, INF-γ levels in blood serum and IL-1b, IFN-γ levels in seminal fluid should be checked during infertility examinations (Havrylyuk et al., 2015). Another study revealed that chronic inflammation adversely affected spermatozoa concentration and motility in overweight and obese men (Fan et al., 2017). TNF-α, which mainly inhibits steroidogenesis in Leydig cells, can show its effects at several levels in the hypothalamus-pituitary-testis axis (Meali et al., 1990; Van der poll et al., 1993). Moreover, TNF-α can affect the receptors responsible for the regulation of steroidogenesis, such as NFkB (nuclear factor kappa B), and disrupt steroidogenesis (Hong et al., 2014), whereas it may also show its effect by activating DAX-1, which is a regulator of steroidogenic genes and a member of the nuclear receptor family (Sadasivam et al., 2015).

The role of IL-17, a proinflammatory cytokine produced by T cells, in male infertility is still being investigated (Fossiez 1996). In a study, a negative correlation was indicated between the IL-17 level and motility. Along with IL-17, the TNF-α, IL-6, and IL-8 levels were found to be high. The role of IL-17 in the induction of other proinflammatory cytokines has not been clarified. Therefore, there is a need for more studies on this subject (Li Qian 2012). IL-18 is one of the proinflammatory cytokines that play a role in innate immunity (Akira 2000). High concentrations of this cytokine in the testicular tissue have been associated with disrupted spermatogenesis (Komsky et al., 2012). In an in-vivo study, a negative correlation was shown between IL-18, spermatozoa concentration and motility. Moreover, the IL-18 level was found to be in a higher concentration in infertile men compared to the fertile group (Matalliotakis et al., 2006).

Cytokine Effects on Testosterone Production

Reduced testosterone production and inflammation have been strongly correlated in the elderly. An increase in proinflammatory cytokines such as IL-6, TNF-α, and IL-1 and a decrease in serum testosterone are characterized by aging (Maggio et al., 2005). In a study conducted on young men, low serum testosterone levels and high levels of proinflammatory cytokines (such as TNF-α, chemokines) were correlated (Bobjer et al., 2013).

In a randomized controlled study, the use of recombinant IL-2 in young and older men was shown to lead to reduced testosterone production by Leydig cells (Veldhuis et al., 2016).

Obesity and Male Infertility

There are many studies indicating a relationship between obesity and male infertility. The effect of obesity on semen parameters has been specifically researched, and it has been proven to be associated with reduced concentration, abnormal morphology, and abnormal motility. This is thought to result from the fact that germ cells are exposed to high aromatase activity for a long time. In a study, it was shown to be influenced by the size of adipocytes rather than aromatase expression (Bekaert et al., 2015). Obesity may induce systemic oxidative stress (Shukla et al., 2014). In this case, the high amount of resulting ROS increases the DNA damage of spermatozoa, reduces the acrosome reaction, and even decreases the probability of embryo implantation after in-vitro fertilization (IVF). There are studies indicating obesity as the cause of low concentrations of FSH, LH, inhibin B and sex hormone-binding globulin (SHBG), which are involved in the regulation of spermatogenesis (Shukla et al., 2014; Du Plessis et al., 2010; Palmer et al., 2012; Tsatsanis et al., 2015). Losing weight results in an increase in anti-Müllerian hormone (AMH), SHBG, testosterone concentration, and free androgen index (FAI) (Schulte et al., 2014).

Adipokines: These are hormones produced by white adipose tissue and involved in inflammation and regulation of the immune system. Leptin, adiponectin, resistin, and visfatin are examples of these hormones. Their major effects are presented in the Table 1.

Table 1. Major effects of adipokines on male infertility

Adiponectin	has a positive effect on the male reproductive system
Leptin	facilitates the secretion of GnRH induces the secretion of FSH and LH inhibits the conversion of progesterone to testosterone
Visfatin	has a positive correlation with the amount of testosterone
Resistin	has an adverse effect on sperm quality

Conclusion

Many studies have suggested that male infertility is based on cytokine changes. On the other hand, the relationship between infertility and cytokines has not been exactly clarified. There is also solid evidence regarding the role of cytokines in male reproduction. The roles of cytokines as biomarkers of male infertility and their potential as therapeutic agents should be clarified. Without doubt, there is a need for a large and wide range of prospective studies to find answers to the questions about the future of cytokines.

References

Al-Daghistani HI, Hamad AWR, Abdel-Dayem M, Al-SwaifiM, ZaidM A(2010). Evaluation of serum testosterone, progesterone, seminal antisperm antibody, and fructose levels among Jordanian males with a history of infertility. *Biochem. Res. Int*. 2010:409640.

Akira S (2000). The role of IL-18 in innate immunity. *Curr. Opin. Immunol.* 12(1):59-63.

Alsaimary IEA (2014). Evaluation of serum levels of pro-inflammatory cytokines (interleukins 2, 6, 8) in fertile and infertile men. *Donnish J. Microbiol. Biotechnol. Res.* 1(2):23-34.

Bobjer J, Katrinaki M, Tsatsanis C, Lundberg Giwercman Y, Giwercman A (2013). Negative association between testosterone concentration and inflammatory markers in young men: a nested cross-sectional study. *PLoS One*8(4):2-9.

Bekaert M, Van Nieuwenhove Y, Calders P, CuvelierC A, BatensA-H, KaufmanJ-M, OuwensD M, RuigeJ B(2015). Determinants of testosterone levels in human male obesity. *Endocrine* 50(1):202-11.

Baker SJ, Rane SG, Reddy EP (2007). Hematopoietic cytokine receptor signaling. *Oncogene* 26(47):6724-37.

Barratt CLR, Björndahl L, De Jonge CJ, Lamb DJ, Osorio Martini F, McLachlan R, Oates RD, van der Poel S, St John B, Sigman M, Sokol R, Tournaye H(2017). The diagnosis of male infertility: an analysis of the evidence to support the development of global WHO guidance-challenges and future research opportunities. *Hum. Reprod. Update* 23(6):660.

Björndahl L, Giwercman A, Tournaye H, Weidner W (2010).Clinical andrology – EAU/ESAUcourse guidelines. *CRC Press*, United States.

Brugh VM 3rd, Lipshultz LI(2004). Male factor infertility: evaluation and management. *Med. Clin. North Am.* 88(2):367.

Camejo MI (2003). Relation between immunosuppressive PGE(2) and IL-10 to pro-inflammatory IL-6 in seminal plasma of infertile and fertile men. *Arch. Androl*. 49:111-116.

Castiglione R, Salemi M, Vicari LO, Vicari E (2013). Relationship of semen hyperviscosity with IL-6, TNF-α, IL-10 and ROS production in seminal plasma of infertile patients with prostatitis and prostato-vesiculitis. *Andrologia* 46(10):1148-55. https://doi.org/10.1111/and.12207.

Cheng CY, Mruk DD (2012). The blood-testis barrier and its implications for male contraception. *Pharmacol. Rev.* 64(1):16-64.

Comhaire F, Bosmans E, Ombelet W, Punjabi U, Schoonjans F (1994). Cytokines in semen of normal men and of patients with andrological diseases. *Am. J. Reprod. Immunol*. 31:99-103.

Comhaire F, Mahmoud A, Depuydt C, Zalata A, Christophe A (1999). Mechanisms and effects of male genital tract infection on sperm quality and fertilizing potential: the andrologist's viewpoint. *Hum. Reprod. Update*5(5):393-8.

Cudicini C, Kercret H, Touzalin AM, Ballet F, Jégou B, (1997). Vectorial production of interleukin 1 and interleukin 6 by rat Sertoli cells cultured in a dual culture compartment system. *Endocrinology* 138:2863-7280.

Depuydt E, Comhaire H (1996). The relation between reactive oxygen species and cytokines in andrological patients with or without male accessory gland infection. *J. Androl.*17(6):699-707.

Dinarello CA (2007). Historical insights into cytokines. *Eur. J. Immunol*. 37(1):34-45.

Du Plessis SS, Cabler S, McAlister DA, Sabanegh E, Agarwal A (2010). The effect of obesity on sperm disorders and male infertility. *Nat. Rev. Urol*.7(3):153-61.

Duan YG, Zhang Q, Liu Y, Mou L, Li G, Gui Y, Cai Z(2014). Dendritic cells in semen of infertile men: association with sperm quality and inflammatory status of the epididymis. *Fertil. Steril.* 101:70-77.

Eggert-Kruse W, Kiefer I, Beck C, Demirakca T, Strowitzki T (2007). Role for tumor necrosis factor alpha (TNF-alpha) and interleukin 1-beta (IL-1beta) determination in seminal plasma during infertility investigation. *Fertil. Steril.* 87:810-823.

Fan W, Xu Y, Liu Y, Zhang Z, Lu L, Ding Z (2017). Obesity or overweight, a chronic inflammatory status in male reproductive system, leads to mice and human subfertility.*Front. Physiol*.8:1117.

Ficarra V, Porcaro AB, Righetti RCerrutoM A, PilloniS, CavalleriS, MalossiniG, ArtibaniW (2002). Antegrade scrotal sclerotherapy in the treatment of varicocele: a prospective study. *BJU Int*. 89:264-268.

Fossiez F (1996). T cell interleukin-17 induces stromal cells to produce proinflammatory and hematopoietic cytokines. *J. Exp. Med.*183(6):2593-603.

Fraczek M, Kurpisz M (2006). Inflammatory mediators exert toxic effects of oxidative stress on human spermatozoa. *J. Androl.* 28(2):325-33.

Fraczek M, Sanocka D, Kamieniczna M, Kurpisz M(2008). Proinflammatory cytokines as an intermediate factor enhancing lipid sperm membrane peroxidation in in vitro conditions. *J. Androl.* 29:85-92.

Fraczek M, Czernikiewicz A, Kurpisz M (2012).*Cytokines and Oxidative Stress in the Germ Line*. In: Agarwal A et al. (eds) Studies on Men's Health and fertility, Oxidative Stress in Applied Basic research and Clinical Practice. Springer Science + Business Media, LLC, p 179-205.

Fraczek M, Szumala-Kakol A, Dworacki G, Sanocka D, Kurpisz M (2013). In vitro reconstruction of inflammatory reaction in human semen: effect on sperm DNA fragmentation. *J. Reprod. Immunol.* 100:76-85.

Friebe K, Bohring C, Skrzypek J, Krause W (2003). Levels of interleukin-6 and interleukin-8 in seminal fluid of men attending an andrological clinic. *Andrologia* 35:126-129.

Fujita Y, Mihara T, Okazaki T, Shitanaka M, Kushino R, Ikeda C, NegishiHZ, RichardsJ S, ShimadaM(2011). Toll-like receptors (TLR) 2 and 4 on human sperm recognize bacterial endotoxins and mediate apoptosis. *Hum. Reprod.* 26(10):2799-806.

Furuya Y, Akashi T, Fuse H (2003). Soluble Fas and interleukin-6 and interleukin-8 levels in seminal plasma of infertile men. *Arch. Androl.* 49:449-452.

Gruschwitz MS, Brezinschek R, Brezinschek HP (1996). Cytokine levels in the seminal plasma of infertile males. *J. Androl.* 17:158-163.

Havrylyuk A, Chopyak V, Boyko Y, Kril I, Kurpisz M (2015). Cytokines in the blood and semen of infertile patients. *Cent. Eur. J. Immunol.*3(3):337-44.

Hedger MP (1997). Testicular leukocytes: what are they doing? *Rev. Reprod.*2:38-47.

Hedger M, Klug J, Fröhlich S, MüllerR, MeinhardtA(2005). Regulatory cytokine expression and interstitial fluid formation in the normal and inflamed rat testis are under Leydig cell control. *J. Androl.* 26:379-386.

Hedger MP (2011). Toll-like receptors and signalling in spermatogenesis and testicular responses to inflammation – a perspective. *J. Reprod. Immunol.*88(2):130-41.

Heidargholizadeh S, Aydos SE, Yukselten Y, Ozkavukcu S, Sun- guroglu A, Aydos K (2017). A differential cytokine expression profile before and after rFSH treatment in Sertoli cell cultures of men with nonobstructive azoospermia. *Andrologia* 49(4):e12647.

Hong CY, Park JH, Ahn RS, ImS Y, ChoiH-S, SohJ, MellonS H, LeeK(2004). Molecular mechanism of suppression of testicular steroidogenesis by proinflammatory cytokine tumor necrosis factor alpha. *Mol. Cell Biol.*24(7):2593-604.

Huleihel M, Lunenfeld E (2004). Regulation of spermatogenesis by paracrine/autocrine testicular factors. *Asian J. Androl.* 6:259-268.

Hussenet F, Dousset B, Cordonnier JL, Jacob C, Foliguet B, Grignon G, Nabet P (1993). Tumour necrosis factor alpha and interleukin 2 in normal and infected human seminal fluid. Hum Reprod 8:409-411.

Ishikawa T, Fujioka H, Ishimura T, Takenaka A, Fujisawa M (2007) Increased testicular 8-hydroxy-2′ -deoxyguanosine in patients with varicocele. BJU Int100(4):863-6

Jacobo P, Guazzone VA, Theas MS, Lustig L (2011). Testicular autoimmunity. *Autoimmun. Rev.*10(4):201-4.

Jaiswal D, Trivedi S, Agrawal NK, Singh R, Singh K (2013). Association of interleukin- 1beta C + 3953T gene polymorphism with human male infertility. *Syst. Biol. Reprod. Med.* 59:347-351.

Ji G, Long Y, Zhou Y, Huang C, Gu A, WangX(2012). Common variants in mis-match repair genes associated with increased risk of sperm DNA damage and male infertility. *BMC Med.* 10:49.

Jungwirth A, Giwercman A, Tournaye H, Diemer T, Kopa Z, Dohle G, Krausz C(2012). European Association of Urology guidelines on Male Infertility: the 2012 update. *Eur. Urol.* 62(2):324.

Kohchi C, Inagawa H, Nishizawa T, Soma GI (2009). ROS and innate immunity. *Anticancer Res.*29(3):817-22.

Koçak I, Yenisey C, Dündar M, Okyay P, Serter M (2002). Relationship between seminal plasma interleukin-6 and tumor necrosis factor alpha levels with semen parameters in fertile and infertile men. *Urol. Res.* 30:263-267.

Kokab A, Akhondi MM, Sadeghi MR, ModarresiM H, AarabiM,JenningsR, PaceyA A, EleyA(2010). Raised inflammatory markers in semen from men with asymptomatic chlamydial infection. *J. Androl.* 31:114-120.

Komsky A, Huleihel M, Ganaiem M, KastersteinE, KomorovskyD, BernO, RazielA, FriedlerS, Ron-ElR, StrassburgerD(2012). Presence of IL-18 in testicular tissue of fertile and infertile men. *Andrologia* 44(1):1-8.

Kopa Z, Wenzel J, Papp GK, Haidl G (2005). Role of granulocyte elastase and interleukin-6 in the diagnosis of male genital tract inflammation. *Andrologia* 37:188-194.

Kruger TF, Acosta AA, Simmons KF, Swanson RJ, Matta JF, Oehninger S (1988). Predictive value of abnormal sperm morphology in in vitro fertilization. *Fertil. Steril*. 49(1):112.

Kursh ED (1987). What is the incidence of varicocele in a fertile population? *Fertil. Steril*. 48: 511.

La Vignera S, Condorelli R, Vicari E, D'AgataR,Calogero A E(2012). High frequency of sexual dysfunction in patients with male accessory gland infections. *Andrologia* 44:438–446.

Li Q (2012). The relationship between IL-17 and male infertility: semen analysis. *African J. Microbiol. Res*. 6(27):5672-5677.

Lotti F, Maggi M (2013). Interleukin 8 and the male genital tract. *J. Reprod. Immunol*. 100:54-65.

Lui WY, Cheng CY (2007). Regulation of cell junction dynamics by cytokines in the testis – A molecular and biochemical perspective. *Cytokine Growth Factor Rev*. 18(3–4):299-311.

Maegawa M, Kamada M, Irahara M, Yamamoto S, Yoshikawa S, Kasai Y, OhmotoY, Gima H, ThalerC J, AonoT(2002). A repertoire of cytokines in human seminal plasma. *J. Reprod. Immunol*. 54:33-42.

Maggio M, Basaria S, Ceda GP, BleA, LingS M, BandinelliS, ValentiG, FerrucciL(2005). The relationship between testosterone and molecular markers of inflammation in older men. *J. Endocrinol. Invest*.28(11):116-9.

Martinez-Prado E, Camejo Bermúdez MI (2010). Expression of IL-6, IL-8, TNF-alpha, IL-10, HSP-60, anti-HSP-60 anti-bodies, and anti-sperm antibodies, in semen of men with leukocytes and/or bacteria. *Am. J. Reprod. Immunol*. 63:233-243.

Matalliotakis I, Kiriakou D, Fragouli I, Sifakis S, Eliopoulos G, Koumantakis E (1998). Interleukin-6 in seminal plasma of fertile and infertile men. *Arch. Androl*. 41:43-50.

Matalliotakis IM, Cakmak H, Fragouli Y, Kourtis A, Arici A, Huszar G (2006). Increased IL-18 levels in seminal plasma of infertile men with genital tract infections. *Am. J. Reprod. Immunol*. 55:428-433.

Mealy K, Robinson B, Millette CF, Majzoub J, Wilmore DW (1990). The testicular effects of tumor necrosis factor. *Ann. Surg*.211:470-475.

Moraes AJ, Bonfa E, Cocuzza M, BorgesC T L, SaitoO, SilvaC A A(2010). Gonad evaluation in male dermatomyositis. A pilot study. *Clin. Exp. Rheumatol*. 28:441-442.

Moraes AJ, Pereira RM, Cocuzza M, CasemiroR,SaitoO, SilvaC A A(2008). Minor sperm abnormalities in young male postpubertal patients with juvenile dermatomyositis. *Braz. J. Med. Biol. Res*. 41:1142-1147.

Naz RK, Evans L (1998). Presence and modulation of interleukin-12 in seminal plasma of fertile and infertile men. *J. Androl*. 19:302-307.

O'Bryan MK, Hedger MP (2008). Inflammatory networks in the control of spermatogenesis: chronic inflammation in an immunologically privileged tissue? Adv. Exp. Med. Biol. 636:92-114.

Ochsendorf FR (1999). Infections in the male genital tract and reactive oxygen species. *Hum. Reprod. Update* 5:399-420.

Oh YS, Jo NH, Park JK, Gye MC (2016). Changes in inflammatory cytokines accompany deregulation of Claudin-11, resulting in inter-Sertoli tight junctions in varicocele rat testes. *J. Urol*. 196(4):1303-12.

Palmer NO, Bakos HW, Fullston T, Lane M (2012). Impact of obesity on male fertility, sperm function and molecular composition. *Spermato- genesis* 2(4):253-63.

Papadimas J, Goulis DG, Sotiriades A, Daniilidis M, Fleva A, Bontis JN, Tourkantonis A (2002). Interleukin-1 beta and tumor necrosis factor-alpha in normal/infertile men. *Arch. Androl*. 48:107-113.

Paradisi R, Mancini R, Bellavia E, Beltrandi E, Pession A, Venturoli S, Flamigni C(1997). T- helper 2 type cytokine and soluble interleukin-2 receptor levels in seminal plasma of infertile men. *Am. J. Reprod. Immunol*. 38:94-99.

Pasqualotto FF, Sundaram A, Sharma RK, Borges Jr E, PasqualottoE B, AgarwalA(2008). Semen quality and oxidative stress scores in fertile and infertile patients with varicocoele. Fertil. Steril. 89:602-607.

Politch JA, Tucker L, Bowman FP, Anderson DJ (2007). Concentrations and significance of cytokines and other immunologic factors in semen of healthy fertile men. *Hum. Reprod*. 22:2928-2035.

Punab M, Poolamets O, Paju P, Vihljajev V, Pomm K, Ladva R, Korrovits P, Laan M (2017). Causes of male infertility: a 9-year prospective monocentre study on 1737 patients with reduced total sperm counts. *Hum. Reprod.* 32(1):18.

Qian L, Sun G, Zhou B, Wang G, Song J, He H (2011). Study on the relationship between different cytokines in the semen of infertility patients. *Am. J. Reprod. Immunol.* 66:157-161.

Remes Lenicov F, Rodriguez Rodrigues C, Sabatté J, Cabrini M, Jancic C, Ostrowski M, Merlotti A, Gonzalez H, Alonso A, Pasqualini R A, Davio C, Geffner J, Ceballos A(2012). Semen promotes the differentiation of tolerogenic dendritic cells. *J. Immunol.* 189:4777-4786.

Sadasivam M, Ramatchandirin B, Balakrishnan S, Prahalathan C (2015). TNF--mediated suppression of Leydig cell steroidogenesis involves DAX-1. *Inflamm. Res.*64(7):549-56.

Sakamoto Y, Ishikawa T, Kondo Y, Yamaguchi K, Fujisawa M (2008). The assessment of oxidative stress in infertile patients with varicocele. *BJU Int.*101(12):1547-52.

Sanocka D, Jedrzejczak P, Szumała-Kakol A, Fraczek M, Kurpisz M (2003). Male genital tract inflammation: The role of selected interleukins in regulation of pro-oxidant and antioxidant enzymatic substances in seminal plasma. *J. Androl.* 24:448-455.

Schuppe H-C, Meinhardt A, Allam JP, Bergmann M, Weidner W, Haidl G (2008). Chronic orchitis: a neglected cause of male infertility? *Andrologia*40(2):84-91.

Schulte DM, Hahn M, Oberhauser F, MalchauG, SchubertM, HeppnerC, MüllerN,GüdelhöferH,FaustM, KroneW,LaudesM(2014) Caloric restriction increases serum testosterone concentrations in obese male subjects by two distinct mechanisms. *Horm. Metab. Res.*46(4):283-6.

Seshadri S, Bates M, Vince G, Jones DI (2009). The role of cytokine expression in different subgroups of subfertile men. *Am. J. Reprod. Immunol.* 62:275-282.

Shoskes DA, Albakri Q, Thomas K, Cook D (2002). Cytokine polymorphisms in men with chronic prostatitis/chronic pelvic pain syndrome: association with diagnosis and treatment response. *J. Urol.* 168:331-335.

Shukla KK, Chambial S, Dwivedi S, Misra S, Sharma P (2014). Recent scenario of obesity and male fertility. *Andrology*2(6):809-18.

Silva CA, Bonfa E, Ostensen M (2010). Maintance of fertility in patients with rheumatic diseases needing anti-inflammatory and immunosupressive drugs. *Arthritis Care Res.* (Hoboken) 62:1682-1690.

Silva CA, Hallak J, Pasqualotto FF, BarbaM F, SaitoM I, KissM H B(2002). Gonadal function in male adolescents and young males with juvenile onset systemic lupus erytematosus. *J. Rheumatol.* 29:2000-2005.

Silva CA, Cocuzza M, Borba EF, Bonfa E (2012). Cutting-Edge Issues in Autoimmune Orchitis. *Clinic Rev. Allerg. Immunol.* 42:256-263.

Suchiro RM, Borba EF, Bonfa E, BonfaE, OkayT S, CocuzzaM, SoaresP M F, SilvaC A A(2008). Testicular Sertoli cell function in male systemic lupus erythematosus. *Reumatology* (Oxford) 47:1692-1697.

Tsatsanis C, Dermitzaki E, Avgoustinaki P, Malliaraki N, Mytaras V, Margioris AN. (2015) The impact of adipose tissue-derived factors on the hypothalamic-pituitary-gonadal (HPG) axis. *Hormones*14(4):549-62.

Tung KSK, Harakal J, Qiao H, RivalC,LiJ C H, PaulA G A, WheelerK, PramoonjagoP,GraferC M, SunW,SampsonR D, WongE W P, ReddiP P, DeshmukhU S, HardyD M, TangH, ChengC Y, GoldbergE(2017). Egress of sperm autoantigen from seminiferous tubules maintains systemic tolerance. *J. Clin. Invest.*127(3): 1046-60.

Van der Poll T, Romijn JA, Endert E, Sauerwein HP (1993). Effects of tumor necrosis factor on the hypothalamic-pituitary-testicular axis in healthy men. *Metabolism*42(3):303-7.

Veldhuis J, Yang R, Roelfsema F, Takahashi PP (2016). roinflammatory cytokine infusion attenuates lh's feedforward on testosterone secretion: modulation by age. *J. Clin. Endocrinol. Metab.*101(2):539-49.

Ventimiglia E, Capogrosso P, Boeri L, Ippolito S, Scano R, Moschini M, Gandaglia G, Papaleo E, Montorsi F, Salonia A(2016). Validation of the American Society for Reproductive Medicine guidelines/recommendations in white European men presenting for couple's infertility. *Fertil. Steril.* 106(5):1076.

Veräjäkorva E, Laato M, Pöllänen P (2002). CD 99 and CD 106 (VCAM-1) in human testis. *Asian J. Androlgy*4(4):243-8.

Vogt PH(2005). Azoospermia factor (AZF) in Yq11: towards a molecular understanding of its function for human male fertility and spermatogenesis. *Reprod. Biomed. Online* 10(1):81.

Winters BR, Walsh TJ(2014). The epidemiology of male infertility. *Urol. Clin. North Am.* 41(1):195.

Wu H, Shi L, Wang Q, ChengL, ZhaoX, ChenQ, JiangQ, FengM, LiQ, HanD(2016). Mumps virus-induced innate immune responses in mouse Sertoli and Leydig cells. *Sci. Rep.*6(1):19507.

Xia W, Mruk DD, Lee WM, Cheng CY (2005). Cytokines and junction restructuring during spermatogenesis – A lesson to learn from the testis. *Cytokine Growth Factor Rev.*16(4–5):469-93.

Yan HHN, Mruk DD, Lee WM, Cheng CY (2008). Blood-testis barrier dynamics are regulated by testosterone and cytokines *via* their differential effects on the kinetics of protein endocytosis and recycling in Sertoli cells. *FASEB J.*22(6):1945-59.

Zalata A, Atwa A, El-Naser Badawy A, Aziz A, El-Baz R, Elhanbly S, Mostafa T(2013). Tumor necrosis factor-α gene polymorphism relationship to seminal variables in infertile men. *Urology* 81:962-966.

Zhang JM, An J (2007). Cytokines, inflammation and pain. *Int. Anesthesiol. Clin.*45(2):27-37.

Zhao S, Zhu W, Xue S, Han D (2014). Testicular defense systems: immune privilege and innate immunity. *Cell Mol. Immunol.*11(5):428-37.

Chapter 23

Cytokines and Surgery

Muhammet Ali Yılmaz[*], MD
Department of Thoracic Surgery, Muhammet Ali Yılmaz Clinic, Samsun, Turkey

Abstract

All cells are in communication with each other via hormones and cytokines. Unlike hormones, cytokines are not stored in any form. Their rapid attendance after injury indicates the stimulated cell's active gene transcription and translation (Dinarello 2000). Cytokines are small peptides that cannot pass the cellular membrane (Holtman 1995). They bind to specific receptors at the cellular membrane that activate intracellular receptor-mediated signalling pathways and adjust gene transcription. Cytokines released in this way control the activity of the immune system, cellular proliferation, and survival. These peptides are in complex interaction with each other, which may either enhance (proinflammatory) or decrease (anti-inflammatory) the inflammatory response (Alazawi 2016).

Keywords: cytokines, systemic inflammatory response syndrome (SIRS), multiple organ failure (MOF), multiple organ dysfunction syndrome (MODS), persistent inflammatory catabolic syndrome (PICS), surgical trauma

Introduction

Cytokines are essential mediators to regulate the inflammatory response against infection or injury, and they are crucial agents for appropriate wound healing. However, the overstated production of proinflammatory cytokines from a local insult area has acute or chronic systemic consequences like hemodynamic instability in septic shock or muscle wasting in metabolic derangements (Lin 2000). Every surgical intervention may trigger overstated proinflammatory cytokine responses that can cause systemic inflammatory response syndrome (SIRS, Table 1) and end-organ injury, leading to multiple organ failure (MOF) and death (Baue 2006). Some of the surviving MOF patients have a prolonged intensive care unit stay, and many of them

[*] Corresponding Author's Email: yilmaz.m.a@gmail.com.

In: Cytokines and Diseases
Editors: Kenan Demir, Selim Görgün and Bahar Uslu
ISBN: 979-8-88697-214-6

progress to newly defined persistent inflammatory catabolic syndrome (PICS) (Mira 2017). The manifestation of anti-inflammatory cytokines may lead to lessening the overstated inflammatory response. However, extreme anti-inflammatory cytokine release can cause patients to be immune-compromised and sensitive to infectious morbidity, defined as compensatory anti-inflammatory response syndrome (CARS) (Bone 1996). Collectively with cytokines, reactive oxygen species (ROS), reactive nitrogen species (RNS), and nitric oxide (NO) play indispensable roles in the pathogenesis of SIRS, and all of them are in interaction with cytokines (Chalhoub 2011).

Table 1. SIRS is present if 2 of the below criteria are met (Accp/Sccm 1992)

Findings	Values
Temperature	< 36°C or > 38°C
Heart rate	> 90/min
Respiratory rate	> 20/min or PaCO2 < 32 mmHg
WBC	< 4000/mm3, >> 12,000/mm3, or ≥ 10% bands

Surgical trauma causes the liberation of endogen sourced damage-associated molecular patterns (DAMPs), also called alarmins (Akira 2004). Alarmins bind to toll-like receptors (TLRs) expressed on the various cellular membranes, which may trigger the expression of proinflammatory and anti-inflammatory cytokines. Some authors define this condition as "sterile inflammation" (Zindel 2020). Ischemia-reperfusion injury is another mechanism of sterile inflammation in surgical patients triggered by DAMPs (Herron & Ciesla 2018).

Following surgery, the dysregulated cytokine response could result in significant morbidity and mortality from SIRS, infection, and sepsis, but another cause of SIRS is infection. This situation creates conflict in predicting the etiology of SIRS (Dąbrowska et al., 2014). A differential diagnosis between surgery-associated inflammation with surgery-related infection or other causes of the condition is a crucial challenge in the postoperative management of surgical patients. Managing these similar clinical situations is also different (Margraf 2020).

Table 2. Preoperative and Perioperative factors influencing the inflammatory response in surgical patients

Preoperative	Perioperative
Infection	Duration (>4 h)
Leukocyte and/or platelet counts	Type of surgery (open/minimally invasive/multiple organs)
Comorbidities	Intensity of tissue trauma/size of wounding
Smoking status	Multihits (multiple injury sites or types of injury)
Anti-inflammatory medication	Heat injury (cauterization)
Anesthetic premedication	Extracorporeal support (dialysis, ECMO)
	Ischemia-reperfusion injury/clamping
	Blood loss and transfusion
	Invasive high-pressure ventilation
	Anesthetic management

BW, body weight; ECMO, extracorporeal membrane oxygenation.
Adopted from Margraf et al., 2020.

Unfortunately, the current medical literature does not have any data about the optimum level of inflammation for surgical patients. On the other hand, we do not have any tool to hold inflammation in balance or at any predicted level. All should be done for patients who develop SIRS, MODS, and MOF like inflammatory disturbances in supportive measures. This situation increases the importance of early diagnosis that defines high-risk groups (Table 2). Every surgical intervention could trigger dysregulated cytokine release. Major surgical procedures already have a greater risk, but minimally invasive surgical procedures that limit tissue damage cannot be altogether abolished.

The patient's age, comorbidities, gender, and surgical or anesthetic factors could affect the incidence of postoperative inflammatory complications and mortality. Still, we do not have enough data to use them as predictors of inflammatory complications and mortality in routine clinical practice (Dąbrowska & Słotwiński 2014).

The most studied cytokines in the surgical viewpoint are tumor necrosis factor-alpha (TNF-α), type 1 interferon, interleukin 1 (IL-1), interleukin 6 (IL-6), interleukin 10 (IL-10), and interleukin 12 (IL-12). When TNF-α and IL-6 are applied together at low doses, they interact synergistically and cause the deterioration of hemodynamics at low doses. In contrast, when administered alone, higher doses are required to achieve this effect. It has been suggested that IL-6 is a major inflammatory cytokine in the early postoperative period and an early predictor of SIRS risk (Fink-Neuboeck 2016). IL-10 suppresses the immune response and cytokine production. Gérard et al. have demonstrated that administration of IL-10 during endotoxemia decreases monocyte TNF-α production and mortality rate (Gérard 1993). In an experimental study on mice with fecal peritonitis, it was observed that mortality increased, and wound healing was impaired when IL-12 was neutralized with polyclonal IL-12 antibodies (Steinhauser 1999). TNF-α is an archetypal inflammatory cytokine that activates multiple defense mechanisms, including acute phase response, phagocytosis, and chemotaxis. Inappropriate or excessive production can be harmful. TNF-α is among the earliest and most potent mediators of subsequent host responses after acute injury or infections. The half-life of TNF-α is less than 20 minutes; this brief appearance is sufficient to evoke mediators distally in the cytokine cascade and marked metabolic and hemodynamic changes (Alazawi 2016).

Conclusion

The effects of trauma on the body have similar properties to surgery, but there are some differences. Surgery is usually a planned procedure if not performed in an emergency condition. Most of the time, surgery is achieved with local or general anesthesia in the operation room. The operation room has all the resources, including trained medical staff, to support patients in any predicted or unpredicted circumstances in a clean medium. In addition, anesthetic drugs and mechanical ventilation could affect the cytokine response of the patient. As trauma cases are usually healthy individuals before the insult, elective surgery cases have one or more comorbidities. These differences could cause different cytokine responses between elective surgery and trauma cases.

On the other hand, some trauma cases need surgical interference like open fractures or internal hemorrhages, which could be a second impulse for cytokine production. Any surgeon aims to reduce mortality and morbidity in surgical treatments and achieve a faster return to daily life with lower hospital costs. Although cytokines are necessary to achieve these goals, their uncontrolled release is one of the biggest threats.

References

Akira S, Takeda K (2004). Toll-like receptor signalling. *Nature reviews Immunology* 4(7):499–511.

Alazawi W, Pirmadjid, N (2016). Inflammatory and Immune Responses to Surgery and Their Clinical Impact. *Annals of Surgery* 264(1):73–80.

American College of Chest Physicians/Society of Critical Care Medicine (ACCP/SCCM) Consensus Conference: definitions for sepsis and organ failure and guidelines for the use of innovative therapies in sepsis (1992) *Critical care medicine* 20(6):864–874.

Baue A E (2006). MOF, MODS, and SIRS: what is in a name or an acronym? *Shock* (Augusta, Ga.) 26(5):438–449.

Bone R C (1996). Sir isaac newton, sepsis, SIRS, and CARS. *Critical care medicine*, 1;24(7):1125-8.

Dąbrowska AM, Słotwiński R (2014) The immune response to surgery and infection. *Central-European journal of immunology* 39(4):532–537.

Dinarello C A (2000). Proinflammatory Cytokines. *Chest* 118:503–508.

Gérard C, Bruyns C (1993). Interleukin 10 reduces the release of tumor necrosis factor and prevents lethality in experimental endotoxemia. *The Journal of experimental medicine*, 177(2):547–550.

Herron T J, Ciesla D J (2018). SIRS/Sepsis/Septic Shock/MOSF. In: Salim A, Brown C, (eds.) *Surgical Critical Care Therapy*, 1st edn. Springer International Publishing, p 391–398.

Holtmann H, Resch K (1995). Cytokines. *Die Naturwissenschaften* 82(4):178–187.

Lin E, Calvano S E (2000). Inflammatory cytokines and cell response in surgery. *Surgery* 127(2):117–126.

Margraf A Ludwig, N (2020). Systemic Inflammatory Response Syndrome After Surgery: Mechanisms and Protection. *Anesthesia & Analgesia* 131(6):1693–1707.

Steinhauser M L, Hogaboam C M (1999). Multiple roles for IL-12 in a model of acute septic peritonitis. *Journal of immunology* (Baltimore, Md.:1950) 162(9):5437–5443.

Zindel J, Kubes P (2020). DAMPs, PAMPs, and LAMPs in Immunity and Sterile Inflammation. *Annual review of pathology* 15:493–518 https://doi.org/10.1146/annurev-pathmechdis-012419-032847.

Chapter 24

Cytokines in Cerebrospinal Fluid of Patients with Acute COVID

Uma Jalloh[1] and Ivana Kawikova[2,*], MD, PhD

[1]Translational Brain Imaging Program, Yale University School of Medicine, New Haven, CT, USA

[2]Department of Biology School of Arts and Sciences, University of Hartford, West Hartford, CT, USA

Abstract

Infection with acute respiratory syndrome-coronavirus type 2 (SARS-CoV-2) strain of coronavirus, or for short COVID-19, is known for its severe impact on pulmonary and cardiovascular functions. Many COVID-19 patients also suffer neurological symptoms that may vary from headaches to stroke, meningoencephalitis or seizures in the central nervous system and may also cause neuropathies of peripheral nerves. Brain imaging or analyses of cerebrospinal fluid can assess inflammatory responses in the brain. Among measured cytokines, interleukin-6 (IL-6) elevation in cerebrospinal fluid appears to be the most consistent finding. IL-6 is a proinflammatory cytokine known as a "suppressor of suppression." It is feasible to inhibit the proinflammatory effects of IL-6 by several clinically available anti-IL-6 biologics. The inhibition has been shown to benefit the long-term survival of severely ill COVID-19 patients, but the treatment was also reported to have severe side effects, especially in immune-compromised patients. More studies need to be performed to determine when and how potent inhibition of IL-6 could be safe and beneficial to administer to manage neurological symptoms related to COVID-19 infection.

Keywords: COVID-19, nervous system, cerebrospinal fluid, cytokines, interleukins, interleukin-6

Introduction

The severe acute respiratory syndrome-coronavirus type 2 (SARS-CoV-2) strain of coronavirus, more commonly known as COVID-19, while first identified in China's Wuhan, soon spread internationally in 2020 and continues to affect millions of people

* Corresponding Author's Email: kawikova@hartford.edu.

In: Cytokines and Diseases
Editors: Kenan Demir, Selim Görgün and Bahar Uslu
ISBN: 979-8-88697-214-6

worldwide. When researchers at Northwestern Medicine investigated the first 509 patients hospitalized within their medical centers, they found that 82% developed a neurological or psychiatric manifestation (Graham et al. 2021), in addition to common respiratory and vascular symptoms. Some neurological manifestations result from septic shock and increased coagulability, that cause hypoxic encephalopathy or embolic stroke, respectively. The most common central nervous system (CNS) manifestations were headaches, dizziness, stroke, disturbances in consciousness and/or mental status, stroke, meningoencephalitis and seizures (Xiong et al. 2020; Helms et al. 2020; Favas et al. 2020; Mao et al. 2020), while the most common peripheral nervous system (PNS) manifestations were disturbances in taste and smell, polyneuropathy and demyelinating conditions (Mao et al. 2020; Montalvan et al. 2020; Orru et al. 2020).

Imaging as a Tool to Identify Brain Inflammation

Given that there are only a few objective markers to diagnose neuropsychiatric conditions, the data from structural and functional neuroimaging of patients infected with SARS-CoV-2 are quite valuable. The most common structural brain imaging techniques used in these patients is structural magnetic resonance imaging (MRI) and computed tomography (CT) scans. The most frequent finding in the patients with clinical neurological manifestations was cerebral microhemorrhages (Chougar et al. 2020; Coolen et al. 2020; Fitsiori et al. 2020; Helms et al. 2020; Paterson et al. 2020; Xiong et al. 2020), especially in the splenium of the corpus callosum (Kremer et al. 2020). A few authors say that they believe this injury to the splenium is because this area of the corpus callosum is particularly vulnerable to cytokine-induced injury because of the high density of cytokine, glutamate, as well as other receptors present (Starkey et al. 2017; Kimura et al. 2008; Hassel et al. 2003). In more severe cases, neurological manifestations such as acute/subacute infarct (Chougar et al. 2020; Coolen et al. 2020; Fitsiori et al. 2020; Helms et al. 2020; Paterson et al. 2020; Xiong et al. 2020), spontaneous acute intracranial hemorrhage (Chougar et al. 2020; Coolen et al. 2020; Fitsiori et al. 2020; Helms et al. 2020; Paterson et al. 2020; Xiong et al. 2020), and encephalitis/encephalopathy (Chougar et al. 2020; Fitsiori et al. 2020; Helms et al. 2020; Paterson et al. Tuma et al. 2020) to name a few.

Functional neuroimaging studies were more limited in comparison. They revealed abnormalities in blood-oxygen level dependent (BOLD) activation in the olfactory system (Ismail & Gad 2020) and hypometabolism in various parts of the brain, such as the bilateral gyrus rectus (Guedj et al. 2020), prefrontal and orbitofrontal cortices, and the cerebellar vermis (Delorme et al. 2020).

Cerebrospinal Fluid Analyses in Patients with COVID-19 Infection

A substance of particular interest when analyzing the CSF of these COVID-19 patients is inflammatory markers. Proinflammatory cytokines are a type of signaling molecule secreted from cells of the immune system, like glial cells in the brain or circulating, and possibly brain tissue infiltrating, T lymphocytes, macrophage, granulocytes.

Perrin and colleagues (2021) examined the CSF of five COVID-19 patients with severe cases, meaning these patients required extensive lab characterization and neuroimaging. They performed brain imaging and the CSF was drawn during ongoing infection, as opposed to being drawn during post-COVID complications. Of the substances they measured in CSF, which include markers of inflammation, cytokine release syndrome (CRS), cell lysis, coagulation and thrombotic microangiopathy were measured, three markers were found to be elevated in three out of the five patients: C-reactive protein (CRP), interleukin-6 (IL-6), and lactate dehydrogenase (LDH).

Helms et al. (2020) analyzed the CSF of twenty-five COVID-19 patients defined as severe when referred to the ICU for acute respiratory distress syndrome from March 3, 2020 to May 5, 2020. Of those patients that were referred, they performed further investigation in those that presented with neuropsychological manifestations, such as encephalopathies and delirium. CSF alone was assessed and similarly to Perrin et al. the CSF was drawn during the ongoing infection. Of the inflammatory markers they measured, they found that 6 out of the 25 patients had elevated levels of IL-6, and 2 out of the 25 patients had elevated levels of interleukin-10 (IL-10).

The following is the data found by Chougar et al. (2020): CSF was drawn during ongoing infection in thirty-five patients with severe COVID cases referred to the ICU. Once the CSF was assessed, they found that 72.7% of patients exhibited a mild increase of IL-6. IL-10 was measured in these patients as well, however, they did not find an elevation as in the previous studies.

Keller and colleagues (2020) investigated the CSF of eight COVID patients with severe cases during ongoing infection. After analyzing the CSF of these patients, they found that IL-6 levels were elevated in all but one.

A case series study was done by Benaumeur et al. (2020) looking at the CSF of three patients with severe COVID-19 cases, which was drawn during ongoing infection. They assessed levels of interleukin-1α (IL-1α), interleukin-1β (IL-1β), interleukin- 2 (IL-2), interleukin 4 (IL-4), IL-6, interleukin-7 (IL-7), interleukin-8 (IL-8), interleukin-9 (IL-9), IL-10, interleukin-12-p40 (IL12-p40) and interleukin-12-p70 (IL12-p70), interferon-gamma–induced protein 10 (IP-10), monocyte chemoattractant protein 1 (MCP-1), macrophage-derived chemokine (MDC), fractalkine (CX3CL1), and tumor necrosis factor α (TNF-α). Of these cytokines, patients with COVID-19 accompanied by neurologic symptoms had increased CSF levels of IL-6, IL-8, IL-10, IP-10, and TNF-α.

Tuma et al. (2020) asked whether cytokine levels in CSF to severity of patient's encephalopathy. The investigators analyzed sixty-six COVID-19 patients12 had suffered no encephalopathies, 12 had mild encephalopathy, 18 had moderate encephalopathy, and 13 had severe encephalopathy. IL-6 was elevated in 50% of the moderate encephalopathy cases, and that IL-6 was elevated in 100% of the severe encephalopathy cases.

In summary, the data of these studies shows that among cytokines elevated in the CSF of COVID-19 patients, the pro-inflammatory marker IL-6 appears to be the most common finding.

Interleukin-6 as a Predominant Cytokine in CSF Of COVID-19 Patients with Neurological Symptoms

IL-6 is a cytokine with a significant proinflammatory impact (Tanaka et al. 2014). Already two decades ago, IL-6 was shown to mediate suppression of regulatory T cells by microbial induction of Toll-like receptor, that some call "suppression of suppression" (Pasare and Medzhitov 2003). Later, it was also identified as a key factor that determines whether CD4 cells develop in the presence of tumor growth factor-beta into regulatory T cells with suppressive function (in the absence of IL-6), or proinflammatory T-helper 17 cells (in the presence of IL-6) (Veldhoen et al. 2006). With this said, the question of what we can predict about the immune response associated with it comes into play. IL-6 is transiently and promptly made as a result of tissue injury, or infections in this case, and helps in processes such as hematopoiesis, acute phase responses, and immune reactions (Tanaka et al. 2014).

Once IL-6 targets its specific receptor, it will initiate a cascade of signaling events associated primarily with the JAK/STAT3 activation pathway (Wang et al. 2013), which promotes the transcription of many downstream genes associated with cellular signaling processes, such as cytokines, adaptor proteins, receptors, and protein kinases. IL-6 is thought to be involved in the progression of several viral infections. IL-6 is considered to be one of the most important cytokines during an infection. In fact, animal studies using IL-6 deficient mice have given evidence that the cytokine is necessary for the survival of the rodents from the influenza virus by promoting the regulation of inflammatory resolution, T-cell response, tissue repair, and more (Yang et al. 2017; Lauder et al. 2013).

Because IL-6 is a prominent cytokine in severe infection, it isn't surprising that it was the most common cytokine found in CSF investigation of COVID-19 patients. Current research going into the novel virus suggests that COVID-19-associated infections include inflammation, pathologic coagulation, cytokine storm, and more. There is a debate about a widely accepted single definition for cytokine storm, but it is currently considered an umbrella term encompassing several disorders of immune dysregulation characterized by systemic inflammation and multiorgan dysfunction that can lead to multiorgan failure (Fajgenbaum & June 2020), which in turn can disturb the blood-brain barrier. Patients of the SARS-CoV virus had low levels of suppressor of cytokine signaling-3, a regulator and stimulator of the negative feedback mechanism of IL-6 (Okabayashi et al. 2004). With the SARS-CoV virus and the novel SARS-CoV-2 virus both being coronaviruses, some think this implication may be similar. Similarly, a study by Wan et al. (2020) found that IL-6 levels were elevated in severe COVID-19 patients, which may be used as a predicting factor for the transition from a mild case to a more severe case. This implication has also been supported by the CSF analysis studies discussed prior.

Pro-inflammatory actions of IL-6 may also have deleterious effects through inappropriately high activation of cellular immune response against viral infection. For example, potential mechanisms that involve the cytokine may be critical for viral clearance.

Table 1. List of cytokines found elevated in CSF of COVID-19 patients expressed as percentages of patients who showed the elevated concentrations

	References					
Elevated Cytokine Levels Found in CSF (% of patients)	**Perrin et al. 2021**	**Helms et al. 2020**	**Chougar et al. 2020**	**Keller et al. 2020**	**Benameur et al. 2020**	**Tuma et al. 2020**
CRP	20	-	-	-	-	-
IL-6	20	24	72.7	87.5	66.7	50
IL-8	-	-	-	-	66.7	-
IL-10	-	8	0	-	66.7	-
IP-10	-	-	-	-	66.7	-
LDH	20	-	-	-	-	-
MCP-1	-	-	-	-	0	-
TNF-α	0	-	-	-	66.7	-

Cells with dashes (-) in them represent one of the following: a) the author did not measure said cytokine, or b) the author did not disclose measuring said cytokine.

Anti-IL6 Treatment in COVID Patients

That a careful navigation between benefits versus detrimental effects of IL-6 is necessary is becoming evident from studies that employed anti-IL-6 treatment. Biologics, such as toculizumab and sarilumab, are used clinically to stop the activity of the proinflammatory cytokine IL-6. On hand, toculizumab treatment was associated with disseminated mucormycosis. Other side effects include elevated liver enzymes, risk of infections like tuberculosis and bacterial or other fungal infections, and bowel perforation. On the other hand, in a multi-site study, toculizumab improved 90-day survival of critically ill COVID patients (Gordon et al. 2021).

One thing of interest with regards to anti-IL-6 biologics in COVID-19 is if there are any recorded cases in which anti-IL6 is given to long-COVID patients (patients with post-infectious sequela). As of now, it appears that data in that realm is slim.

Conclusion

In summary, inflammatory responses in COVID patients occur in the CNS as evident from both brain imaging studies and analyses of CSF. These responses include elevated levels of multiple cytokines, among which the most consistently elevated cytokine is IL-6. The NIH currently does not recommend the use of anti-IL6 biologics for COVID treatment. Further studies need to be performed in patients with chronic post-COVID sequela where toculizumab or other anti-IL6 biologics may be considered, especially if low doses turn to have less serious side effects.

References

Benameur, K., Agarwal, A., Auld, S. C., Butters, M. P., Webster, A. S., Ozturk, T., Howell, J. C., Bassit, L. C., Velasquez, A., Schinazi, R. F., Mullins, M. E., & Hu, W. T. (2020) Encephalopathy and Encephalitis Associated with Cerebrospinal Fluid Cytokine Alterations and Coronavirus Disease, Atlanta, Georgia, USA, 2020. *Emerg. Infect. Dis.* 26(9):2016-2021. https://doi.org/10.3201/eid2609.202122.

Choi, Y., Lee, M. K. (2020) Neuroimaging findings of brain MRI and CT in patients with COVID-19: A systematic review and meta-analysis. *Eur. J. Radiol.* 133:109393. https://doi.org/10.1016/j.ejrad.2020.109393.

Chomarat, P., Banchereau, J., Davoust, J., Palucka, A. K. (2000) IL-6 switches the differentiation of monocytes from dendritic cells to macrophages. *Nat. Immunol.* 1(6):510-514. https://doi.org/10.1038/82763.

Chougar, L., Shor, N., Weiss, N., Galanaud, D., Leclercq, D., Mathon, B., Belkacem, S., Ströer, S., Burrel, S., Boutolleau, D., Demoule, A., Rosso, C., Delorme, C., Seilhean, D., Dormont, D., Morawiec, E., Raux, M., Demeret, S., Gerber, S., ... For the CoCo Neurosciences Study Group. (2020) Retrospective Observational Study of Brain MRI Findings in Patients with Acute SARS-CoV-2 Infection and Neurologic Manifestations. *Radiology* 297(3):E313-E323. https://doi.org/10.1148/radiol.2020202422.

Delorme, C., Paccoud, O., Kas, A., Hesters, A., Bombois, S., Shambrook, P., Boullet, A., Doukhi, D., Le Guennec, L., Godefroy, N., Maatoug, R., Fossati, P., Millet, B., Navarro, V., Bruneteau, G., Demeret, S., Pourcher, V., the CoCo-Neurosciences study group and COVID SMIT PSL study group, Delorme, C., Houot, M. (2020) COVID-19-related encephalopathy: a case series with brain FDG-positron-emission tomography/computed tomography findings. *Eur. J. Neurol.* 27(12):2651-2657. https://doi.org/10.1111/ene.14478.

Diener, H. C., Berlit, P., Masjuan, J. (2020) COVID-19: patients with stroke or risk of stroke. *Eur. Heart J.* Suppl. 22(Suppl Pt t):P25-P28. https://doi.org/10.1093/eurheartj/suaa174.

Dienz, O., Rincon, M. (2009) The effects of IL-6 on CD4 T cell responses. *Clin. Immunol.* 130(1):27-33. https://doi.org/10.1016/j.clim.2008.08.018.

Fajgenbaum, D. C., June, C. H. (2020) Cytokine Storm. *N. Engl. J. Med.* 383(23):2255-2273. https://doi.org/10.1056/NEJMra2026131.

Favas, T. T., Dev, P., Chaurasia, R. N., Chakravarty, K., Mishra, R., Joshi, D., Mishra, V. N., Kumar, A., Singh, V. K., Pandey, M., & Pathak, A. (2020) Neurological manifestations of COVID-19: a systematic review and meta-analysis of proportions. *Neurol. Sci.* 41(12):3437-3470. https://doi.org/10.1007/s10072-020-04801-y.

Fitsiori, A., Pugin, D., Thieffry, C., Lalive, P., Vargas, M. I. (2020) COVID-19 is Associated with an Unusual Pattern of Brain Microbleeds in Critically Ill Patients. *J. Neuroimaging* 30(5):593-597. https://doi.org/10.1111/jon.12755.

Gordon, C. A., Mouncey, P. R., Al-Beidh, F., et al. (2021) Interleukin-6 receptor antagonists in critically ill patients with Covid-19. *N. Engl. J. Med.* 384(16):1491-1502. https://doi.org/10.1056/NEJMoa2100433.

Graham, E. L., Clark, J. R., Orban, Z. S., Lim, P. H., Szymanski, A. L., Taylor, C., DiBiase, R. M., Jia, D. T., Balabanov, R., Ho, S. U., Batra, A., Liotta, E. M., & Koralnik, I. J. (2021) Persistent neurologic symptoms and cognitive dysfunction in non-hospitalized Covid-19 "long haulers." *Annals of Clinical and Translational Neurology* 8(5):1073-1085. https://doi.org/10.1002/acn3.51350.

Guedj, E., Million, M., Dudouet, P., Tissot-Dupont, H., Bregeon, F., Cammilleri, S., & Raoult, D. (2021) ^{18}F-FDG brain PET hypometabolism in post-SARS-CoV-2 infection: substrate for persistent/delayed disorders? *Eur. J. Nucl. Med. Mol. Imaging* 48(2):592-595. https://doi.org/10.1007/s00259-020-04973-x.

Hassel, B., Boldingh, K. A., Narvesen, C., Iversen, E. G., Skrede, K. K. (2003) Glutamate transport, glutamine synthetase and phosphate-activated glutaminase in rat CNS white matter. A quantitative study. *J. Neurochem.* 87(1):230-237. https://doi.org/10.1046/j.1471-4159.2003.01984.x.

Helms, J., Kremer, S., Merdji, H., Schenck, M., Severac, F., Clere-Jehl, R., Studer, A., Radosavljevic, M., Kummerlen, C., Monnier, A., Boulay, C., Fafi-Kremer, S., Castelain, V., Ohana, M., Anheim, M., Schneider, F., & Meziani, F. (2020) Delirium and encephalopathy in severe COVID-19: a cohort analysis of ICU patients. *Crit. Care* 24(1):491. https://doi.org/10.1186/s13054-020-03200-1.

Helms, J., Kremer, S., Merdji, H., Clere-Jehl, R., Schenck, M., Kummerlen, C., Collange, O., Boulay, C., Fafi-Kremer, S., Ohana, M., Anheim, M., Meziani, F. (2020) Neurologic features in severe SARS-COV-2 infection. *N Engl. J. Med.* 382(23):2268-2270.

Hermine, O., Mariette, X., Tharaux, P. L., et al. (2021) Effect of Tocilizumab vs Usual Care in Adults Hospitalized With COVID-19 and Moderate or Severe Pneumonia: A Randomized Clinical Trial. *JAMA Intern. Med.* 181(1):32-40. https://doi.org/10.1001/jamainternmed.2020.6820.

Ismail, I. I., Gad, K. A. (2021) Absent Blood Oxygen Level-Dependent Functional Magnetic Resonance Imaging Activation of the Orbitofrontal Cortex in a Patient with Persistent Cacosmia and Cacogeusia after COVID-19 Infection. *JAMA Neurol.* 78(5):609-610. https://doi.org/10.1001/jamaneurol.2021.0009.

Keller, E., Brandi, G., Winklhofer, S., Imbach, L. L., Kirschenbaum, D., Frontzek, K., Steiger, P., Dietler, S., Haeberlin, M., Willms, J., Porta, F., Waeckerlin, A., Huber, M., Abela, I. A., Lutterotti, A., Stippich, C., Globas, C., Varga, Z., & Jelcic, I. (2020) Large and Small Cerebral Vessel Involvement in Severe COVID-19: Detailed Clinical Workup of a Case Series. *Stroke.* 51(12):3719-3722. https://doi.org/10.1161/strokeaha.120.031224.

Kimura, E., Okamoto, S., Uchida Yuji, Hirahara, T., Ikeda, T., Hirano, T., Uchino, M. (2008) A reversible lesion of the corpus callosum splenium with adult influenza-associated encephalitis/encephalopathy: A case report. *Journal of Medical Case Reports* 2:220. https://doi.org/10.1186/1752-1947-2-220.

Kremer, S., Lersy, F., de Sèze, J., Ferré, J.-C., Maamar, A., Carsin-Nicol, B., Collange, O., Bonneville, F., Adam, G., Martin-Blondel, G., Rafiq, M., Geeraerts, T., Delamarre, L., Grand, S., Krainik, A., For the SFNR-COVID Group, Kremer, S., Adam, G., Alleg, M., Cotton, F. (2020) Brain MRI Findings in Severe COVID-19: A Retrospective Observational Study. *Radiology* 297(2):E242-E251. https://doi.org/10.1148/radiol.2020202222.

Lauder, S. N., Jones, E., Smart, K., Bloom, A., Williams, A. S., Hindley, J. P., Ondondo, B., Taylor, P. R., Clement, M., Fielding, C., Godkin, A. J., Jones, S. A., & Gallimore, A. M. (2013) Interleukin-6 limits influenza-induced inflammation and protects against fatal lung pathology. *Eur. J. Immunol.* 43(10):2613-2625. https://doi.org/10.1002/eji.201243018.

Radosa, J. C., Mertke, P., Radosa, C. G., Brucker, S., Taran, F. A., Kommoss, S., Ulrich, U., Hackethal, A., Deeken, M., Radosa, M. P., Juhasz-Bãss, I., & Solomayer, E.-F. (2020) New onset acute symptomatic seizure and risk factors in coronavirus disease 2019: A retrospective multicenter study. *Epilepsia* 61(6):e49-e53. https://doi.org/10.1111/epi.16524.

Mao, L., Jin, H., Wang, M., et al. (2020) Neurologic Manifestations of Hospitalized Patients With Coronavirus Disease 2019 in Wuhan, China. *JAMA Neurol.* 77(6):683-690. https://doi.org/10.1001/jamaneurol.2020.1127.

Montalvan, V., Lee, J., Bueso, T., De Toledo, J., Rivas, K. (2020) Neurological manifestations of COVID-19 and other coronavirus infections: A systematic review. *Clin. Neurol. Neurosurg.* 194:105921. https://doi.org/10.1016/j.clineuro.2020.105921.

Okabayashi, T., Kariwa, H., Yokota, S., Iki, S., Indoh, T., Yokosawa, N., Takashima, I., Tsutsumi, H., & Fujii, N. (2006) Cytokine regulation in SARS coronavirus infection compared to other respiratory virus infections. *J. Med. Virol.* 78(4):417-424. https://doi.org/10.1002/jmv.20556.

Orrù, G., Conversano, C., Malloggi, E., Francesconi, F., Ciacchini, R., Gemignani, A. (2020) Neurological Complications of COVID-19 and Possible Neuroinvasion Pathways: A Systematic Review. *Int. J. Environ. Res. Public Health* 17(18):6688. https://doi.org/10.3390/ijerph17186688.

Pasare, C., Medzhitov, R. (2003) Toll pathway-dependent blockade of CD4+CD25+ T cell-mediated suppression by dendritic cells. *Science* 299:(5609):1033-6. https://doi.org/ 10.1126/science.1078231.

Perrin, P., Collongues, N., Baloglu, S., Bedo, D., Bassand, X., Lavaux, T., Gautier-Vargas, G., Keller, N., Kremer, S., Fafi-Kremer, S., Moulin, B., Benotmane, I., & Caillard, S. (2021) Cytokine release syndrome-associated encephalopathy in patients with COVID-19. *European Journal of Neurology* 28(1):248-258. https://doi.org/ 10.1111/ene.14491.

Rossi, B., Nguyen, L. S., Zimmermann, P., Boucenna, F., Dubret, L., Baucher, L., Guillot, H., Bouldouyre, M. A., Allenbach, Y., Salem, J. E., Barsoum, P., Oufella, A., & Gros, H. (2021) Tocilizumab in Hospitalized Patients with Severe Covid-19 Pneumonia. *N Engl. J. Med.* 384(16):1503-1516. https://doi.org/10.1056/NEJMoa2028700.

Salama, C., Han, J., Yau, L., Reiss, W. G., Kramer, B., Neidhart, J. D., Criner, G. J., Kaplan-Lewis, E., Baden, R., Pandit, L., Cameron, M. L., Garcia-Diaz, J., Chávez, V., Mekebeb-Reuter, M., Lima de Menezes, F., Shah, R., González-Lara, M. F., Assman, B., Freedman, J., & Mohan, S. V. (2021) Tocilizumab in patients hospitalized with COVID-19 pneumonia. *N Engl. J. Med.* 384(1):20-30.

Salvarani, C., Dolci, G., Massari, M., et al. (2021) Effect of Tocilizumab vs Standard Care on Clinical Worsening in Patients Hospitalized with COVID-19 Pneumonia: A Randomized Clinical Trial. *JAMA Intern. Med.* 181(1):24-31. https://doi.org/10.1001/jamainternmed.2020.6615.

Starkey, J., Kobayashi, N., Numaguchi, Y., Moritani, T. (2017) Cytotoxic Lesions of the Corpus Callosum That Show Restricted Diffusion: Mechanisms, Causes, and Manifestations. *Radiographics* 37(2):562-576. https://doi.org/10.1148/rg.2017160085.

Stone, J. H., Frigault, M. J., Serling-Boyd, N. J., Fernandes, A. D., Harvey, L., Foulkes, A. S., Horick, N. K., Healy, B. C., Shah, R., Bensaci, A. M., Woolley, A. E., Nikiforow, S., Lin, N., Sagar, M., Schrager, H., Huckins, D. S., Axelrod, M., Pincus, M. D., Fleisher, J., Mansour, M. K. (2020) Efficacy of Tocilizumab in Patients Hospitalized with Covid-19. *N Engl. J. Med.* 383(24):2333-2344. https://doi.org/10.1056/NEJMoa2028836.

Tanaka, T., Narazaki, M., Kishimoto, T. (2014) IL-6 in inflammation, immunity, and disease. *Cold Spring Harb. Perspect. Biol.* 6(10):a016295. https://doi.org/10.1101/cshperspect.a016295.

The REMAP-CAP Investigators (2021) Interleukin-6 receptor antagonists in critically ill patients with covid-19. *New England Journal of Medicine* 384(16):1491-1502. https://doi.org/10.1056/nejmoa2100433.

Tuma, R. L., Guedes, B. F., Carra, R., Iepsen, B., Rodrigues, J., Camelo-Filho, A. E., Kubota, G., Ferrari, M., Studart-Neto, A., Oku, M. H., Terrim, S., Lopes, C. C. B., Passos Neto, C. E. B., Fiorentino, M. D., Souza, J. C. C., Baima, J. P. S., Silva, T., Perissinotti, I., Martin, M. da G. M., Castro, L. H. (2021) Clinical, cerebrospinal fluid, and neuroimaging findings in COVID-19 encephalopathy: a case series. *Neurological Sciences: Official Journal of the Italian Neurological Society and of the Italian Society of Clinical Neurophysiology* 42(2):479-489. https://doi.org/10.1007/s10072-020-04946-w.

Veiga, V. C., Prats, J. A. G. G., Farias, D. L. C., et al. (2021) Effect of tocilizumab on clinical outcomes at 15 days in patients with severe or critical coronavirus disease 2019: randomised controlled trial. *BMJ* 372:n84-n84.

Veldhoen, M., Hocking, R. J., Atkins, C. J., Locksley, R. M., Stockinger, B. (2006) TGFbeta in the context of an inflammatory cytokine milieu supports de novo differentiation of IL-17-producing T cells. *Immunity* 24(2):179-189. https://doi.org/ 10.1016/j.immuni.2006.01.001.

Wang, Y., van Boxel-Dezaire, A. H., Cheon, H., Yang, J., Stark, G. R. (2013) STAT3 activation in response to IL-6 is prolonged by the binding of IL-6 receptor to EGF receptor. *Proc. Natl. Acad. Sci. USA* 110(42):16975-16980. https://doi.org/10.1073/pnas.1315862110.

Wan, S., Yi, Q., Fan, S., et al. (2020) Characteristics of lymphocyte subsets and cytokines in peripheral blood of 123 hospitalized patients with 2019 novel coronavirus pneumonia (NCP). *J. Infect. Dis.* 221(11):1762-1769. https://doi.org/10.1093/infdis/jiaa150.

Yang, M. L., Wang, C. T., Yang, S. J., Leu, C. H., Chen, S. H., Wu, C. L., & Shiau, A. L. (2017) IL-6 ameliorates acute lung injury in influenza virus infection. *Sci. Rep.* 7:43829. https://doi.org/10.1038/srep43829.

Valentine, K. M., Hoyer, K. K. (2019) CXCR5+ CD8 T Cells: Protective or Pathogenic? *Front. Immunol.* 10:1322. https://doi.org/10.3389/fimmu.2019.01322.

Chapter 25

Do Therapeutics for Treatment-Resistant Depression Alter Cytokine Profiles?

Caitlin Sullivan and Ivana Kawikova*, MD, PhD
Graduate Neuroscience Program, Department of Biology, School of Arts and Sciences, University of Hartford, West Hartford, CT, USA

Abstract

About 30% of patients with major depressive disorder remain resistant to pharmacological treatment even though attempts to treat with at least two different classes of anti-depressant medications were completed at a sufficient dose for a sufficient length of time. The mechanism of treatment-resistant depression is not yet understood. Inflammatory molecules are often increased in patients with major depressive disorder. One possibility is that the inflammatory processes contribute to the resistance to treatment with anti-depressants that affect neuronal circuitries by elevating levels of norepinephrine or serotonin in neuronal synapses. The role of inflammation in the pathogenesis of depression is supported by randomized, double-blind clinical trials that tested inhibitors of cyclooxygenase or cytokine blockers and showed additive effects of the anti-inflammatory medications to a classical anti-depressant. Therapeutic interventions in treatment-resistant depression include electroconvulsive therapy, ketamine, and psilocybin. All the interventions have anti-inflammatory properties, but little is known about psilocybin, whose impact on inflammation was tested only in vitro. Till today, there is no direct comparison of inflammatory markers in individuals that are treatment-sensitive versus treatment-resistant. Such comparisons will establish whether the addition of anti-inflammatory medication may assist in the therapeutic effect.

Keywords: treatment-resistant depression, inflammation, cyclooxygenase, cytokines, interleukins, electroconvulsive therapy, ketamine, psilocybin

Introduction

Major depressive disorder (MDD) affects 4.7% of the global population (Ferrari et al., 2013). Since diagnosis of MDD is based on symptoms and no biological markers are available, it

* Corresponding Author's Email: kawikova@hartford.edu.

In: Cytokines and Diseases
Editors: Kenan Demir, Selim Görgün and Bahar Uslu
ISBN: 979-8-88697-214-6

remains unclear whether MDD represents mechanistically one or several different conditions (Souery et al., 1999). The latter appears more likely since 30% of individuals affected by MDD do not respond to most effective antidepressant medications (Al-Harbi 2012; Joffe et al., 1996). These patients are then said to suffer treatment resistant depression (TRD) that is defined as a failure to improve after two mechanistically distinct medications that were given at adequate doses and duration (Gaynes et al., 2020). Alternative approaches to treat patients with TRD include electroconvulsive treatment, and more recently also ketamine and psilocybin (Pandarakalam 2018).

In recent years, significant evidence suggests a role of immune mechanisms in pathogenesis of MDD. A meta-analysis uncovered a significant increase in proinflammatory cytokines IL-6 and TNF-α in depressed subjects compared to healthy controls (Dowlati et al., 2010). An evaluation of cytokine and chemokine panel that included MIP-1α, IL-1α, IL-1β, IL-6, IL-8, IL-10, Eotaxin, GM-CSF, and IFNγ demonstrated a significant increase in those with MDD compared to the healthy controls (Simon et al., 2008). Similarly in postmortem studies, the mRNA and protein expression levels cytokines IL-6, IL-β and TNFα in the prefrontal cortex of teenage suicide victims revealed a significant increase of these three cytokines in Brodmann's area 10 of the suicide victims compared to the healthy controls (Pandey et al., 2012). There is, however, no direct comparison of cytokines in patients with MDD versus TRD.

We asked here whether treatments with anti-inflammatory medications have any beneficial effects in treating depression, and whether some of the alternative treatment approaches to manage TRD affect inflammatory cytokine profiles of the patients.

Do Anti-Inflammatory Medications Improve Depressive Symptoms?

Elevated levels of prostaglandins were observed in patients with depression (Linnoila et al., 1983), which motivated clinical trials on effects of inhibition of prostaglandin synthesis by non-steroidal anti-inflammatory drugs (NSAIDs) that blocking cyclooxygenase (COX). A prospective, double blind clinical trial employed a COX-2 inhibitor, celecoxib, that is particularly effective at sites of induced inflammation. Forty patients with acute depressive episode received either reboxetine alone (a norepinephrine reuptake inhibitor; 4-10 mg) or reboxetine plus celecoxib (400 mg) for six weeks. Over this period, both groups improved, but celecoxib showed significantly greater improvement on Hamilton Depression Rating Score (Ham-D) (Muller et al., 2006). In another randomized, double-blind, placebo-controlled study, celecoxib (400mg) was/or was not added to sertraline (200mg) treatment for six weeks. In addition to Ham-D scores, IL-6 concentrations were measured at the beginning and the end of this study. The patients who received celecoxib and sertraline achieved greater reduction of Ham-D scores, as well as IL-6 levels in comparison to patients who received a placebo plus sertraline. The Ham-D scores corelated with IL-6 serum concentration at week 6 of the therapy (Abbasi et al., 2012). Consistently, an experimental study that tested a commonly-used NSAID, Ibuprofen, in male rats exposed to chronic restraint stress for 21 days revealed less depressed symptoms, better memory and higher wait gain compared to the vehicle control (Nozari et al., 2020).

Besides prostaglandins, also various cytokines are known to be elevated in patients with MDD. In double blind study of 618 patients with moderate psoriasis who were treated with anti-tumor necrosis factor alpha (TNF α) antibody, etanercept, revealed not only alleviation of the skin symptoms, but also, as secondary outcome, significant improvements on the Ham-D scale and the Beck depression inventory (BDI) at week 12 of treatment as compared to placebo (Tyring et al., 2006). A study investigating the IL-12 and IL-23 inhibitor ustekinumab showed also significant improvements in their Hospital Anxiety and Depression Scale-Depression and Hospital Anxiety and Depression Scale (Kohler et al., 2014; Muller et al., 2006; Tyring et al., 2006).

In summary, anti-inflammatory medications resulted in improvement of depressive syndrome suggesting that inflammation may be an ongoing phenomenon in major depressive disorder and its inhibition has a functional impact on improvement of MDD symptoms. Given that immune-based therapies have significant side effects, it will be important to establish their risk-to- benefit ratio in comparison to traditional anti-depressant medications.

Do Alternative Approaches to TRD Affect Cytokine Levels?

Electroconvulsive Therapy

Electroconvulsive therapy (ECT) is considered the gold standard for treating those with TRD. (Rasmussen 2002) However, its neuro-physical mechanism of action remains unknown. (Kato 2009). ECT is delivered as high frequency pulses to the right hemisphere and vertex (unilateral ECT) or bitemporal (bitemporal ECT). Bitemporal Standard Pulse ECT is the most commonly used with a response rate up to 75%. The Right Unilateral Ultrabrief is less responsive but it's still highly effective.(Lisanby 2007; Voineskos et al., 2020) A study done by The Consortium for Research in ECT (CORE) reported 79% of the 217 participants that completed the acute ECT course showed a sustained antidepressant response and 75% of those participants went into remission (Autry et al., 2011). A meta-analysis done by the UK ECT Review Group revealed that Real ECT was significantly more effective than stimulated ECT, treatment with ECT was slightly more effective than medication and that bilateral ECT was more effective that Unipolar ECT (Group 2003).

The impact of ECT on cytokines levels remains equivocal. Kruse and colleagues measured cytokine difference in serum samples (Kruse et al., 2018). Kranaster and colleagues measured cytokine levels in CSF and in serum (Kranaster et al., 2018), and Allen and colleagues measured cytokine levels in saliva and whole blood (Allen et al., 2018). Kruse and colleagues found CRP and IL-6 levels increased from baseline to after 2nd treatment of ECT and then significantly decreased after ECT treatment. They did not find any significant different in levels of TNF-α and IL-8 (Kruse et al., 2018). However, Kranaster and colleagues and Allen and colleagues did not find any significant difference in cytokine levels between their treatment groups. (Allen et al., 2018; Kranaster et al., 2018) (Table 2).

Ketamine

Ketamine is a glutamate NMDA-R antagonist that has been used as an anesthetic since the 1960s. It has since seen a recent surge of interest at subanesthetic levels as an antidepressant due to its efficacy, and both rapid and long-lasting effects (Berman et al., 2000). Ketamine was shown to be efficacious in as little as 4 hours and more effective than active placebos (i.e., Midazolam) (Berman et al., 2000; Diazgranados et al., 2010; Murrough et al., 2013). Ketamine is typically administered through intravenous injection (IV), however new emerging studies are showing similar efficacy through intranasal (Lapidus et al., 2014) and intramuscular routes (Chilukuri et al., 2014). There are currently no studies on optimal dose of ketamine, however it is typically given at 0.5mg/kg (Table 1).

Three studies assessed the impact of ketamine on at cytokines in serum (Chen et al., 2018; Kiraly et al., 2017; Yang et al., 2015) and one investigated cytokines in a whole blood analysis (Zhan et al., 2020). Each study revealed higher IL-6 levels compared to baseline. Kiraly and colleagues found no significant difference between healthy control and the treatment group for cytokines IL-1α, IL-1β and TNF-α at baseline (Kiraly et al., 2017), whereas, Yang and colleagues found that their responders and non-responders of the ketamine treatment had significantly higher levels of IL-1β and TNF-α compared to the controls and their responders had significantly higher levels of IL-1β and IL-6 compared to the controls and non-responders at baseline (Yang et al., 2015). Kiraly and colleagues and Yang and colleagues both found significant decreases in certain cytokine levels post treatment. Kiraly and colleagues found significantly lower IL-6 and IL-1α levels 4 hours post treatment (Kiraly et al., 2017). Yang and colleagues found significantly lower IL-6 levels in the responder group at 230min and 3 days post infusion and significantly lower IL-1β levels 230min and one day post infusion (Kiraly et al., 2017). Interestingly, Kiarly and colleagues did not find significant differences between cytokine levels before and after treatment after 24hrs (Kiraly et al., 2017). Chen and colleagues looked at the differences in dose and cytokine levels. They found that the 0.2 mg/kg and 0.5mg/kg of ketamine group both showed significant decreases of IL-6 and TNF-α, whereas IL-6 showed a significant decrease at 240 minutes compared to post infusion day 3 and 7 and TNF-α showed significant decreases at 40 minutes compared to post infusion day 3 and 7 (Chen et al., 2018). Zhan and colleagues investigated the effects of 6 infusions of ketamine in a 12-day period. They looked at 20 different cytokines and found the levels of IL-10, IL-12p70, IL-17A, IL-1β, IL-2, IL-4, IL-23, IL-5, IL6, IL-7, GM-CSF, IFN-γ fractalkine, and TNF-α were significantly lower on day 26 than at baseline (Zhan et al., 2020) (Table 2).

Psilocybin

The clinical effects of psilocybin in comparison to ketamine are summarized in Table 1. Psilocybin is a classical hallucinogen that acts as an agonist against serotonergic receptors 5-HT1A, 5-HT1D, 5-HT2A and 5-HT2C. It has its high affinity to 5-HT2A and 5-HT1A (Creese et al., 1975). Psilocybin is mainly taken orally, and the effects begin to appear between 10-40 minutes after ingestion (Hasler et al., 1997). A John Hopkins study found that the ideal dosage for a positive and long-term effect is 20 mg/70 kg of body weight (Johnson et al., 2012). When given in a sportive setting, psilocybin has shown to be efficacious in treating major depressive disorder, existential anxiety, and substance abuse disorders (Johnson & Griffiths 2017). An opened label pilot study revealed that after two sessions of psilocybin (session one 10mg/kg; session 2 25 mg/kg), depression symptoms decreased significantly at 1 week and 3 months post

Table 1. Differences and similarities in clinical effects of ketamine and psilocybin

Treatment	Pharmacokinetics	Mechanism of Action	Use	Adverse Events
Ketamine	Administration • Primarily intravenously • Intramuscularly • Trandermally • Subcutaneously • Intranasally • intrarectally • orally Bioavailability: • Intravenously 100% • Orally 20% • Half-life: • 2.5-3 hours	• NMDA receptor antagonist • Disinhibits pyramidal cells leading to increase in glutamate • Activates AMPA receptors • Blocks excitotoxic extra synaptic NMDA receptors • Activates synaptogenetic intracellular signaling (MTORC1, BDNF)	• TRD • MDD • Bipolar • Substance abuse disorder • Post-traumatic stress disorder • Obsessive compulsive disorder	• If administered at 0.05mg/kg, common side effects include: • Dissociation • Transient perceptual disturbances • Dysphoria • Euphoria • Anxiety • Dizziness • Nausea • increase in blood pressure and heart rate.
Psilocybin	Administration: • primarily orally • Intravenous • Half-life: • Intravenously -74 minutes • Orally- 163 minutes • Bioavailability: • Orally- 52.7%	Agonist for 5-HT1A, 5-HT1D, 5-HT2A and 5-HT2C.	• MDD • TRD • OCD • PTSD • Substance abuse disorder	• Prolonged psychosis • Increase in blood pressure • Anxiety • Confusion • Transient headaches

References: (Abdallah et al., 2016; Autry et al., 2011; Bloch et al., 2012; Creese et al., 1975; Dakwar et al., 2014; Diazgranados et al., 2010; Feder et al., 2014; Hasler et al., 1997; Homayoun & Moghaddam 2007; Johnson et al., 2008; Johnson & Griffiths 2017; Johnson et al., 2012; Li et al., 2010; Liu et al., 2012; Maeng et al., 2008; Mion & Villevieille 2013; Romeo et al., 2015; Thomas et al., 2017; Zhao et al., 2012)

Table 2. The impact of TRD therapeutic approaches on inflammatory markers

Intervention	Cytokines Measured	Cytokine Levels at Baseline	Changes in Cytokine Levels Post Treatment	Reference
Electroconvulsive Therapy	IL-1β, IL-6, IL-8, TNF-α and CRP (Plasma)	N/A	CRP ↓(p < 0.001) IL-6 ↓ (p < 0.01) TNF-α and IL-8 not sig.	(Kruse et al., 2018)
	IL-6, neopterin, sCD14, sCD163 MIF and MCP1 (CSF and Serum)	N/A	IL-6, neopterin, sCD14, sCD163, MIF and MCP not sig. MIF ↓ sCD14 ↓ in remitters group	(Kranaster et al., 2018)
	IL-6, IL-8, IL-10, and IFN-γ (Saliva and whole blood)	IL-6, IL-8, IL-10, and IFN-γ not sig. but were in saliva samples in ECT group (p =0.006)	•Not sig. in either groups	(Allen et al., 2018)
Ketamine	IL-6, IL-1α, IL-1β, TNF-α (serum)	• TRD IL-6 ↑ compared to HC at (p= 0.01)	• IL-6 (p < 0.05)↓ • IL-1α (p < 0.05) ↓ • Not sig. • after 24 hours	(Kiraly et al., 2017)
	IL-6, IL-1β, TNF-α (serum)	• R and NR ↑ IL-1β and TNF-α (p < .001) • R↑ IL-1β and IL-6 compared to NR and HC (p < 0.001)	• R IL-1β ↓ (p= 0.013) • R group IL-6 ↓ (p < 0.001)	(Yang et al., 2015)
	CRP, IL-6, TNF-α (serum)	N/A	• CRP levels (p = 0.472) • IL-6 ↓ (p =0.002) • TNF-α ↓(p = 0.001) • 0.5mg/kg group TNF-α levels ↓ (p< 0.05)	(Chen et al., 2018)
	ITAC, GM-CSF, fractalkine, IFN-γ, IL-10, MIP-3α, IL-12p70, IL-13, IL-17A, IL-1β, IL-2, IL-4, IL-23, IL-5, IL-6, IL-7, IL-8, MIP-1β, and TNF-α (Whole Blood)	N/A	• IL-10, IL-12p70, IL-17A, IL-1β, IL-2, IL-4, IL-23, IL-5, IL6, IL-7, GM-CSF, IFN-γ fractalkine, and TNF-α ↓(p < 0.05)	(Zhan et al., 2020)
Psilocybin	IL-6, IL-10, IL-1β, TNF-α	N/A	• TNF-α ↓(p <0.001), • IL-1β↓ (p < 0.05) • IL-6 ↓ (p< 0.05)	(Nkadimeng et al., 2021)

Notes: Interleukin (IL); Tumor Necrosis Factor- alpha (TNF-α); C-Reactive Protein; Soluble CD (sCD); Macrophage Migration Inhibitory Factor (MIF); Monocyte Chemoattractant Protein (MCP); Interferon gamma (IFN-γ); granulocyte-macrophage colony-stimulating factor (GM-CSF); CSF cerebral spinal fluid; ECT- Electroconvulsive therapy; R= Responder, NR= Nonresponder; HC= Healthy Control; ↑ = increase; ↓= decrease treatment for those with TRD (Carhart-Harris et al., 2016). A recent study looked into participants with moderate to severe, long standing MDD. In this study psilocybin and escitalopram were compared on their efficacy. The study found no significant differences on their efficacy between either drug however, the participants tended to favored psilocybin over escitalopram (Carhart-Harris et al., 2021).

One study was found that investigated psilocybin effects on inflammation. In this study four different psilocybin containing mushrooms, *Panaeolus cyanescens, Psilocybe natalensis, Psilocybe cubensis* and *Psilocybe cubensis leucistic A+ strain,* were extracted with boiling water and examined in vitro on 15-lipoxygenase activity(15-LOX), and on lipopolysaccharide (LPS)-induced inflammation in human U937 macrophage cells. IL-6, IL-1β, TNF-α, IL-10 and COX-2 concentrations were also determined. Results from the study revealed that all four strains of mushroom had low inhibition properties on LOX-15. When human U937 macrophage cells were stimulated with LPS, the COX-2 levels increased significantly when compared to non-stimulated controls ($p = 0.009$). However, when treated with the four extracts, COX-2 significantly decreased ($p = 0.039$). LPS stimulated cells increased the levels of TNF-α ($p = 0.003$), IL-1β ($p < 0.001$), IL-6 ($p = 0.010$). When treated with each of the four stains, TNF-α significantly decreased ($p < 0.001$), IL-1β ($p < 0.05$) and IL-6 however these changes were only seen with *P. natalensis* stain at 25 and 50 μg/mL ($p = 0.025$ and $p = 0.015$ respectively) and *P. cubensis* strain at 50 μg/mL ($p = 0.040$). IL-10 decreased with the stimulation LPS cells; however, this was found to be not significant, and the production of IL-10 increased non significantly with each treatment in LPS induced cells (Nkadimeng et al., 2021).

Conclusion

Interventional studies in MDD suggest that an addition of anti-inflammatory medications, such as ibuprofen, celocoxib or enterecept, improve anti-depressive effects of classical medications. Concerning therapeutic approaches to TRD, ketamine appears to have anti-inflammatory properties, which likely contribute to its anti-depressive impact. Concerning electroconvulsive therapy, inflammatory molecules appear to drop after a second treatment. Finally, psilocybin does have anti-inflammatory effects in vitro, but whether this effect will correspond to an inhibition of depressive symptoms in vivo is yet to be determined. In summary, existing data suggest that inhibition of inflammation is a beneficial add-on treatment, and that approaches that appear effective in TRD may at least in part work due to their anti-inflammatory effects. More studies are needed to directly compare inflammatory markers in TRD versus treatment-sensitive depression.

References

Abbasi S H, Hosseini F, Modabbernia A, Ashrafi M, Akhondzadeh S (2012) Effect of celecoxib add-on treatment on symptoms and serum IL-6 concentrations in patients with major depressive disorder: randomized double-blind placebo-controlled study. *J. Affect. Disord.* 141(2-3):308-314. https://doi.org/10.1016/j.jad.2012.03.033.

Abdallah C G, Adams T G, Kelmendi B, Esterlis I, Sanacora G, Krystal J H (2016) Ketamine's Mechanism of Action: A Path to Rapid-Acting Antidepressants. *Depress. Anxiety* 33(8):689-697. https://doi.org/10.1002/da.22501.

Al-Harbi K S (2012) Treatment-resistant depression: therapeutic trends, challenges, and future directions. *Patient Prefer Adherence* 6:369-388. https://doi.org/10.2147/PPA.S29716.

Allen A P, Naughton M, Dowling J, Walsh A, O'Shea R, Shorten G, . . . Dinan TG (2018) Kynurenine pathway metabolism and the neurobiology of treatment-resistant depression: Comparison of multiple ketamine infusions and electroconvulsive therapy. *J. Psychiatr. Res.* 100:24-32. https://doi.org/10.1016/j.jpsychires.2018.02.011.

Autry A E, Adachi M, Nosyreva E, Na E S, Los MF, Cheng P F, . . . Monteggia L M (2011) NMDA receptor blockade at rest triggers rapid behavioural antidepressant responses. *Nature* 475(7354):91-95. https://doi.org/10.1038/nature10130.

Berman R M, Cappiello A, Anand A, Oren D A, Heninger G R, Charney D S, Krystal J H (2000) Antidepressant effects of ketamine in depressed patients. *Biol. Psychiatry* 47(4):351-354. https://doi.org/10.1016/s0006-3223(99)00230-9.

Bloch M H, Wasylink S, Landeros-Weisenberger A, Panza KE, Billingslea E, Leckman J F, . . . Pittenger C (2012) Effects of ketamine in treatment-refractory obsessive-compulsive disorder. *Biol. Psychiatry* 72(11):964-970. https://doi.org/10.1016/j.biopsych.2012.05.028.

Carhart-Harris R, Giribaldi B, Watts R, Baker-Jones M, Murphy-Beiner A, Murphy R, . . . Nutt DJ (2021) Trial of Psilocybin versus Escitalopram for Depression. *N. Engl. J. Med.* 384(15):1402-1411. https://doi.org/10.1056/NEJMoa2032994.

Carhart-Harris R L, Bolstridge M, Rucker J, Day CM, Erritzoe D, Kaelen M, . . . Nutt DJ (2016) Psilocybin with psychological support for treatment-resistant depression: an open-label feasibility study. *Lancet Psychiatry* 3(7):619-627. https://doi.org/10.1016/S2215-0366(16)30065-7.

Chen M H, Li C T, Lin W C, Hong C J, Tu P C, Bai Y M, . . . Su TP (2018) Rapid inflammation modulation and antidepressant efficacy of a low-dose ketamine infusion in treatment-resistant depression: A randomized, double-blind control study. *Psychiatry Res.* 269:207-211. https://doi.org/10.1016/j.psychres.2018.08.078.

Chilukuri H, Reddy N P, Pathapati R M, Manu A N, Jollu S, Shaik A B (2014) Acute antidepressant effects of intramuscular versus intravenous ketamine. *Indian J. Psychol. Med.* 36(1):71-76. https://doi.org/10.4103/0253-7176.127258.

Creese I, Burt D R, Synder S H (1975) The dopamine receptor: differential binding of d-LSD and related agents to agonist and antagonist states. *Life Sci.* 17(11):1715-1719. https://doi.org/10.1016/0024-3205(75)90118-6.

Dakwar E, Levin F, Foltin R W, Nunes E V, Hart C L (2014) The effects of subanesthetic ketamine infusions on motivation to quit and cue-induced craving in cocaine-dependent research volunteers. *Biol. Psychiatry* 76(1):40-46. https://doi.org/10.1016/j.biopsych.2013.08.009.

Diazgranados N, Ibrahim L, Brutsche NE, Newberg A, Kronstein P, Khalife S, . . . Zarate CA Jr (2010) A randomized add-on trial of an N-methyl-D-aspartate antagonist in treatment-resistant bipolar depression. *Arch. Gen. Psychiatry* 67(8):793-802. https://doi.org/10.1001/archgenpsychiatry.2010.90.

Dowlati Y, Herrmann N, Swardfager W, Liu H, Sham L, Reim E K., Lanctot KL (2010) A meta-analysis of cytokines in major depression. *Biol. Psychiatry* 67(5):446-457. https://doi.org/10.1016/j.biopsych.2009.09.033.

Feder A, Parides M K, Murrough J W, Perez A M, Morgan J E, Saxena S, . . . Charney DS (2014) Efficacy of intravenous ketamine for treatment of chronic posttraumatic stress disorder: a randomized clinical trial. *JAMA Psychiatry* 71(6):681-688. https://doi.org/10.1001/jamapsychiatry.2014.62.

Ferrari A J, Somerville A J, Baxter A J, Norman R, Patten S B, Vos T, Whiteford HA (2013) Global variation in the prevalence and incidence of major depressive disorder: a systematic review of the epidemiological literature. *Psychol. Med.* 43(3):471-481. https://doi.org/10.1017/S0033291712001511.

Gaynes B N, Lux L, Gartlehner G, Asher G, Forman-Hoffman V, Green J, . . . Lohr KN (2020) Defining treatment-resistant depression. *Depress Anxiety* 37(2):134-145. https://doi.org/10.1002/da.22968.

Group UER (2003) Efficacy and safety of electroconvulsive therapy in depressive disorders: a systematic review and meta-analysis. Lancet 361(9360):799-808. https://doi.org/10.1016/s0140-6736(03)12705-5.

Hasler F, Bourquin D, Brenneisen R, Bar T, Vollenweider FX (1997) Determination of psilocin and 4-hydroxyindole-3-acetic acid in plasma by HPLC-ECD and pharmacokinetic profiles of oral and intravenous psilocybin in man. *Pharm. Acta Helv.* 72(3):175-184. https://doi.org/10.1016/s0031-6865(97)00014-9.

Homayoun H, Moghaddam B (2007) NMDA receptor hypofunction produces opposite effects on prefrontal cortex interneurons and pyramidal neurons. *J. Neurosci.* 27(43):11496-11500. https://doi.org/10.1523/JNEUROSCI.2213-07.2007.

Joffe R T, Levitt AJ, Sokolov S T (1996) Augmentation strategies: focus on anxiolytics. J Clin Psychiatry 57(Suppl 7): 25-31. Avaible via https://www.ncbi.nlm.nih.gov/pubmed/8690693.

Johnson M, Richards W, Griffiths R (2008) Human hallucinogen research: guidelines for safety. *J. Psychopharmacol.* 22(6):603-620. https://doi.org/10.1177/0269881108093587.

Johnson M W, Griffiths R R (2017) Potential Therapeutic Effects of Psilocybin. Neurotherapeutics 14(3):734-740. https://doi.org/10.1007/s13311-017-0542-y.

Johnson M W, Sewell R A, Griffiths R R (2012) Psilocybin dose-dependently causes delayed, transient headaches in healthy volunteers. *Drug Alcohol. Depend.* 123(1-3):132-140. https://doi.org/10.1016/j.drugalcdep.2011.10.029.

Kato N (2009) Neurophysiological mechanisms of electroconvulsive therapy for depression. *Neurosci. Res.* 64(1):3-11. https://doi.org/10.1016/j.neures.2009.01.014.

Kiraly D D, Horn S R, Van Dam N T, Costi S, Schwartz J, Kim-Schulze S, . . . Murrough JW (2017) Altered peripheral immune profiles in treatment-resistant depression: response to ketamine and prediction of treatment outcome. *Transl. Psychiatry* 7(3):e1065. https://doi.org/10.1038/tp.2017.31.

Kohler O, Benros M E, Nordentoft M, Farkouh M E, Iyengar R L, Mors O, Krogh J (2014) Effect of anti-inflammatory treatment on depression, depressive symptoms, and adverse effects: a systematic review and meta-analysis of randomized clinical trials. *JAMA Psychiatry* 71(12):1381-1391. https://doi.org/10.1001/jamapsychiatry.2014.1611.

Kranaster L, Hoyer C, Aksay S S, Bumb J M, Müller N, Zill P, . . . Sartorius A (2018) Antidepressant efficacy of electroconvulsive therapy is associated with a reduction of the innate cellular immune activity in the cerebrospinal fluid in patients with depression. *World J. Biol. Psychiatry* 19(5):379-389. https://doi.org/10.1080/15622975.2017.1355473.

Kruse J L, Congdon E, Olmstead R, Njau S, Breen E C, Narr K L, . . . Irwin M R (2018) Inflammation and Improvement of Depression Following Electroconvulsive Therapy in Treatment-Resistant Depression. *J. Clin. Psychiatry* 79(2):17m11597. https://doi.org/10.4088/JCP.17m11597.

Lapidus K A, Levitch C F, Perez A M, Brallier J W, Parides M K, Soleimani L, . . . Murrough JW (2014) A randomized controlled trial of intranasal ketamine in major depressive disorder. *Biol. Psychiatry* 76(12):970-976. https://doi.org/10.1016/j.biopsych.2014.03.026.

Li N, Lee B, Liu R J, Banasr M, Dwyer J M, Iwata M, . . . Duman RS (2010) mTOR-dependent synapse formation underlies the rapid antidepressant effects of NMDA antagonists. *Science* 329(5994):959-964. https://doi.org/10.1126/science.1190287.

Linnoila M, Whorton A R, Rubinow D R, Cowdry RW, Ninan P T, Waters R N (1983) CSF prostaglandin levels in depressed and schizophrenic patients. *Arch. Gen. Psychiatry* 40(4):405-406. https://doi.org/10.1001/archpsyc.1983.01790040059008.

Lisanby S H (2007) Electroconvulsive therapy for depression. *N. Engl. J. Med.* 357(19):1939-1945. https://doi.org/10.1056/NEJMct075234.

Liu R J, Lee FS, Li X Y, Bambico F, Duman R S, Aghajanian G K (2012) Brain-derived neurotrophic factor Val66Met allele impairs basal and ketamine-stimulated synaptogenesis in prefrontal cortex. *Biol. Psychiatry* 71(11):996-1005. https://doi.org/10.1016/j.biopsych.2011.09.030.

Maeng S, Zarate C A Jr, Du J, Schloesser R J, McCammon J, Chen G, Manji H K (2008) Cellular mechanisms underlying the antidepressant effects of ketamine: role of alpha-amino-3-hydroxy-5-methylisoxazole-4-propionic acid receptors. *Biol. Psychiatry* 63(4):349-352. https://doi.org/10.1016/j.biopsych.2007.05.028.

Mion G, Villevieille T (2013) Ketamine pharmacology: an update (pharmacodynamics and molecular aspects, recent findings) *CNS Neurosci. Ther.* 19(6):370-380. https://doi.org/10.1111/cns.12099.

Muller N, Schwarz M J, Dehning S, Douhe A, Cerovecki A, Goldstein-Muller B, . . . Riedel M (2006) The cyclooxygenase-2 inhibitor celecoxib has therapeutic effects in major depression: results of a double-blind, randomized, placebo controlled, add-on pilot study to reboxetine. *Mol. Psychiatry* 11(7):680-684. https://doi.org/10.1038/sj.mp.4001805.

Murrough J W, Perez A M, Pillemer S, Stern J, Parides M K, aan het Rot M, . . . Iosifescu DV (2013) Rapid and longer-term antidepressant effects of repeated ketamine infusions in treatment-resistant major depression. *Biol. Psychiatry* 74(4):250-256. https://doi.org/10.1016/j.biopsych.2012.06.022.

Nkadimeng S M, Steinmann C M L, Eloff J N (2021) Anti-Inflammatory Effects of Four Psilocybin-Containing Magic Mushroom Water Extracts in vitro on 15-Lipoxygenase Activity and on Lipopolysaccharide-Induced Cyclooxygenase-2 and Inflammatory Cytokines in Human U937 Macrophage Cells. *J. Inflamm. Res.* 14:3729-3738. https://doi.org/10.2147/JIR.S317182.

Nozari M, Nahavandi A, Zeinivand M, Eslami Gharaati M, Godarzi M, Ahmadi M, Jamali-Raeufy N (2020) Ibuprofen Protection Against Restrained Chronic Stress-induced Depression in Male Rats. *Basic Clin. Neurosci.* 11(4):413-422. https://doi.org/10.32598/bcn.11.4.1775.2.

Pandarakalam J P (2018) Challenges of Treatment-resistant Depression. *Psychiatr. Danub.* 30(3):273-284. https://doi.org/10.24869/psyd.2018.273.

Pandey GN, Rizavi HS, Ren X, Fareed J, Hoppensteadt DA, Roberts RC, . . . Dwivedi Y (2012) Proinflammatory cytokines in the prefrontal cortex of teenage suicide victims. *J. Psychiatr. Res.* 46(1):57-63. https://doi.org/10.1016/j.jpsychires.2011.08.006.

Rasmussen K (2002) The practice of electroconvulsive therapy: recommendations for treatment, training, and privileging (second edition). *J. ECT* 18(1):58-59. https://doi.org/10.1097/00124509-200203000-00015.

Romeo B, Choucha W, Fossati P, Rotge JY (2015) Meta-analysis of short- and mid-term efficacy of ketamine in unipolar and bipolar depression. *Psychiatry Res.* 230(2):682-688. https://doi.org/10.1016/j.psychres.2015.10.032.

Simon N M, McNamara K, Chow C W, Maser R S, Papakostas G I, Pollack M H, . . . Wong K K (2008) A detailed examination of cytokine abnormalities in Major Depressive Disorder. *Eur. Neuropsychopharmacol.*18(3):230-233. https://doi.org/10.1016/j.euroneuro.2007.06.004.

Souery D, Amsterdam J, de Montigny C, Lecrubier Y, Montgomery S, Lipp O, . . . Mendlewicz J (1999) Treatment resistant depression: methodological overview and operational criteria. *Eur. Neuropsychopharmacol.* 9(1-2):83-91. https://doi.org/10.1016/s0924-977x(98)00004-2.

Thomas K, Malcolm B, Lastra D (2017) Psilocybin-Assisted Therapy: A Review of a Novel Treatment for Psychiatric Disorders. *J. Psychoactive Drugs* 49(5):446-455. https://doi.org/10.1080/02791072.2017.1320734.

Tyring S, Gottlieb A, Papp K, Gordon K, Leonardi C, Wang A, . . . Krishnan R (2006) Etanercept and clinical outcomes, fatigue, and depression in psoriasis: double-blind placebo-controlled randomised phase III trial. *Lancet* 367(9504):29-35. https://doi.org/10.1016/S0140-6736(05)67763-X.

Voineskos D, Daskalakis Z J, Blumberger DM (2020) Management of Treatment-Resistant Depression: Challenges and Strategies. Neuropsychiatr Dis Treat 16:221-234. https://doi.org/10.2147/NDT.S198774.

Yang JJ, Wang N, Yang C, Shi JY, Yu HY, Hashimoto K (2015) Serum interleukin-6 is a predictive biomarker for ketamine's antidepressant effect in treatment-resistant patients with major depression. *Biol .Psychiatry* 77(3):e19-e20. https://doi.org/10.1016/j.biopsych.2014.06.021.

Zhan Y, Zhou Y, Zheng W, Liu W, Wang C, Lan X, . . . Ning Y (2020) Alterations of multiple peripheral inflammatory cytokine levels after repeated ketamine infusions in major depressive disorder. *Transl. Psychiatry* 10(1):246. https://doi.org/10.1038/s41398-020-00933-z.

Zhao X, Venkata S L, Moaddel R, Luckenbaugh D A, Brutsche NE, Ibrahim L, . . . Wainer IW (2012) Simultaneous population pharmacokinetic modelling of ketamine and three major metabolites in patients with treatment-resistant bipolar depression. *Br. J. Clin. Pharmacol.* 74(2):304-314. https://doi.org/10.1111/j.1365-2125.2012.04198.x.

Chapter 26

Cytokines and Neuroinflammation/Neurodegeneration

Esra Yalçın, MD, Hacer İşler*, MD and Zeynep Köksal, MD
Samsun Gazi State Hospital Department of Neurology, Samsun, Turkey
University of Health Sciences, Samsun Training and Research Hospital, Department of Medical Microbiology, Samsun, Turkey
Samsun Gazi State Hospital Department of Medical Microbiology, Samsun, Turkey

Abstract

Neuroinflammation is defined as the response of brain cells to infections and other causes of cell death, as well as to altered homeostasis of reactive central nervous system (CNS) elements, whose passage by cells of the innate and adaptive immune systems into the brain and spinal cord is affected from inside or outside the CNS. It includes all neurological diseases that are ischemic, inflammatory, traumatic, metabolic and developmentally contagious, neoplastic, toxic and neurodegenerative diseases. Microglial cells, astrocytes, oligodendrocytes, and NG2+ glia together with the blood-brain barrier (BBB), cytokines, and cytokine signaling, form the main reactive components of the CNS. This process is often referred to as neuroinflammation. The microglia are at the center of this process where some important cytokines have an effect on some immunological events related to the central nervous system. In this context, the etiopathogenic effects of IL-17 and IL-6 are particularly important. IL-17 is an important autoimmune agent, especially in stroke and multiple sclerosis. IL-6 is a factor in the etiology of experimental autoimmune encephalomyelitis (EAE). Fractalkin has important roles in neuroinflammation and neurodegeneration. In diseases with neurodegeneration, activated microglia are observed in the lesions and their relationship with proinflammatory cytokines has been determined.

Keywords: neuroinflammation, cytokines, neurodegeneration

Introduction

It provides cells with the ability to communicate with each other and regulate complex multicellular behavior. In proteinopathies, cytokines produced by cells in the CNS cause tissue damage in the central nervous system. Such as multiple sclerosis and encephalitis, in

* Corresponding Author's Email: hacerturkisler@gmail.com.

In: Cytokines and Diseases
Editors: Kenan Demir, Selim Görgün and Bahar Uslu
ISBN: 979-8-88697-214-6

degenerative illness proinflammatory cytokines are importantly released by leukocytes that infest the tissue. In degenerative diseases such as multiple sclerosis and encephalitis, proinflammatory cytokines released by leukocytes invade tissue, providing cells with the ability to communicate with each other and regulate complex multicellular behaviors (Becher et al., 2017). The most common examples of typical proteinopathies are Alzheimer's illness and Parkinson's illness. In the healthy brain, those proteins are in the physiological monomer form. In those diseases, unstructured proteins endure change that leads to small oligomers that will finally aggregate into higher-order structures (Bayer 2015).

In the last few decades, the concept of neuroinflammation has been defined as the response of brain cells to infections and other causes of cell death, as well as the transition of reactive central nervous system (CNS) elements to the brain and spinal cord by cells of the innate and adaptive immune systems, altered and imposed from inside or outside the CNS. It is defined as the response to homeostasis and characterizes all neurological diseases, including developmental, traumatic, ischemic, inflammatory, metabolic and infectious, toxic, neoplastic and neurodegenerative diseases. Microglial cells, astrocytes, oligodendrocytes, and NG2+ glia (also called polydendrocytes or oligodendrocyte progenitor cells), together with the blood-brain barrier (BBB), cytokines, and cytokine signaling, form the main reactive components of the CNS. Cytokines are substances in a peptide or glycoprotein structure with a weight of 20-30 kD synthesized by stimulated lymphocytes, monocytes, macrophages and some other somatic cells. Their molecular weights are quite low. They are active even at 10-15 molar concentrations and effective in soluble form (Weber et al., 2017).

Chemokines are small proteins that are involved in cellular migration and intercellular communication. They weigh between 8 and 12 kDa. Chemokines and their receptors are found in the glia and neurons in the brain. These receptors are located in the hypothalamus, hippocampus, thalamus, cortex, limbic system, and cerebellum in the brain. They are also known as neurotransmitters, neuromodulators, neuropeptides and neurohormones such as CX3CL1 (Fractalkin), CCL2 (MCP-1), CXCL12 (SDF 1α), CCL3 (MIP1α), CXCL10 (IP10) and CCL5 (RANTES), chemokines that are often localized in the neurons and glia in the brain. These named molecules affect not only neuronal activity, but also the regulation of the pathological and hemostatic state of the brain and nervous system (Niemir et al., 1995).

Neurotransmitters play a role in interneuronal communication and transmission of the message between the neuron and the effector. Endogenous molecules are synthesized and secreted presynaptically. They qualify synaptic activity, regulate contagion, and play a role in the secondary message system. Neurohormones have intrinsic activity and are responsible for regulating the functions of both neuronal and non-neuronal cells and the molecules released from them (Compston et al., 1998).

Fractalkin is a chemokine, a small protein of 373 amino acids from the CX3C group. It is first released from neuronal cells in the brain. Fractalkin receptors (CX3CR1) are expressed in the microglia. The fractalkin synthesized in the microglia and astrocytes is stimulated by TNFα and IFNγ (Imaizumi et al., 2004). The soluble form of fractalkin, a glycoprotein weighing 95 kDa in its membranous form, plays a potent chemoattractive activator role for T cells, NK cells and monocytes. They inhibit the activation of the microglia by inhibiting TNFα secretion from the activated microglia. Activation of the microglia triggers the release of proinflammatory cytokines, NO and peroxynitrite. NO and peroxynitrite have toxic effects on the neuronal cells. Fractalkin, on the other hand, protects neurons by inhibiting these effects (Ormerod and McDonald 1984). It is involved in chemotactic reactions, leukocyte movement and TNF alpha formation through CX3CR1 receptors localized on the microglia, monocytes, and NK and T cells. While its soluble form activates monocytes, and NK and T cells, it increases the synthesis of other cytokines (Dimberg et al., 2007; Ormerod and McDonald 1984).

Fractalkin stimulated by TNFα and IFNγ is synthesized in the microglia and astrocytes (Imaizumi et al., 2004). The soluble form of fractalkin, a glycoprotein weighing 95 kDa in its membranous form, plays a potent chemoattractive activator role for T cells, NK cells and monocytes. They inhibit the activation of microglia by inhibiting TNFα secretion from activated microglia. Activation of microglia causes the release of proinflammatory cytokines, NO and peroxynitrite, and these molecules have toxic effects on neuronal cells. In the last few decades, the concept of neuroinflammation has been defined as the response of brain cells to infections and other causes of cell death, as well as the transition of reactive central nervous system (CNS) elements to the brain and spinal cord by cells of the innate and adaptive immune systems, altered and imposed from inside or outside the CNS. It is defined as the response to homeostasis and characterizes all neurological diseases, including developmental, traumatic, ischemic, inflammatory, infectious, toxic, metabolic, neoplastic and neurodegenerative illness. Microglial cells, oligodendrocytes, astrocytes, the blood-brain barrier (BBB), cytokines, and cytokine signaling, form the gross reactive components of the CNS (Alliot et al., 1999).

The adaptive immune system also affects neuroinflammation. T cells institute immune responses through fundamental dendritic cells. However, in normal brain parenchyma, there are no cells that can take up the antigen for presentation, exit the CNS, and enter a local lymphatic system on their way to a lymph node (Matyszak 1998). This key difference defends the cellular basis of the immune dispensation of the CNS.

Central memory CD4+ T cells complete the immune surveillance. Those cells enter the CSF via the choroid plexus and meningeal veins and ascend to the deep cervical lymph nodes mostly via the cribriform plate (Louveau et al., 2015; Andres et al., 1987). Leukocyte migration, which is an integral component of many neuroinflammatory reactions, turns on the leukocyte-endothelial cell bonds constituent with selectins/carbohydrate bonds; chemokines and other G protein-coupled receptor ligands and their receptors; and integrins/cellular adhesion molecules initiate physiological and pathological events (Von Andrian and Mackay 2000; Leick et al., 2014).

B cells produce antibodies after antigen presentation to the CNS, which, unlike cellular immunity, can initiate humoral adaptive immune reactions within the CNS. B cells that can discriminate plasma cells and plasmablasts source the construction of contentious cytokines and the activation of T cells (Gordon et al., 1992).

CD40 excitation is important in the formation of IL-6 and IL-10 by stimulating B cells in pathogenic (IL-6) and regulatory (IL-10) functions in vivo. IL-6 is incremented by CD40 stimulation while IL-10 is inhibited. It suggests that B cells that correspond to TLRs become regulatory, and that T cells help B cells to purport inflammation by secreting IL-6 (Burdin et al., 1995). IL-6 appears to inhibit Ig secretion for B cells triggered by the simultaneous neutralization of IL-10, CD40 Ag and AgR (65-75%). Ingeniously produced IL-6 and IL-10 are proved in CD40-activated B-cell differentiation which demonstrates that B-cell deficiency therapy (BCDT) can effectively rebate disease evolution in regression-distributing multiple sclerosis (RR-MS) and empirical autoimmune encephalomyelitis (Bar-Or et al., 2008; Hauser et al., 2008; Matsushita et al., 2008).

In both patients and mice, the rebated illness severity after B-cell reduction was attended by a reduction in an autoreactive Th17 reply, meaning that B cells make an essential donation to the boosting of IL-6-dependent pathogenic Th17 separation (Betteli et al., 2006).

Inhibiting the function of the IL-17 family of cytokines, where IL-6 has many other effects on the pathology in autoimmune or chronic inflammatory conditions, may have a beneficial effect on pathogenic conditions in the CNS (Neurath and Finotto 2011), i.e., elevated IL-17 levels. There is evidence linking depression as a common comorbidity with various inflammatory diseases, as well as different types of infection of the CNS, suggesting that B cells may also secrete other proinflammatory cytokines in MS (Duddy et al., 2007; Bar-Or et al., 2010).

Inflammation has been recognized as playing a central role in many CNS diseases. IFN-γ is a pleiotropic cytokine. The role of inflammation, and particularly IFN-γ, in modulating NSPC functions is being actively studied. IFNγ is a variable that influences how NSPCs respond in inflammatory conditions. Here, studies in Alzheimer's disease, multiple sclerosis and viral neurotropic infection models are plentiful (Wyss et al., 2021).

Neurodegenerative diseases are an important health problem today and basically neuron death takes place (Przedborski 2008). Neurodegeneration can be explained as the cells in the nervous system losing their structures and therefore their functions in a certain process. Many factors are blamed for the resulting diseases. In studies on this subject, it has been understood that unwanted protein accumulation, and endogenous and exogenous factors play a role in the etiology of neurodegeneration (Kwon and Koh 2020). Alzheimer's disease can be given as an example for these etiopathologies. The main problem here is the accumulation of amyloid beta proteins, which are cut by proteosomes but cannot be removed by protease enzymes, like senile plaques between neurons (Tobore 2019). After tau proteins become hyperphosphorylated, they accumulate in neurons and neurofibrillary tangles are formed. When the etiopathogenesis of Parkinson's disease is followed, a different process is followed. This time alpha-synuclein (Lewy) deposits accumulate inside the neuron (Gomez-Benito et al., 2020).

Inflammation, which has been shown to cause neurodegeneration, creates oxidative stress. This results in the collection of Lewy-like structures in the intraneuronal region (Hickman et al., 2018). The neuroimmune system takes care of the normal functioning, aging, development, and injury of the central nervous system with the microglia. It has the ability to damage and kill neurons as a result of neuroinflammation. In diseases such as Alzheimer's disease, the mechanism is driven by injury to neurons, dysregulation of the defense function and neuroinflammation (Hickman et al., 2008). The neuroimmune system is involved in the development, normal functioning, aging, and injury of the central nervous system. Microglia are one of the most essential parts of this system. Microglia are the focal point for any discussion of neuroinflammation. The microglial cells' innate immune cells perform the primary immune surveillance and macrophage-like activities of the CNS, including the production of cytokines and chemokines. Indeed, much of the inherent immune capacity of the CNS is mediated by the microglia. They also control Cx3cr1 and Trem2, the progranulin pathways, which act as immune checkpoints to keep the microglial inflammatory reply under control, and the scrounge receptor pathways, which promote clearance of injurious stimuli. Peripheral interference from systemic inflammation or the gut microbiome can also alter the evolvement of such injury. Microglial cells trigger other immune elements through cytokines. Proinflammatory cytokine (interleukin (IL)-1β), with tumor necrosis factor (TNF)α and IL-6 emerging, CNS cells, chemokines (CCL2, CXCL1, CCL5) secondary messengers (NO and prostaglandins), and reactive oxygen species are relevant in neuroinflammation (DiSabato et al., 2016).

Under normal circumstances, neuroinflammation acts as a neuroprotection, neural plasticity and tissue repair process. This situation can be accepted as a defensive act of normal brain tissue against all exogen and endogen factors. However, irritation can also give rise to the exertion of immune cells, edema, and tissue damage. When the whole process is prolonged and becomes chronic the cytokines result in catastrophic circumstances on potential cell death (Norden et al., 2016). Moreover, the degree of neuroinflammation depends on the context, duration, and course of the primary stimulus.

The formation of chronic inflammation in the brain is directly proportional to the uptake of certain immune elements and the release of certain cytokines. It has also been observed that single point mutations (SNPs) in some disease-related genes induce a maladaptive primary immune response. The fact that the maladaptive primary immune response is also associated with aging and epigenetic changes reveals the link between neurodegeneration and aging (Gan et al., 2018).

There are many other cytokines responsible for the etiopathogenesis of diseases in the central nervous system. In these, IL-17 is thought to be particularly effective in stroke and multiple sclerosis (Waisman et al., 2015). The IL-17-related cytokine family is located in the space between tissue cells and immune cells. IL-17 is a cytokine that has been extensively studied in the last decade and it belongs to a very large family. The functions of cytokines, which have been defined so far from IL-17 A to IL-17 F, are quite different from one to other (Duddy et al., 2007). IL-17 A and IL-17 F are synthesized by a special group of lymphoid defense cells such as Th17 and γδ T cells. Basically, while other members of the IL-17 family have a stimulating effect on the immune system, IL-17 E, on the contrary, has a suppressive effect on the inflammatory process. In some studies, even in diseases such as rheumatoid arthritis with chronic inflammation, IL-17 levels in the CNS are high (Barr et al., 2012). One of the main mediators providing communication between tissue and immune cells in the CNS is IL-17. The disease most closely associated with Th17 cells and IL-17 in the CNS is multiple sclerosis (MS) (Compston and Coles 2008). Immunological mechanisms have been widely discussed in the etiopathogenesis and treatment of MS disease. In some previous experimental studies, it has been shown that B-cell depletion therapy (BCDT) effectively slows down the progression of the disease and experimental autoimmune encephalomyelitis (IEM) (Fillatreau et al., 2002). In this context, B cells are thought to support the inflammatory response in MS, in addition to their known regulatory role and capacity. Polymorphism in genes that control T-cell stimulation commonly in RR-MS is observed as a very common problem (Bettelli et al., 2006). However, although it is known that the tissue damage caused by B cells in RR-MS disease is caused by the production of autoantibodies, the other mechanisms responsible for the etiopathology are not fully understood.

In the clinic, it is known that BCDT administration significantly changes the course of autoimmune diseases independent of autoantibody levels. This shows that the mechanism of action of BCDT is not fully understood (Fillatreau et al., 2008). In fact, new evidence is emerging that IL-6 acquisition is markedly raised in RR-MS patients and is a part of the B-cell-mediated inflammatory process. Rituximab treatment is effective in these patients by reducing the level of IL-6, which is produced in high amounts by B cells (Hauser et al., 2008). After treatment, the IL-6 level produced by B cells is observed as normal in these patients. The supportive effect of interventions on IL-6 levels and activation on Th17 in MS treatment is remarkable (Eugster et al., 1998). In animal experiments, there is a decrease in the Th17 autoreactive response, especially due to the decrease in the efficiency of B cells.

Another defense cell, Th1, is also implicated in the etiopathogenesis of EAE and MS. These cells are thought to provide for the progression of the illness. In the presence of IL-6, IL-17 A stimulates T-cell migration, especially by stimulating astrocytes (Lee et al., 2011). However, IL-17 A alone cannot produce such an effect. In fact, IL-6, which is synthesized by B cells, is an agent that has a role in many other autoimmune or chronic inflammatory pathologies, although its mechanism of action has not been fully elucidated (Neurath and Finotto 2011). IL-6 controls the proliferation of activated T cells and their resistance to apoptosis, which affects T cell functions (Scheller et al., 2006). The development of Th17 cells as well as myelin-specific Th1 in EAE can be attributed to this condition. Although it is frequently emphasized that the main contribution of B cells to MS disease is via IL-6, it is hoped that this process will be understood in more detail in the future (Alatab et al., 2011). B cells that respond to TLRs directly or indirectly act as a regulator for T cells and support the inflammatory response with IL-6. Human B cells' IL-10 can also be increased by CD40 stimulation. For example, it has recently been understood that IL-10 is derived from naive B cells in contrast to activated/mind B cells in patients with RR-MS, and the reverse is true for inflammatory cytokines such as TNF and lymphotoxin (Yen et al., 2015). In future studies, it will be important to identify the urging that induces the in-vivo IL-6 definition. Definition studies are needed regarding the signals that turn on different B-cell cytokine reactions in vivo during illness selection.

Conclusion

As summarized above, neuroinflammation has a very important role in many diseases involving the CNS. With the studies to be done on this subject, effective methods can be developed that can have a positive effect on the clinical condition of the patients and control neuroinflammation.

References

Alatab S, Maghbooli Z, Hossein-Nezhad A, Khosrofar M, Mokhtari F (2011) Cytokine profile, Foxp3 and nuclear factor-kB ligand levels in multiple sclerosis subtypes. *Minerva Med.* 102(6):461-8.

Alliot F, Godin I, Pessac B (1999) Microglia derive from progenitors, originating from the yolk sac, and which proliferate in the brain. *Brain Res. Dev. Brain Res.* 117:145–152 https://doi.org/10.1016/S0165-3806(99)00113-3.

Alliot F, Lecain E, Grima B, Pessac B (1991) Microglial progenitors with a high proliferative potential in the embryonic and adult mouse brain. *Proc. Natl. Acad. Sci. USA* 88:1541–1545 https://doi.org/10.1073/pnas.88.4.1541.

Anderson K L, Smith K A, Conners K, McKercher S R, Maki R A, Torbett B E (1998) Myeloid development is selectively disrupted in PU.1 null mice. *Blood* 91:3702–3710.

Angelov D N, Arnhold S, Andressen C, Grabsch, Puschmann M, Hescheler J et al. (1998) Temporospatial relationships between macroglia and microglia during in vitro differentiation of murine stem cells. *Dev. Neurosci.* 20:42–51.

Andres K H, Von Düring M, Muszynski K, Schmidt R F (1987) Nerve fibers and terminals of the dura mater encephaly of rats. *Anat. Embryol.* (Berl) 175:289-301. https://doi.org/10.1007/BF00309843.

Ashwell K (1990) Microglia and cell death in the developing mouse cerebellum. *Brain Res. Dev. Brain Res.* 55:219–230.

Barr T A, Shen P, Brown S et al. (2012) B cell depletion therapy ameliorates autoimmune disease through ablation of IL-6–producing B cells. *J. Exp. Med.* 209(5):1001–1010.

Bayer TA (2015) Proteinopathies, a core concept for understanding and ultimately treating degenerative disorders? European neuropsychopharmacology: *the journal of the European College of Neuropsychopharmacology* 25(5):713–724.

Becher B, Spath S, Goverman J (2017) Cytokine networks in neuroinflammation. *Nature reviews Immunology* 17(1):49–59. https://doi.org/10.1038/nri.2016.123.

Bettelli E, Carrier Y, Gao W, Korn T, Strom TB, Oukka M, Weiner HL, Kuchroo VK (2006). Reciprocal developmental pathways for the generation of pathogenic effector TH17 and regulatory T cells. *Nature* 441:235–238. https://doi.org/10.1038/nature04753.

Bilimoria P M, Stevens B (2014) Microglia function during brain development: New insights from animal models. *Brain Res.* 1617:7-17.

Burdin N, Van Kooten C, Galibert L, Abrams JS, Wijdenes J, Banchereau J, Rousset F (1995) Endogenous IL-6 and IL-10 contribute to the differentiation of CD40-activated human B lymphocytes. *Journal of immunology* (Baltimore, Md:1950) 154(6):2533–2544.

Compston A, Coles A (2008) Multiple sclerosis. *Lancet Oct.* 372(9648):1502-17. https://doi.org/10.1016/S0140-6736(08)61620-7.

Davalos D, Grutzendler J, Yang G, et al. (2005) ATP mediates rapid microglial response to local brain injury in vivo. *Nat. Neurosci.* 8:752–758. https://doi.org/10.1038/nn1472.

Di Sabato DJ, Quan N, Godbout JP (2016) Neuroinflammation: The Devil is in the Details. *Journal of Neurochemistry* (139):136-153. https://doi.org/10.1111/jnc.13607.

Duddy M, Niino M, Adatia F, Hebert S, Freedman M, Atkins H, Kim HJ, Bar-Or A (2007) Distinct effector cytokine profiles of memory and naive human B cell subsets and implication in multiple sclerosis. *J. Immunol.* 178:6092–6099.

Eugster HP, Frei K, Kopf M, Lassmann H., Fontana A (1998) IL-6-deficient mice resist myelin oligodendrocyte glycoprotein-induced autoimmune encephalomyelitis. *Eur. J. Immunol.* 28:2178–2187.

Fillatreau S, Gray D, Anderton S M (2008) Not always the bad guys: B cells as regulators of autoimmune pathology. *Nat. Rev. Immunol.* 8:391–397. https://doi.org/10.1038/nri2315.

Fillatreau S, Sweenie C H, McGeachy M J, Gray D, Anderton S M (2002) B cells regulate autoimmunity by provision of IL-10. *Nat. Immunol.* 3:944–950. https://doi.org/10.1038/ni833.

Galea I, Bechmann I, Perry V H (2007) What is immune privilege (not)? *Trends Immunol.* 28(1):12–18. https://doi.org/10.1016/j.it.11.004.

Gan L, Cookson M R, Petrucelli L. et al. (2018) Converging pathways in neurodegeneration, from genetics to mechanisms. *Nat. Neurosci.* 21:1300–1309. https://doi.org/10.1038/s41593-018-0237-7.

Goldmann J, Kwidzinski E, Brandt C, Mahlo J, Richter D, Bechmann I (2006) T cells provide traffic flow from the brain to the cervical lymph nodes via the cradle plate and nasal mucosa. *J. Leukoc. Biol.* 80:797-801. https://doi.org/10.1189/jlb.0306176.

Gomez-Benito M, Granado N, Garcia-Sanz P et al. (2020) Modeling Parkinson's Disease with the Alpha-Synuclein Protein. *Front Pharmacol.* 11:356. https://doi.org/10.3389/fphar.2020.00356.

Gordon L B, Knopf P M, Cserr H F (1992) Ovalbumin is more immunogenic than eacerebral when administered to the brain or cerebrospinal fluid. *J. Neuroimmunol.* 4:81-87. https://doi.org/10.1016/0165-5728(92)90215-7.

Hauser S L Waubant E, Arnold D L, Vollmer, Antel J, Fox R J, Bar-Or A, Panzara M, Sarkar N, Agarwal S, Langer-Gould, Smit C, HERMES Trial Group (2008) B-cell depletion with rituximab in relapsing-remitting multiple sclerosis. *The New England journal of medicine* 358(7):676–688. https://doi.org/10.1056/NEJMoa0706383.

Hickman S E, Allison E K, El Khoury J (2008) Microglial dysfunction and defective beta-amyloid clearance pathways in aging Alzheimer's disease mice. *J. Neurosci.* 28:8354–8360.

Hickman S, Izzy S, Sen P et al. (2018) Microglia in neurodegeneration. Nature Neuroscience 21:1359–1369.

Hirsch EC, Vyas S, Hunot S (2012) Neuroinflammation in Parkinson's disease. *Parkinsonism Association Disorder* 18(appendix 1):210–212.

Kwon H S, Koh S-H (2020) Neuroinflammation in neurodegenerative disorders: the roles of microglia and astrocytes. Translational Neurodegeneration 9(1):42. https://doi.org/10.1186/s40035-020-00221-2.

Lee SK et al. (2011) B cell priming for extrafollicular antibody responses requires Bcl-6 expression by T cells. *J. Exp. Med.* 208:1377–1388.

Leick M, Azcutia V, Newton G, Luscinskas F W (2014) Leukocyte recruitment in inflammation: fundamental concepts and new mechanistic insights based on new models and microscopic imaging technologies. *Cell Tissue Res.* 355:647–656. https://doi.org/10.1007/s00441-014-1809-9.

Louveau A, Smirnov I, Keyes T J, et al. (2015) Structural and functional features of central nervous system lymphatic vessels. *Nature* 523:337–341. https://doi.org/10.1038/nature14432.

Matyszak M K (1998) Inflammation in the CNS: the balance between immunological privilege and immune responses. *Prog. Neurobiol.* 56:19–35. https://doi.org/10.1016/S0301-0082(98)00014-8.

Mattson M P (2000) Apoptosis in neurodegenerative disorders. Nat Rev Mol Cell Biol 1:120–130.

McKercher SR, Torbett BE, Anderson KL et al. (1996) Targeted disruption of the PU.1 gene results in multiple hematopoietic abnormalities. *EMBO J.* 15:5647-5658.

Neurath M, Finotto S (2011) IL-6 signaling in autoimmunity, chronic inflammation and inflammation-associated cancer. *Cytokine Growth Factor Rev.* 22(2):83-9. https://doi.org/10.1016/j.cytogfr.2011.02.003.

Nimmerjahn A, Kirchhoff F, Helmchen F (2005) Resting microglial cells are highly dynamic observers of the brain parenchyma in vivo. *Science* 308:1314-1318. https://doi.org/10.1126/science.1110647.

Norden D M, Trojanowski P J, Villanueva E, Navarro E, Godbout J P (2016) Sequential activation of microglia and astrocyte cytokine expression precedes increased iba-1 or GFAP immunoreactivity following systemic immune challenge. *Glia* 64:300–316.

Paloneva J, Manninen T, Christman G, et al. (2002) Mutations in two genes encoding different subunits of a receptor signaling complex result in an identical disease phenotype. *Am. J. Hum. Genet.* 71:656-662. https://doi.org/10.1086/342259.

Przedborski S (2008) Neurodegeneration. In: Gendelman HE, Ikezu T (eds) *Neuroimmune Pharmacology.* Springer, Boston, p 229-237. https://doi.org/10.1007/978-0-387-72573-4_17.

Scheller J, Ohnesorge N, Rose-John S (2006) Interleukin-6 trans-signalling in chronic inflammation and cancer. *Scand. J. Immunol.* 63(5):321-329. https://doi.org/10.1111/j.1365-3083.2006.01750.x.

Tobore T O (2019) On the Etiopathogenesis and Pathophysiology of Alzheimer's Disease: A Comprehensive Theoretical Review. *J. Alzheimers Dis.* 68(2):417-437. https://doi.org/10.3233/JAD-181052.

Von Andrian UH, Mackay CR (2000) T-cell function and migration. Two sides of the same coin. *N. Engl. J. Med.* 34:1020–1034. https://doi.org/10.1056/NEJM200010053431407.

Waisman A, Hauptmann J, Regen T (2015) The role of IL-17 in CNS diseases. *Actaneuropathologica* 129(5):625–637. https://doi.org/10.1007/s00401-015-1402-7.

Walker L, Thresholds GJ (2012) Inflammation and epilepsy: foundations of a new therapeutic approach in epilepsy? Epilepsy Curr 12(1):8–12.

Werner C, Engelhard K (2007) Pathophysiology of traumatic brain injury. *Br. J. Anaesth.* 99:4– 9.

Wyss-Coray T, Rogers J (2012) Inflammation in Alzheimer disease-a brief review of the basic science and clinical literature. *Cold Spring Harbor perspectives in medicine* 2(1):a006346. https://doi.org/10.1101/cshperspect.a006346.

Yen J H, Kong W, Emig F, Rahbari K M, Kuo P C, Scofield B A, Ganea D (2015). Differential effects of IFN-β on IL-12, IL-23, and IL-10 expression in TLR-stimulated dendritic cells. *J. Leukoc. Biol. J. Leukoc. Biol.* 98(5):689-702. https://doi.org/10.1189/jlb.3HI0914-453R.

Chapter 27

Pregnancy and Cytokines

Nazan Yurtcu[1,*], MD and Sevgi Durna Dastan[2], PhD

[1]Sivas Cumhuriyet University, Faculty of Medicine, Department of Obstetrics and Gynecology, Sivas, Turkey

[2]Sivas Cumhuriyet University, Faculty of Science, Department of Biology, Sivas, Turkey

Abstract

Pregnancy is a physiological state designated as the regional immune tolerance of the mother organism against paternal sourced antigens found in embryonic cells. While the paternal heritage makes up half of the embryo, mammals bear their embryos in the uterus. There are defined immunological mechanisms for the embryo to survive and develop in the uterus. The mother's immune system must work healthy for the pregnancy to be shaped, continued, and terminated normally. It is a common view valid in all mammals that the cellular immunity reactions are suppressed for the duration of pregnancy, while humoral immunity continues to operate. At this point, cytokines such as T-regulator (Treg) cells, and the interleukin (IL)-10 they secrete, and tumor growth factors (TGFs) play an essential role. Treg cells are crucial in immune tolerance toward the fetus during pregnancy, especially in T-helper 2 (Th-2) cell polarization. In this respect, the negativities that may occur in Treg and Th2 cells, and the cytokines they secrete may lead to various pregnancy pathologies, premature births, and abortions. It is necessary to monitor the activities of these cells and cytokines to be protected from such negativities or to determine the cause of the disorders that may occur.

Keywords: pregnancy, cytokines, fetus, immunological mechanism

Introduction

Cytokines function as part of an intricate system of interrelated proteins called the cytokine network and signal transduction (Bamberg et al., 2012; Akdogan and Yontem 2018). This signal transduction is forming highly complicated cellular interactions according to the perceived signals, which results in heterogeneous responses toward the same cytokine. Such

* Corresponding Author's Email: nyurtcu58@gmail.com.

In: Cytokines and Diseases
Editors: Kenan Demir, Selim Görgün and Bahar Uslu
ISBN: 979-8-88697-214-6

signaling is critically selective in differentiating responses to form either protective or damaging results (Bamberg et al., 2012). A single cytokine has the ability to regulate other cytokines by affecting the production of cytokines at various levels such as pathways, where they can enhance or repress the production. Yet again, cytokines have mutually exclusive behavior modifications on other cytokines, which might translate into antagonism, addition, or synergism. While cytokines are generally not stored, they are readily synthesized by the direct influence of gene expression, which in turn results in short-lived mRNAs. Overall, they are produced only when needed by a diverse array of cells that have roles in both innate and acquired immunity (Akdogan and Yontem 2018). Specific cytokines act on many cell types. Although cytokine expression and its effects on the immune system are crucial issues, it should not be forgotten that cytokines affect other parts of the body. The intricate connections formed by cytokines are remarkable, and they show overlapping sequences and related links between each other (Boshtam et al., 2017). Within this network, a cytokine can enhance or repress itself or others along with receptors and can be antagonized or synergized with other cytokines (Risvanli and Godekmerdan 2015; Mutluay and Oner 2016).

It is known that the maternal immune system plays a prominent role in the formation of pregnancy (Izgi and Sur 2009; Bamberg et al., 2012). A sizeable number of scientific studies have produced information about the pregnancy process that have supported and/or rejected each other in the historical course (Wilczyński et al., 2003; Mutluay and Oner 2016; Dos Santos Fagundes et al., 2021). It has been shown in various studies that fetal cells can activate the immune system. However, ectopic pregnancies have dispelled the view that the uterus is an immune-tolerant region. Again, the definition of a phenomenon called micro-chimerism, which expresses bidirectional cell transfer between the mother and offspring, invalidated the claim that the placenta is a barrier preventing cell traffic (Trowsdale and Betz 2006; Izgi and Sur 2009; Risvanli and Godekmerdan 2015). As a result, for the continuation of a successful pregnancy, either the maternal immune system is prevented from perceiving the fetal tissues as foreign substances, or the attachment of the maternal immune system cells to the fetal cells to develop an immune reaction is prevented (De Lemos 2003; Izgi and Sur 2009). Rejection of the offspring by the mother, that is, maternal tolerance deficiency, is held responsible for infertility events encountered without any pathological cause (Trowsdale and Betz 2006; Izgi and Sur 2009). The development of maternal immune tolerance initially depends on maternal factors. Progesterone hormone, which has an immunosuppressive effect, begins to be secreted from the ovaries in the secretion phase of the cycle. While implantation is characterized by the release of cytokines, cytokines are also secreted from other leukocytes, including neutrophils and macrophages. In this way, the mother is stimulated for implantation (Hunt 2006; Izgi and Sur 2009). Cytokines, which act as immunomodulators during pregnancy, are responsible for determining the immune response (Wilczyński et al., 2003; Halari et al., 2021). For a healthy pregnancy to proceed, cytokines involved in the pregnancy pose vital importance (Mutluay and Oner 2016). Cytokines can be designated as hormones regulating the immune system due to their pleiotropic traits, which enable their regulatory functions (Raghupathy 2001). Both the cells of the immune system and other cells that are not part of the immune system directly synthesize these molecules with the effect of a stimulus and generally affect more than one mechanism by binding to their specific target cell receptors (Mutluay and Oner 2016). As lightweight polypeptides, cytokines have a wide array of functions, namely, cyclic corpus luteum protection, adhesion and invasion of the fetus, implantation, and certain regulations in immune responses (Wilczyński et al., 2003). Communication-associated cytokines are produced by the embryo; however, PBLs (peripheral blood lymphocytes), macrophages, and cells of the oviduct and endometrium can also produce them (Schäfer-Somi 2003). The immune system of the mother maintains its ability to effectively fight off the immunogens during the pregnancy, but at the same time tolerates the antigens presented by the fetus, which is tightly balanced by cytokine networking. Cytokines are also vital in physiological reproduction processes that are implantation, placentation, and trophoblast invasion. As a general opinion, it has been suggested that the Th2 immune response is necessary for a successful pregnancy, but the Th1 response is harmful to the fetus. In addition, it has been shown that the balance in Th1/Th2 activity in a physiological pregnancy is in the direction of Th2. Studies on Th1/Th2 have shown that a Th1/Th2 partnership is necessary for healthy reproduction. In this book chapter, the functional possibilities of cytokines in the pregnancy period were investigated and focused on understanding the role and mechanisms of cytokines during pregnancy (Wilczyński et al., 2003; Mutluay and Oner 2016; Dos Santos Fagundes et al., 2021).

Cytokine Activity in Pregnancy Conditions

Interactions between cytokines, which are secreted during pregnancy, have important roles in ensuring the control of the maternal immune system and maintaining the survival of the embryo. While IL-2, interferon-gamma, and TNF-alpha cytokines secreted from Th1 cells are considered to be in the group of cytokines that are harmful to the embryo; IL-4, IL-5, IL-6, IL-10, and leukemia inhibitory factor cytokines secreted from Th2 cells are considered to be cytokines that work for the benefit of pregnancy (Kanellopoulos-Langevin et al., 2003; Bulla et al., 2004; Bamberg et al., 2012).

The environmental conditions must be suitable for the mother to accept the embryo (Risvanli and Godekmerdan 2015; Mutluay and Oner 2016; Miko et al., 2021). First, the maternal-fetal space and uterine tissue must be in proper physiological regulation. Cytokines are primarily produced by CD4 T cells (Lash and Ernerudh 2015; Mutluay and Oner 2016). Cytokine-producing lymphocyte CD4 cells are involved in the antibody responses and associated regulations together with cytotoxicity (Aris et al., 2008; Nakamura 2009). Cytokines during pregnancy can be classified according to their functions as proinflammatory and anti-inflammatory cells and Th1, Th2, Th17, and Treg cells, which are related to Th cells (Lash and Ernerudh 2015). Th1 mainly produces IL-1 and 2, IL-18/15, and IL-12 interleukin molecules, IFN-gamma, and TNF-alpha molecules, while Th2 cells produce IL-4, 5, 6, 13, and granulocyte-macrophage colony-stimulating factor (Wilczyński et al., 2003; Wilczyński 2005; Bamberg et al., 2012). Th17 cells are the source of IL-17A and IL-17E (Raghupathy 2001). Cellular immunity depends on the Th1 cellular activity. Being vital elements of innate immunity, both macrophages and the NK (natural killer) cells express specific cytokines to recruit and direct CD4 cells to hot spots, which require IFN-y and IL-12 coupled with IL-4 for T-helper 2 responses (Röcken et al., 1996; Mutluay and Oner 2016). Studies have shown that IL-10 and TGF-P increase during immune suppression and have important functions during pregnancy (Aluvihare et al., 2004; Wilkes et al., 2021). Th17 cells produce IL-17A, which is pro-inflammatory, and they are important in the initiation of inflammation and acute transplantation rejection. In the current literature, when normal pregnant women are compared with those with idiopathic recurrent miscarriage, it has been found that the amount of Th17 cells in the peripheral circulation and decidua increases (Wang et al., 2010; Zhu et al., 2015; Guo et al., 2020).

During pregnancy, the endometrium produces a wide variety of cytokines. Studies have shown that these cytokines are effective in the differentiation of the uterus during the establishment of gestation, uterine development for the physiological implantation, and its proper structure, and the formation of a healthy placenta (Lash and Ernerudh 2015; Mutluay and Oner 2016). During pregnancy, cytokine-producing sites are stated to be decidua epithelia, stromal cells, and syncytiotrophoblast, chorion, amnion, and Hofbauer cells. It is observed that cytokines originating from these regions are effective in initiating maternal tolerance, regulating local immunity against infective factors, and in tissue regeneration and placental hormonal production during trophoblast invasion (Wilczyński 2005). Various cells can produce T-helper-associated cytokines, including trophoblasts, stromal cells, epithelia, maternal T cells, macrophages, NK cells, and other leukocytes of the maternal line (Vince and Johnson 2000; Kanellopoulos-Langevin et al., 2003; Nakamura 2009). Therefore, it is known that the cytokines seen in the maternal-fetal space affect the provision of the appropriate physiological conditions for gestation, which include implantation, development of the placenta, proliferation of cytotrophoblast, angiogenesis, arterial restructuring, and cell growth – apoptosis balance (Lash and Ernerudh 2015). Endometrial decidualization is shown *in vitro* to be negatively affected by the T-helper 1 functions (IL-1, TNF-α). Reduced serum levels of IL-4, IL-6, and IL-10 cytokines were seen in women with multiple implantation failures (Wilczyński et al., 2003; Staun-Ram et al., 2004; Bamberg et al., 2012). It is reported that during implantation, the embryo actively regulates its interaction with the decidua by decreasing Th1 secretion and increasing the production of Th2 cytokines (Mutluay and Oner 2016). In addition, it has been reported that the embryo can secrete IL-10, and TGF-P in an autocrine way, suppress the trophoblast invasion and inhibit the maternal proinflammatory TNF-α and IFN-gamma cytokines through the paracrine way (Anteby et al., 2004; Qiu et al., 2004).

In the case of an increase in IL-2, IL-12, TNF-a, and IFN-gamma cytokines, trophoblast development is also interrupted and this causes fetal losses. Th2 cells, which are dominant in the pregnant uterus, are closely associated with the healthy maintenance of pregnancy (Nakamura 2009; Bamberg et al., 2012). In both the endometrial tissue and the decidua, the IL-10 cytokine should be expressed by Treg cells in the first phases of gestation, which is primarily responsible for decidual proliferation and TNF-α synthesis (Viganò et al., 2002). It is shown that there is a significant increase in the level of IL-10 during early pregnancy in women, and it remains elevated just before the onset of labor during the third trimester (Wilczyński et al., 2003; Thaxton and Sharma 2010; Robertson et al., 2013). The TGF-3 cytokine, on the other hand, is critically important for the immune tolerance of the mother, which is especially striking in the implantation, and in the formation of morphological changes associated with implantation, i.e., VEGF (vascular endothelial growth factor), MMP-9 (matrix metalloproteinase-9), and IGFBP-1 (insulin-like growth factor binding protein-1) (Kulkarni and Karlsson 1993; Herrler et al., 2003; Dimitriadis et al., 2005). It is stated in the literature that the immune suppression required in maternal tissues during pregnancy occurs by synchronous co-inhibition of the following cytokines; IL-10, TGFs, proinflammatory T-helper 1 cytokines, IFN-ɣ, and TNF-α (Jenkins et al., 2000; Wilczyński et al., 2003; Costeas et al., 2004). When the cytokine profiles of women who are not pregnant and have a history of recurrent miscarriage and healthy women are examined, it is seen that Th1 cytokines are primarily produced in women with a history of recurrent miscarriage, while Th2 cells are produced at a higher rate in healthy women (Jenkins et al., 2000; Lim et al., 2000; Costeas et al., 2004; Piccinni et al., 2021). It has been reported that IL-1, IL-3, TNF-alpha, IL-8, and prostaglandins limit proinflammatory effects (Mutluay and Oner 2016). It has been determined that cytotrophoblasts in humans also produce IL-4 cytokine (Schäfer-Somi 2003). In humans, it was shown that activated T cells are for elimination by CRH (corticotrophin-releasing hormone), which is primarily secreted by trophoblasts and placental decidua cells. This hormone is also responsible for gestation continuation (Makrigiannakis et al., 2001; Piccinni et al., 2021). During both the menstrual cycle and decidual formation, the IL-6 is observed in humans (Tabibzadeh et al., 1995; Costeas et al., 2004; Salamonsen et al., 2007; Fedorka et al., 2021; Piccinni et al., 2021).

It has been reported that IL-1 and IL-18 cytokines are substantial in the invasion, neoangiogenesis, and implantation occurring in embryonic-endometrial communication (Huang 2006; De Oliveira et al., 2010). Other cytokines such as IL-1P, IL-6, and TNF-a play an important role in the regulation of the ovarian cycle and the growth and development of the ovarian follicle (Vital Reyes et al., 2005). It has been observed that increased production of TNF-alpha and IFN-gamma cytokines resulted in infertility and repeated unplanned abortions (Reid et al., 2001; Wysocka et al., 2021). TNF-a cytokine is a multifunctional proinflammatory molecule that affects lipid metabolism, coagulation, insulin resistance, and the endothelium (El-Far et al., 2009; Guzeloglu-Kayisli et al., 2009; Sehring and Jeelani 2021). Studies have found that serum TNF-a levels are high in cases with recurrent miscarriage and reproductive disorders (Wilson et al., 2004; El-Far et al., 2009). While IFN-gamma production was low in women with recurrent miscarriages, production of IL-10 and IL-4 cytokines was found to be high. It has been found in various studies that there is no significant difference in terms of TNF-α levels, particularly between patients that have successful labor and patients with repeated cases of miscarriage. However, patients with a repeated miscarriage history exhibited striking decreases in TNF-α levels (Wegmann et al., 1993; Bates et al., 2002; Wu et al., 2021). IL-1 cytokine is a signal molecule that comes from the blastocyst and affects the endometrium (Viganò et al., 2002; Staun-Ram and Shalev 2005; Wu et al., 2021). IL-1 cytokine stimulates trophoblastic MMP-9 activation and endometrial stroma gene expression (Staun-Ram and Shalev 2005). In the luteal phase of the menstrual cycle, it was observed that the mRNA expressions of IL-4 and IL-6 cytokines in endometrial cells increased compared to the expressions of IL-2, IL-12, and IFN-gamma cytokines (Lim et al., 2000; Piccinni et al., 2021). It has been shown that co-operation between IL-4 and TGF promotes two essential processes of trophoblast invasion and endometrium decidualization (Arici et al., 1996; Jauniaux et al., 1996; Peng et al., 2021). It has also been shown that IFN-gamma suppresses the growth of trophoblast cells, while cytotoxic T cells are activated by IL-2 and induce apoptosis and fetal losses in trophoblasts (Jauniaux et al., 1996; Ikeda et al., 2021; Peng et al., 2021). It was stated that IFN-gamma secreted from the uterus is necessary to maintain decidual cell viability, change the maternal endothelia, and trophoblast inhibition after the growth threshold (Mahdi 2011).

It is known that the platelet-activating factor (PAF) molecule is also crucial in maintaining gestation. Considerable amounts of PAF are known to be secreted from embryos prior to implantation, and from the decidua, and it is widely believed that PAF secretion and embryonic development stimulate cytokine synthesis from endometrial stromal cells. It has been suggested for healthy gestation that increases in the amount of the PAF local cytokine are essential (Aboussahoud et al., 2021; Fiorenza et al., 2021; Halari et al., 2021; Arosh et al., 2022). It has been observed that the Th1/Th2 balance becomes dominant in the direction of Th2 during pregnancy in humans, and the Th1/Th2 balance in the circulation mostly stays the same in the early phases (Bertoja et al., 2005; Saito et al., 2007). It has been shown that if Th1 cytokines are dominant in the blood, this negatively affects embryo development and placental growth (Hill and Choi 2000).

Conclusion

As a result, the balance between Th1 and Th2 has critical importance in the formation of healthy reproductive functions (Costeas et al., 2004). It has been stated that physiological pregnancy is achieved due to the low-index Th1/Th2 immune response (Raghupathy 2001). The negativity of Th1 immune responses and the positive effects of the Th2 immune responses for the gestation was suggested after the discovery of the binary opposition of the Th1/Th2 balance (Wegmann et al., 1993; Ghaebi et al., 2017). However, it has been shown that Th1 cytokines are essential for the continuation of pregnancy. Some studies do not support the effect of the Th1/Th2 ratio but show that the etiological factors are effective in recurrent miscarriages (Thaxton and Sharma 2010; Piccinni et al., 2021). It has also been reported that IFN-gamma is necessary for healthy labor with its association in the terminal phases of gestation, and also for spiral endothelia restructuring (Robson et al., 2012). Pregnancy requires a precise immunologic balance between tolerance and suppression, which makes it a unique immune phenomenon. Maintaining a healthy pregnancy depends on the healthy establishment of the interaction between fetal tissues and the maternal decidua in the early period. Appropriate cytokine expression is required for healthy fetal development. It is seen that the levels of cytokines are effective in pregnancy pathologies such as recurrent pregnancy loss and recurrent miscarriage.

References

Aboussahoud W. S, Smith H., Stevens A., Wangsaputra I., Hunter H. R., Kimber S. J., Seif M. W., Brison D. R. (2021) The expression and activity of Toll-like receptors in the preimplantation human embryo suggest a new role for innate immunity. *Hum Reprod* 36(10):2661-2675.

Akdogan M., Yontem M. (2018) Cytokines. *Online Turk Saglik Dergisi (OTSBD)* 1(3):36-45.

Aluvihare V. R., Kallikourdis M., Betz A. G. (2004) Regulatory T cells mediate maternal tolerance to the fetus. *Nat Immunol* 5(3):266-71.

Anteby E. Y., Greenfield C., Natanson-Yaron S., Goldman-Wohl D., Hamani Y., Khudyak V., Ariel I., Yagel S. (2004) Vascular endothelial growth factor, epidermal growth factor and fibroblast growth factor-4 and -10 stimulate trophoblast plasminogen activator system and metalloproteinase-9. *Mol Hum Reprod* 10(4):229-35.

Arici A., MacDonald P. C., Casey M. L. (1996) Modulation of the levels of interleukin-8 messenger ribonucleic acid and interleukin-8 protein synthesis in human endometrial stromal cells by transforming growth factor-beta 1. *J Clin Endocrinol Metab* 81(8):3004-9.

Aris A., Lambert F., Bessette P., Moutquin J. M. (2008) Maternal circulating interferon-gamma and interleukin-6 as biomarkers of Th1/Th2 immune status throughout pregnancy. *J Obstet Gynaecol Res* 34(1):7-11.

Arosh J. A., Lee J., Banu S. K. (2022) Effects of dual inhibition of AKT and ERK1/2 pathways on endometrial pro-inflammatory, hormonal, and epigenetic microenvironment in endometriosis. *Mol Cell Endocrinol* 539:111446.

Bamberg C., Fotopoulou C., Thiem D., Roehr C. C., Dudenhausen J. W., Kalache K. D. (2012) Correlation of midtrimester amniotic fluid cytokine concentrations with adverse pregnancy outcome in terms of spontaneous abortion, preterm birth, and preeclampsia. *J Matern Fetal Neonatal Med* 25(6):812-7.

Bates M. D., Quenby S., Takakuwa K., Johnson P. M., Vince G. S. (2002) Aberrant cytokine production by peripheral blood mononuclear cells in recurrent pregnancy loss? *Hum Reprod* 17(9):2439-44.

Bertoja A. Z., Zenclussen M. L., Casalis P. A., Sollwedel A., Schumacher A., Woiciechowsky C., Volk H. D., Zenclussen A. C. (2005) Anti-P- and E-selectin therapy prevents abortion in the CBA/J x DBA/2J combination by blocking the migration of Th1 lymphocytes into the foetal-maternal interface. *Cell Immunol* 238(2):97-102.

Boshtam M., Asgary S., Kouhpayeh S., Shariati L., Khanahmad H. (2017) Aptamers Against Pro- and Anti-Inflammatory Cytokines: A Review. *Inflammation* 40(1):340-349.

Bulla R., Fischetti F., Bossi F., Tedesco F. (2004) Feto-maternal immune interaction at the placental level. *Lupus* 13(9):625-9.

Costeas P. A., Koumouli A., Giantsiou-Kyriakou A., Papaloizou A., Koumas L. (2004) Th2/Th3 cytokine genotypes are associated with pregnancy loss. *Hum Immunol* 65(2):135-41.

De Lemos M. A. (2003) How your mother tolerated you for nine months. *Biol Teach Journal* 1:27-30.

De Oliveira L. G., Lash G. E., Murray-Dunning C., Bulmer J. N., Innes B. A., Searle R. F., Sass N., Robson S. C. (2010) Role of interleukin 8 in uterine natural killer cell regulation of extravillous trophoblast cell invasion. *Placenta* 31(7):595-601.

Dimitriadis E., White C. A., Jones R. L., Salamonsen L. A. (2005) 'Cytokines, chemokines and growth factors in endometrium related to implantation. *Hum Reprod Update* 11(6):613-30.

Dos Santos Fagundes I., Brendler E. P., Nunes Erthal I., Eder Ribeiro R. J., Caron-Lienert R. S., Machado D. C., Pinheiro da Costa B. E., Poli-de-Figueiredo C. E. (2021) Total Th1/Th2 cytokines profile from peripheral blood lymphocytes in normal pregnancy and preeclampsia syndrome. *Hypertens Pregnancy* 23:1-8.

El-Far M., El-Sayed I. H., El-Motwally A. E., Hashem I. A., Bakry N. (2009) Serum levels of TNF-alpha and antioxidant enzymes and placental TNF-alpha expression in unexplained recurrent spontaneous miscarriage. *J Physiol Biochem* 65(2):175-81.

Fedorka C. E., El-Sheikh Ali H., Walker O. F., Scoggin K. E., Dini P., Loux S. C., Troedsson M. H. T., Ball B. A. (2021) The imbalance of the Th17/Treg axis following equine ascending placental infection. *J Reprod Immunol* 144:103268.

Fiorenza M. F., Amaral C. D. S., da Anunciação A. R. A., Portela V. V. M., Marey M. A., Miyamoto A., Antoniazzi A. Q. (2021) Possible impact of neutrophils on immune responses during early pregnancy in ruminants. *Anim Reprod* 18(3):e20210048.

Ghaebi M., Nouri M., Ghasemzadeh A., Farzadi L., Jadidi-Niaragh F., Ahmadi M., Yousefi M. (2017) Immune regulatory network in successful pregnancy and reproductive failures. *Biomed Pharmacother* 88:61-73.

Guo Z., Xu Y., Zheng Q., Liu Y., Liu X. (2020) Analysis of chromosomes and the T helper 17 and regulatory T cell balance in patients with recurrent spontaneous abortion. *Exp Ther Med* 19(4):3159-3166.

Guzeloglu-Kayisli O., Kayisli U. A., Taylor H. S. (2009) The role of growth factors and cytokines during implantation: endocrine and paracrine interactions. *Seminars in reproductive medicine* 27(1):62-79.

Halari C. D., Renaud S. J. and Lala P. K. (2021) Molecular mechanisms in IL-1β-mediated decorin production by decidual cells. *Mol Hum Reprod* 27(12).

Herrler A., von Rango U., Beier, H. M. (2003) Embryo-maternal signalling: how the embryo starts talking to its mother to accomplish implantation. *Reprod Biomed Online* 6(2):244-56.

Hill J. A. 3rd, Choi BC (2000) Immunodystrophism: evidence for a novel alloimmune hypothesis for recurrent pregnancy loss involving Th1-type immunity to trophoblast. *Semin Reprod Med* 18(4):401-5.

Huang H. Y. (2006) The cytokine network during embryo implantation. *Chang Gung Med J* 29(1):25-36.

Hunt J. S. (2006) Stranger in a strange land. *Immunol Rev* 213:36-47.

Ikeda R., Ushio N., Abdou A. M., Furuoka H., Nishikawa Y. (2021) Toll-Like Receptor 2 is Involved in Abnormal Pregnancy in Mice Infected with Toxoplasma gondii During Late Pregnancy. *Front Microbiol* 12:741104.

Izgi M., Sur E. (2009) Maternal Tolerance. *Ataturk Universitesi Vet Bil Derg* 4(2):123-132.

Jauniaux E., Gulbis B., Schandene L., Collette J., Hustin J. (1996) Distribution of interleukin-6 in maternal and embryonic tissues during the first trimester. *Mol Hum Reprod* 2(4):239-43.

Jenkins C., Roberts J., Wilson R., MacLean M. A., Shilito J., Walker J. J. (2000) Evidence of a T(H) 1 type response associated with recurrent miscarriage. *Fertil Steril* 73(6):1206-8.

Kanellopoulos-Langevin C., Caucheteux S. M., Verbeke P., Ojcius D. M. (2003) Tolerance of the fetus by the maternal immune system: role of inflammatory mediators at the feto-maternal interface. *Reprod Biol Endocrinol* 1:121.

Kulkarni A. B., Karlsson S. (1993) Transforming growth factor-beta 1 knockout mice. A mutation in one cytokine gene causes a dramatic inflammatory disease. *Am J Pathol* 143(1):3-9.

Lash G. E., Ernerudh J. (2015) Decidual cytokines and pregnancy complications: focus on spontaneous miscarriage. *J Reprod Immunol* 108:83-9.

Lim K. J., Odukoya O. A., Ajjan R. A., Li T. C., Weetman A. P., Cooke I. D. (2000) The role of T-helper cytokines in human reproduction. *Fertil Steril* 73(1):136-42.

Mahdi B. M. (2011) Role of Some Cytokines on Reproduction. *Middle East Fertility Society* 16:220-223.

Makrigiannakis A., Zoumakis E., Kalantaridou S., Coutifaris C., Margioris A. N., Coukos G., Rice K. C., Gravanis A., Chrousos G. P. (2001) Corticotropin-releasing hormone promotes blastocyst implantation and early maternal tolerance. *Nat Immunol* 2(11):1018-24.

Miko E., Barakonyi A., Meggyes M., Szereday L. (2021) The Role of Type I and Type II NKT Cells in Materno-Fetal Immunity. *Biomedicines* 9(12):1901.

Mutluay D., Oner J (2016) Role of cytokines during pregnancy. *Ann Med Res* 23(1):126-131.

Nakamura O. (2009) Children's immunology, what can we learn from animal studies (1): Decidual cells induce specific immune system of feto-maternal interface. *J Toxicol Sci* 34(Suppl 2): SP331-9.

Peng L., Chelariu-Raicu A., Ye Y., Ma Z., Yang H., Ishikawa-Ankerhold H., Rahmeh M., Mahner S., Jeschke U., von Schönfeldt V. (2021) Prostaglandin E2 Receptor 4 (EP4) Affects Trophoblast Functions via Activating the cAMP-PKA-pCREB Signaling Pathway at the Maternal-Fetal Interface in Unexplained Recurrent Miscarriage. *Int J Mol Sci* 22(17):9134.

Piccinni M. P., Raghupathy R., Saito S., Szekeres-Bartho J. (2021) Cytokines, Hormones and Cellular Regulatory Mechanisms Favoring Successful Reproduction. *Front Immunol* 12:717808.

Qiu Q., Yang M., Tsang B. K., Gruslin A. (2004) EGF-induced trophoblast secretion of MMP-9 and TIMP-1 involves activation of both PI3K and MAPK signalling pathways. *Reproduction* 128(3):355-63.

Raghupathy R. (2001) Pregnancy: success and failure within the Th1/Th2/Th3 paradigm. *Semin Immunol* 13(4):219-27.

Reid J. G., Simpson N. A., Walker R. G., Economidou O., Shillito J., Gooi H. C., Duffy S. R., Walker J. J. (2001) The carriage of pro-inflammatory cytokine gene polymorphisms in recurrent pregnancy loss. *Am J Reprod Immunol* 45(1):35-40.

Risvanli A., Godekmerdan A. (2015) The Effects of Post-Mating Administration of Anti-IL-10 and Anti-TGFß on Conception Rates in Mice. *Int J Fertil Steril* 9(1):65-70.

Robertson S. A., Prins J. R., Sharkey D. J., Moldenhauer L. M. (2013) Seminal fluid and the generation of regulatory T cells for embryo implantation. *Am J Reprod Immunol* 69(4):315-30.

Robson A., Harris L. K., Innes B. A., Lash G. E., Aljunaidy M. M., Aplin J. D., Baker P. N., Robson S. C., Bulmer J. N. (2012) Uterine natural killer cells initiate spiral artery remodeling in human pregnancy. *FASEB J* 26(12):4876-85.

Röcken M., Racke M., Shevach E. M. (1996) IL-4-induced immune deviation as antigen-specific therapy for inflammatory autoimmune disease. *Immunol Today* 17(5):225-31.

Saito S., Shiozaki A., Sasaki Y., Nakashima A., Shima T., Ito M. (2007) Regulatory T cells and regulatory natural killer (NK) cells play important roles in feto-maternal tolerance. *Semin Immunopathol* 29(2):115-22.

Salamonsen L. A., Hannan N. J., Dimitriadis E. (2007) Cytokines and chemokines during human embryo implantation: roles in implantation and early placentation. *Semin Reprod Med* 25(6):437-44.

Schäfer-Somi S. (2003) Cytokines during early pregnancy of mammals: a review. *Anim Reprod Sci* 75(1-2):73-94.

Sehring J., Jeelani R. (2021) Human implantation: The complex interplay between endometrial receptivity, inflammation, and the microbiome. *Placenta* 117:179-186.

Staun-Ram E., Goldman S., Gabarin D., Shalev E. (2004) Expression and importance of matrix metalloproteinase 2 and 9 (MMP-2 and -9) in human trophoblast invasion. *Reprod Biol Endocrinol* 2:59.

Staun-Ram E., Shalev E. (2005) Human trophoblast function during the implantation process. *Reprod Biol Endocrinol* 3:56.

Tabibzadeh S., Kong Q. F., Babaknia A., May L. T. (1995) Progressive rise in the expression of interleukin-6 in human endometrium during menstrual cycle is initiated during the implantation window. *Hum Reprod* 10(10):2793-9.

Thaxton J. E., Sharma S. (2010) Interleukin-10: a multi-faceted agent of pregnancy. *Am J Reprod Immunol* 63(6):482-91.

Trowsdale J., Betz A. G. (2006) Mother's little helpers: mechanisms of maternal-fetal tolerance. *Nat Immunol* 7(3):241-6.

Viganò P., Somigliana E., Mangioni S., Vignali M., Vignali M., Di Blasio A. M. (2002) Expression of interleukin-10 and its receptor is up-regulated in early pregnant versus cycling human endometrium. *J Clin Endocrinol Metab* 87(12):5730-6.

Vince G. S., Johnson P. M. (2000) Leucocyte populations and cytokine regulation in human uteroplacental tissues. *Biochem Soc Trans* 28(2):191-195.

Vital Reyes V. S., Téllez Velasco S., Hinojosa Cruz J. C., Ortiz Romero Mde J., Chavarría Olarte M. E., Reyes Fuentes A. (2005) Serum levels of IL-1beta, IL-6 and TNF-alpha in infertile patients with ovarian dysfunction. *Ginecol Obstet Mex* 73(11):604-10.

Wang W. J., Hao C. F., Yi-Lin, Yin G. J., Bao S. H., Qiu L. H., Lin Q. D. (2010) Increased prevalence of T helper 17 (Th17) cells in peripheral blood and decidua in unexplained recurrent spontaneous abortion patients. *J Reprod Immunol* 84(2):164-70.

Wegmann T. G., Lin H., Guilbert L., Mosmann T. R. (1993) Bidirectional cytokine interactions in the maternal-fetal relationship: is successful pregnancy a TH2 phenomenon? *Immunol Today* 14(7):353-6.

Wilczyński J. R., Tchórzewski H., Głowacka E., Banasik M., Szpakowski M., Wieczorek A., Wilczyński J. (2003) *In vitro* cytokine secretion by peripheral blood and decidual lymphocytes during the third trimester of normal pregnancy. *Gynecol Obstet Invest* 55(2):68-72.

Wilczyński J. R. (2005) Th1/Th2 cytokines balance - yin and yang of reproductive immunology. *Eur J Obstet Gynecol Reprod Biol* 122(2):136-143.

Wilkes M. C., Shibuya A., Sakamoto K. M. (2021) Signaling Pathways That Regulate Normal and Aberrant Red Blood Cell Development. *Genes* 12(10).

Wilson R., Jenkins C., Miller H., McInnes I. B., Moore J., McLean M. A., Walker J. J. (2004) Abnormal cytokine levels in non-pregnant women with a history of recurrent miscarriage. *Eur J Obstet Gynecol Reprod Biol* 115(1):51-54.

Wu Z., Wang M., Liang G., Jin P., Wang P., Xu Y., Qian Y., Jiang X., Qian J., Dong M. (2021) Pro-Inflammatory Signature in Decidua of Recurrent Pregnancy Loss Regardless of Embryonic Chromosomal Abnormalities. *Front Immunol* 12:772729.

Wysocka U., Sakowicz A., Jakubowski L., Pinkier I., Rybak-Krzyszkowska M., Alaszewski W., Dudarewicz L., Gach A. (2021) Association between idiopathic recurrent pregnancy loss and genetic polymorphisms in cytokine and matrix metalloproteinase genes. *Ginekolo pol* 92(6):440-445.

Zhu L. Y., Chen X., Xu Z. Z., Xu L., Mao T., Zhang H. (2015) Changes and clinical significance of peripheral blood helper T lymphocyte and natural killer (NK) cells in unexplained recurrent spontaneous abortion (URSA) patients after abortion and successful pregnancy. *Clinical and experimental obstetrics & gynecology* 42(1):62-66.

Chapter 28

Infertility and Cytokines

Serkan Oral*, MD

Halic University, Department of Obstetrics and Gynecology, Istanbul, Turkey

Abstract

Infertility problems are seen in 8-12% of the reproductive age population worldwide. Although infertility is seen in both men and women due to various factors, the cause of infertility cannot be explained in some cases. Cytokines, in the protein and glycoprotein structure, play an important role in the inflammation process. An increase or decrease in cytokine secretion in imbalances in proinflammatory and anti-inflammatory pathways may cause infertility for both sexes, prevent attachment of the formed fetus, and cause growth retardation and spontaneous abortion. In this section, the effects of cytokines on infertility are examined.

Keywords: infertility, cytokine, immunity, endometriosis, PCOS, unexplained infertility

Introduction

Despite recent advances in assisted reproductive technologies (ART), persistent infertility continues. As a global problem, infertility affects more than 15% of couples, 30% of men, and about 40% of women (Ghaebi et al., 2019). Infertility, which is a complex disorder, has various etiological factors. There are difficulties in the treatment due to physical and psychosocial reasons, and medical and surgical treatments can be used according to the patient's condition (Stentz et al., 2020).

Recognizing the fetus as an antigen, with the embryo and decidualized endometrium in a complex relationship, is essential for implantation success, and this creates an immune tolerance that prevents the rejection of the fetus from the body. Changes in the decidua mediated by immune cells, cytokines, and chemokines are required for maternal immune tolerance (Guzeloglu-Kayisli et al., 2009). The immune system consisting of autoantibodies and cytokines plays an important role in female fertility and infertility (Erlebacher 2013).

* Corresponding Author's Email: drserkanoral@gmail.com.

In: Cytokines and Diseases
Editors: Kenan Demir, Selim Görgün and Bahar Uslu
ISBN: 979-8-88697-214-6

Cytokines and growth factors are either protein or glycoprotein structures. They show autocrine or paracrine effects by being released to the extracellular environment and regulate reactions such as chemotaxis, mitosis, and angiogenesis (Kawamura et al., 2007). The interaction of cytokines, which has an important function for the reproductive system and pregnancy, affects uterine function through implantation, pregnancy and childbirth (Orsi and Tribe 2008). The cytokine interactions are a complex and dynamic process regulated by the hormones released during pregnancy.

This section will evaluate the effects of inflammatory cytokines on male and female infertility.

Male Infertility

This is a multi-step process regulated by the endocrine and immune system of the male reproductive system, which begins with the production of germ cells in the testicles and the transport of sperm to the sperm-egg binding site in the fallopian tube.

With inflammation of a male reproductive system that can cause changes in cytokine levels, cytokines are released from different immune cells found in the male reproductive tract in response to foreign antigens, pathogens and chronic inflammation (Ochsendorf 1999). To combat infection of the reproductive system, the innate host defense begins with the secretion of cytokines.

Orchitis is one of the common causes of infertility. Studies on autoimmune orchitis show an increase in proinflammatory cytokines such as IL-1 and TNF-a in the initial stage of inflammation (Lysiak 2004). Examining cytokines in semen showed high levels of cytokines in the semen, including IL-1b, IL-6, and IL-8, which are often associated with inflammation and infection of the male reproductive system (Fraczek and Kurpisz 2015; Syriou et al., 2018).

An evaluation of male infertility and its relationship with cytokines will be examined in detail in other sections.

Female Infertility

Endometriosis-Related Infertility

Endometriosis is a disease that is informed as the placement and spread of endometrial tissue outside the uterine cavity, and its definitive diagnosis is made after surgery (Bulun 2009). The true prevalence rate of endometriosis is unknown since surgery is performed only on examining patients with suspected or symptomatic endometriosis. It is seen in approximately 10-15% of women of reproductive age and 9-50% of the infertile population (de Ziegler et al., 2010). This rate rises to 50% in adolescents with chronic pelvic pain and dysmenorrhea (Cramer and Missmer 2002).

Cytokines and growth factors contribute to the pathogenesis of endometriosis by stimulating the implantation of endometriotic cells, their adhesion to the peritoneal surface, spreading, and angiogenesis. Young women have infertility problems as well as chronic pain. In cases with endometriosis, the infertility problem may be associated with pelvic adhesions, tubal ostium occlusions, decreased folliculogenesis, and mechanical deterioration (Tanbo and Fedorcsak 2017). As chronic inflammation in the peritoneum increases cytokine synthesis, the oocyte-sperm union is affected, and fertility may decrease.

With the introduction of the highly sensitive enzyme-linked immunosorbent assay (ELISA), the number of cytokines in the peritoneal fluid could be measured. The main cytokines are IL-1, IL-4, IL-5, IL-6, IL-8, IL-10, IL-12, IL-13, interferon-gamma (IFN-g), tumor necrosis factor-alpha (TNF-α), regulated on activation, normal T-cell expressed, and secreted RANTES, monocyte chemotactic protein-1 (MCP-1), macrophage colony-stimulating factor (MCSF), transforming growth factor TGF-beta and vascular endothelial growth factor (VEGF) (Harada et al., 2001).

Studies show that cytokine levels increase in the peritoneal fluid of endometriosis patients. While cytokines regulate the effects of leukocytes in the peritoneum, they also contribute to the pathogenesis of endometriosis by affecting ectopic endometrial cells (Betjes et al., 1993). The macrophages that originate from the bone marrow and are found as monocytes in the circulation are the ones that produce the most cytokines. Chemotactic substances such as monocyte chemotactic protein-1, RANTES, and IL-8 are involved in the accumulation of macrophages in the peritoneal fluid. Lymphocytes also contribute to cytokine release, although less so than macrophages. T helper cells from T lymphocytes, divided into two groups as T helper 1 and T helper 2. T helper 1 cells increase cellular immunity by increasing the production of IL-2, IL-12, IFN-gamma, while T helper 2 cells suppress cellular immunity by the production of IL-4, IL-5, IL-10, and IL-13. In endometriosis patients, a change is observed in the distribution of cytokines made by Th1 and Th2, and the greater predominance of cytokines made by Th2 contributes to the pathogenesis of endometriosis by suppressing cellular immunity (Hsu et al., 1997).

Unlike women with tubal infertility, it has been shown that follicular fluid TNF-α, granulocyte-macrophage colony-stimulating factor (GM-CSF), and IL-15 levels are increased, while IL-10 levels are significantly decreased in women with endometriosis-related infertility. In addition, it was determined that IL-6 levels in the follicular fluid did not increase in these patients (Falconer et al., 2009; Tseng et al., 1996).

IL-6 supports the acute-phase inflammatory response by effectively differentiating B cells and cytotoxic T cells (Kang et al., 2014). IL-6 can cause infertility because it restricts sperm motility. IL-6 is also thought to play a role in preeclampsia and preterm labor (Prins Gomez-Lopez and Robertson 2012).

IL-1 disrupts endometrial decidualization. It also changes signaling pathways by affecting estrogen and progesterone receptors (Yu et al., 2019).

It was determined that TNF-a and IL-6 levels in the peritoneal fluid obtained from women who underwent surgery for reasons such as pain, tubal ligation and endometriosis were significantly elevated (Gori et al., 2011). On the other hand, it has been stated that higher IL-8 levels in the peritoneal fluid are associated with TNF-a induction (Miller et al., 2017).

As a result of increased levels of proinflammatory cytokines in the peritoneal fluid, a decrease in the quality of the oocyte and, consequently, of the embryos can be observed. Various mechanisms involved in endometriosis-related infertility include impaired adhesion, implantation, and angiogenesis (Halis and Arici 2004).

Polycystic Ovary Syndrome-Related Infertility

Polycystic ovary syndrome (PCOS) is a condition that affects 4-18% of women and causes infertility. The diagnosis is made by oligo-ovulation, hyperandrogenism, polycystic ovaries, and the exclusion of other explicable causes ("Revised 2003 consensus on diagnostic criteria and long-term health risks related to polycystic ovary syndrome," 2004). Clinical manifestations of the disease include an irregular menstrual cycle, oligomenorrhea, hirsutism, multiple cysts or polycystic ovaries, insulin resistance, and hyperandrogenism. The disease is related to infertility and has long-term health consequences due to its association with insulin resistance and metabolic syndrome (Dahan and Reaven 2019).

In recent years, extensive research has been carried out on signaling pathways concerning treatment. Cytokines are elevated in most inflammatory diseases and can be used as potential targets for treatment. The IL-6 family of proteins includes cytokines such as IL-6, IL-27, IL-11, cardiotrophin-1 (CT-1), oncostatin M (OSM), and neuropoietin (NP-1) (Rose-John et al., 2006).

Studies in numerous murine models and humans show elevated cytokines, particularly IL-6, with PCOS. The proinflammatory release of adipose tissue and adipokines in PCOS has been shown in many studies. Ghowsi et al., evaluated the expression of IL-6 and the role of resveratrol on PCOS in the adipose tissue of 15 Wistar rats divided into three groups (Ghowsi et al., 2018). Control rats expressed a lower concentration of IL-6 from adipose tissue than the PCOS group.

A significant decrease in IL-6 expression was observed in the resveratrol-treated group. It is thought that the anti-inflammatory effect reduces the level of IL-6.

In many clinical studies, the relationship of IL-6 levels with PCOS, insulin resistance, and metabolic syndrome has been evaluated. IL-6 levels were significantly higher in almost all studies, especially in PCOS cases with the obese phenotype. The decrease in IL-6 levels with weight loss supports that adiposity and infertility in PCOS are associated with inflammation (Mannerås et al., 2008).

Increased IL-1 levels are observed in patients with PCOS (González et al., 2014). Ex-vivo experimental studies have determined that IL-1 signaling in the dominant follicle may represent an alternative pathway for the LH surge that will trigger ovulation. This pro-ovulatory effect is thought to be mediated by the IL-1-induced production of prostaglandins. However, IL-1 inhibits plasminogen activators that are not useful for ovulation (Brännström et al., 1993). Furthermore, IL-1 has been consistently shown to have adverse effects on different fertility measures such as the fertilized oocyte count, oocyte maturation, and pregnancy rates (Uri-Belapolsky et al., 2017).

Unexplained Infertility

Among the explainable causes of female infertility are ovulation disorders, and endometrial and tubal problems. Apart from these reasons, some uncertain conditions are called unexplained infertility (UI) (Hull et al., 1985). About 15% of female infertility has no explicable cause (Aboulghar et al., 2003). The diagnosis of unexplained infertility is made by evaluating the tubal patency and proving the absence of hormonal and endometrial disorders (Gelbaya et al., 2014).

The decidua secretes proinflammatory cytokines during early pregnancy to create an anti-inflammatory environment for placental support. IL-35 from these secreted cytokines inhibits the development of Th-17 cells (Mao et al., 2013). Imbalance in cytokine release can cause pregnancy loss and infertility, including UI.

A recent study comparing female patients with UI and fertile women found a higher ratio of TNF-α/IL-10, IFN-γ/IL-10, and IFN-γ/IL-4 and a lower IL-35/IL-17 (Ozkan et al., 2014). High IL-4 levels were reported in women with UI in this study.

As a result, changes during pregnancy to ensure maternal immune tolerance against the fetus sometimes cause imbalances, and this negativity in the inflammatory process is thought to cause UI (Ehsani et al., 2019).

Wang et al., evaluated the effect of the adoptive transfer of trichostatin-induced CD4+ CD25+ FOXP3+ Treg cells on recurrent spontaneous abortions in CBA/J mice and demonstrated the high secretion of TGF-beta and IL-10 in successful pregnancy mice (Wang et al., 2019).

Recurrent Pregnancy Loss-Related Infertility

Th2-type cytokines (IL-10, IL-4) are in normal values in pregnancies resulting in a live birth, and deficiency in these cytokines can cause poor placentation, fetal growth retardation, and possibly even fetal death (Agarwal et al., 2003; Raghupathy 1997).

Th1 inflammatory cytokines (IFN-γ, TNF-α, IL-2) are harmful to pregnancy and may cause harmful effects on the fetus by direct embryotoxic activity or damage to the placental trophoblast (Raghupathy et al., 2000). These cytokines may also act by inducing NK and lymphokine-activated killer cells (Chaouat et al., 2003).

Recent studies have investigated the presence of other cytokines that play a role in recurrent pregnancy loss. IL-18 appears to be Th1-like in the presence of IL-12 in the decidua, but in the absence of IL-12, IL-18 has Th2-inducing properties. IL-12 plus IL-18 causes abnormal NK cell function and causes abortion in preeclampsia (Chaouat et al. 2003). In addition, T-cell activation, persistent TNF-α production, and oxidative stress have been associated with abortion.

Conclusion

In preclinical and clinical studies, it has been observed that imbalances in proinflammatory and anti-inflammatory pathways in diseases involved in the etiology of infertility affect cytokine release, and this situation causes infertility and recurrent pregnancy loss. More extensive clinical studies are needed to better understand the role of cytokines in male and female infertility.

References

Aboulghar M A, Mansour R T, Serour G I, Al-Inany H G (2003). Diagnosis and management of unexplained infertility: an update. *Arch. Gynecol. Obstet.* 267(4):177-188. https://doi.org/10.1007/s00404-002-0300-0.

Agarwal A, Saleh R A, Bedaiwy M A (2003). Role of reactive oxygen species in the pathophysiology of human reproduction. *Fertil. Steril.* 79(4):829-843. https://doi.org/10.1016/s0015-0282(02)04948-8.

Betjes M G, Tuk C W, Struijk D G, Krediet R T, Arisz L, Hart M, Beelen R H (1993). Interleukin-8 production by human peritoneal mesothelial cells in response to tumor necrosis factor-alpha, interleukin-1, and medium conditioned by macrophages cocultured with Staphylococcus epidermidis. *J. Infect. Dis.* 168(5):1202-1210. https://doi.org/10.1093/infdis/168.5.1202.

Brännström M, Wang L, Norman R J (1993). Ovulatory effect of interleukin-1 beta on the perfused rat ovary. *Endocrinology* 132(1):399-404. https://doi.org/10.1210/endo.132.1.8419137.

Bulun S E (2009). Endometriosis. *N. Engl. J. Med.* 360(3):268-279. https://doi.org/10.1056/NEJMra0804690.

Chaouat G, Ledee-bataille N, Zourbas S, Dubanchet S, Sandra O, Martal J, Frydman R (2003). Implantation: can immunological parameters of implantation failure be of interest for preeclampsia? *J. Reprod. Immunol.* 59(2):205-217. https://doi.org/10.1016/s0165-0378(03)00048-2.

Chaouat G, Lédée-Bataille N, Zourbas S, Ostojic S, Dubanchet S, Martal J, Frydman R (2003). Cytokines, implantation and early abortion: re-examining the Th1/Th2 paradigm leads to question the single pathway, single therapy concept. *Am. J. Reprod. Immunol.* 50(3):177-186. https://doi.org/10.1034/j.1600-0897.2003.00080.x

Cramer D W, Missmer S A (2002). The epidemiology of endometriosis. *Ann. N. Y. Acad. Sci.* 955:11-22, discussion 34-16:396-406. https://doi.org/10.1111/j.1749-6632.2002.tb02761.x.

Dahan M H, Reaven G (2019). Relationship among obesity, insulin resistance, and hyperinsulinemia in the polycystic ovary syndrome. *Endocrine* 64(3):685-689. https://doi.org/10.1007/s12020-019-01899-9.

de Ziegler D, Borghese B, Chapron C (2010). Endometriosis and infertility: pathophysiology and management. *Lancet* 376(9742):730-738. https://doi.org/10.1016/s0140-6736(10)60490-4.

Ehsani M, Mohammadnia-Afrouzi M, Mirzakhani M, Esmaeilzadeh S, Shahbazi M (2019). Female Unexplained Infertility: A Disease with Imbalanced Adaptive Immunity. *J. Hum. Reprod. Sci.* 12(4):274-282. https://doi.org/10.4103/jhrs.JHRS_30_19.

Erlebacher A (2013). Immunology of the maternal-fetal interface. *Annu. Rev. Immunol.* 31:387-411. https://doi.org/10.1146/annurev-immunol-032712-100003.

Falconer H, Sundqvist J, Gemzell-Danielsson K, von Schoultz B, D'Hooghe T M, Fried G (2009). IVF outcome in women with endometriosis in relation to tumour necrosis factor and anti-Müllerian hormone. *Reprod. Biomed. Online* 18(4):582-588. https://doi.org/10.1016/s1472-6483(10)60138-1.

Fraczek M, Kurpisz M (2015). Cytokines in the male reproductive tract and their role in infertility disorders. *J. Reprod. Immunol.* 108:98-104. https://doi.org/10.1016/j.jri.2015.02.001

Gelbaya T A, Potdar N, Jeve Y B, Nardo L G (2014). Definition and epidemiology of unexplained infertility. *Obstet. Gynecol. Surv.* 69(2):109-115. https://doi.org/10.1097/ogx.0000000000000043.

Ghaebi M, Abdolmohammadi-Vahid S, Ahmadi M, Eghbal-Fard S, Dolati S, Nouri M, Yousefi M (2019). T cell Subsets in Peripheral Blood of Women with Recurrent Implantation Failure. *J. Reprod. Immunol.* 131:21-29. https://doi.org/10.1016/j.jri.2018.11.002.

Ghowsi M, Khazali H, Sisakhtnezhad S (2018). Evaluation of TNF-α and IL-6 mRNAs expressions in visceral and subcutaneous adipose tissues of polycystic ovarian rats and effects of resveratrol. *Iran. J. Basic Med. Sci.* 21(2):165-174. https://doi.org/10.22038/ijbms.2017.24801.6167.

González F, Sia C L, Shepard M K, Rote N S, Minium J (2014). The altered mononuclear cell-derived cytokine response to glucose ingestion is not regulated by excess adiposity in polycystic ovary syndrome. *J. Clin. Endocrinol. Metab.* 99(11):E2244-2251. https://doi.org/10.1210/jc.2014-2046.

Gori I, Pellegrini C, Staedler D, Russell R, Jan C, Canny G O (2011). Tumor necrosis factor-α activates estrogen signaling pathways in endometrial epithelial cells via estrogen receptor α. *Mol. Cell Endocrinol.* 345(1-2):27-37. https://doi.org/10.1016/j.mce.2011.06.043.

Guzeloglu-Kayisli O, Kayisli U A, Taylor H S (2009). The role of growth factors and cytokines during implantation: endocrine and paracrine interactions. *Semin. Reprod. Med.* 27(1):62-79. https://doi.org/10.1055/s-0028-1108011.

Halis G, Arici A (2004). Endometriosis and inflammation in infertility. *Ann. N. Y. Acad. Sci.* 1034:300-315. https://doi.org/10.1196/annals.1335.032.

Harada T, Iwabe T, Terakawa N (2001). Role of cytokines in endometriosis. *Fertil. Steril.* 76(1):1-10. https://doi.org/10.1016/s0015-0282(01)01816-7.

Hsu C C, Yang B C, Wu M H, Huang K E (1997). Enhanced interleukin-4 expression in patients with endometriosis. *Fertil. Steril.* 67(6):1059-1064. https://doi.org/10.1016/s0015-0282(97)81439-2.

Hull M G, Glazener C M, Kelly N J, Conway D I, Foster P A, Hinton R A, Desai K M (1985). Population study of causes, treatment, and outcome of infertility. *Br. Med. J.* (Clin Res Ed) 291(6510):1693-1697. https://doi.org/10.1136/bmj.291.6510.1693.

Kang Y J, Jeung I C, Park A, Park Y J, Jung H, Kim T D, Yoon S R (2014). An increased level of IL-6 suppresses NK cell activity in peritoneal fluid of patients with endometriosis via regulation of SHP-2 expression. *Hum. Reprod.* 29(10):2176-2189. https://doi.org/10.1093/humrep/deu172.

Kawamura K, Kawamura N, Kumagai J, Fukuda J, Tanaka T (2007). Tumor necrosis factor regulation of apoptosis in mouse preimplantation embryos and its antagonism by transforming growth factor alpha/phosphatidylinositol 3-kinase signaling system. *Biol. Reprod.* 76(4):611-618. https://doi.org/10.1095/biolreprod.106.058008.

Lysiak J J (2004). The role of tumor necrosis factor-alpha and interleukin-1 in the mammalian testis and their involvement in testicular torsion and autoimmune orchitis. Reprod Biol Endocrinol 2:9. https://doi.org/10.1186/1477-7827-2-9.

Mannerås L, Jonsdottir I H, Holmäng A, Lönn M, Stener-Victorin E (2008). Low-frequency electro-acupuncture and physical exercise improve metabolic disturbances and modulate gene expression in adipose tissue in rats with dihydrotestosterone-induced polycystic ovary syndrome. *Endocrinology* 149(7):3559-3568. https://doi.org/10.1210/en.2008-0053.

Mao H, Gao W, Ma C, Sun J, Liu J, Shao Q, Qu X (2013). Human placental trophoblasts express the immunosuppressive cytokine IL-35. *Hum. Immunol.* 74(7):872-877. https://doi.org/10.1016/j.humimm.2013.04.010.

Miller J E, Ahn S H, Monsanto S P, Khalaj K, Koti M, Tayade C (2017). Implications of immune dysfunction on endometriosis associated infertility. *Oncotarget* 8(4):7138-7147. https://doi.org/10.18632/oncotarget.12577.

Ochsendorf F R (1999). Infections in the male genital tract and reactive oxygen species. *Hum. Reprod. Update* 5(5):399-420. https://doi.org/10.1093/humupd/5.5.399.

Orsi N M, Tribe R M (2008). Cytokine networks and the regulation of uterine function in pregnancy and parturition. *J. Neuroendocrinol.* 20(4):462-469. https://doi.org/10.1111/j.1365-2826.2008.01668.x.

Ozkan Z S, Deveci D, Kumbak B, Simsek M, Ilhan F, Sekercioglu S, Sapmaz E (2014). What is the impact of Th1/Th2 ratio, SOCS3, IL17, and IL35 levels in unexplained infertility? *J. Reprod. Immunol.* 103:53-58. https://doi.org/10.1016/j.jri.2013.11.002.

Prins J R, Gomez-Lopez N, Robertson S A (2012). Interleukin-6 in pregnancy and gestational disorders. *J. Reprod. Immunol.* 95(1-2):1-14. https://doi.org/10.1016/j.jri.2012.05.004.

Raghupathy R (1997). Th1-type immunity is incompatible with successful pregnancy. *Immunol. Today* 18(10):478-482. https://doi.org/10.1016/s0167-5699(97)01127-4.

Raghupathy R, Makhseed M, Azizieh F, Omu A, Gupta M, Farhat R (2000). Cytokine production by maternal lymphocytes during normal human pregnancy and in unexplained recurrent spontaneous abortion. *Hum. Reprod.* 15(3):713-718. https://doi.org/10.1093/humrep/15.3.713.

Revised 2003 consensus on diagnostic criteria and long-term health risks related to polycystic ovary syndrome (2004) *Fertil. Steril.* 81(1):19-25. https://doi.org/10.1016/j.fertnstert.2003.10.004.

Rose-John S, Scheller J, Elson G, Jones S A (2006). Interleukin-6 biology is coordinated by membrane-bound and soluble receptors: role in inflammation and cancer. *J. Leukoc. Biol.* 80(2):227-236. https://doi.org/10.1189/jlb.1105674.

Stentz N C, Koelper N, Barnhart K T, Sammel M D, Senapati S (2020). Infertility and mortality. *Am. J. Obstet. Gynecol.* 222(3):251.e251-251.e210. https://doi.org/10.1016/j.ajog.2019.09.007.

Syriou V, Papanikolaou D, Kozyraki A, Goulis D G (2018). Cytokines and male infertility. *Eur. Cytokine Netw.* 29(3):73-82. https://doi.org/10.1684/ecn.2018.0412.

Tanbo T, Fedorcsak P (2017). Endometriosis-associated infertility: aspects of pathophysiological mechanisms and treatment options. *Acta Obstet. Gynecol. Scand.* 96(6):659-667. https://doi.org/10.1111/aogs.13082.

Tseng J F, Ryan I P, Milam T D, Murai J T, Schriock E D, Landers D V, Taylor R N (1996). Interleukin-6 secretion in vitro is up-regulated in ectopic and eutopic endometrial stromal cells from women with endometriosis. *J. Clin. Endocrinol. Metab.* 81(3):1118-1122. https://doi.org/10.1210/jcem.81.3.8772585.

Uri-Belapolsky S, Miller I, Shaish A, Levi M, Harats D, Ninio-Many L, Shalgi R (2017). Interleukin 1-alpha deficiency increases the expression of Follicle-stimulating hormone receptors in granulosa cells. *Mol. Reprod. Dev*. 84(6):460-467. https://doi.org/10.1002/mrd.22799.

Wang J, Yang J, Yan Y, Zhu Z, Mu Y, Wang X, Chi Y (2019). Effect of adoptive transfer of CD4(+)CD25(+)Foxp3(+) Treg induced by trichostatin A on the prevention of spontaneous abortion. *J. Reprod. Immunol*. 131:30-35. https://doi.org/10.1016/j.jri.2018.12.002.

Yu J, Berga S L, Zou W, Taylor R N (2019). Interleukin-1β inhibits estrogen receptor-α, progesterone receptors A and B and biomarkers of human endometrial stromal cell differentiation: implications for endometriosis. *Mol. Hum. Reprod*. 25(10):625-637. https://doi.org/10.1093/molehr/gaz045.

Chapter 29

Cytokines and Endometriosis

Halenur Bozdağ*, **MD**

Department of Obstetrics and Gynecology, Bahçeşehir University, Faculty of Medicine, Göztepe, Istanbul, Turkey

Abstract

Endometriosis represents a chronic inflammatory gynecological disease that is described as the growth of endometrial tissue outside the uterine cavity. The immune system plays a significant part in the formation and progression of endometriosis. Immunological dysfunction causes endometrial cells to survive in the pelvic peritoneum, adhering, implanting, invading and finally progressing to endometriotic lesions. Endometriosis constitutes an inflammatory microenvironment. As part of the inflammatory process, cytokines take part in endometriosis pathophysiology and make a contribution to developing endometriosis-associated infertility and pelvic pain.

Keywords: cytokines, endometriosis, infertility, pelvic pain

Introduction

Endometriosis represents a benign chronic inflammatory disease during which the endometrial gland and stromal cells are present outside the uterine cavity. It commonly influences females of reproductive age and is related to chronic pelvic pain, dysmenorrhea, dyspareunia, and infertility. In females of reproductive age, the estimated prevalence of endometriosis is about 10-15% (Giudice and Kao 2004; Kvaskoff et al. 2015). Globally, about 176 million women aged between 15 and 49 suffer from endometriosis (Adamson et al. 2010). There is an association between endometriosis and work productivity loss. In the United States of America, the total annual healthcare costs related to endometriosis were estimated at US $69.4 billion in 2009 (Nnoaham et al. 2011). For European countries, they were estimated in the range of 0.8 million to 12.5 billion euros (Simoens et al. 2012). In addition to the economic burden, endometriosis significantly affects women's health and well-being in their social and sexual relationships and work life.

* Corresponding Author's Email: halenurbozdag@hotmail.com.

In: Cytokines and Diseases
Editors: Kenan Demir, Selim Görgün and Bahar Uslu
ISBN: 979-8-88697-214-6

In this chapter, the present knowledge about the pathogenesis of endometriosis is consolidated with a particular point of view on the correlation between cytokines and endometriosis. Endometriosis-related infertility and chronic pelvic pain are also evaluated from a cytokine perspective.

Theories on the Etiopathogenesis of Endometriosis

Endometriosis has a heterogeneous nature. A unifying theory about the etiopathogenesis of the disease has not been established. Most theories related to the pathogenesis have taken into account the tissue from which endometriosis originates. The sources of endometriosis can come from Müllerian or non-Müllerian stem cells. Endometriosis has also been categorized as implants that arise from uterine endometrial cells and implants that originate from cells of other tissues (Vercellini et al. 2013).

Origin of Endometriosis

Theories about the origin of endometriosis have been categorized as the transplantation theory and the in-situ theory.

According to the in-situ theory, the endometrial stromal cells and glands of endometriosis arise from the embryological remnants or the local tissues by metaplasia. During embryonic life, embryonic cell residues reside in the migration track of the Müllerian ducts. The "Müllerianosis" or "in-situ" theory suggests that endometrial-like tissue can develop because of the differentiation and proliferation of these cell residues (Batt et al. 2013). This hypothesis may explain why endometriosis frequently attacks the Douglas pouches, the uterosacral ligaments, and the medial leaf of the broad ligaments. Furthermore, the fact that endometriosis may exist in women with vaginal and uterine agenesis, in adolescents, and even in human female fetuses supports the above-mentioned hypothesis (Batt et al. 2003; Troncon et al. 2014).

During the embryonic period, the mesothelial cells of the serosa and the epithelial layer of the inside of the Müllerian ducts arise from the coelomic epithelium. The thesis that endometriosis arises from the metaplastic transformation of the coelomic epithelium constitutes the basis of the coelomic metaplasia hypothesis. Inflammatory processes, hormonal influences, and endogenous biochemical or immunological agents can induce the metaplasia of the mesenchyme into the endometrial epithelial cells and glands (Sourial et al. 2014). In-situ theories clarify the presence of endometriosis in females without menstruation or an endometrium and the existence of endometriosis throughout the body.

The transplantation theory is established on the fact that the eutopic endometrium can be the origin of the stroma cells and glands of endometriosis. Sampson presented the word endometriosis in 1927. Sampson proposed that eutopic endometrial fragments spread into the peritoneum via the fallopian tubes in the course of menstruation and growth in the peritoneum and/or on the ovary. The dissemination of the eutopic endometrium to the pelvic cavity creates a benign metastasis, in which the transition develops from the endometrium to endometriosis. Nevertheless, Sampson suggested that the reflux of menstruation was not capable of describing all forms of endometriosis, and he proposed that dissemination with the venous flow or metaplasia was an alternative hypothesis (Sampson 1940).

The retrograde menstruation theory has been supported by an increase in documented evidence in recent years. The tubal reflux of menstrual tissue was demonstrated in 76-90% of females with intact fallopian tubes (Burney and Giudice 2012). During the peri-menstrual period, 90% of females having patent tubes and 15% with occluded tubes had blood in their peritoneal cavity. In the early proliferative phase, endometrial epithelial cells were also found in peritoneal fluid. Moreover, isolated endometrial cells and glands in the menstrual reflux have been demonstrated as viable (Koks et al. 1997). Endometriotic lesions are frequently present on the left side of the hemipelvis and the right side of the diaphragm consistent with the counter-clockwise flow of peritoneal fluid. The correlation between the counter-clockwise flow of peritoneal fluid and the anatomical location of endometriosis supports the "retrograde menstruation" theory (Vercellini et al. 2007; Bricou et al. 2008). Nevertheless, the transplantation theory cannot clarify the existence of endometriosis in females without menses or endometrium (i.e., Mayer–Rokitansky–Küster–Hauser syndrome), adolescents, and males.

Although the initiator alterations related to endometriosis have not been clearly elucidated, they may be inherited, including immunologic, inflammatory, epigenetic, and genetic changes, or they may be acquired, e.g., the recurrent peritoneal menstrual reflux and exogenous chemical factors. It is clear that a single etiopathogenetic model is inadequate to clarify the complicated pathology of endometriosis.

Despite the prevalent observation of endometrial-like tissue in the resected pelvic tissue and small lesions in females of reproductive age, endometriosis develops as a destructive disease in only a subset of women. To identify the endometriosis origin and elucidate how it develops, numerous studies and in-vivo and in-vitro analyses have been conducted. The starting points of much of the research are, why endometrial tissue shedding with retrograde menstruation is transplanted into the peritoneum; how the endometrial stromal cells and glands shedding into the pelvic cavity can adhere to the peritoneal matrix and degrade it and then induce neo-angiogenesis to survive; why this process evolves into endometriosis instead of spontaneous resolution; and how Müllerian tissue or non-Müllerian stem cells differentiate into endometriosis (Evers 1994; Koninckx 1994; Donnez et al. 2003).

Role of Hormones in Endometriosis

The endometrial cells can be regenerated cyclically under the effect of estrogen, which is followed by estrogen/progesterone stimulation. However, the impairment in the regulation of hormonal pathways and numerous inherited and acquired interconnected factors potentially seem to take a key part in the development of endometriosis from endometrial stem cells (Garai et al. 2006).

Endometriosis has an estrogen-dependent nature. The local biosynthesis of estradiol, the expression of nuclear estrogen receptors (ERs), and ER signaling are changed by an aberrant immune-endocrine microenvironment in endometriotic tissue.

The reflux of the basal endometrial layer into the peritoneal cavity may trigger inflammatory activity and induce tissue injury and repair (TIAR) mechanisms. The local generation of estradiol is activated by TIAR mechanisms, contributing to the infiltrative growth and proliferation of endometrial cells. Estradiol represents a potent proliferative factor for endometrial implants and a direct stimulator for angiogenesis (Mueller et al. 2000).

Endometriosis is characterized by an estradiol-rich microenvironment. Deterioration in the enzymatic activity assures an important contribution to this milieu. The aromatase enzyme catalyzes the conversion of androstenedione to estrone and of testosterone to estradiol. An increase in the expression of the aromatase enzyme in endometriotic tissue provides a source of estrogens in endometriosis. The potent 17β-estradiol is converted to the weak estrone by 17β-hydroxysteroid dehydrogenase (17β-HSD) type 2, which modulates the estrogenic exposure. Because of enzymatic deficiency in endometriosis, the 17β-HSD loss has protective action in the local production of estrogens. Increased estrogen production triggers the cyclooxygenase type 2 (COX-2) enzyme, causing a rise in the level of prostaglandin E2, which leads to the stimulation of the aromatase activity (Bulun et al. 2002).

The estrogenic microenvironment activates macrophages resulting in the secretion of tumor necrosis factor-α (TNF-α) and interleukin-1β (IL-1β), stimulating nuclear factor kappa B (NFkB) activation. Moreover, the expression of vascular endothelial growth factor (VEGF) is induced by this activation cascade (Agic et al. 2009).

Estrogen receptors mediate the duty of estrogens in endometriotic tissue development and survival. The suppression of estrogen receptors (ERα or ERβ) prevents endometriotic tissue development. The overexpression of ERβ causes the estrogen-induced ectopic endometrial tissue development and suppresses the TNF-α-triggered apoptosis signaling. ERβ also takes part in the direct activation of the NFkB tract in which nuclear factor kappa B (NF-κB) signaling makes a contribution not only to immunity but also inflammation and the function of the nervous system (Han et al. 2015).

Progesterone has anti-inflammatory activity in uterine cells. Ectopic implants are characterized by a decrease in progesterone receptor (PR) expression and progesterone action. Decreasing progesterone activity causes a rise in local proinflammatory cytokines (Patel et al. 2015). NF-κB proteins can control the genes associated with cell proliferation, apoptosis, adhesion, and inflammation. Progesterone exhibits suppressor activity on NF-κB signaling networks. Progesterone resistance causes a rise in NF-κB activity and contributes to a proinflammatory state in the endometriotic tissue (Guo 2007). Tumor necrosis factor-α and IL-1β take a direct part in progesterone resistance by decreasing the levels of both PR isoforms and disrupting the receptor function (Wu et al. 2008). In turn, all factors related to progesterone resistance lead to impairment in decidualization and the establishment of ectopic endometrial implants (Grandi et al. 2017).

Role of Cytokines in Endometriosis

The most popular theory of endometriosis development is Sampson's retrograde menstruation theory. Retrograde menstruation is a frequent finding in 76 to 90% of asymptomatic females (Halme et al. 1984). An insignificant number of them have endometriosis. The shedding of endometrial tissue fragments into the peritoneal cavity is not enough to explain the disease development.

The insufficient removal of refluxed menstrual debris triggers the initiation of peritoneal inflammation that results in the accumulation and activation of innate and humoral immune cells. Immune system cells attack the pelvic peritoneal cavity in females with endometriosis. Lymphocytes, macrophages, ectopic endometrial implants, and mesothelial cells of the peritoneum are the major components of the inflammatory peritoneal environment. T and B cells, regulatory T cells, and natural killer cells also take part in the immune response. Different growth factors, complement components, cytokines, hydrolytic enzymes, and prostanoids are synthesized and secreted by recruited cell groups (Podgaec et al. 2012; Gupta et al. 2016; Nisenblat et al. 2016). Changes in the peritoneal environment are important to become receptive of pelvic tissue for endometrial fragments. The implantation and proliferation of endometrial cells may be influenced by immune factors, e.g., increased inflammatory response, impaired immune recognition, and defective apoptotic activity (Liu 2016).

Cytokines called interleukins are cell-to-cell messengers. Structurally, they are polypeptides, proteins, and glycoproteins. Their members are numbered from IL-1 to IL-38. They have an important role in tissue local homeostasis, such as growth, cellular activation, development, differentiation, and interaction with other body tissues and organs. Cytokines show their activity by influencing neighboring cells, called paracrine action, or by affecting cells that have generated them, named autocrine action.

Cytokine secretion into the microenvironment is induced by following external provocation and is not generally continuous. Their secretion can be regulated by a simple negative feedback mechanism. However, these regulations may be destroyed under some pathophysiological conditions, including endometriosis, and their levels may exceed physiological levels.

The action of most cytokines is confined to a short distance (with exceptions, e.g., IL-1, IL-6, TNF). Cytokines show their effects by binding to their receptors localized on the target cells. Cytokine-receptor interaction can cause either a rapid reaction resulting in chemotaxis of target cells or slow action following new protein synthesis in the target cells. Chemotaxis can cause the accumulation of the other defensive cells. The synthesis of intracellular, membrane, or secretory proteins makes the target cells more responsive to other cytokines. Moreover, the production of novel intracellular molecules is capable of promoting tissue survival by regulating growth or by altering the regulation of apoptosis through activating specific proteases, named caspases.

Cytokines are capable of influencing the production and regulation of different stimulant factors responsible for the activation of the single line of cells (i.e., stem cell factor (SCF), granulocyte-CSF (G-CSF), colony-stimulating factor (CSF), macrophage-CSF (M-CSF), etc.), or the specific tissues (epidermal growth factors (EGF), fibroblast growth factors (FGF), platelet-derived growth factor (PDGF), vascular endothelial growth factors (VEGF), endothelin, nerve growth factors (NGF), etc.) or across all the body (i.e., TNF-α and TNF-β, TGF-β) (Dembic 2015).

Immunomodulatory cytokines are associated with endometriosis disease, either as a cause or result of the disease. Cytokines seem to be responsible for all or part of the pathophysiology and symptomatology of endometriosis disease. They take part in the adhesion of endometrial cells to the peritoneum and the angiogenesis and proliferation of endometriotic lesions (Lebovic et al. 2001; Rakhila et al. 2016).

During endometriosis formation, the accumulated inflammatory cells secrete various growth factors and cytokines. Macrophages are an essential source of IL-1 family factors, IL-6, and tumor necrosis factor-α (TNF-α). Mast cells secrete IL-2, IL-3, IL-6, IL-7, IL-9, IL-10, and IL-25. The release of IL-8, IL-17, and IL-17α is promoted by neutrophils. Moreover, other inflammatory cells are capable of secreting MCP1, IL-33, IL-10, and IL-4 in addition to the other cytokines. Peritoneal fluid (PF) taken from subjects with endometriosis contains higher TNFα, IL-8, and IL-10 concentrations than PF derived from healthy controls (Bedaiwy et al. 2002; Pizzo et al. 2002; Akoum et al. 2008). Increased IL-1β, IL-6, and TNFα concentrations were also demonstrated in females with endometriosis compared to healthy controls (Barcz et al. 2012).

Endometrial fragments shedding into the peritoneal cavity can trigger a strong inflammatory response. Endometriotic lesions may be created by a decreased capacity of immune cells to clear the said fragments or a possible autoimmune condition, leading to higher sensitivity of peritoneal resident immune cells to endogenous damage signals. Some studies revealed that the peritoneal fluid of females with endometriosis has higher levels of inflammatory and angiogenic cytokines generated by immune cells, mesothelial cells, and/or the lesion itself.

Interleukin-1 (IL-1)

IL-1 represents a cytokine monomeric polypeptide. IL-1 is one of the proinflammatory cytokines and also has an immune regulatory, angiogenic, and hematopoietic effect. However, it can be produced by all nucleated cells. The main source of IL-1 is activated macrophages. The IL-1 family comprises seven ligands exhibiting agonist activity (IL-1, IL-1β, IL-18, IL-33, IL-36α, IL36β, and IL36γ), three receptor antagonists (IL-1Rα, IL-36Rα, and IL-38), and an anti-inflammatory cytokine (IL-37) (Garlanda et al. 2013a).

The best-known of these are IL-1α and IL-1β. They are synthesized as precursor proteins and then processed by caspase-1(interleukin-1-converting enzyme "ICE") to convert into an active form. Active forms of IL-1α and IL-1β exert binding impacts to mainly two receptors, such as the functional signaling receptor type 1 (IL-1R1) and "decoy" receptor type 2 (IL-1R2). IL-1R2 has inhibitor activity for IL-1β. The soluble form (sIL-1R2) of the "decoy" receptor captures IL-1β and inhibits its binding to IL-1R1 (Boraschi et al. 2013; Garlanda et al. 2013b). IL-1α and IL-1β are secreted from the cells at the very early stage in inflammation and induce the first localized inflammation. Their action causes the increased amount of circulating acute-phase proteins, the differentiation of B cells, and the development of the Th17 phenotype of helper T cells (Ma 2016).

IL-1 takes part in the pathogenesis of various acute and chronic inflammatory diseases, e.g., endometriosis. It has been reported that the peritoneal fluid levels of IL-1β, ICE, and proIL-1β in females with endometriosis are higher than in the control group. The lower mean peritoneal fluid sIL-1R2 level was detected in females with endometriosis rather than controls (Sikora et al. 2016).

An increase in IL-1β and proIL-1β secretion can cause inflammation in the peritoneal cavity. The reduced IL-1R2 expression can be the reason for an increase in endometrial cell responsiveness to IL-1β (Hou et al. 2008; Lawson et al. 2008). A prospective case-control study revealed a positive correlation between plasma IL-1β levels and an increase in the risk of laparoscopically confirmed endometriosis (Mu et al. 2018). IL-1β also takes a significant part in the angiogenesis of endometriotic lesions by stimulating the secretion of IL-6 and vascular endothelial growth factor in the endometriotic stromal cells (Lebovic et al. 2000).

There are conflicting results about IL-1 concentrations in the peritoneal fluid at various endometriosis stages. Akoum et al. reported higher concentrations at the early disease stage (Akoum et al. 2008). However, Kondera-Anasz et al. found higher peritoneal fluid and serum IL-1 levels at the advanced stage (Kondera-Anasz et al. 2005). Jiang et al. reported that the serum and peritoneal fluid levels of IL-1β in females with endometriosis did not differ significantly from those of healthy females (Jiang et al. 2019). IL-1 is one of the first secreted cytokines during inflammation. At the acute stage of endometriosis, it may be secreted abundantly rather than at the late chronic inflammation stage. Different results among studies on IL-1 and IL-1β may be linked with the stage of the disease.

Interleukin-6 (IL-6)

Interleukin-6 (IL-6) represents a pleiotropic cytokine. Macrophages secrete IL-6, whose action can cause endometrial cell proliferation and angiogenesis in endometriosis (Symons et al. 2018). Furuya et al. reported that the mean IL-6 levels in the peritoneal fluid were considerably higher in endometriosis cases than those without endometriosis. They also speculated that the presence of endometriosis considerably affected the specific and characteristic alterations of intraperitoneal cell-mediated immunity (Furuya et al. 2003). In endometriosis cases, a significantly increased concentration of IL-6 was found not only in the peritoneal fluid but also in the serum, and it was reported to be positively correlated with the disease stage (Mosbah et al. 2016).

However, Jiang et al. suggested the possible use of IL-6 and IL-37 as diagnostic biomarkers for endometriosis (Jiang et al. 2019). A systematic review based on a meta-analysis reported that IL-6 had no diagnostic value as a biomarker in endometriosis (Nisenblat et al. 2016).

Interleukin-8 (IL-8)

Interleukin-8 is called a chemokine. It has a chemotactic property and a potent angiogenic activity. It is also a strong chemoattractant for neutrophils. Its chemotactic impacts on neutrophils result in transforming acute to chronic inflammation (Sikora et al. 2017; Marí-Alexandre et al. 2018). IL-8 is generated by the vast majority of cell types, e.g., monocytes, endothelial cells, fibroblasts, mesothelial cells, and endometrial stromal cells. It can make a contribution to the pathogenesis of endometriosis both by attracting and activating neutrophils and stimulating new blood vessel formation. Interleukin-8 also facilitates endometrial cell adhesion, invasion, and implantation. Females with endometriosis have elevated IL-8 levels in the peritoneal fluid. It contributes to the growth and maintenance of the endometriotic tissue by inducing endometrial cell proliferation and protecting endometriotic cells against apoptosis (Sikora et al. 2017).

Interleukin-17

Interleukin-17 (IL-17) has a proinflammatory nature and is secreted from Th17 cells, NK cells, neutrophils, and mast cells. The IL-17 family consists of six similar members (IL-17A-F).

The recruitment of neutrophils into the endometriotic environment causes an increase in the secretion of IL-17 (Takamura et al. 2012; Hirata et al. 2011; Ahn et al. 2015). IL-17 also represents the main cytokine product of Th17 cells. It is increased in the peritoneal fluid and plasma of endometriosis patients, and may contribute to endometriosis progression as a result of stimulating the formation of cytokines, which cause inflammation and angiogenesis (Ahn et al. 2015; Hirata et al. 2011). Cell adhesion is promoted by the above-mentioned process. Cell adhesion induces TNF-α, TNF-β1, and IL-1 expression through the signaling pathways and makes a contribution to VEGF and IL-8 expression (Wang et al. 2017). The said impacts promote the proliferation of endometrial stromal cells and angiogenesis. IL-17 concentrations are higher in females who suffer from endometriosis and infertility. It is speculated that IL-17 is involved in the pathogenesis of early endometriosis and endometriosis-related infertility (Zhang et al. 2005).

IL-17A represents a member of the IL-17 family believed to be primarily produced by T-helper 17 cells (Song and Qian 2013). Endometriotic lesions and the eutopic endometrium in females with endometriosis are also capable of producing IL-17A. The plasma IL-17A levels obtained from females with endometriosis were reported to be significantly higher in comparison with healthy controls. Moreover, serum IL-17A concentrations decreased after the surgical removal of lesions. The stimulation of different cell cultures with IL-17A causes the increased generation of angiogenic and chemotactic cytokines and increased expression of proinflammatory and chemotactic cytokines, e.g., IL-1β, IL-8, and IL-9. IL-17A makes a contribution to the pathogenesis of endometriosis as a result of triggering angiogenic growth factors and proinflammatory cytokines (Ahn et al. 2015). IL-17A promotes the secretion of COX-2 and IL-8 and contributes to the proliferation of endometrial stromal cells (Saito et al. 2011; Hirata et al. 2011).

Interleukin-37

Cytokines take part in the pathogenesis of endometriosis, with their inflammatory and anti-inflammatory activity. Interleukin (IL)-37 represents a member of the IL-1 family, a natural inhibitor of proinflammatory cytokines (Cavalli and Dinarello 2018) and a suppressor of innate immunity (Nold et al. 2010). In endometriosis, high IL-37 levels were found in the serum and peritoneal fluid compared to the control group, and this was associated with the endometriosis stage (Jiang et al. 2019).

In-vitro and in-vivo research in mice has shown that IL-37 overexpression considerably suppresses the adhesion, proliferation, invasion, and migration of endometrial stromal cells. Moreover, the treatment of mice with endometriosis using recombinant human IL-37 has alleviated the endometriotic-like lesion and suppressed the expression of TNF-α, IL-1β, IL-6, IL-10, soluble intercellular adhesion molecule-I (ICAM-I), and vascular endothelial growth factor (VEGF) in the peritoneal fluid (Jiang et al. 2018). However, there is no exact knowledge about the mechanism of IL-37 interference with local and systemic immune responses in females with endometriosis. The inhibitor effect of IL-37 on nuclear factor-κB may cause the suppression of inflammatory mediators (Xie et al. 2016; Kaabachi et al. 2017).

Tumor Necrosis Factor (TNF)

The structure of TNF represents a molecular triangle created by three monomers. TNF has a membrane-bound form. Metalloproteases (named sheddases or metallopeptidases (ADAM1-17)) or TNF converting enzyme (TACE) is capable of cleaving and secreting extracellular portions of TNF. Sheddases act as a notch factor, influencing the development and growth of the cell.

TNF can be produced by all nucleated cells in an organism. However, macrophages, Th1 cells, and NK cells mainly produce and activate it. TNF-α exerts similar effects and acts synergistically with IL-1. Both of them cause the activation of the canonical NF-κB inflammatory pathway. Harada et al. indicated that the TNF-α level in the peritoneal fluid of females with endometriosis was increased and there was a positive association of TNF-α concentrations with the endometriotic lesion size (Harada et al. 1997). Higher TNF-α levels have also been reported in the endometrium and peritoneal fluid of females with endometriosis but only at the mild or early disease stage, suggesting that TNF-α plays a part in the early endometriosis stages during lesion formation (Cheong et al. 2002; Pizzo et al. 2002).

Moreover, TNF-α and IL-1 induce the expression of the cyclooxygenase-2 (COX-2) enzyme, regulating prostaglandin E2 (PGE2) synthesis. PGE2 itself can induce the expression of COX-2. This positive feedback cycle results in the overproduction of PGE2. PGE2 promotes inflammation, cell proliferation, local estrogen synthesis, angiogenesis, and pain. It can also enhance macrophages' cytotoxicity (Wu et al. 2010).

A prospective study showed that higher blood TNF-α levels were related to the increased risk of endometriosis in females under 40 years of age (Mu et al. 2018). TNF-α is capable of inducing the proliferation of human endometriotic stromal cells by causing the expression of the interleukin-8 gene and protein (Iwabe et al. 2000).

Vascular endothelial growth factor (VEGF) represents an angiogenic factor and it is responsible for angiogenesis in the endometrial tissue. Experimental studies demonstrated that tumor necrosis factor α (TNF-α) and interleukin 6 (IL-6) increased VEGF secretion after the implantation of endometrial tissue into the peritoneum (Lin et al. 2006).

Cytokines in Endometriosis-Related Infertility

The prevalence of endometriosis is about 50% in infertile females (Mishra et al. 2017). Furthermore, infertility is detected in 37% of subjects with endometriosis (Eisenberg et al. 2018).

Endometriosis creates a detrimental microenvironment containing inflammatory mediators in peritoneal and follicular fluids. The inflammatory content of the peritoneal fluid can deteriorate the fertilization process at various levels and cause the impairment of reproductive conditions (Macer and Taylor 2012). Potential factors related to the deterioration of reproductive function in endometriosis are reported as decreased oocyte quality (Da Broi and Navarro 2016; Sanchez et al. 2018), impairment of sperm and oocyte interaction (Hsu et al. 2015), and deterioration in the quality of the embryo and its implantation and development (Stilley et al. 2012).

Some research has shown that intrafollicular cytokine levels are changed in subjects with endometriosis (Sarapik et al. 2012; Singh et al. 2016). Elevated cytokine levels in the peritoneal fluid and serum of subjects with endometriosis are also documented. IL-1 with a strong proinflammatory activity is involved in endometriosis-related infertility. The peritoneal fluid IL-1 level was stated to be considerably higher in infertile females with endometriosis in comparison with controls (Akoum et al. 2008; Michaud et al. 2011). The follicular fluid IL-1 level obtained from infertile patients was also found to be higher in females with endometriosis than in females without endometriosis (Singh et al. 2016; Wu et al. 2017).

IL-6 represents a multifunctional cytokine known to be a regulator of the immune response, inflammation, and angiogenesis. IL-6 concentrations in the peritoneal fluid and follicular fluid were detected to be higher in endometriosis-associated infertility than non-endometriosis subjects (Yi et al. 2000; Singh et al. 2016; Wu et al. 2017). On the contrary, some researchers stated there was no significant difference in the peritoneal fluid (Furuya et al. 2003) and follicular fluid IL-6 levels between infertile subjects with endometriosis and controls (Wunder et al. 2006).

IL-8 represents a proinflammatory cytokine, a powerful regulator of angiogenesis, and a growth-promoting factor. Its properties can make a contribution to the pathogenesis of endometriosis-related infertility. In comparison with infertile women without endometriosis, significantly higher IL-8 concentrations were found in the peritoneal fluid (Skrzypczak et al. 2005) and the follicular fluid and serum of the endometriosis group (Singh et al. 2016). The researchers also reported a negative relationship between IL-8 concentrations and oocyte maturity and embryo quality. However, IL-8 levels in the follicular fluid did not differ significantly between the two study groups (Wunder et al. 2006; Wu et al. 2017). A meta-analysis reported a correlation between increased IL-6 and/or IL-8 concentrations in the serum and endometriosis-related infertility (Malvezzi et al. 2019).

Significantly elevated concentrations of proinflammatory cytokines (TNF-α, IL-1β, IL-2, IL-8, and IL-12) and anti-inflammatory cytokines (IL-4, IL-6, and IL-10) were detected in the serum and follicular fluid of infertile females with endometriosis in comparison with controls. Furthermore, IL-8 and IL-12 levels in the follicular fluid of females with endometriosis were reported to be negatively correlated with embryo quality and oocyte maturity (Singh et al. 2016).

The peritoneal fluid of females with endometriosis has an elevated level of Th1 cytokines, e.g., IL-1β, TNF-α, IFN-γ, IL-6, and IL-12. The toxic impacts of the said inflammatory cytokines on the female reproductive system, sperm, or embryo may lead to infertility or subfertility in females with endometriosis (Gomez-Torres et al. 2002).

IL-17 and IL-23 are inflammatory cytokines related to the Th17 subset. It is reported that IL-17 and IL-23 concentrations in the peritoneal fluid have been found to be not considerably different between infertile endometriosis and non-endometriosis fertile women (Tarokh et al. 2019). No association has been shown between the serum and peritoneal fluid IL-23 concentrations and infertility in subjects with endometriosis and controls (Andreoli et al. 2011). The peritoneal fluid or serum IL-17 concentrations did not differ significantly between subjects with endometriosis and controls (Zhang et al. 2005; Andreoli et al. 2011). Nevertheless, Zhang et al. indicated that the IL-17 level in the peritoneal fluid was significantly higher in infertile subjects than in fertile subjects with endometriosis (Zhang et al. 2005).

With respect to IL-18, two groups of researchers found an increased concentration in the peritoneal fluid of infertile subjects with endometriosis in comparison with controls (Arici et al. 2003; Oku et al. 2004). With respect to IL-15, no difference was detected in the peritoneal fluid concentration (Wunder et al. 2006), and one study found no IL-15, either in the follicular fluid or serum of infertile females with endometriosis (Wu et al. 2017).

Deteriorated endometrial decidualization represents a pathophysiological condition that is related to decreased implantation rates (Gellersen and Brosens 2014) and it is also a detrimental component of endometriosis (Aghajanova et al. 2011). IL-1β and TNFα deteriorate the decidualization of human endometrial stromal cells (Yu 2017). The prolonged stimulation of endometrial stromal cells with TNFα and IL-1β may cause an insufficient response to progesterone in patients with endometriosis and create progesterone resistance (Patel et al. 2017). Alterations in the decidualization of the endometrium may disrupt successful embryo implantation and contribute to endometriosis-related infertility.

Cytokines in Endometriosis-Related Pelvic Pain

The prevalence of endometriosis reaches 73% among women with chronic pelvic pain (Ballard et al. 2008). The exact mechanism of endometriosis-related pain still remains unclear. The vast majority of neurotrophins, particularly brain-derived neurotrophic factor and nerve growth (NGF) factor, are related to endometriosis-associated pain. The elevation of brain-derived neurotrophic factor and NGF in the endometriotic microenvironment enhances the total nerve fiber density and leads to persistent inflammatory pain (Coxon et al. 2018; Tai et al. 2018). The production of brain-derived neurotrophic factor by the eutopic endometrial stromal cells is stimulated by IL-1β via an IL-1 receptor-dependent action. Hence, it aggravates endometriosis-related pain and inflammation (Yu et al. 2018; Ding et al. 2018). IL-1β and TNF-α also upregulate the secretion of NGF from inflammatory cells (Mita et al. 2014). The overexpression of IL-1β and NGF in the peritoneal fluid may lead to a surplus of neuropeptide substance P-positive nerve fibers. Moreover, IL-1β decreases the mechanical nociceptor threshold and causes the activation of the nociceptive nerve (Arnold et al. 2012). IL-6 and IL-33 are two cytokines positively correlated with dysmenorrhea (Velasco et al. 2010; Santulli et al. 2012).

The loss of sympathetic nerve fibers constitutes a hallmark of the transition from acute to chronic inflammatory processes. This leads to an elevation in the concentration of proinflammatory peptide substance-P, which may lead to the secretion of proinflammatory cytokines, such as IL-6, IL-8, and TNF (Coxon et al. 2018).

Various groups of researchers studied the correlation between interleukins (IL-1, IL-2, IL-4, IL-6, IL-8, IL-18, and IL-33) and endometriosis-associated pelvic pain (Rapkin et al. 2000; Arici et al. 2003a; 2003b; Manero and Alcazar 2010; Velasco et al. 2010; Drosdzol-Cop et al. 2012; Malhotra et al. 2012; Santulli et al. 2012). Most of the above-mentioned research indicated a relationship between endometriosis-related pain and cytokine concentration in subjects with endometriosis in comparison with controls. Just two of the said studies reported similar associations between pain and serum cytokine levels in both patient groups (Drosdzol-Cop et al. 2012; Santulli et al. 2012).

Changes in inflammatory factors and the interaction with the autonomic nervous system (ANS) may be responsible for pain. Increases in nerve growth factor (NGF), IL-1β, IL-6, IL-8, immune cells, and the vast majority of inflammatory factors can contribute to endometriosis-related pelvic pain, dysmenorrhea, and dyspareunia (Tai et al. 2018).

Ectopic endometrium implants consist of sympathetic, parasympathetic, and sensory nerve fibers. Furthermore, endometriotic lesions represent various abnormal innervations consisting of the increasing number of total intact nerve fibers, the constitution of cholinergic and unmyelinated nerve fibers (Wang et al. 2009), and the decreasing sympathetic nerve fiber density (NFD) (Arnold et al. 2012).

Conclusion

The present evidence demonstrates that innate and humoral immunity contribute considerably to endometriosis pathogenesis. Endometrial cells are precursors of endometriotic lesions. However, it is still unclear how endometriotic lesions develop from endometrial cells. A dysfunctional immune response can cause endometriotic lesions to implant and survive through the up-regulation of inflammatory pathways. This process is managed by using cytokines and chemokine signaling. Due to pleiotropic effects, cytokines have specific effects on the interactions between cells, intercellular communication, or intracellular actions. Because of these properties, cytokines take part in endometriosis pathogenesis and contribute to the inflammatory environment in the pelvic peritoneum. Endometriosis creates a toxic microenvironment with high levels of inflammatory cytokines that affect the female reproductive system, sperm or embryo, resulting in infertility or subfertility in endometriotic women. Additionally, endometriotic lesions may also cause the expression of inflammatory mediators, including cytokines and pain-associated substances. The mentioned process may result in endometriosis-associated pain and inflammation.

References

Adamson GD, Kennedy S and Hummelshoj L (2010) Creating Solutions in Endometriosis: Global Collaboration through the World Endometriosis Research Foundation. *Journal of Endometriosis* 2(1):3–6.

Agic A, Djalali S, Diedrich K, Hornung D (2009). Apoptosis in Endometriosis. *Gynecologic and Obstetric Investigation* 68(4):217–223.

Aghajanova L, Giudice LC (2010) Molecular Evidence for Differences in Endometrium in Severe Versus Mild Endometriosis. *Reproductive Sciences* 18(3):229–251.

Ahn SH, Edwards AK Singh SS, Young SL, Lessey BA, Tayade C (2015) IL-17A Contributes to the Pathogenesis of Endometriosis by Triggering Proinflammatory Cytokines and Angiogenic Growth Factors. *The Journal of Immunology* 195(6):2591–2600.

Akoum A, Al-Akoum M, Lemay A, Maheux R and Leboeuf M (2008) Imbalance in the peritoneal levels of interleukin 1 and its decoy inhibitory receptor type II in endometriosis women with infertility and pelvic pain. *Fertility and Sterility* 89(6):1618–1624.

Andreoli CG, Genro VK, Souza CA, Michelon T, Bilibio JP, Scheffel C, Cunha-Filho JS (2011) T helper (Th)1, Th2, and Th17 interleukin pathways in infertile patients with minimal/mild endometriosis. *Fertility and Sterility* 95(8):2477–2480.

Arici A, Matalliotakis I, Goumenou A, Koumantakis G, Vassiliadis S, Mahutte NG (2003a) Altered expression of interleukin-18 in the peritoneal fluid of women with endometriosis. *Fertility and Sterility* 80(4):889–894.

Arici A (2003b) Increased levels of interleukin-15 in the peritoneal fluid of women with endometriosis: inverse correlation with stage and depth of invasion. *Human Reproduction* 18(2):429–432.

Arnold J, Barcena de Arellano ML, Rüster C, Vercellino GF, Chiantera V, Schneider A, Mechsner S (2012) Imbalance between sympathetic and sensory innervation in peritoneal endometriosis. *Brain, Behavior, and Immunity* 26(1):132–141.

Barcz E, Milewski Ł, Dziunycz P, Kamiński P, Płoski R, Malejczyk J (2012) Peritoneal cytokines and adhesion formation in endometriosis: an inverse association with vascular endothelial growth factor concentration. *Fertility and Sterility* 97(6):1380-1386.

Ballard K, Seaman H, de Vries C, Wright J (2008) Can symptomatology help in the diagnosis of endometriosis? Findings from a national case-control study-Part 1. *BJOG: An International Journal of Obstetrics & Gynaecology* 115(11):1382–1391.

Batt RE, Mitwally MFM (2003) Endometriosis from thelarche to midteens: pathogenesis and prognosis, prevention and pedagogy. *Journal of Pediatric and Adolescent Gynecology* 16(6):337–347.

Batt RE, Yeh J (2013) Müllerianosis. *Reproductive Sciences* 20(9):1030–1037.

Bedaiwy MA (2002) Prediction of endometriosis with serum and peritoneal fluid markers: a prospective controlled trial. *Human Reproduction* 17(2):426–431.

Boraschi D, Tagliabue A (2013) The interleukin-1 receptor family. *Seminars in Immunology* 25(6):394–407.

Bricou A, Batt RE, Chapron C (2008) Peritoneal fluid flow influences anatomical distribution of endometriotic lesions: Why Sampson seems to be right. *European Journal of Obstetrics & Gynecology and Reproductive Biology* 138(2):127–134.

Burney RO, Giudice LC (2012) Pathogenesis and pathophysiology of endometriosis. *Fertility and Sterility* 98(3):511–519.

Bulun SE, Gurates B, Fang Z, Tamura M, Sebastian S, Zhou J, Amin S, Yang S (2002) Mechanisms of excessive estrogen formation in endometriosis. *Journal of Reproductive Immunology* 55(1-2):21–33.

Cavalli G, Dinarello CA (2018) Suppression of inflammation and acquired immunity by IL-37. *Immunological Reviews* 281(1):179–190.

Cheong YC (2002) IL-1, IL-6 and TNF-alpha concentrations in the peritoneal fluid of women with pelvic adhesions. *Human Reproduction* 17(1):69–75.

Coxon L, Horne AW, Vincent K (2018) Pathophysiology of endometriosis-associated pain: A review of pelvic and central nervous system mechanisms. *Best Practice & Research Clinical Obstetrics & Gynaecology* 51:53–67.

Da Broi MG, Navarro PA (2015) Oxidative stress and oocyte quality: ethiopathogenic mechanisms of minimal/mild endometriosis-related infertility. *Cell and Tissue Research* 364(1):1–7.

Dembic Z (2015) *The cytokines of the immune system: the role of cytokines in disease related to immune response*. Academic Press, p 1-16.

Ding S, Zhu T, Tian Y, Xu P, Chen Z, Huang X, Zhang X (2018) Role of Brain-Derived Neurotrophic Factor in Endometriosis Pain. *Reproductive Sciences* 25(7):1045–1057.

Donnez J, Squifflet J, Casanas-Roux F, Pirard C, Jadoul P, Van Langendonckt A (2003) Typical and subtle atypical presentations of endometriosis. *Obstetrics and Gynecology Clinics of North America* 30(1):83–93.

Drosdzol-Cop A, Skrzypulec-Plinta V, Stojko R (2012) Serum and Peritoneal Fluid Immunological Markers in Adolescent Girls with Chronic Pelvic Pain. *Obstetrical & Gynecological Survey* 67(6):374–381.

Eisenberg V, Weil C, Chodick G, Shalev V (2017) Epidemiology of endometriosis: a large population-based database study from a healthcare provider with 2 million members. *BJOG: An International Journal of Obstetrics & Gynaecology* 125(1):55–62.

Evers JLH (1994) Is mild endometriosis a disease: Endometriosis does not exist; all women have endometriosis. *Human Reproduction* 9(12):2206–2209.

Furuya K, Murakami M, Makimura N, Matsuda H, Ikou K, Saito K, Kawakami Y, Shibazaki T, Fukui U, Mizumoto Y, Tokuoka S, Nagata I, Kikuchi Y (2003) Immunological and endocrinological studies on lymphocyte subpopulation and medical treatment for infertility in patients with endometriosis. *Molecular and Cellular Endocrinology* 202(1-2):195–199.

Garai J (2006) Endometriosis: harmful survival of an ectopic tissue. *Frontiers in Bioscience* 11(1):595.

Garlanda C, Dinarello CA, Mantovani A (2013a) The Interleukin-1 Family: Back to the Future. *Immunity* 39(6):1003–1018.

Garlanda C, Riva F, Bonavita E, Mantovani A (2013b) Negative regulatory receptors of the IL-1 family. *Seminars in Immunology* 25(6):408–415.

Gellersen B, Brosens JJ (2014) Cyclic Decidualization of the Human Endometrium in Reproductive Health and Failure. *Endocrine Reviews* 35(6):851–905.

Giudice LC, Kao LC (2004) Endometriosis. *The Lancet* 364(9447):1789–1799.

Gomez-Torres MJ, Acien P, Campos A, Velasco I (2002) Embryotoxicity of peritoneal fluid in women with endometriosis. Its relation with cytokines and lymphocyte populations. *Human Reproduction* 17(3):777–781.

Grandi G, Mueller MD, Bersinger NA, Facchinetti F, McKinnon BD (2017) The association between progestins, nuclear receptors expression and inflammation in endometrial stromal cells from women with endometriosis. *Gynecological Endocrinology* 33(9):712–715.

Guo SW (2006) Nuclear Factor-κB (NF-κB): An Unsuspected Major Culprit in the Pathogenesis of Endometriosis That Is Still at Large? *Gynecologic and Obstetric Investigation* 63(2):71–97.

Gupta D, Hull ML, Fraser I, Miller L, Bossuyt PM, Johnson N, Nisenblat V (2016) Endometrial biomarkers for the non-invasive diagnosis of endometriosis. *Cochrane Database of Systematic Reviews* 4(4):CD012165. https://doi.org/10.1002/14651858.CD012165.

Han S, Jung S, Wu SP, Hawkins Shannon M, Park M, Kyo S, Qin J, Lydon John P, Tsai Sophia Y, Tsai MJ, DeMayo Francesco J, O'Malley Bert W (2015) Estrogen Receptor β Modulates Apoptosis Complexes and the Inflammasome to Drive the Pathogenesis of Endometriosis. *Cell* 163(4):960–974.

Harada T, Yoshioka H, Yoshida S, Iwabe T, Onohara Y, Tanikawa M, Terakawa N (1997) Increased interleukin-6 levels in peritoneal fluid of infertile patients with active endometriosis. *American Journal of Obstetrics and Gynecology* 176(3):593–597.

Hirata T, Osuga Y, Takamura M, Saito A, Hasegawa A, Koga K, Yoshino O, Hirota Y, Harada M, Taketani Y (2011) Interleukin-17F increases the secretion of interleukin-8 and the expression of cyclooxygenase 2 in endometriosis. *Fertility and Sterility* 96(1):113–117.

Hou Z, Zhou J, Ma X, Fan L, Liao L, Liu J (2008) Role of interleukin-1 receptor type II in the pathogenesis of endometriosis. *Fertility and Sterility* 89(1):42–51.

Hsu AL, Townsend PM, Oehninger S, Castora FJ (2015) Endometriosis may be associated with mitochondrial dysfunction in cumulus cells from subjects undergoing in vitro fertilization-intracytoplasmic sperm injection, as reflected by decreased adenosine triphosphate production. *Fertility and Sterility* 103(2):347-352.

Iwabe T, Harada T, Tsudo T, Nagano Y, Yoshida S, Tanikawa M, Terakawa N (2000) Tumor Necrosis Factor-α Promotes Proliferation of Endometriotic Stromal Cells by Inducing Interleukin-8 Gene and Protein Expression. *The Journal of Clinical Endocrinology & Metabolism* 85(2):824–829.

Jiang J, Yu K, Jiang Z, Xue M (2018) IL-37 affects the occurrence and development of endometriosis by regulating the biological behavior of endometrial stromal cells through multiple signaling pathways. *Biological Chemistry* 399(11):1325–1337.

Jiang J, Jiang Z, Xue M (2019) Serum and peritoneal fluid levels of interleukin-6 and interleukin-37 as biomarkers for endometriosis. *Gynecological Endocrinology* 35(7):571–575.

Kaabachi W, Kacem O, Belhaj R, Hamzaoui A, Hamzaoui K (2017) Interleukin-37 in endometriosis. *Immunology Letters* 185:52–55.

Koks CAM, Dunselman GAJ, de Goeij AFPM, Arends, JW, Evers JLH (1997) Evaluation of a menstrual cup to collect shed endometrium for in vitro studies. *Fertility and Sterility* 68(3):560–564.

Kondera-Anasz Z, Sikora J, Mielczarek-Palacz A, Jońca M (2005) Concentrations of interleukin (IL)-1α, IL-1 soluble receptor type II (IL-1 sRII) and IL-1 receptor antagonist (IL-1 Ra) in the peritoneal fluid and serum of infertile women with endometriosis. *European Journal of Obstetrics & Gynecology and Reproductive Biology* 123(2):198–203.

Koninckx PR (1994) Is mild endometriosis a disease? Is mild endometriosis a condition occurring intermittently in all women? *Human Reproduction* 9(12):2202–2205.

Kvaskoff M, Mu F, Terry KL, Harris HR, Poole EM, Farland L, Missmer SA (2015) Endometriosis: a high-risk population for major chronic diseases? *Human Reproduction Update* 21(4):500–516.

Lawson C, Bourcier N, Al-Akoum M, Maheux R, Naud F, Akoum A (2008) Abnormal interleukin 1 receptor types I and II gene expression in eutopic and ectopic endometrial tissues of women with endometriosis. *Journal of Reproductive Immunology* 77(1):75–84.

Lebovic DI, Bentzien F, Chao VA, Garrett EN, Meng YG, Taylor RN (2000) Induction of an angiogenic phenotype in endometriotic stromal cell cultures by interleukin-1. *Molecular Human Reproduction* 6(3):269–275.

Lebovic DI, Mueller MD, Taylor RN (2001) Immunobiology of endometriosis. *Fertility and Sterility* 75(1):1–10.

Lin YJ, Lai MD, Lei HY, Wing LYC (2006) Neutrophils and Macrophages Promote Angiogenesis in the Early Stage of Endometriosis in a Mouse Model. *Endocrinology* 147(3):1278–1286.

Liu Z (2016) Inflammation and endometriosis. *Frontiers in Bioscience* 21(5):941–948.

Ma X (ed.) (2016) *Regulation of cytokine gene expression in immunity and diseases*. Springer Netherlands, p 21-26.

Macer ML, Taylor HS (2012) Endometriosis and Infertility. *Obstetrics and Gynecology Clinics of North America* 39(4):535–549.

Malhotra N, Karmakar D, Tripathi V, Luthra K, Kumar S (2011) Correlation of angiogenic cytokines-leptin and IL-8 in stage, type and presentation of endometriosis. *Gynecological Endocrinology* 28(3):224–227.

Malvezzi H, Hernandes C, Piccinato C, Podgaec S (2019) Interleukin in endometriosis-associated infertility-pelvic pain: systematic review and meta-analysis. *Reproduction* 158(1):1-12.

Manero MG, Alcazar JL (2010) Interleukin-8 serum levels do not correlate with pelvic pain in patients with ovarian endometriomas. *Fertility and Sterility* 94(2):450–452.

Marí-Alexandre J, Barceló-Molina M, Belmonte-López E, García-Oms J, Estellés A, Braza-Boïls A, Gilabert-Estellés J (2018) Micro-RNA profile and proteins in peritoneal fluid from women with endometriosis: their relationship with sterility. *Fertility and Sterility* 109(4):675-684.

Matsuzaki S, Gremeau AS, Pouly JL (2020) Impaired pathogen-induced autophagy and increased IL-1β and TNFα release in response to pathogenic triggers in secretory phase endometrial stromal cells of endometriosis patients. *Reproductive BioMedicine Online* 41(5):767–781.

Michaud N, Al-Akoum M, Gagnon G, Girard K, Blanchet P, Rousseau JA, Akoum A (2011) Decreased concentrations of soluble interleukin-1 receptor accessory protein levels in the peritoneal fluid of women with endometriosis. *Journal of Reproductive Immunology* 92(1-2):68–73.

Mishra VV, Bandwal P, Agarwal R, Aggarwal R (2016) Prevalence, Clinical and Laparoscopic Features of Endometriosis Among Infertile Women. *The Journal of Obstetrics and Gynecology of India* 67(3):208–212.

Mita S, Shimizu Y, Sato A, Notsu T, Imada K, Kyo S (2014) Dienogest inhibits nerve growth factor expression induced by tumor necrosis factor-α or interleukin-1β. *Fertility and Sterility* 101(2):595-601.

Mosbah A, Nabiel Y, Khashaba E (2016) Interleukin-6, intracellular adhesion molecule-1, and glycodelin A levels in serum and peritoneal fluid as biomarkers for endometriosis. *International Journal of Gynecology & Obstetrics* 134(3):247–251.

Mu F, Harris HR, Rich-Edwards JW, Hankinson SE, Rimm EB, Spiegelman D, Missmer SA (2017). A Prospective Study of Inflammatory Markers and Risk of Endometriosis. *American Journal of Epidemiology* 187(3):515–522.

Mueller MD, Vigne JL, Minchenko A, Lebovic DI, Leitman DC, Taylor RN (2000) Regulation of vascular endothelial growth factor (VEGF) gene transcription by estrogen receptors alpha and beta. *Proceedings of the National Academy of Sciences* 97(20):10972–10977.

Nisenblat V, Bossuyt PM, Shaikh R, Farquhar C, Jordan V, Scheffers CS, Mol BWJ, Johnson N, Hull ML (2016) Blood biomarkers for the non-invasive diagnosis of endometriosis. *Cochrane Database of Systematic Reviews* 2016(5):CD012179.

Nnoaham KE, Hummelshoj L, Webster P, d'Hooghe T, de Cicco Nardone F, de Cicco Nardone C, Jenkinson C, Kennedy SH, Zondervan KT (2011) Impact of endometriosis on quality of life and work productivity: a multicenter study across ten countries. *Fertility and Sterility* 96(2):366-373.

Oku H (2004) Role of IL-18 in pathogenesis of endometriosis. *Human Reproduction* 19(3):709–714.

Patel B, Elguero S, Thakore S, Dahoud W, Bedaiwy M, Mesiano S (2014) Role of nuclear progesterone receptor isoforms in uterine pathophysiology. *Human Reproduction Update* 21(2):155–173.

Patel BG, Rudnicki M, Yu J, Shu Y, Taylor RN (2017) Progesterone resistance in endometriosis: origins, consequences and interventions. *Acta Obstetricia et Gynecologica Scandinavica* 96(6):623–632.

Pizzo A, Salmeri FM, Ardita FV, Sofo V, Tripepi M, Marsico S (2002) Behaviour of cytokine levels in serum and peritoneal fluid of women with endometriosis. *Gynecologic and Obstetric Investigation* 54(2):82–87.

Podgaec S, Rizzo LV, Fernandes LFC, Baracat EC, Abrao MS (2012) CD4+CD25highFoxp3+ Cells Increased in the Peritoneal Fluid of Patients with Endometriosis. *American Journal of Reproductive Immunology* 68(4):301–308.

Rakhila H, Al-Akoum M, Bergeron M-E, Leboeuf M, Lemyre M, Akoum A, Pouliot M (2016) Promotion of angiogenesis and proliferation cytokines patterns in peritoneal fluid from women with endometriosis. *Journal of Reproductive Immunology* 116:1–6.

Rapkin A, Morgan M, Bonpane C, Martinez-Maza O (2000) Peritoneal fluid interleukin-6 in women with chronic pelvic pain. *Fertility and Sterility* 74(2):325–328.

Saito S, Nakashima A, Ito M, Shima T (2011) Clinical implication of recent advances in our understanding of IL-17 and reproductive immunology. *Expert Review of Clinical Immunology* 7(5):649–657.

Sanchez AM, Vanni VS, Bartiromo L, Papaleo E, Zilberberg E, Candiani M, Orvieto R, Viganò P (2017) Is the oocyte quality affected by endometriosis? A review of the literature. *Journal of Ovarian Research* 10(1):43.

Santulli P, Borghese B, Chouzenoux S, Vaiman D, Borderie D, Streuli I, Goffinet F, de Ziegler D, Weill B, Batteux F, Chapron C (2012) Serum and peritoneal interleukin-33 levels are elevated in deeply infiltrating endometriosis. *Human Reproduction* 27(7):2001–2009.

Sampson JA (1940) The development of the implantation theory for the origin of peritoneal endometriosis. *American journal of obstetrics and gynecology* 40:549–557.

Sarapik A, Velthut A, Haller-Kikkatalo K, Faure GC, Béné M-C, de Carvalho Bittencourt M, Massin F, Uibo R, Salumets A (2012) Follicular Proinflammatory Cytokines and Chemokines as Markers of IVF Success. *Clinical and Developmental Immunology* 2012:1–10.

Sikora J, Mielczarek-Palacz A, Kondera-Anasz Z (2016) Association of the Precursor of Interleukin-1β and Peritoneal Inflammation-Role in Pathogenesis of Endometriosis. *Journal of Clinical Laboratory Analysis* 30(6):831–837.

Sikora J, Smycz-Kubańska M, Mielczarek-Palacz A, Kondera-Anasz Z (2017) Abnormal peritoneal regulation of chemokine activation-The role of IL-8 in pathogenesis of endometriosis. *American Journal of Reproductive Immunology* 77(4):p.e12622.

Simoens S, Dunselman G, Dirksen C, Hummelshoj L, Bokor A, Brandes I, Brodszky V, Canis M, Colombo GL, DeLeire T, Falcone T, Graham B, Halis G, Horne A, Kanj O, Kjer JJ, Kristensen J, Lebovic D, Mueller M, Vigano P (2012) The burden of endometriosis: costs and quality of life of women with endometriosis and treated in referral centres. *Human Reproduction* 27(5):1292–1299.

Singh AK, Dutta M, Chattopadhyay R, Chakravarty B, Chaudhury K (2016) Intrafollicular interleukin-8, interleukin-12, and adrenomedullin are the promising prognostic markers of oocyte and embryo quality in women with endometriosis. *Journal of Assisted Reproduction and Genetics* 33(10):1363–1372.

Skrzypczak J, Szczepańska M, Puk E, Kamieniczna M and Kurpisz M (2005) Peritoneal fluid cytokines and sICAM-1 in minimal endometriosis: search for discriminating factors between infertility and/or endometriosis. *European Journal of Obstetrics & Gynecology and Reproductive Biology* 122(1):95–103.

Song X, Qian Y (2013) IL-17 family cytokines mediated signaling in the pathogenesis of inflammatory diseases. *Cellular Signalling* 25(12):2335–2347.

Sourial S, Tempest N, Hapangama DK (2014) Theories on the Pathogenesis of Endometriosis. *International Journal of Reproductive Medicine* 2014:1–9.

Stilley JAW, Birt JA, Sharpe-Timms KL (2012) Cellular and molecular basis for endometriosis-associated infertility. *Cell and Tissue Research* 349(3):849–862.

Symons LK, Miller JE, Kay VR, Marks RM, Liblik K, Koti M, Tayade C (2018) The Immunopathophysiology of Endometriosis. *Trends in Molecular Medicine* 24(9):748–762.

Tai F-W, Chang C, Chiang J-H, Lin W-C, Wan L (2018) Association of Pelvic Inflammatory Disease with Risk of Endometriosis: A Nationwide Cohort Study Involving 141,460 *Individuals. Journal of Clinical Medicine* 7(11): 379.

Takamura M, Osuga Y, Izumi G, Yoshino O, Koga K, Saito A, Hirata T, Hirota Y, Harada M, Hasegawa A, Taketani Y (2012) Interleukin-17A is present in neutrophils in endometrioma and stimulates the secretion of growth-regulated oncogene–α (Gro-α) from endometrioma stromal cells. *Fertility and Sterility* 98(5):1218-1224.

Tarokh M, GhaffariNovin M, Poordast T, Tavana Z, Nazarian H, Norouzian M, Gharesi-Fard B (2019) Serum and peritoneal fluid cytokine profiles in infertile women with endometriosis. *Iranian Journal of Immunology* 16(2):151-162.

Troncon JK, Zani ACT, Vieira ADD, Poli-Neto OB, Nogueira AA, Rosa-e-Silva JC (2014) Endometriosis in a Patient with Mayer-Rokitansky-Küster-Hauser Syndrome. *Case Reports in Obstetrics and Gynecology* 2014:1–4.

Velasco I, Acién P, Campos A, Acién MI, Ruiz-Maciá E (2010) Interleukin-6 and other soluble factors in peritoneal fluid and endometriomas and their relation to pain and aromatase expression. *Journal of Reproductive Immunology* 84(2):199–205.

Vercellini P, Abbiati A, Vigano P, Somigliana ED, Daguati R, Meroni F, Crosignani PG (2007) Asymmetry in distribution of diaphragmatic endometriotic lesions: evidence in favour of the menstrual reflux theory. *Human Reproduction* 22(9):2359–2367.

Vercellini P, Viganò P, Somigliana E, Fedele L (2013) Endometriosis: pathogenesis and treatment. *Nature Reviews Endocrinology* 10(5):261–275.

Wang G, Tokushige N, Markham R, Fraser IS (2008) Rich innervation of deep infiltrating endometriosis. *Human Reproduction* 24(4):827–834.

Wang X-Q, Zhou W-J, Luo X-Z, Tao Y, Li D-J (2017) Synergistic effect of regulatory T cells and proinflammatory cytokines in angiogenesis in the endometriotic milieu. *Human Reproduction* 32(6):1304–1317.

Wu Y, Starzinski-Powitz A, Guo S-W (2008) Prolonged stimulation with tumor necrosis factor-α induced partial methylation at PR-B promoter in immortalized epithelial-like endometriotic cells. *Fertility and Sterility* 90(1):234–237.

Wu M-H, Lu C-W, Chuang P-C, Tsai S-J (2010) Prostaglandin E2: the master. *Exp Biol Med* (Maywood) 235(6):668-677.

Wu G, Bersinger NA, Mueller MD, von Wolff M (2017) Intrafollicular inflammatory cytokines but not steroid hormone concentrations are increased in naturally matured follicles of women with proven endometriosis. *Journal of Assisted Reproduction and Genetics* 34(3):357–364.

Wunder DM, Mueller MD, Birkhäuser MH, Bersinger NA (2006) Increased ENA-78 in the follicular fluid of patients with endometriosis. *Acta Obstetricia Et Gynecologica Scandinavica* 85(3):336–342.

Xie Y, Li Y, Cai X, Wang X, Li J (2016) Interleukin-37 suppresses ICAM-1 expression in parallel with NF-κB down-regulation following TLR2 activation of human coronary artery endothelial cells. *International Immunopharmacology* 38:26–30.

Yi L, Lilan L, Haibo Z (2000) Changes of cytokines levels in peritoneal fluids of patients with endometriosis and its effect on reproductive activity. *Journal of Tongji Medical University* 20(2):163–165.

Yu J, Berga SL, Zou W, Yook DG, Pan JC, Andrade AA, Zhao L, Sidell N, Bagchi IC, Bagchi MK, Taylor RN (2017) IL-1β Inhibits Connexin 43 and Disrupts Decidualization of Human Endometrial Stromal Cells Through ERK1/2 and p38 MAP Kinase. *Endocrinology* 158(12):4270–4285.

Yu J, Francisco AMC, Patel BG, Cline JM, Zou E, Berga SL, Taylor RN (2018) IL-1β Stimulates Brain-Derived Neurotrophic Factor Production in Eutopic Endometriosis Stromal Cell Cultures. *The American Journal of Pathology* 188(10):2281–2292.

Zhang X, Xu H, Lin J, Qian Y, Deng L (2005) Peritoneal fluid concentrations of interleukin-17 correlate with the severity of endometriosis and infertility of this disorder. *BJOG: An International Journal of Obstetrics & Gynaecology* 112(8):1153–1155.

Chapter 30

Cytokines and Chronic Pelvic Pain

Zehra Yilmaz*, MD

Department of Obstetrics and Gynecology, Zehra Yilmaz Clinic, Samsun, Turkey

Abstract

Chronic pelvic pain (CPP) is a serious problem that triggers the depressive mood of women and reduces their quality of life. There are some challenges in diagnosis and treatment for both the patient and the physician. As the disease has a wide differential diagnosis, it is diagnosed late, and treatment interventions fail. There are contradictions between the results obtained with respect to the relationship between CPP and cytokines. It is still not clear whether and how cytokines take part in the pathophysiology of pelvic pain. In this article, there will be an attempt to explain the relationship between the common causes of CPP and cytokines.

Keywords: chronic pain, pelvic pain, cytokine

Introduction

Chronic pelvic pain (CPP) is described as severe pain in the pelvic region, which lasts for more than six months, is not associated with the menstrual cycle, pregnancy, local trauma, or pelvic operations, and leads to limitation of functions. It is more common in women at a frequency between 3% and 10%. Due to this pain, loss of workdays in about 15%, and a performance decrease in about 45% of women have been reported (Grinberg et al., 2020). The pathophysiology has not been clearly revealed and is associated with allodynia, hyperesthesia, and pelvic floor dysfunction. It is usually observed with symptoms indicating genital, lower urinary system, bowel, myofascial, pelvic floor, and gynecological dysfunction in addition to adverse behavioral, cognitive, sexual, and emotional consequences (ACOG 2020). In a prospective observational study conducted at a referral gynecology center, the most common diagnoses determined respectively for CPP were irritable bowel syndrome, adhesions, musculoskeletal causes, and endometriosis (Lamvu et al., 2006). Studies have attempted to

* Corresponding Author's Email: z.a.yilmaz@gmail.com.

In: Cytokines and Diseases
Editors: Kenan Demir, Selim Görgün and Bahar Uslu
ISBN: 979-8-88697-214-6

demonstrate the relationship between CPP and cytokines, and some relationships have been identified between the causes of CPP and cytokines. It is still not clear whether and how cytokines take part in the pathophysiology of pelvic pain.

The entire series of complex electrochemical events taking place between tissue injury and the perception of pain is called nociception. Pain is a perception event in nociception. On the other hand, painful stimuli are called noxious stimuli. Severe noxious stimulation leads to measurable metabolic, biochemical, and electrophysiological changes in the dorsal horn. This condition, which turns acute pain into chronic pain, is defined as "neuroplastic change." Neuroplastic change activates the N-methyl-D-aspartate receptors of the dorsal horn and thus triggers a process that results in a loss of inhibition in neurons. Loss of inhibition in neurons ends in a process in which the sense of "pain" is continuously transmitted and never "comes to an end." Accordingly, the slightest noxious stimulation brings about the clinical picture characterized by a sense of "pain" perceived as exaggerated and never alleviated. In the clinical context, this physiopathological process is referred to as "allodynia" and then "hyperalgesia" (Prato et al., 2017). Briefly, noxious stimulation that triggers the "acute pain," which is normally supposed to last for a short time, turns into "chronic pain" with neuroplastic change and activation of the receptors in the dorsal horn.

The urogenital and gastrointestinal systems are evaluated comprehensively in CPP patients. Screening questionnaires are also part of the evaluation. Specific diagnoses are established by paying attention to the history and physical examination findings of patients. Postmenopausal bleeding and the onset of pain, unexplained weight loss, pelvic mass, hematuria, and postcoital bleeding necessitate careful examination in respect of malignancy. The differential diagnosis of CPP is quite wide. For convenience, it will be appropriate to perform the visceral, neuromuscular, and psycho-social evaluations. Visceral causes (gynecological) include endometriosis, adenomyosis, pelvic adhesion, vulvodynia, vestibulitis, ovarian remnant syndrome, chronic pelvic inflammatory disease, leiomyoma, and pain after tubal ligation. Visceral causes (GIS) are as follows: irritable bowel syndrome, gastrointestinal cancer and colorectal cancer, diverticular colitis, celiac disease, and inflammatory bowel disease. Visceral causes (urological) involve interstitial cystitis (painful bladder syndrome), chronic cystitis, radiation cystitis, urethral syndrome, and chronic urolithiasis. Neuromuscular causes are fibromyalgia, myofascial pain syndrome, postural syndrome, hypertonic pelvic floor syndrome, coccydynia, and pelvic congestion syndrome. Psycho-social causes include abuse (physical, emotional, sexual), depressive disorders, anxiety disorders, somatic symptom disorders, and substance addictions (ACOG 2020).

A detailed history of the patient should be taken. All conditions that contribute to pain and reduce the quality of life should be investigated. Adopting a multidisciplinary approach will be more appropriate for these patients. The patient should be enabled to localize the pain on a visual body map. In this way, the patient can describe the areas of pain and reveal a dermatome extension indicating a non-visceral source of pain. Pain and its severity should be questioned during menstruation, sexual activity, urination, and defecation. The response to previous treatments should be identified. In CPP, physical examination is a significant part of the evaluation. However, this can be stressful and painful for patients. The aim of the examination is to determine the dermatome, tissue, nerve, muscle, and organs where the patient has pain symptoms. The examination should be performed systematically, softly, and with good communication to alleviate stress. It should be explained how the examination will be performed, and it is necessary to perform the examination slowly. The patient's pain should be questioned starting from the least painful area, and the anatomical regions where the pain increases should be described. The pelvis, abdomen, back and extremities should be examined in detail. The patient should be examined for any trigger points, surgical scars, and masses in the abdomen and pelvis. Palpation, as well as a cotton swab, can be preferred during the examination. A cotton swab may be useful to find the source of cutaneous pain (Nasr-Esfahani et al., 2013). External genital infectious findings and inflammatory dermatological findings should be evaluated in terms of vulvar cancers and neurological etiology. Tenderness and hypertonicity should be checked in pelvic floor muscles. Tenderness and pain during the palpation of the lumbar region, pubic symphysis, or sacroiliac joints may indicate that the etiology originates from the musculoskeletal system. The Carnett test is frequently used in chronic pelvic pain. During the palpation on the patient in the supine position, the clinician places his finger on the sensitive area of the patient's abdomen and asks the patient to lift both legs from the stretcher. If the patient's pain escalates during this maneuver, the test is considered as positive. A positive test suggests that the pain is associated with abdominal wall pathologies. This situation may be linked with hematoma, hernia, or anterior abdominal wall muscles (Ortiz et al., 2008). In CPP, no standardized imaging studies or laboratory tests are available. Laboratory tests have limited values. The history, physical examination, and clinical suspicion are the most important elements in diagnosis. Laboratory tests and imaging studies are conducted according to anamnesis and physical examination results. In sexually active women, microbiological tests should be requested for sexually transmitted diseases (chlamydia, gonorrhea, trichomonas), and a complete urine test and urinary culture should be requested to exclude urinary tract infection. To exclude the chronic infectious or inflammatory process and pregnancy, the complete blood count, pregnancy test, erythrocyte sedimentation rate, and CRP tests can be requested. To investigate the metabolic causes of abdominal pain, glucose, creatinine, and serum electrolytes can be requested. Liver function tests should be requested in patients with upper abdominal pain. Ultrasonography is the first diagnostic method following physical examination and inspection. Uterine pathologies such as adnexal pathologies (endometrioma), adenomyosis, and myoma uteri can be identified. Moreover, in the case of a suspected endometriotic focus in the sacrouterine ligaments during a physical examination in patients with deep endometriosis, ultrasonography can also detect the focus if the person performing it is experienced. In soft tissue pathologies, magnetic resonance imaging is superior to ultrasonography. Its diagnostic power is high in detecting deep endometriosis and nodules, and adenomyosis. In the presence of severe pain, a diagnostic laparoscopy can be performed on the patient if the diagnosis is not clear after initial evaluations. With laparoscopy, pathologies such as endometriosis, and pelvic or abdominal adhesions can be diagnosed and treated. There is a controversial relationship between CPP and pelvic adhesions (Hammoud et al., 2004). It is of limited relevance in the treatment of CPP.

Endometriosis is the growth of the endometrial gland and stroma outside the uterus. In CPP, it can be diagnosed at an approximate rate of 33%. Endometriosis can be observed in 15-80% of patients who undergo a diagnostic laparoscopy for CPP (Barbiery et al., 1990). Different research groups have studied the relationship between IL-1, IL-2, IL-4, IL-6, IL-8, IL-18, or IL-33 and endometriosis-associated pelvic pain (Rapkin et al., 2000; Arici et al., 2008; Oku et al., 2003; Manero et al., 2010; Velasco et al., 2010; Michaud et al., 2011; Drosdzol-Cop et al., 2012; Malhotra et al., 2012; Malhotra et al., 2012; Santulli at al. 2012). Most of these studies reported increased interleukin levels in the peritoneal fluid in patients with endometriosis compared to control participants and revealed a relationship between endometriosis-associated pain and cytokine concentration. Only two of these studies state similar significant relationships for serum cytokine levels in patients compared to control participants (Drosdzol et al., 2012; Malhotra et al., 2012; Santulli et al., 2012). In all of the studies addressed, IL-1 and IL-18 were increased from the peritoneal fluid, IL-4 from the peritoneal fluid and serum, and IL-33 from the serum (Arici et al., 2008; Oku et al., 2003; Michaud et al., 2011; Drosdzol et al., 2012; Santulli at al. 2012). However, in endometriosis patients, a positive correlation between IL-6 and dysmenorrhea and pelvic pain could only be reached in one study (Velasco et al., 2010) and between IL-33 and dysmenorrhea in one study alone (Santulli et al., 2012). Research on IL-6 and IL-8 has revealed inconsistent results, although they are perhaps the most studied interleukins in endometriosis. Some authors have obtained significantly higher concentrations in patients with endometriosis (Manero et al.,; 2010; Velasco et al., 2010; Drosdzol et al., 2012), but others reported no difference in patients and control participants, independent of the fluid evaluated (Rapkin et al., 2000). Since endometriosis is an inflammatory disease, the current evidence indicates that a local peritoneal inflammatory reaction caused by ectopic endometrial implants leads to endometriosis-associated pelvic pain (Izumi and Ahn et al., 2018). Local angiogenesis and secretion of growth factors and cytokines, especially peritoneal neutrophils and macrophages, can help to maintain the viability of the endometriotic focus after its attachment to the peritoneum (Izumi and Koga et al., 2018). Not all endometrial cells in the peritoneal cavity may be eliminated by the macrophages and natural killer (NK) cells of patients with endometriosis, and this is known to result in abnormal cytokine secretion and inflammation (Izumi and Koga et al., 2018). Macrophages and epithelial cells release IL-8, a powerful chemokine for neutrophils. IL-6 is rapidly produced by many cell types and activated macrophages in response to injury. Th17 lymphocytes, which act in multiple chronic inflammatory diseases, are considered to be proinflammatory cytokines involved in the maintenance of inflammation and activation. All these complex interactions and inflammation lead to significant abdominal pain in patients with endometriosis.

Cytokines play a crucial role in the immunopathogenesis of inflammatory bowel disease (IBD), in which they direct and regulate several aspects of bowel inflammation. The disease progresses and tissue damage occurs due to the imbalance between proinflammatory and anti-inflammatory cytokines that emerge in IBD. Thus, the resolution of inflammation is restricted. Cytokines have been studied extensively due to their roles in initiating, mediating, maintaining, and controlling bowel inflammation and tissue injury and because they are critical in the pathogenesis of IBD and can be potential therapeutic targets (Neurath et al., 2014; Chen et al., 2016). Antibodies against TNF, IL-12/IL-23p40, IFN-γ, IL-6R, IL-11, IL-13, IL-17A, integrin, and recombinant IL-10 and IFN-β have been tested or applied in clinics to treat IBD patients (Neurath et al., 2014).

Irritable bowel syndrome (IBS) is a functional gastrointestinal (GI) disorder characterized by varying bowel habits, accompanied by recurrent abdominal pain or discomfort and often abdominal bloating and/or distension (Chey et al., 2015). Some studies asserted the unbalanced cytokine signaling as an important pathogenetic factor of IBS. However, the changes were inconsistent (Bashashati et al., 2014; Bashashati et al., 2012). Previous studies have specifically demonstrated high systemic levels of IL-6, IL-8, and TNF-α in IBS patients compared to healthy control participants (Bashashati et al., 2012; Rana et al., 2012; Seyedmirzaee et al., 2016; Scully et al., 2016). In another study, no difference was observed in these levels between healthy control participants and IBS patients. Interestingly, a 3-week low-carbohydrate diet decreased the serum levels of proinflammatory IL-6 and IL-8 (Hustoft et al., 2017). IL-10 and IL-12 obtained from the peripheral blood of IBS patients were compared to those of healthy control participants, and an abnormal IL-10/IL-12 ratio was observed, which indicated the proinflammatory status (O'Mahony et al., 2005).

The International Society for the Vulvovaginal Disease describes vulvodynia as a condition of chronic pain or discomfort which involves the vulva, lasts for more than 3 months, and does not have a clear etiology (32 Bornstein et al., 2015). Clinically, vulvar pain syndrome (VPS) is accepted as a complex gynecological disorder mainly characterized by different levels of pain, sexual dysfunction, and psychological distress (Moyal-Barracco et al., 2003). It has been revealed that several cytokines and growth factors involved in inflammatory processes are significantly correlated with VPS and proven that vulvodynia might be a cytokine-mediated pain syndrome (Zhang et al., 2011; Micheletti et al., 2014). Recently, neuro-inflammation has been discussed extensively as a pathogenetic component in vulvodynia (Micheletti et al., 2014). A few studies have suggested an increase in specific proinflammatory expression in women with vestibulodynia and associated this increase with neuroinflammatory cytokines, including IL-1b and IL-6 (Chalmers et al., 2016; Eliavet al., 2009).

Pain felt in the whole body is an important clinical characteristic in individuals with chronic pain. Since the individual feels pain in the whole body, this may cause greater pain for the patient and difficulties in finding successful treatment options. Fibromyalgia is a chronic pain condition characterized by widespread body pain. Studies on fibromyalgia reveal the role of IL-8, which is a proinflammatory cytokine (Karshikoff et al., 2021). High TNFα levels have been associated with greater fatigue in women with chronic pelvic pain. TNFα levels have been found to be unassociated with depression scores or pain severity. No association with IL-6 has been observed (Karshikoff et al., 2021).

Interstitial cystitis/bladder pain syndrome (IC/BPS) is a chronic inflammatory disease of the bladder, which is characterized by urinary frequency, urgency, nocturia, and bladder pain associated with sterile urine (Homma et al., 2009). A study which analyzed IL-33 and galectin-3 (Gal-3) in 24-hour urine samples taken from patients with IC/BPS and healthy subjects reported that IL-33 and Gal-3 levels increased substantially in IC/BPS (Kochiashvili et al., 2014). In a study comparing the urinary chemokine and IL-4 levels of patients with interstitial cystitis to those of the healthy control group, the chemokine and IL-4 levels of patients with interstitial cystitis were observed to be significantly higher (Abernethy et al., 2017). In other studies, these two proinflammatory cytokines were found to increase (Tyagi et al., 2012; Lamale et al., 2006).

Conclusion

There is a need for more studies on interleukins and chronic pelvic pain. The available evidence indicates there are increased cytokine concentrations in patients but, it is still not clear whether and how cytokines, especially interleukins, take part in the physiopathology of pelvic pain. More studies are needed on this subject.

References

Abernethy M G, Rosenfeld A, White J R, Mueller M G, Lewicky-Gaupp C, Kenton K (2017) Urinary Microbiome and Cytokine Levels in Women with Interstitial Cystitis. *Obstet. Gynecol.* 129(3):500-506.

American College of Obstetricians and Gynecologists (ACOG) (2020) Chronic pelvic pain: ACOG practice bulletin, Number 218. *Obstetrics and gynecology* 135:98-109.

Arici A, Matalliotakis I, Goumenou A, Koumantakis G, Vassiliadis S, Mahutte NG (2003a) Altered expression of interleukin-18 in the peritoneal fluid of women with endometriosis. *Fertil. Steril.* 80(4):889-94.

Arici A, Matalliotakis I, Goumenou A, Koumantakis G, Vassiliadis S, Selam B, Mahutte NG (2003b) Increased levels of interleukin-15 in the peritoneal fluid of women with endometriosis: inverse correlation with stage and depth of invasion. *Human Reproduction* 18:429–432.

Barbieri RL (1990) Etiology and epidemiology of endometriosis. *American journal of obstetrics and gynecology* 162(2):565-567.

Bashashati M, Rezaei N, Andrews CN, et al. (2012) Cytokines and irritable bowel syndrome: where do we stand? *Cytokine* 57:201– 209.

Bashashati M, Rezaei N, Shafieyoun A, et al. (2014) Cytokine imbalance in irritable bowel syndrome: a systematic review and meta-analysis. *Neurogastroenterol. Motil.* 26:1036– 1048.

Bornstein J, Goldstein AT, Stockdale CK, Bergeron S, Pukall C, Zolnoun D, et al. (2015) ISSVD, ISSWSH, and IPPS consensus terminology and classification of persistent vulvar pain and vulvodynia. *Obstet. Gynecol.* 127(4):745-751.

Chalmers KJ, Madden VJ, Hutchinson MR, Moseley GL (2016) Local and systemic inflammation in localized, provoked vestibulodynia: a systematic review *Obstet. Gynecol.* 128(2):337-347.

Chen ML, Sundrud MS (2016) Cytokine networks and T-cell subsets in inflammatory bowel diseases. *Inflammatory Bowel Diseases* 22(5):1157–1167.

Chey WD, Kurlander J, Eswaran S (2015) Irritable bowel syndrome: a clinical review. *JAMA* 313:949– 958.

Cystitis Guideline Committee (2009) Clinical guidelines for interstitial cystitis and hypersensitive bladder syndrome. *Int. J. Urol.* 16:597–615.

Drosdzol-Cop A, Skrzypulec-Plinta V (2012) Selected cytokines and glycodelin A levels in serum and peritoneal fluid in girls with endometriosis. *Journal of Obstetrics and Gynaecology Research* 38:1245–1253

Drosdzol-Cop A, Skrzypulec-Plinta V, Stojko R (2012) Serum and peritoneal fluid immunological markers in adolescent girls with chronic pelvic pain. *Obstetrical and Gynecological Survey* 67:374–381.

Eliav E, Benoliel R, Herzberg U, Kalladka M, Tal M (2009) The role of IL-6 and IL-1beta in painful perineural inflammatory neuritis. *Brain Behav. Immun.* 23 (4):474-484.

Grinberg K, Sela Y, Nissanholtz-Gannot R (2020) New insights about chronic pelvic pain syndrome (CPPS). *International journal of environmental research and public health* 17(9):3005.

Hammoud A, Gago LA, Diamond MP (2004) Adhesions in patients with chronic pelvic pain: a role for adhesiolysis? *Fertil. Steril.* 82(6):1483-91.

Homma Y, Ueda T, Tomoe H, Lin AT, Kuo HC, Lee MH, Lee JG, Kim DY, Lee KS; Interstitial cystitis guideline committee (2009) Clinical guidelines for interstitial cystitis and hypersensitive bladder syndrome. *Int. J. Urol.* 16(7):597-615.

Hustoft TN, Hausken T, Ystad SO, Valeur J, Brokstad K, Hatlebakk JG, Lied GA (2017). Effects of varying dietary content of fermentable short-chain carbohydrates on symptoms, fecal microenvironment, and cytokine profiles in patients with irritable bowel syndrome. *Neurogastroenterol. Motil.* 29(4). https://doi.org/10.1111/nmo.12969.

Izumi G, Koga K, Takamura M, Makabe T, Satake E, Takeuchi A, Taguchi A, Urata Y, Fujii T, Osuga Y 2018 Involvement of immune cells in the pathogenesis of endometriosis. *Journal of Obstetrics and Gynaecology Research* 44:191–198.

Izumi JE, Ahn SH, Monsanto SP, Khalaj K, Koti M, Tayade C (2017) Implications of immune dysfunction on endometriosis associated infertility. *Oncotarget* 8:7138–7147.

Karshikoff B, Martucci KT, Mackey S (2021) Relationship Between Blood Cytokine Levels, Psychological Comorbidity, and Widespreadness of Pain in Chronic Pelvic Pain. *Front Psychiatry* 12:651083.

Kochiashvili G, Kochiashvili D (2014) Urinary IL-33 and galectin-3 increase in patients with interstitial cystitis/bladder pain syndrome (review). *Georgian Med. News* (232-233):12-5.

Lamale LM, Lutgendorf SK, Zimmerman MB, Kreder KJ (2006) Interleukin-6, histamine and methylhistamine as diagnostic markers for interstitial cystitis. *Urology* 68:702–706.

Lamvu G, Williams R, Zolnoun D, Wechter ME, Shortliffe A, Fulton G, Steege JF (2006) Long-term outcomes after surgical and nonsurgical management of chronic pelvic pain: one year after evaluation in a pelvic pain specialty clinic. *Am. J. Obstet. Gynecol.* 195(2):591-600.

Lewicky-Gaupp C, Kenton K (2017) Urinary Microbiome and Cytokine Levels in Women with Interstitial Cystitis. *Obstetrics & Gynecology* 129(3):500-506.

Malhotra N, Karmakar D, Tripathi V, Luthra K, Kumar S (2012) Correlation of angiogenic cytokines-leptin and IL-8 in stage, type and presentation of endometriosis. *Gynecological Endocrinology* 28:224–227

Manero MG, Alcazar JL (2010) Interleukin-8 serum levels do not correlate with pelvic pain in patients with ovarian endometriomas. *Fertility and Sterility* 94:450–452.

Michaud N, Al-Akoum M, Gagnon G, Girard K, Blanchet P, Rousseau JA, Akoum A (2011) Decreased concentrations of soluble interleukin-1 receptor accessory protein levels in the peritoneal fluid of women with endometriosis. *Journal of Reproductive Immunology* 92:68–73.

Micheletti L, Radici G, Lynch PJ (2014) Provoked vestibulodynia: inflammatory, neuropathic or dysfunctional pain? A neurobiological perspective. *J. Obstet. Gynaecol. 34(4):285-288.*

Moyal-Barracco M, Lynch PJ (2003) ISSVD terminology and classification of vulvodynia: a historical perspective. *J. Reprod. Med.* 49(10):772-777.

Nasr-Esfahani M, Jarrell J (2013) Cotton-tipped applicator test: validity and reliability in chronic pelvic pain. *Am. J. Obstet. Gynecol.* 208(1):52.e1-5.

Neurath MF (2014) Cytokines in inflammatory bowel disease. *Nature Reviews Immunology* 14(5):329–342.

Oku H, Tsuji Y, Kashiwamura SI, Adachi S, Kubota A, Okamura H & Koyama K (2004) Role of IL-18 in pathogenesis of endometriosis. *Human Reproduction* 19:709–714.

O'Mahony L, McCarthy J, Kelly P, Hurley G, Luo F, Chen K, O'Sullivan GC, Kiely B, Collins JK, Shanahan F, Quigley EM (2005) Lactobacillus and bifidobacterium in irritable bowel syndrome: symptom responses and relationship to cytokine profiles. *Gastroenterology* 128(3):541-51.

Ortiz D D (2008) Chronic pelvic pain in women. *Am. Fam. Physician.* 77(11):1535-42.

Prato V, Taberner F J, Hockley J R F, Callejo G, Arcourt A, Tazir B, Hammer L, Schad P, Heppenstall P A, Smith ES, Lechner SG (2017) Functional and Molecular Characterization of Mechanoinsensitive "Silent" Nociceptors. *Cell Rep.* 21(11):3102-3115.

Rana SV, Sharma S, Sinha SK, Parsad KK, Malik A, Singh K (2012) Pro-inflammatory and anti-inflammatory cytokine response in diarrhoea-predominant irritable bowel syndrome patients. *Trop. Gastroenterol.* 33:251–256.

Rapkin A, Morgan M, Bonpane C, Martinez-Maza O (2000) Peritoneal fluid interleukin-6 in women with chronic pelvic pain. *Fertility and Sterility* 74:325–328.

Santulli P, Borghese B, Chouzenoux S, Vaiman D, Borderie D, Streuli I, Goffinet F, de Ziegler D, Weill B, Batteux F et al. (2012) Serum and peritoneal interleukin-33 levels are elevated in deeply infiltrating endometriosis. *Human Reproduction* 27:2001–2009.

Scully P, McKernan DP, Keohane J, et al. (2010) Plasma cytokine profiles in females with irritable bowel syndrome and extra-intestinal co-morbidity. *Am. J. Gastroenterol.* 105:2235–2243.

Seyedmirzaee S, Hayatbakhsh MM, Ahmadi B, et al. (2016) Serum immune biomarkers in irritable bowel syndrome. *Clin. Res. Hepatol. Gastroenterol.* 40(5):631-637.

Tyagi P, Killinger K, Tyagi V, Nirmal J, Chancellor M, Peters KM (2012) Urinary chemokines as noninvasive predictors of ulcerative interstitial cystitis. *J. Urol.* 187:2243–8.

Velasco I, Acién P, Campos A, Acién M I, Ruiz-Maciá E (2010) Interleukin-6 and other soluble factors in peritoneal fluid and endometriomas and their relation to pain and aromatase expression. *Journal of Reproductive Immunology* 84:199–205.

Zhang Z, Zolnoun D A, Francisco EM, Holden JK, Dennis RG, Tommerdahl M (2011) Altered central sensitization in subgroups of women with vulvodynia. *Clin. J. Pain.* 27(9):755-763.

Chapter 31

Dysmenorrhea and Cytokines

Selim Gülücü[1,*], MD and Sebahattin Çelik[2], MD

[1]Gaziosmanpasa University, Department of Obstetrics and Gynecology, Tokat, Turkey
[2]Balikesir Ozel Sevgi Hospital, Department of Obstetrics and Gynecology, Balikesir, Turkey

Abstract

Dysmenorrhea may negatively affect the daily activity, physical performance, and quality of life in women of reproductive age, causing loss of workdays among women who are working and attending school. The cause of primary dysmenorrhea has not been fully understood. In the literature, different results have been shown among publications investigating the relationship between dysmenorrhea and cytokines. In this article, we will try to explain the relationship between dysmenorrhea and cytokines.

Keywords: dysmenorrhea, menstrual cycle, cytokine, IL-6, prostaglandin

Introduction

Dysmenorrhea represents a frequently observed gynecological problem in reproductive-age females and is characterized by severe cramping pain in the lower abdomen in the course of menstruation. The pain may radiate to the thighs or lower spine. Symptoms such as headache, back pain, vomiting, and diarrhea may accompany lower abdominal pain. Menstrual pain begins at the time of menstruation or a few hours before (Dawood 2006). It reduces women's daily activity, performance and quality of life and has socio-economic effects. Dysmenorrhea is examined under two headings as primary and secondary dysmenorrhea. Primary dysmenorrhea defines painful menstruation, although there is no underlying pelvic pathology. Clinical examination findings are characterized by pain from pathological uterine contraction (Coco 1999). Acquired lesions (leiomyoma, adenomyosis, endometriosis, chronic pelvic inflammation), involving the reproductive organs' functional and anatomical abnormalities (Coco 1999; Lacovides et al. 2015), lead to secondary dysmenorrhea. The pathomechanism of dysmenorrhea is not completely comprehended, and the immunological features underlying

* Corresponding Author's Email: selim.gulucu@gop.edu.tr.

In: Cytokines and Diseases
Editors: Kenan Demir, Selim Görgün and Bahar Uslu
ISBN: 979-8-88697-214-6

this condition are remarkable. Prostaglandins play an essential part in the pathomechanism of dysmenorrhea (Barcikowska 2020). The generation of pain during menstruation by prostaglandins is frequently studied.

The menstrual cycle is a feedback system in the hypothalamic-pituitary-gonadal axis. This system includes the regular and sequential release of luteinizing hormone (LH) and follicle-stimulating hormone (FSH) from the pituitary gland. This release occurs as a reaction to gonadotropin-releasing hormone from the hypothalamus. The follicle growth in the ovary, oocyte maturation, and the secretion of progesterone and estrogen are the results of this cycle (Ryan 2017; Messinis et al. 2014). The follicular phase constitutes the first half of the menstrual cycle. In the follicular phase, an increase in estrogen concentration and then menstruation occur. The progesterone peak occurs in the luteal phase, which represents the second half of the menstrual cycle. If fertilization does not occur, the progesterone level decreases sharply three days before menstruation in the luteal phase (Draper et al. 2018). If there is no fertilization, the corpus luteum, which is responsible for progesterone production, is destroyed, and the progesterone level decreases. Lytic enzymes and acid phosphatase found in lysosomes are released into the cytoplasm with the decreasing progesterone level. The release of prostaglandins is caused by these enzyme digesting cells. Moreover, the lowering progesterone level causes the inflammatory response that induces menstrual bleeding and the flaking of the endometrium (Dawood 2006). Cyclic changes in ovarian hormone concentrations are the primary cause of the menstrual cycle. Hence, uterine contractile activity and changes in the prostaglandin level are the consequences of cyclic changes (Bulletti 2000). Prostaglandins cause not only the constriction of blood vessels feeding the uterus but also the abnormal contraction of the uterus. Ischemia, an increase in the sensitivity of nerve endings, and uterine hypoxia are the other effects of prostaglandins (Coco 1999; Ryan 2017).

Pickles et al. showed the elevated premenstrual prostaglandin concentration among the factors involved in dysmenorrhea (Pickles et al. 1965). The overproduction of prostaglandins in dysmenorrhea has also been demonstrated in other studies (Lundström and Green 1978). Another study suggested that menstruation could be considered as an inflammatory condition since the invasion of leukocytes and the consequent generation of inflammatory mediators were detected during menstruation (Finn, 1986). Before menstruation, the endometrial tissue becomes red and edematous and acquires inflammatory properties. The local increase in the generation of chemokines, involving proinflammatory cytokines (IL-1, IL-6, TNF), interleukin 8 (IL-8), and leukocyte efflux cause endometrial edema (Maybin and Critchley 2011).

There was a significant increase in the expression levels of proinflammatory cytokine genes (IL-1B, IL-6, TNF, and IL-8) on the first menstruation day. However, anti-inflammatory cytokines (IL-5 and IL-11) were significantly decreased in comparison with unaffected controls (Ma et al. 2013). A lot of research has reported that proinflammatory cytokines are capable of stimulating the synthesis or release of PGF2α and oxytocin, causing uterine hypercontractility, reducing the endometrial blood flow, and leading to pain. The administration of IL-1b and TNF-α to cultured endometrial stromal cells increased PGF2α production, which was related to the increased COX-2 protein expression (Skarzynski et al., 2000; Huang et al. 1998). Moreover, proinflammatory cytokines increase oxytocin/Ca+2 signaling. This signaling plays an essential part in myometrial contractions (Friebe-Hoffmann et al. 2001) and IL-6-regulated uterine oxytocin receptor mRNA expression and binding capacity in human smooth muscle cells via tyrosine and serine phosphorylation pathways (Rauk et al. 2001). TNF-α increased oxytocin-stimulated Ca+2 shifts in human myometrial cells, which were effectively abolished by progesterone (Thompson et al. 2004). This clearly shows that the differential expression of cytokine genes in peripheral blood mononuclear cells (PBMCs) among women with and without dysmenorrhea takes place not only during the menstrual phase; it also occurs throughout the entire menstrual cycle (Harel 2006). In the cyclic changes of the endometrium, inflammatory responses differ and are hormonally regulated. Proinflammatory cytokines (TNF-α and IL-1b) are incorporated in endometrial decidualization during the secretory phase. Via the cAMP pathway, PGE2, which was induced by proinflammatory cytokines, significantly increased decidualization (Skarzynski et al. 2000; Arcuri et al. 2009; Strakova et al. 2002). Proinflammatory cytokines did not induce an abnormal increase in the inflammatory response in the endometrium because progesterone was present.

Progesterone efficiently prevented TNFα-induced PGF2a and oxytocin release and considerably suppressed metalloproteinase expression and activation via NF-kB in the endometrial tissue (Jabbour et al. 2006). The decreasing progesterone level terminates the deactivation of the inflammatory response in the perimenstrual phase. In this phase, a cascade of inflammatory mediators (PGF2α, TNF-α, MMPs, etc.) is activated, causing cytokines to break down the endometrial extracellular matrix and leading to subsequent menstrual bleeding. The resolution of inflammation occurs following menstruation. Then a weak inflammatory response makes a partial contribution to endometrial repair through PGE2 (Henriet et al. 2012; Maybin et al. 2011). The local mechanisms of inflammation recovery in the proliferative phase have not been defined yet. One research study demonstrated that more PGF2α was induced by TNF-α from decidual cells than from normal epithelial cells following pretreating with E2/P4 (Szo'stek et al. 2011). This suggests that decidual tissue can represent the primary resource of inflammatory mediators. In the case of expelling the decidualized endometrium from the uterus, there is a possibility of the natural evolvement of the strong inflammatory response into a weaker one. Moreover, members of the growth factor TGF-β family take part in decidualization. Decidualization can be facilitated by up-regulated proinflammatory and down-regulated TGF-β family member genes (Ma et al. 2013). Since decidual cells have been reported to secrete more PGF2a following pretreating with E2/P4 compared to normal epithelial cells without E2/P4 pretreating, there is a possibility that excessive decidual transformation in the secretory phase causes pain in the menstrual phase via the increased production of inflammatory mediators.

Progesterone has an anti-inflammatory impact and prevents the release and activation of metalloproteinases in the secretory phase. It also influences the regulation and synthesis of leukocytes and prostaglandins (Maybin and Critchley 2011). The secretion of leukotrienes and prostaglandins leads to uterine contractions. Discomforts, e.g., headache, nausea, vomiting, and bloating, are the other consequences of this secretion. The metabolization of arachidonic acid occurs in two ways, the cyclooxygenase and 5-lipoxygenase pathways. The cyclooxygenase pathway generates prostaglandins (PGF2α and PGE2), thromboxane, and prostacyclins. Leukotrienes are composed in the 5-lipoxygenase pathway. Arachidonic acid metabolites, including cyclooxygenase and PGF2α prostaglandin, lead to vasoconstriction. The contraction of uterine smooth muscles causes ischemia, reducing the pain threshold and leading to pain (Harel 2006). Via the action of cyclooxygenase COX-2 and lipoxygenase, arachidonic acid represents a precursor in the generation of prostacyclins, prostaglandins, leukotrienes, and thromboxane (Evans and Salamonsen 2012). The constriction of arcuate vessels is mediated by PGF2α, causing the local hypoxia of endometrial tissues. The stimulation of smooth muscle contraction, promoting menstrual bleeding, is another function of PGF2α. The receptor type determines the action of PGE2, which can relax endometrial blood vessels and act to recruit leukotrienes by increasing edema. However, prostaglandins have important roles in creating other growth factors and chemokines that take part in the inflammatory response or postmenstrual repair. Additionally, prostaglandins can enhance the neutrophil and leukocyte migration to the endometrium (Evans and Salamonsen 2012).

A study compared the prostaglandin levels of females with dysmenorrhea to those of healthy controls. Its metabolites and PGF2α were evaluated in the endometrium and plasma. Endometrial samples were taken before and on the first menstruation day, whereas plasma samples were collected on the first menstruation day. It was detected that the concentration of the PGF2α prostaglandin metabolites in the plasma differed significantly between the dysmenorrhea and control groups. Furthermore, women with dysmenorrhea had a significantly higher prostaglandin concentration in the endometrium. However, there was no similar difference when evaluating the prostaglandin concentration in the endometrium before menstruation. The researchers defined the correlation of uterine contractions with prostaglandin levels. It has been indicated that females with high prostaglandin levels in both the plasma and endometrium experience severe uterine contractions (Lundström and Green 1978). Similar results were obtained in a study comparing vasopressin levels and prostaglandin metabolites in women with and without premenstrual pain or dysmenorrhea (Strömberg et al. 1984). However, another study investigating the level of PGF2α prostaglandin metabolites found no considerable difference between females with dysmenorrhea and females with painless menstruation (Liedman et al. 2008). It has been shown that females with higher prostaglandin levels in both the endometrium and plasma experience severe uterine contractions (Lundström and Green 1978). PGF2α and PGE2 generated by the myometrium take part in synthesizing numerous proteins, including cytokines (Xu et al. 2015). Cytokines take part in regulating the reproductive process, menstrual cycle, and pregnancy and mediate the body's immune response (Strömberg et al., 1984; Xu et al. 2015). In the process of implanting the embryo, which ensures normal pregnancy, the role of cytokines was emphasized. When there is no pregnancy, cytokines take part in the cyclic transformation of uterine tissues (Critchley et al. 1999).

Activated macrophages procreate proinflammatory cytokines such as IL-1, IL-6, TNFα, etc., which are involved in regulating inflammatory responses (Ma et al. 2013; Kannan et al. 2019). It has been shown that the said mediators initiate the synthesis or release of prostaglandin (Kannan et al. 2019; Leimert et al. 2019) and cause the sore contraction of the uterine, leading to the ischemic pain of primary dysmenorrhea. The plasma levels of proinflammatory cytokines, such as IL6 and TNFα, were lower in females without menstrual disorders than in females with dysmenorrhea (Ma et al. 2013). In addition, TNFα represents a cytokine inducing apoptosis accountable for the inhibition of endometrial proliferation. Previous research has shown that endometrial cells procreate higher TNFα concentrations in the course of menstruation (Ciebiera et al. 2018). IL-6 represents a pleiotropic cytokine having multiple impacts on innate and adaptive immune system cells. The primary duty of IL-6 is the initiation and regulation of the acute inflammatory response. Furthermore, it facilitates the developing and targeting of the acquired response. IL-6 has proinflammatory and anti-inflammatory characteristics and is currently regarded as a significant target for clinical interventions (Hunter and Jones 2015). A study involving females without menstrual disorders revealed significant variability in plasma cytokine levels (Whitcomb et al. 2014). The level of a number of factors was elevated in the course of ovulation and then peaked in the course of menstruation, which is regarded as a proinflammatory event (King and Critchley 2010). IL-6, IL-8, and IL-1β levels were adversely related to progesterone and estradiol levels, further supporting the immune response relationship of the menstrual cycle (Bertone-Johnson et al. 2014). However, in another study, they showed the increased IL-6 concentration in the follicular phase in the case of an increase in the estradiol level. In the luteal phase, the progesterone level increased by 10 times, while the plasma IL6 level decreased by 1.5-4.4 times. The IL-6 level rose again in the next cycle (Angstwurm et al. 1977). A lot of research has detected a high level of IL-6 concentration in females having dysmenorrhea (Yeh et al. 2004; Konecna et al. 2000). They showed that the IL-6 level was statistically significantly higher in the luteal phase than in the follicular phase (Konecna et al. 2000).

Non-steroidal anti-inflammatory drugs (NSAIDs) represent the first-line therapy in dysmenorrhea. Cyclooxygenase (COX), which is the enzyme involved in the synthesis of prostaglandins, is inhibited by NSAIDs. Reducing the production of prostaglandins has been demonstrated to decrease the strength of uterine contractions, thereby reducing women's discomfort. NSAID therapy has been shown to be the most effective if started several days prior to the beginning of menstruation (Harel 2012). Women whose dysmenorrhea cannot be reduced by NSAIDs can receive hormone therapy during a minimum of three menstrual cycles (Harel 2012). Thereby, another possibility for treating menstrual pain may be found in hormonal contraceptives and, in particular, combined oral contraceptives (Yu 2014). Combined hormonal contraceptives, involving oral contraceptives, contraceptive rings and patches, limit the endometrium growth.

Conclusion

More studies are needed on cytokines and dysmenorrhea. Contemporary results are insufficient regarding how cytokines are involved in the pathophysiology of dysmenorrhea, although current evidence points to increased cytokine concentrations in dysmenorrhea patients. Especially PGF2α, IL-6, IL-8, and IL-10 are the substances that work most frequently in this area. As the findings of studies on cytokines are presented, the pathophysiology of this disease may be identified more clearly.

References

Angstwurm MW, Gärtner R, Ziegler-Heitbrock HW (1997) Cyclic plasma IL-6 levels during normal menstrual cycle. *Cytokine* 9(5):370-374.

Arcuri F, Toti P, Buchwalder L, Casciaro A, Cintorino M, Schatz F, Rybalov B, Lockwood CJ (2009) Mechanisms of leukocyte accumulation and activation in chorioamnionitis: interleukin 1 beta and tumor necrosis factor alpha enhance colony stimulating factor 2 expression in term decidua. *Reproductive Sciences* (Thousand Oaks, Calif) 16(5):453-461.

Barcikowska Z, Rajkowska-Labon E, Grzybowska ME, Hansdorfer-Korzon R, Zorena K (2020) Inflammatory Markers in Dysmenorrhea and Therapeutic Options. *International Journal of Environmental Research and Public Health* 17(4):1191.

Bertone-Johnson ER, Ronnenberg AG, Houghton SC, Nobles C, Zagarins SE, Takashima-Uebelhoer BB, Faraj JL, Whitcomb BW (2014) Association of inflammation markers with menstrual symptom severity and premenstrual syndrome in young women. *Human Reproduction* (Oxford, England) 29(9):1987-1994.

Bulletti C, de Ziegler D, Polli V, Diotallevi L, Del Ferro E, Flamigni C (2000) Uterine contractility during the menstrual cycle. *Human Reproduction* (Oxford, England) 15(Suppl 1):81-89.

Ciebiera M, Włodarczyk M, Zgliczyńska M, Łukaszuk K, Męczekalski B, Kobierzycki C, Łoziński T, Jakiel G (2018) The Role of Tumor Necrosis Factor α in the Biology of Uterine Fibroids and the Related Symptoms. *International Journal of Molecular Sciences* 19(12):3869.

Coco AS (1999) Primary dysmenorrhea. *American Family Physician* 60(2):489-496.

Critchley HO, Jones RL, Lea RG, Drudy TA, Kelly RW, Williams AR, Baird DT (1999) Role of inflammatory mediators in human endometrium during progesterone withdrawal and early pregnancy. *The Journal of Clinical Endocrinology and Metabolism* 84(1):240-248.

Dawood MY (2006) Primary dysmenorrhea: advances in pathogenesis and management. *Obstetrics and Gynecology* 108(2):428-441.

Draper CF, Duisters K, Weger B, Chakrabarti A, Harms AC, Brennan L, Hankemeier T, Goulet L, Konz T, Martin FP, Moco S, van der Greef J (2018) Menstrual cycle rhythmicity: metabolic patterns in healthy women. *Scientific Reports* 8(1):14568.

Evans J, Salamonsen LA (2012) Inflammation, leukocytes and menstruation. *Reviews in Endocrine & Metabolic Disorders* 13(4):277-288.

Finn CA (1986) Implantation, menstruation and inflammation. *Biological Reviews of the Cambridge Philosophical Society* 61(4):313-328.

Friebe-Hoffmann U, Chiao JP, Rauk PN (2001) Effect of IL-1beta and IL-6 on oxytocin secretion in human uterine smooth muscle cells. *American Journal of Reproductive Immunology* (New York: 1989) 46(3):226-231.

Harel Z (2006) Dysmenorrhea in adolescents and young adults: etiology and management. *Journal of Pediatric and Adolescent Gynecology* 19(6):363-371.

Harel Z (2012) Dysmenorrhea in adolescents and young adults: an update on pharmacological treatments and management strategies. *Expert Opinion on Pharmacotherapy* 13(15):2157-2170.

Henriet P, Gaide Chevronnay HP, Marbaix E (2012) The endocrine and paracrine control of menstruation. *Molecular and Cellular Endocrinology* 358(2):197-207.

Huang JC, Liu DY, Yadollahi S, Wu KK, Dawood MY (1998) Interleukin-1 beta induces cyclooxygenase-2 gene expression in cultured endometrial stromal cells. *The Journal of Clinical Endocrinology and Metabolism* 83(2):538-541.

Hunter CA, Jones SA (2015) IL-6 as a keystone cytokine in health and disease. *Nature Immunology* 16(5):448-457.

Lacovides S, Avidon I, Baker FC (2015) What we know about primary dysmenorrhea today: a critical review. *Human Reproduction Update* 21(6):762-778.

Jabbour HN, Kelly RW, Fraser HM, Critchley HO (2006). Endocrine regulation of menstruation. *Endocrine Reviews* 27(1):17-46.

Kannan P, Cheung KK, Lau BW (2019) Does aerobic exercise induced-analgesia occur through hormone and inflammatory cytokine-mediated mechanisms in primary dysmenorrhea? *Medical Hypotheses* 123:50-54.

King AE, Critchley HO (2010) Oestrogen and progesterone regulation of inflammatory processes in the human endometrium. *The Journal of Steroid Biochemistry and Molecular Biology* 120(2-3):116-126.

Konecna L, Yan MS, Miller LE, Schölmerich J, Falk W, Straub RH (2000) Modulation of IL-6 production during the menstrual cycle *in vivo* and *in vitro*. *Brain, Behavior, and Immunity* 14(1):49-61.

Leimert KB, Verstraeten B, Messer A, Nemati R, Blackadar K, Fang X, Robertson SA, Chemtob S, Olson DM (2019) Cooperative effects of sequential PGF2α and IL-1β on IL-6 and COX-2 expression in human myometrial cells. *Biology of Reproduction* 100(5):1370-1385.

Liedman R, Hansson SR, Howe D, Igidbashian S, McLeod A, Russell RJ, Akerlund M (2008) Reproductive hormones in plasma over the menstrual cycle in primary dysmenorrhea compared with healthy subjects. *Gynecological Endocrinology: the Official Journal of the International Society of Gynecological Endocrinology* 24(9):508-513.

Lundström V, Gréen K (1978) Endogenous levels of prostaglandin F2alpha and its main metabolites in plasma and endometrium of normal and dysmenorrheic women. *American Journal of Obstetrics and Gynecology* 130(6):640-646.

Ma H, Hong M, Duan J, Liu P, Fan X, Shang E, Su S, Guo J, Qian D, Tang Y (2013) Altered cytokine gene expression in peripheral blood monocytes across the menstrual cycle in primary dysmenorrhea: a case-control study. *Plos One* 8(2):55200.

Maybin JA, Critchley HO (2011) Progesterone: a pivotal hormone at menstruation. *Annals of the New York Academy of Sciences* 1221:88-97.

Maybin JA, Critchley HO, Jabbour HN (2011) Inflammatory pathways in endometrial disorders. *Molecular and Cellular Endocrinology* 335(1):42-51.

Messinis IE, Messini CI, Dafopoulos K (2014) Novel aspects of the endocrinology of the menstrual cycle. *Reproductive Biomedicine Online* 28(6):714-722.

Pickles VR, Hall WJ, Best FA, Smith GN (1965) Prostaglandins in Endometrium and Menstrual Fluid from Normal and Dysmenorrhoeic Subjects. *The Journal of Obstetrics and Gynaecology of the British Commonwealth* 72:185-192.

Rauk PN, Friebe-Hoffmann U, Winebrenner LD, Chiao JP (2001) Interleukin-6 up-regulates the oxytocin receptor in cultured uterine smooth muscle cells. *American Journal of Reproductive Immunology* (New York: 1989) 45(3):148-153.

Ryan SA (2017) The Treatment of Dysmenorrhea. *Pediatric clinics of North America* 64(2):331-342.

Skarzynski DJ, Miyamoto Y, Okuda K (2000) Production of prostaglandin f(2alpha) by cultured bovine endometrial cells in response to tumor necrosis factor alpha: cell type specificity and intracellular mechanisms. *Biology of Reproduction* 62(5):1116-1120.

Strakova Z, Srisuparp S, Fazleabas AT (2002) IL-1beta during in vitro decidualization in primate. *Journal of Reproductive Immunology* 55(1-2):35-47.

Strömberg P, Akerlund M, Forsling ML, Granström E, Kindahl H (1984) Vasopressin and prostaglandins in premenstrual pain and primary dysmenorrhea. *Acta obstetricia et gynecologica Scandinavica* 63(6):533-538.

Szóstek AZ, Siemieniuch MJ, Deptula K, Woclawek-Potocka I, Majewska M, Okuda K, Skarzynski DJ (2011) Ovarian steroids modulate tumor necrosis factor-α and nitric oxide-regulated prostaglandin secretion by cultured bovine oviductal epithelial cells. *Domestic Animal Endocrinology* 41(1):14-23.

Thompson M, Barata da Silva H, Zielinska W, White TA, Bailey JP, Lund FE, Sieck GC, Chini EN (2004) Role of CD38 in myometrial Ca2+ transients: modulation by progesterone. *American Journal of Physiology. Endocrinology and Metabolism* 287(6):1142-1148.

Whitcomb BW, Mumford SL, Perkins NJ, Wactawski-Wende J, Bertone-Johnson ER, Lynch KE, Schisterman EF (2014) Urinary cytokine and chemokine profiles across the menstrual cycle in healthy reproductive-aged women. *Fertility and Sterility* 101(5):1383-1391.

Xu C, Liu W, You X, Leimert K, Popowycz K, Fang X, Wood SL, Slater DM, Sun Q, Gu H, Olson DM, Ni X (2015) PGF2α modulates the output of chemokines and pro-inflammatory cytokines in myometrial cells from term pregnant women through divergent signaling pathways. *Molecular Human Reproduction* 21(7):603-614.

Yeh ML, Chen HH, So EC, Liu CF (2004). A study of serum malondialdehyde and interleukin-6 levels in young women with dysmenorrhea in Taiwan. *Life Sciences* 75(6):669-673.

Yu A (2014) Complementary and alternative treatments for primary dysmenorrhea in adolescents. *The Nurse Practitioner* 39(11):1-12.

Chapter 32

Cytokines and Polycystic Ovary Syndrome

Yaşam Kemal Akpak[1,*], MD, Alper Şişmanoğlu[2], MD and Serkan Oral[3], MD

[1]University of Health Sciences, Tepecik Training and Research Hospital, Department of Obstetrics and Gynecology, Izmir, Turkey
[2]Altınbas University, Department of Obstetrics and Gynecology, Istanbul, Turkey
[3]Halic University, Department of Obstetrics and Gynecology, Istanbul, Turkey

Abstract

Polycystic ovary syndrome (PCOS) is the most common endocrine disorder in the reproductive age. Unfortunately, since the etiopathogenesis and the molecular pathways involved cannot be clarified, a consensus has not yet been established in the diagnosis and treatment. The clinical picture followed by menstrual irregularity, anovulation, infertility, and hair growth leaves its place to cardiovascular diseases and diabetes mellitus due to the increased metabolic deterioration in the future. It is important for PCOS to first understand cytokines, the main component of chronic inflammation, which is thought to occur in obesity and hyperandrogenism, and then evaluate them in treatment.

Keywords: insulin resistance, inflammation, hyperandrogenism, cytokines, obesity, polycystic ovary syndrome

Introduction

Cytokines are substances in a peptide or glycoprotein structure with a weight of 20-30 kD synthesized by cells such as stimulated lymphocytes, monocytes, and macrophages to increase the activities of cells participating in the immune or inflammatory response. Although cytokines are similar to hormones, they are not exactly hormones. Although the cells in which they were secreted were not identified initially, they were called lymphokines and monokines, but it was observed that they were secreted by many other cells, and the name cytokine began to be used more often. Their molecular weights are quite low, and they are effective in soluble form. They

* Corresponding Author's Email: drykakpak@gmail.com.

In: Cytokines and Diseases
Editors: Kenan Demir, Selim Görgün and Bahar Uslu
ISBN: 979-8-88697-214-6

regulate immune and inflammatory events, including inflammation, cell growth, healing, and the systemic response to injury. It has been determined that they are involved in many malignancies due to these effects. They are non-storage proteins secreted from stimulated cells in a very short time. They generally move over short distances, in short time intervals, and at very low intensity. Cytokines show their effects by binding to specific receptors on the target cell, as in polypeptide hormones. They act by binding to specific membrane receptors that signal cells with secondary messengers, mostly tyrosine kinases, to change their behavior. Responses to cytokines involve the release of effector molecules through the increase or decrease of membrane proteins. They can show agonist and antagonist effects as autocrine, paracrine, and endocrine (Carvalho et al., 2018).

Let us look at their functions in the body. They ensure the proliferation and differentiation of some other cells, especially in the lymphoid system, activate cells involved in inflammation and attract them to the area of inflammation, thus ensuring wound healing, take a role in embryogenesis and especially provide the development of the nervous system, and participate in hematopoietic regulation by acting on the bone marrow. They may cause fever, muscle pain, and soreness after the acute-phase response. However, they can cause shock and death in high concentrations and show antiviral activity (Escobar-Morreale et al., 2011).

Polycystic ovary syndrome (PCOS) is an important social health problem with reproductive, metabolic, and psychological effects. Polycystic ovaries and polycystic ovary syndrome are entirely different concepts. The polycystic ovary condition is the presence of multiple small cysts with a 2-8 mm diameter on ultrasonographic ovarian examination. On the other hand, polycystic ovary syndrome expresses a heterogeneous disorder accompanied by metabolic deterioration in which androgens increase and ovulation is impaired. Although it shows ethnic differences, it is a complex of diseases observed in 5-10% of those of reproductive age (Sirmans and Pate 2013).

Today, it is important to develop effective diagnosis and treatment methods for PCOS to prevent conditions that may shorten patients' lives, such as diabetes, cancer, and cardiovascular diseases. Although the etiology of PCOS is not clear, there are links to familial inheritance based on genetics. Insulin resistance is more common in families with PCOS, and men are also affected by this condition. Studies have shown that low β-cell functioning in families of women with PCOS is genetically inherited (Diamanti-Kandarakis and Dunaif 2012). The genes associated with PCOS development are the CYP17A gene encoding the cytochrome P450c-17α enzyme, the CYP11A gene encoding the P450 side chain-breaking enzyme, and the insulin gene. Polymorphisms in the TNF-R (tumor necrosis factor receptor) and PPAR (peroxisome proliferator-activated receptor-gamma) genes are associated with PCOS (Legro 2002). In addition to these, it was determined that the expression of the aldehyde dehydrogenase 6, retinol dehydrogenase 2, and transcription factor GATA6 (GATA binding protein 6) genes increased significantly when PCOS theca cells were compared with normal theca cells (Wild et al., 2000). Although the clinical picture has a mechanism mediated by cytokines, the expression of genes belonging to many molecular signaling pathways in women with PCOS changes and causes functional disorders in the ovaries (Amato and Simpson 2004).

When we look at the diagnosis history of the disease, we can see that the confusion created by the mechanisms mentioned above is also reflected in the diagnostic criteria. Stein and Leventhal first reported the association of menstrual irregularity, hirsutism, and ovaries containing many small follicles in their article, which they prepared by collecting the diagnostic criteria of the syndrome in 1935 and suggested that wedge resection may have a place in the treatment of these cases (Stein and Leventhal 1935). In the following years, after many publications on these diagnostic criteria and this clinical picture, in 1990, it was stated in the "National Institute of Health/National Institute of Child Health and Human Development" criteria that the association of clinical and/or biochemical hyperandrogenism with menstrual dysfunction is necessary. However, the main factor in these diagnostic criteria is the fact that there is an exclusion criterion, and the emphasis is on the need to evaluate the existing diagnostic criteria after excluding certain diseases. The most important addition compared to the past is that the polycystic appearance in the ovaries observed on ultrasound has no diagnostic value (Huang et al., 2010). In the light of these criteria, PCOS has been defined as a syndrome characterized by increased androgen levels and as having an ovarian etiology.

The developed ultrasonographic technology was also included in the diagnostic criteria at the Rotterdam "European Society of Human Reproduction and Embryology" (ESHRE) and "American Society of Reproductive Medicine" (ASRM) meeting in 2003. The new system introduced is called the Rotterdam criteria. The Rotterdam criteria conclude that PCOS can be diagnosed in the presence of at least two of the three clinical features: Oligo/anovulation; clinical and/or biochemical hyperandrogenism; and polycystic ovary morphology. In addition to these criteria, it is also necessary to exclude all other known diseases that may cause hyperandrogenemia. At this conference, it was thought that PCOS has a broader spectrum than that determined by the NIH criteria. Considering that polycystic ovary is an indicator of ovarian dysfunction, it has been stated that if a woman with regular menstrual bleeding has polycystic ovary and signs of hyperandrogenism, a diagnosis of PCOS should be made, and its treatment should be shaped according to this diagnosis (PCOS Consensus Workshop Group 2004).

In 2006, "Androgen Excess and PCOS Society" (AEPCOS) criteria were proposed, stating that only hyperandrogenemia cases can be diagnosed with PCOS (Azziz et al., 2009). These criteria have emerged in the light of suspicion that the prevalence may be calculated as higher than it should be due to the relatively expanded diagnostic criteria and in the light of new studies. Accordingly, the diagnosis of PCOS is made according to the presence of two clinical features: Hyperandrogenism (hirsutism and/or hyperandrogenemia) and ovarian dysfunction (oligo/anovulation and/or a demonstration of PCOM). Again, all other possible factors must be excluded together with these criteria. The most important difference brought by the AE-PCOS criteria compared to the Rotterdam criteria is the emphasis on hyperandrogenism.

On the contrary, it has been suggested that patients who do not show signs of hyperandrogenism in the presence of oligo/anovulation and polycystic ovary should be considered as a different syndrome. In the last report on "AE-PCOS Criteria" published in 2009, it was stated that the diagnostic criteria of PCOS could go through many evolutionary stages. It has been underlined that it is possible to act according to the aims of the researches or personal preferences regarding which criteria will be used. With the knowledge that a more objective and detailed definition of PCOS, which many associations and organizations try to define from their perspectives, is a clear requirement, the "2018 International Evidence-Based PCOS Evaluation and Management Guideline" (2018 PCOS Guideline), with the partnership of the "European Society of Human Reproduction and Embryology" (ESHRE) and "American Society of Reproductive Medicine" (ASRM), has been published very recently (Teede et al., 2018). Since PCOS is a multisystemic disease and heterogeneous, the need for consensus on a specific diagnostic criterion has been seen as inevitable.

Many diagnostic criteria and an unclear algorithm state exist because the syndrome's pathophysiology has not yet been clarified. At the same time, this makes the treatment very difficult or incomplete. The role of cytokines in PCOS formation will provide more opportunities to manage this disease in both diagnosis and treatment.

PCOS and Cytokine Relationship

Specific cytokines are increased in women with PCOS. However, no consensus exists on which cytokines are increased. Also, it has not been revealed whether the relationship between PCOS and cytokines arises from the disease itself or from obesity and insulin resistance that develop due to the syndrome (Samy et al., 2009).

PCOS can be a metabolic disorder characterized by visceral obesity, glucose intolerance, insulin resistance, and dyslipidemia. A low-grade chronic inflammatory condition may be linked with the metabolic effects and cardiovascular complications in PCOS (Xiong et al., 2011; Ebejer and Calleja-Agius 2013).

It has been suggested that androgens facilitate the development of visceral type obesity by stimulating the differentiation of pre-adipocytes into adipocytes. The incidence of this situation can be as high as 90%. Adipocyte hypertrophy is important since it causes adipose tissue hypoperfusion after hypertrophy in the stromal vessels. The increased angiotensin level creates hypertension in the patient and worsens the circulation of adipose tissue after peripheral vasoconstriction (Deligeoroglou et al., 2012).

Deepening adipose tissue hypoxia stimulates an immune response, which is very important in inducing the production and release of cytokines involved in the inflammatory process. Some of the cytokines that are part of this process are tumor necrosis factor-alpha (TNF-α), transforming growth factor-beta (TGF-β), interferon-gamma, and interleukins. This process results in the recruitment of macrophages and lymphocytes into the adipose tissue, which does not allow the inflammation to heal, impairs the fat cell function, and eventually leads to cellular necrosis. As the inflammation deepens, the vicious circle is not broken and continues to increase insulin resistance. In particular, the studied cytokines were detected at a higher rate in PCOS patients than in the control groups. Although this situation was observed in patients without insulin resistance or in non-obese patients, this difference was higher in patients with insulin resistance and those who were obese, and this is due to the cascade of inflammation in the adipose tissue, which enters this vicious circle (Ebejer and Calleja-Agius 2013).

In this case, the question of whether PCOS is a result, or a cause arises. Lean women with PCOS have an altered pattern of central fat distribution, defined as visceral obesity. Normal weight patients with PCOS have a higher visceral fat deposition and less subcutaneous fat in the gluteofemoral region, and this concludes that a PCOS patient does not have to have a high BMI to exhibit an inflammatory condition (Sathyapalan and Atkin 2010). Also, hyperandrogenism in PCOS increases mononuclear cell sensitivity to ingested glucose, and cells become activated. The increase in mononuclear cell sensitivity to glucose has stimulated an inflammatory response by encouraging mononuclear cells to release TNF-α and IL-6. This inflammation caused by glucose, in turn, further increases the production of androgens by the ovarian theca cells (Escobar-Morreale et al., 2011; Ebejer and Calleja-Agius 2013).

Hyperinsulinemia and insulin resistance increase androgen secretion in women, putting PCOS in a vicious circle. Especially in PCOS patients receiving insulin-sensitizing therapy, with the decrease in fasting insulin levels, androgen amounts decrease, and ovulation improves.

This shows that insulin triggers the secretion of gonadotropin hormones. In women with PCOS, insulin tends to significantly increase the sensitivity of the adrenal cortex to ACTH activation by accelerating androgen production. Particularly, higher insulin rates are associated with lower levels of sex hormone-binding globulin (SHBG), which further increases the availability of androgens (Pauli et al., 2011; Abraham Gnanadass et al., 2021). It indirectly blocks the production of SHBG via fructose and provides the glucose-induced blocking of hepatocyte nuclear factor 4 alpha (HNF-4α). In addition, insulin suppresses the activity of insulin-like growth factor-binding protein-1 (IGFBP-1) and increases the availability of insulin-like growth factor 1 (IGF-1). This triggers insulin activity in the ovaries and liver, leading to decreased SHBG levels (Wallace et al., 2013; Abraham Gnanadass et al., 2021). Insulin aggravates steroidogenesis-related gene levels and elevates testosterone and progesterone levels in PCOS patients. High testosterone concentration and significantly lower SHBG concentration were independently associated with insulin resistance. Females with PCOS have a considerably higher chance of glucose tolerance and insulin resistance for comparable weight and age without PCOS (Abraham Gnanadass et al., 2021).

C-Reactive Protein (CRP)

C-reactive protein (CRP) is increased in the bloodstream in tissue damage and inflammation. Studies have determined that it is increased in colon cancer, cardiovascular diseases, peritoneal cancers, and ovarian carcinogenesis (Carvalho et al., 2018). CRP is increased in the case of PCOS. In particular, this increase is observed independently of obesity (Escobar-Morreale et al., 2011). In addition, ever-increasing CRP concentrations increase the chances of acquiring type 2 diabetes mellitus and cardiovascular diseases (Legro 2002).

Tumor Necrosis Factor (TNF)

Tumor necrosis factor-α is a potent proinflammatory cytokine secreted from myeloid cells. This cytokine is also detected in follicular fluid, theca cells, oocytes, and granulosa cells during ovulation (Kaipa et al., 1996). In animal experiments, it has been observed that it triggers follicular apoptosis and plays a role in follicular atresia. TNF-α contributes to ovarian cancer by participating in metastasis, angiogenesis, and invasion (Dobrzycka et al., 2009). In PCOS, there is a positive relationship between insulin resistance and hyperandrogenism. In addition, insulin receptors are functionally and genetically normal. The presence of insulin resistance in PCOS results from defective insulin signaling due to the post-receptor defect. This defect leads to increased receptor serine phosphorylation and decreased receptor autophosphorylation in insulin binding. TNF-α causes an increase in serine phosphorylation and is, therefore, a mediator of insulin resistance (Samy et al., 2009; Ebejer and Calleja-Agius, 2013). It also affects glucose transport by reducing the activity of glucose transporter type-4 (GLUT-4). Thus, the proinflammatory state in PCOS may be responsible for initiating insulin resistance, with TNF-α possibly acting as the triggering cytokine (Lorenzo et al., 2008). Many scientific studies have demonstrated that TNF-α expression is increased in adipose tissue, especially in obese people and experimental diabetes and obesity models. It has been reported that TNFR60 and

TNFR80 mRNA expressions, and TNF receptors in adipose tissue, are increased in obese women with glucose tolerance (Hube et al., 1999).

Interferon-γ

Interferon-γ is a cytokine involved in innate and adaptive immune responses (Schoenborn and Wilson 2007). Interferon-γ plays an important role in the autoimmune pathogenesis of type 1 diabetes. This type of interferon suppresses the differentiation of adipocytes and decreases insulin sensitivity by mediating activation of the JAK-STAT1 pathway (McGillicuddy et al., 2009). It provokes weight gain by increasing the inflammatory response in obesity. It increases insulin resistance by stimulating cytokine signal suppressor isoforms in adipocytes.

Interleukins

Interleukin-1α (IL-1α)

Interleukin-1α is an intracellular transcriptional and regulatory cytokine with a proinflammatory effect (Barksby et al., 2007). Interleukin-1α gene expression is associated with lipid metabolism and atherogenesis. It inhibits insulin signaling by phosphorylation of insulin receptor substrate-1 in adipocytes. Thus, it creates insulin resistance (He et al., 2006). Studies show that increased serum IL-1α concentration can be an important marker of metabolic syndrome (Mirhafez et al., 2015). It has been reported that IL-1α production in peripheral blood mononuclear cell culture obtained from obese women is higher than in normal-weight women (Raymond et al., 2000).

Interleukin-1β (IL-1β)

IL-1β is a proinflammatory cytokine that increases the expression of adhesion molecules in endothelial cells and triggers the acute-phase response (Barksby et al., 2007). Interleukin-1β plays a regulatory role in the formation or increase of fatty liver in obesity by triggering inflammation in adipose tissue. Interleukin-1β plays a role with other cytokines in developing insulin resistance in adipocytes by decreasing the expression of insulin receptor substrate-1 by an ERK-dependent mechanism and impairing the effect of insulin signaling (Jager et al., 2007). Long-term IL-1β administration plays a role in diabetes mellitus through triggering insulin resistance by reducing the synthesis of adiponectin, a specific protein known to increase insulin sensitivity (Lagathu et al., 2006). Recently, studies have also revealed the role of progesterone as an immunomodulator. The binding of progesterone to its receptor leads to a series of events that include binding to nuclear factor-kappa B (NF-kB) and activator protein 1 (AP-1), leading to decreased expression of the proinflammatory cytokines TNF-a and IL-1β. Therefore, the progesterone in combined oral contraceptives used in PCOS treatment aims to address hormonal abnormalities and correct the chronic low-grade inflammatory state by reducing proinflammatory cytokine production (Tait et al., 2008; Banaszewska et al., 2011; Ebejer and Calleja-Agius 2013).

Interleukin-6 (IL-6)

The primary function of interleukin-6 is to differentiate monocytes into macrophages, and this regulates the secretion of gonadal steroids, implantation, corpus luteum function, and embryonic development (Nilsson et al., 2005; Abraham Gnanadass et al., 2021). The activity of IL-6 is induced by specific inflammation-promoting molecules such as TNFα, interferon-y, and interleukin-1. IL-6 is involved in inflammation, angiogenesis, and infiltration of tumors (Łukaszewicz et al., 2007). It induces the formation of other signaling molecules. Previous studies show that serum IL-6 is elevated in ovarian hyperstimulation syndrome (OHSS) (Bersinger et al., 2014). Adipocytes in the subcutaneous adipose tissue are the primary storage source and play a role in forming insulin resistance.

For this reason, they are also used as markers of metabolic syndrome. IL-6, which is high in lean PCOS patients, increases even more if the patient is PCOS and obese. In addition, IL-6, which was also studied in infertile PCOS patients, was significantly higher than in the control groups (Samy et al., 2009).

Interleukin-7 (IL-7)

On the other hand, this cytokine provides the transformation of T and B lymphocytes by stimulating the release of cytokines from monocytes and macrophages. It contributes to the increase of the adipose tissue mass and the development of insulin resistance by being secreted more in the adipose tissue of obese people. It also causes atherosclerosis by increasing the movement of monocytes and macrophages to the endothelium (Li et al., 2012).

Interleukin-8 (IL-8)

Interleukin-8 (IL-8) functions specifically as a neutrophil activator. It helps to regulate oocyte maturation, ovulation, and follicular development. It is observed at high levels in ovarian malignancies and endometriomas (Goto et al., 2002). Its increased expression increases proliferation, angiogenesis, and adhesion. Although few studies reveal the relationship between IL-8 and PCOS, studies show a positive correlation between the blood level and PCOS. Recent publications shed light on the working mechanism of IL-8 by showing that IL-8 increases but decreases after treatment with metformin and pioglitazone, especially in women with PCOS (Ali et al., 2019). It has been suggested that there is a correlation between the circulating IL-8 level and characteristic obesity parameters such as body mass index, waist circumference, IL-6, and HDL-cholesterol, and that IL-8 mediates metabolic complications such as atherosclerosis and diabetes (Kim et al., 2006).

Interleukin-10 (IL-10)

Interleukin-10 (IL-10) is a cytokine that reduces inflammation and has an immunosuppressant effect. Suppressing the effects of T helper lymphocytes is one of its main tasks. In addition to this reproductive effect, it contributes to the continuation of pregnancy by providing the maturation of the corpus luteum with progesterone synthesis (Moore et al., 2001). A low IL-10 concentration is associated with metabolic syndrome and obesity. It has been determined that plasma IL-10 levels increase after calorie restriction and an exercise program and weight loss in obese people (Jung et al., 2008). It was observed that plasma IL-10 decreased in PCOS patients, whereas clomiphene citrate increased IL-10 and helped to increase the pregnancy rate and ovulation rate in women with PCOS (Sylus et al., 2018).

Interleukin-12 (IL-12)

Increased serum IL-12 levels concerning body mass index, insulin, proinsulin, and HDL-cholesterol have been reported in patients with type 2 diabetes compared to healthy people (Wegner et al., 2008). In obese individuals, an increased IL-12 concentration has been reported in association with obesity markers such as body mass index, body fat percentage, serum glucose, triglyceride, and TNF-α levels (Suárez-Álvarez et al., 2013).

Interleukin-18 (IL-18)

Interleukin-18 (IL-18) is a signaling molecule that promotes inflammation and activates other inflammatory cytokines. Initially, pro-IL-18 (the inactive precursor of IL-18) is degraded by caspase-1; IL-18 induces the stimulation of NF-kB and activates the cascade of inflammation-promoting cytokines such as IL-1β and TNFα. It plays a role in the pathophysiology of OHSS and ovarian malignancy (Gutman et al., 2004; Abraham Gnanadass et al., 2021). Serum levels of the proinflammatory cytokine IL-18 are significantly higher in women with PCOS. With or without insulin resistance, women with PCOS have a higher serum concentration of IL-18. Compared with controls, serum levels of IL-18 are increased in women with PCOS, regardless of BMI. However, obese women with PCOS show higher levels of IL-18 compared to lean women with PCOS (Zhang et al., 2006).

Interleukin-33 (IL-33)

IL-33 is a signaling cytokine. It is a nuclear protein because it has a nucleotide-binding domain, and it controls the regulation of unacquired immunity and T helper cells. It is found in ovarian theca cells and plays a fundamental role in ovulation (Bonilla et al., 2012). It also plays a fundamental role in the pathophysiology of preeclampsia and endometriosis (Santunni et al., 2012; Granne et al., 2011). Studies show that hyperandrogenism is associated with high serum IL-33 levels, which play an active role in insulin resistance and coronary atherosclerosis in PCOS patients (Zhang et al., 2012).

Conclusion

Elucidating the molecular basis of PCOS and finding out which genes are affected in these pathways are important for a better understanding of PCOS mechanisms, especially for the development of diagnosis and treatment methods. However, with their newly discovered roles, cytokines will play an important role both in our understanding of the mechanism and in improving the treatment.

References

Abraham Gnanadass S, Divakar Prabhu Y, Valsala Gopalakrishnan A (2021). Association of metabolic and inflammatory markers with polycystic ovarian syndrome (PCOS): an update. *Arch. Gynecol. Obstet.* 303(3):631-643.

Ali D E S, Shah M, Ali A, Malik M O, Rehman F, Badshah H, Ehtesham E, Vitale S G (2019). Treatment with metformin and combination of metformin plus pioglitazone on serum levels of IL-6 and IL-8 in polycystic ovary syndrome: a randomized clinical trial. *Horm. Metab. Res.* 51:714-722.

Amato P, Simpson J L (2004). The genetics of polycystic ovary syndrome. *Best Pract. Res. Clin. Obstet. Gynaecol.* 18(5):707-718.

Azziz R, Carmina E, Dewailly D, Diamanti-Kandarakis E, Escobar-Morreale H F, Futterweit W, Janssen O E, Legro R S, Norman R J, Taylor A E, Witchel S F (2009). Task Force on the Phenotype of the Polycystic Ovary Syndrome of The Androgen Excess and PCOS Society the Androgen Excess and PCOS Society criteria for the polycystic ovary syndrome: the complete task force report. *Fertil. Steril.* 91(2):456-488.

Banaszewska B, Spaczynski R Z, Ozegowska K, Pawelczyk L (2011). The influence of low-dose oral contraceptive pill on clinical and metabolic parameters in young women with polycystic ovary syndrome. *Ginekolog Polska* 82:430-435.

Barksby H E, Lea S R, Preshaw P M, Taylor J J (2007). The expanding family of interleukin-1 cytokines and their role in destructive inflammatory disorders. *Clin. Exp. Immunol.* 149(2):217-225.

Bersinger N A, Kollmann Z, Von Wolff M (2014). Serum but not follicular fluid cytokine levels are increased in stimulated versus natural cycle IVF: a multiplexed assay study. *J. Reprod. Immunol.* 106:27-33.

Bonilla W V, Fröhlich A, Senn K, Kallert S, Fernandez M, Johnson S, Kreutzfeldt M, Hegazy A N, Schrick C, Fallon P G, Klemenz R, Nakae S, Adler H, Merkler D, Löhning M, Pinschewer D D (2012). The alarmin interleukin-33 drives protective antiviral CD8+ T cell responses. *Science* 335:984-989.

Carvalho L M L, Dos Reis F M, Candido A L, Nunes F F C, Ferreira C N, Gomes K B (2018). Polycystic Ovary Syndrome as a systemic disease with multiple molecular pathways: a narrative review. *Endocr. Regul.* 52(4):208-221.

Deligeoroglou E, Vrachnis N, Athanasopoulos N, Iliodromiti Z, Sifakis S, Iliodromiti S, Siristatidis C, Creatsas G (2012). Mediators of chronic inflammation in polycystic ovarian syndrome. *Gynecol. Endocrinol.* 28(12):974-978.

Diamanti-Kandarakis E, Dunaif A (2012). Insulin resistance and the polycystic ovary syndrome revisited: an update on mechanisms and implications. *Endocr. Rev.* 33(6):981-1030.

Dobrzycka B, Terlikowski S J, Garbowicz M, Niklińska W, Bernaczyk P S, Nikliński J, Kinalski M, Chyczewski L (2009). Tumor necrosis factor-alpha and its receptors in epithelial ovarian cancer. *Folia Histochem. Cytobiol.* 47:609-613.

Ebejer K, Calleja-Agius J (2013). The role of cytokines in polycystic ovarian syndrome. *Gynecol. Endocrinol.* 29(6):536-540.

Escobar-Morreale H F, Luque-Ramı´rez M, Gonza´lez F (2011). Circulating inflammatory markers in polycystic ovary syndrome: a systematic review and meta-analysis. *Fertil. Steril.* 95:1048-1058.

Goto J, Suganuma N, Takata K, Kitamura K, Asahina T, Kobayashi H, Muranaka Y, Furuhashi M, Kanayama N (2002). Morphological analyses of interleukin-8 effects on rat ovarian follicles at ovulation and luteinization in vivo. *Cytokine* 20:168-173.

Granne I, Southcombe J H, Snider J V, Tannetta D S, Child T, Redman C W G, Sargent I L (2011). ST2 and IL-33 in pregnancy and preeclampsia. *PLoS ONE* 6:e24463.

Gutman G, Soussan-Gutman L, Malcov M, Lessing J B, Amit A, Azem F (2004). Interleukin-18 is high in the serum of IVF pregnancies with ovarian hyperstimulation syndrome. *Am. J. Reprod. Immunol.* 51:381-384.

He J, Usui I, Ishizuka K, Kanatani Y, Hiratani K, Iwata M, Bukhari A, Haruta T, Sasaoka T, Kobayashi M (2006). Interleukin-1alpha inhibits insulin signaling with phosphorylating insulin receptor substrate-1 on serine residues in 3T3-L1 adipocytes. *Mol. Endocrinol.* 20(1):114-124.

Huang A, Brennan K, Azziz R (2010). Prevalence of hyperandrogenemia in the polycystic ovary syndrome diagnosed by the National Institutes of Health 1990 criteria. *Fertil. Steril.* 93(6):1938-1941.

Hube F, Birgel M, Lee Y M, Hauner H (1999). Expression pattern of tumour necrosis factor receptors in subcutaneous and omental human adipose tissue: role of obesity and non-insulin-dependent diabetes mellitus. *Eur. J. Clin. Invest.* 29(8):672-678.

Jager J, Grémeaux T, Cormont M, Le Marchand-Brustel Y, Tanti J F (2007). Interleukin-1beta-induced insulin resistance in adipocytes through down-regulation of insulin receptor substrate-1 expression. *Endocrinology* 148(1):241-251.

Jung S H, Park H S, Kim K S, Choi W H, Ahn C W, Kim B T, Kim S M, Lee S Y, Ahn S M, Kim Y K, Kim H J, Kim D J, Lee K-W (2008). Effect of weight loss on some serum cytokines in human obesity: increase in IL-10 after weight loss. *J. Nutr. Biochem.* 19(6):371-375.

Kaipia A, Chun S-Y, Eisenhauer K, Hsueh A J (1996). Tumor necrosis factor-alpha and its second messenger, ceramide, stimulate apoptosis in cultured ovarian follicles. *Endocrinology* 137:4864-4870.

Kim C S, Park H S, Kawada T, Kim K, Lim D, Hubbard N, Kwon B-S, Erickson K L, Yu R (2006). Circulating levels of MCP-1 and IL-8 are elevated in human obese subjects and associated with obesity-related parameters. *Int. J. Obes.* (Lond) 30(9):1347-1355.

Lagathu C, Yvan-Charvet L, Bastard J P, Maachi M, Quignard-Boulangé A, Capeau J, Caron M (2006). Long-term treatment with interleukin-1beta induces insulin resistance in murine and human adipocytes. *Diabetologia* 49(9):2162-2173.

Legro R S (2002). Diabetes prevalence and risk factors in polycystic ovary syndrome. *Curr. Opin. Endocrinol. Diabetes* 9:451-458.

Li R, Paul A, Ko K W, Sheldon M, Rich B E, Terashima T, Dieker C, Cormier S, Li L, Nour E A, Chan L, Oka K (2012). Interleukin-7 induces recruitment of monocytes/macrophages to endothelium. *Eur. Heart J.* 33(24):3114-3123.

Lorenzo M, Fernández-Veledo S, Vila-Bedmar R, Garcia- Guerra L, De Alvaro C, Nieto-Vazquez I (2008). Insulin resistance induced by tumor necrosis factor-alpha in myocytes and brown adipocytes. *J. Anim. Sci.* 86(14):94-104.

Łukaszewicz M, Mroczko B, Szmitkowski M (2007). Clinical significance of interleukin-6 (IL-6) as a prognostic factor of cancer disease. *Pol. Arch. Med. Wewn.* 117:247-251.

McGillicuddy F C, Chiquoine E H, Hinkle C C, Kim R J, Shah R, Roche H M, Smyth E M, Reilly M P (2009). Interferon gamma attenuates insulin signaling, lipid storage, and differentiation in human adipocytes via activation of the JAK/STAT pathway. *J. Biol. Chem.* 284(46):31936-31944.

Mirhafez S R, Pasdar A, Avan A, Esmaily H, Moezzi A, Mohebati M, Meshkat Z, Mehrad-Majd H, Eslami S, Rahimi H R, Ghazavi H, Ferns G A, Ghayour-Mobarhan M (2015). Cytokine and growth factor profiling in patients with the metabolic syndrome. *Br. J. Nutr.* 113(12):1911-1919.

Moore K W, de Waal M R, Coffman R L, O'Garra A (2001). Interleukin- 10 and the interleukin-10 receptor. *Annu. Rev. Immunol.* 19:683-765.

Nilsson M B, Langley R R, Fidler I J (2005). Interleukin-6, secreted by human ovarian carcinoma cells, is a potent proangiogenic cytokine. *Cancer Res.* 65:10794-10800.

Pauli J M, Raja-Khan N, Wu X, Legro R S (2011). Current perspectives of insulin resistance and polycystic ovary syndrome. *Diabet. Med.* 28:1445-1454.

Raymond N C, Dysken M, Bettin K, Eckert E D, Crow S J, Markus K, Pomeroy C (2000). Cytokine production in patients with anorexia nervosa, bulimia nervosa, and obesity. *Int. J. Eat. Disord.* 28(3):293-302.

Rotter V, Nagaev I, Smith U (2003). Interleukin-6 (IL-6) induces insulin resistance in 3T3-L1 adipocytes and is, like IL-8 and tumor necrosis factor-alpha, overexpressed in human fat cells from insulin resistant subjects. *J. Biol. Chem.* 278(46):45777-45784.

Samy N, Hashim M, Sayed M, Said M (2009). Clinical significance of inflammatory markers in polycystic ovary syndrome: their relationship to insulin resistance and body mass index. *Dis. Marker* 26:163-170.

Santulli P, Borghese B, Chouzenoux S, Vaiman D, Borderie D, Streuli I, Goffinet F, de Ziegler D, Weill B, Batteux F, Chapron C (2012). Serum and peritoneal interleukin-33 levels are elevated in deeply infiltrating endometriosis. *Hum. Reprod.* 27:2001-2009.

Sathyapalan T, Atkin S L (2010). Mediators of inflammation in polycystic ovary syndrome in relation to adiposity. *Mediators Inflammat.* 2010:758656.

Schoenborn J R, Wilson C B (2007). Regulation of interferon-gamma during innate and adaptive immune responses. *Adv. Immunol.* 96:41-101.

Sirmans S M, Pate K A (2013). Epidemiology, diagnosis, and management of polycystic ovary syndrome. *Clin. Epidemiol.* 6:1-13.

Stein F, Leventhal M.L (1935). Amenorrhea associated with bilateral polycystic ovaries. *Am. J. Obstet. Gynecol.* 29:181-191.

Suárez-Álvarez K, Solís-Lozano L, Leon-Cabrera S, González-Chávez A, Gómez-Hernández G, Quiñones-Álvarez M S, Serralde-Zúñiga A E, Hernández-Ruiz J, Ramírez-Velásquez J, Galindo-González F J, Zavala-Castillo J C, De León-Nava M A, Robles-Díaz G and Escobedo G (2013). Serum IL-12 is increased in Mexican obese subjects and associated with lowgrade inflammation and obesity-related parameters. *Mediators Inflamm.* 2013:967067.

Sylus A M, Nandeesha H, Sridhar M G, Chitra T, Sreenivasulu K (2018). Clomiphene citrate increases nitric oxide, interleukin-10 and reduces matrix metalloproteinase-9 in women with polycystic ovary syndrome. *Eur. J. Obstet. Gynecol. Reprod. Biol.* 228:27-31.

Tait A S, Butts C L, Sternberg E M (2008). The role of glucocorticoids and progestins in inflammatory, autoimmune and infectious disease. *J. Leukocyte Biol.* 84:924-31.

Teede H J, Misso M L, Costello M F, Dokras A, Laven J, Moran L, Piltonen T, Norman R J. International PCOS Network (2018) Recommendations from the international evidence-based guideline for the assessment and management of polycystic ovary syndrome. *Hum. Reprod.* 33(9):1602-1618, Erratum in: Hum Reprod 34(2):388. https://doi.org/10.1093/humrep/dey256.

The Rotterdam ESHRE/ASRM-Sponsored PCOS Consensus Workshop Group (2004) Revised 2003 consensus on diagnostic criteria and long-term health risks related to polycystic ovary syndrome. *Fertil. Steril.* 81:19-2.

Wallace I R, McKinley M C, Bell P M, Hunter S J (2013). Sex hormone binding globulin and insulin resistance. *Clin. Endocrinol.* 78:321–329.

Wang Y, Xu R C, Zhang X L, Niu X L, Qu Y, Li L Z, Meng X Y (2012). Interleukin-8 secretion by ovarian cancer cells increases anchorage-independent growth, proliferation, angiogenic potential, adhesion and invasion. *Cytokine* 59:145-155.

Wegner M, Winiarska H, Bobkiewicz-Kozłowska T, Dworacka M (2008). IL-12 serum levels in patients with type 2 diabetes treated with sulphonylureas. *Cytokine* 42(3):312-316.

Wild S, Pierpoint T, McKeigue P, Jacobs H (2000). Cardiovascular disease in women with polycystic ovary syndrome at long-term follow-up: a retrospective cohort study. *Clin. Endocrinol.* 52:595-600.

Xiong Y L, Liang X Y, Yang X, Li Y, Wei L-n (2011) Low-grade chronic inflammation in the peripheral blood and ovaries of women with polycystic ovarian syndrome. *Eur. J. Obstet. Gynecol. Reprod. Biol.* 159:148-150.

Zhang H-F, Xie S-L, Chen Y-X, Mai J-T, Wang J-F, Zhu W-L, Zhu L-G (2012). Altered serum levels of IL-33 in patients with advanced systolic chronic heart failure: correlation with oxidative stress. *J. Transl. Med.* 10:120.

Zhang Y F, Yang Y S, Hong J, Gu W-q, Shen C-f, Xu M, Du P-f, Li X-y, Ning G (2006). Elevated serum levels of interleukin-18 are associated with insulin resistance in women with polycystic ovary syndrome. *Endocrine* 29(3):419-423.

About the Editors

Kenan Demir, MD
Health Sciences University
Samsun Training and Research Hospital
(Samsun Eğitim ve Araştırma Hastanesi),
İlkadım, Turkey
Email: kenandemir@hotmail.com
ORCID ID: 0000-0003-2864-6041

Dr. Selim Görgün, MD
Health Sciences University
Samsun Training and Research Hospital
(Samsun Eğitim ve Araştırma Hastanesi),
İlkadım, Turkey
Email: selimgorgun55@gmail.com
ORCID ID: 0000-0001-5841-591X

Prof. Bahar Uslu, MD, PhD
Department of Histopathology
Faculty of Medicine, Quinnipiac University,
North Haven, CT, USA
Email: Bahar.uslu.md.phd@gmail.com
ORCID ID: 0000-0003-3378-2566

Index

A

B

C

D

E

F

G

H

I

J

K

L

M

R

S

T

U

V

W

Y

γ